Endosonography

Endosonography

Edited by **Robert H. Hawes** MD

Professor of Medicine
Division of Gastroenterology/Hepatology
Digestive Disease Center
Medical University of South Carolina
Charleston, SC, USA

Paul Fockens MD PhD

Professor of Gastrointestinal Endoscopy
Department of Gastroenterology and Hepatology
Academic Medical Center
University of Amsterdam
Amsterdam, Netherlands

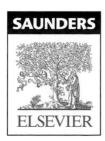

SAUNDERS

ELSEVIER

SAUNDERS
ELSEVIER

An imprint of Elsevier Inc

ISBN-13: 978 1 4160 2953 3
ISBN-10: 1 4160 2953 2

British Library Cataloguing in Publication Data
A catalogue record for this book is available from the British Library

Library of Congress Cataloging in Publication Data
A catalog record for this book is available from the Library of Congress

Notice
Medical knowledge is constantly changing. Standard safety precautions must be followed, but as new research and clinical experience broaden our knowledge, changes in treatment and drug therapy may become necessary or appropriate. Readers are advised to check the most current product information provided by the manufacturer of each drug to be administered to verify the recommended dose, the method and duration of administration, and contraindications. It is the responsibility of the practitioner, relying on experience and knowledge of the patient, to determine dosages and the best treatment for each individual patient. Neither the Publisher nor the author assume any liability for any injury and/or damage to persons or property arising from this publication.

The Publisher

Printed in China
Last digit is the print number: 9 8 7 6 5 4 3 2 1

Commissioning Editor:	**Karen Bowler**
Project Development Manager:	**Sheila Black**
Editorial Assistant:	**Liz Brown**
Project Manager:	**Gemma Lawson**
Design Manager:	**Jayne Jones**
Illustration Buyer:	**Gillian Murray**
Illustrator:	**Gillian Lee**, **Martin Woodward**
Marketing Manager(s):	**Amy Hey** (UK), **Laura Meiskey** (USA)

Contents

Contents

List of Contributors

Jouke T. Annema MD PhD
Chest Physician
Department of Pulmonology
Leiden University Medical Center
Leiden, Netherlands

Promila Banerjee MD
GI Fellow
Department of Gastroenterology
Centre Hospitalier de l'Université de Montréal
Hôpital St Luc
Montreal, Canada

Cynthia Behling MD PhD
Associate Professor, Clinical Pathology
Department of Pathology
University of California School of Medicine
San Diego, CA, USA

Giancarlo Caletti MD
Director of the Master in Advanced Endoscopy;
Director of the Unit of Gastroenterology and
Digestive Endoscopy;
Associate Professor of Gastroenterology
Department of Internal Medicine and
Gastroenterology
University of Bologna
Bologna, Italy

John DeWitt MD
Assistant Professor of Medicine
Division of Gastroenterology
Indiana University Medical Center
Indianapolis, IN, USA

Gidej Durivage MD FRCP(c)
Gastroenterologist
Fédération d'Hépatogastroentérologie
Hôpital Edouard Herriot
Lyons, France

Mohamad A. Eloubeidi MD, MHS, FACP, FACG
Associate Professor of Medicine
Director, Endoscopic Ultrasound Program
Co-director, Pancreatico-biliary Center
University of Alabama at Birmingham
Birmingham, AL, USA

Douglas O. Faigel MD
Associate Professor of Medicine
Director of Endoscopy
Department of Gastroenterology
Oregon Health & Science University
Portland, OR, USA

Paul Fockens MD PhD
Professor of Gastrointestinal Endoscopy
Department of Gastroenterology and Hepatology
Academic Medical Center
University of Amsterdam
Amsterdam, Netherlands

Annette Fritscher-Ravens MD
Consultant Gastroenterologist
Department of Gastroenterology, Endoscopy Unit
St. Mary's Hospital
Homerton University Hospital
London, UK

Pietro Fusaroli MD
Consultant Gastroenterologist
Department of Internal Medicine and
Gastroenterology
University of Bologna
Bologna, Italy

Steve Halligan MB BS MD FRCP FRCR
Professor of Gastrointestinal Radiology
Department of Specialist Radiology
University College Hospital
London, UK

Gavin C. Harewood MD MSc
Associate Professor of Medicine
Division of Gastroenterology
Mayo Clinic
Rochester, MN, USA

Robert H. Hawes MD
Professor of Medicine
Division of Gastroenterology/Hepatology
Digestive Disease Center
Medical University of South Carolina
Charleston, SC, USA

Joo Ha Hwang MD PhD
Acting Assistant Professor of Medicine
Division of Gastroenterology
University of Washington
Seattle, WA, USA

Ann Marie Joyce MD
Instructor of Medicine
Gastroenterology Division
Hospital of the University of Pennsylvania
Philadelphia, PA, USA

Mitsuhiro Kida MD
Assistant Professor
Department of Gastroenterology
Kitasato University East Hospital
Sagamihara-city
Kanagawa, Japan

List of Contributors

Eun Young (Ann) Kim MD PhD
Assistant Professor of Internal Medicine
Gastroenterology Department
Deagu Catholic University Medical Center
Deagu, South Korea

Michael B. Kimmey MD
Professor of Medicine
Division of Gastroenterology
University of Washington Medical Center
Seattle, WA, USA

Michael L. Kochman MD FACP
Professor of Medicine and Surgery
Co-Director Gastrointestinal Oncology
Gastroenterology Division
University of Pennsylvania Health System
Philadelphia, PA, USA

Christine Lefort MD
Gastroenterologist
Fédération d'Hépatogastroentérologie
Hôpital Edouard Herriot
Lyons, France

Anne Marie Lennon PhD MRCP
Specialist Registrar
Gastrointestinal Unit
Western General Hospital
Edinburgh, UK

Michael J. Levy MD
Associate Professor
Division of Gastroenterology and Hepatology
Mayo Clinic
Rochester, MN, USA

Costas Markoglou MD
Gastroenterologist
Fédération d'Hépatogastroentérologie
Hôpital Edouard Herriot
Lyons, France

John Meenan MD PhD FRCPI FRCP
Consultant Gastroenterologist
Department of Gastroenterology
Guy's and St Thomas' Hospital
London, UK

Bertrand Napoléon MD
Gastroenterologist
Department of Gastroenterology
Clinique Sainte Anne Lumière
Lyons, France

Phuong T. Nguyen MD
Associate Clinical Professor of Medicine
Division of Gastroenterology
Department of Medicine
University of California, Irvine Medical Center
Orange, CA, USA

Ian D. Penman MD FRCP (ED)
Consultant Gastroenterologist
Gastrointestinal Unit
Western General Hospital
Edinburgh, UK

Klaus F. Rabe MD PhD
Professor of Medicine
Chairman & Head of Department of Pulmonology
Leiden University Medical Centre
Leiden, Netherlands

Joseph Romagnuolo MD FRCPC MScEpid
Associate Professor of Medicine
Division of Gastroenterology and Hepatology
Medical University of South Carolina
Charleston, SC, USA

Anand V. Sahai MD MSc(Epid) FRCPC
Assistant Professor of Medicine
Department of Gastroenterology
Centre Hospitalier de l'Université de Montréal
Hôpital St Luc
Montreal, Canada

Michael K. Sanders MD
EUS Fellow/Clinical Instructor of Medicine
Division of Gastroenterology and Hepatology
Oregon Helath & Science University
Portland, OR, USA

Thomas J. Savides MD
Professor of Clinical Medicine
University of California,
UCSD Thornton Medical Center
Division of Gastroenterology
La Jolla, CA, USA

Mark Topazian MD
Associate Professor of Medicine
Division of Gastroenterology and Hepatology
Mayo Clinic
Rochester, MN, USA

Charles Vu MB FRACP FAMS
Consultant Gastroenterologist
Department of Gastroenterology
Tan Tock Seng Hospital
Singapore

Preface

It may be surprising to you that, in this day and age of electronic data communication, we decided to create a new textbook on Endoscopic Ultrasonography (EUS). Let us explain.

EUS started its slow but steady entrance into the field of gastrointestinal endoscopy 25 years ago. Doubts, doubts and more doubts surrounded the technique for many years. It seemed to be too difficult to learn and too time consuming for the endoscopist to perform. The equipment was substantially more expensive when compared to other endoscopic procedures. The procedure was too operator dependent and the interpretation of the images too subjective; surgeons and oncologists preferred to rely on standardized images created by computed tomography. Finally, reimbursement was slow to come and, once it was established, was proportionally much lower than that for other endoscopic procedures. Despite these obstacles, EUS remained doggedly on the endoscopic scene and, with the introduction of EUS-guided fine-needle aspiration (EUS-FNA), began steadily to grow. It continues to have a firm grip as the procedure of choice in the detection and assessment of lymph nodes, and remains the only modality capable of visualizing the gut wall layers. Consequently, EUS is now firmly established in the 'culture' of gastrointestinal endoscopy.

So why a textbook? We feel that because EUS has established itself and is still growing, and with the inevitable adoption of the technique by those outside gastrointestinal endoscopy (pulmonologists and thoracic surgeons), there is a need for a resource that combines a basic understanding of the capabilities of EUS with teaching the technique. We believe this can be an enduring product because its emphasis is very strongly on teaching; thus we anticipate it will become a valuable tool for future generations of endosonographers because textbooks remain one of the cornerstones of teaching and learning.

For this book we have invited vibrant leaders in EUS from around the world to write chapters in their respective areas of expertise that will thoroughly cover important information and future trends in their subject. We have not asked them to cover their subject area exhaustively, as this would include many irrelevant or outdated issues, but rather to provide the reader with key information that is important now and will likely continue to be so in the future. This key information will help in learning about EUS as well as aiding in implementing this technique into clinical decision-making and practice. The authors were selected not only because of their knowledge and status in the field, but also because they share a common bond of being active teachers. As a result, they are able to share with us their critical approach to the technique. We have tried to cover the entire field of EUS from the basics of ultrasonography, including how to set up an EUS service, to the future of therapeutic EUS.

We have included a number of unique features in this book that we hope you find interesting and useful. One of these features is that every section of the book starts with a short and simple 'how to' chapter, designed to help those just beginning to perform EUS to learn standard maneuvers for obtaining appropriate images. Every chapter also has a 'key points' box highlighting important issues that are further developed in the text. Where applicable, chapters have an 'examination checklist', which describes those areas that should be examined when performing EUS for a specific diagnosis. We hope that you will find these features helpful as a guide when reading the different chapters of this book. Furthermore every chapter is heavily illustrated with some of the best photographic material in the world.

Perhaps the most important and unique feature of this book is the accompanying DVD. The DVD contains sections showing how to perform EUS following what we call the 'station technique' – a method of teaching that shows how to position the transducer in particular stations and what anatomic structures can be examined from each of these stations. These 'station technique' videos go hand in hand with the 'how to' sections of the text. The DVD also contains case studies that will enhance the presentations in the various chapters and tie into the examination checklists.

We hope, and expect, that this EUS textbook and the DVD will provide a valuable resource to current and future endosonographers. Most importantly, we hope that the use of this textbook will improve the practice of EUS around the world, as we believe this will ultimately lead to improvement in the care of our patients – the final goal for all of us.

Robert H. Hawes, Charleston
Paul Fockens, Amsterdam

Acknowledgements

We are extremely grateful for the support and encouragement we have received from our respective institutions, colleagues and friends.

At the Medical University of South Carolina (MUSC), I owe a great debt of gratitude to Linda K. McDaniel and James C. Webb who did virtually all of the video editing. They have become enormously experienced over the years and have been central figures in all of the electronic educational materials produced by the Digestive Disease Center. I regrettably burdened them, in my usual fashion, by selecting the time codes and presenting the raw tapes for editing at the last minute. Despite this burden, they accomplished their work with great proficiency and constant good cheer.

I also owe a debt of gratitude to the endoscopic ultrasound fellows over the last year and a half during which time the taping was accomplished. MUSC has been blessed with tremendously talented individuals who have come to train in EUS and those directly responsible for assisting in the taping of cases for this DVD include:

Andre Chong	Brandn Hunter	Sarto Paquin
Jason Conway	Rya Kaplan	Rhys Vaughan
Sandra Faias	Inder Maine	

I am also deeply indebted to Brenda Ferguson, who is our principle EUS nurse and endures all of the extra time and attention to detail that is required to do both research as well as develop educational materials. I am similarly indebted to my EUS partners, Brenda Hoffman and Joe Romagnuolo, whose hard work has created the large EUS service from which the patients were selected for presentation on this DVD.

Finally, the constant bright-eyed "can do" force in my professional life is my secretary, Tracy Farber, who has worked hard to help me organize this project as she has all other projects that I have been involved with since coming to MUSC in 1994. Clearly I have been blessed by a tremendously talented and enthusiastic group of co-workers in the Division of Gastroenterology and the Digestive Disease Center, to all of whom I am immensely grateful.

Robert H. Hawes, M.D.

At the Academic Medical Center (AMC), I want to thank my EUS-partners Jacques Bergman, Marco Bruno and (more recently) Sheila Krishnadath. EUS is a lot of fun because it does not only consist of a high-level technical endoscopic procedure but at the same time it exposes us to many different, mostly serious, problems in gastroenterology. It has allowed endosonographers to find a specific niche in gastroenterology and at the same time keep a broad perspective on general gastroenterology with a focus on gastrointestinal oncology. Without a doubt, most of the interesting patients I have seen in the past 15 years have come in through the EUS-door.

Our fellows have been very active supporters of our EUS-program and it has been a pleasure to see them battle for a place in the room. Our nursing staff are led by Monique van den Bergh, who always finds a way to add an extra patient or perform an extra procedure. She is the key factor in motivating our hard-working nurses. Our international exposure at AMC is channeled through the European Postgraduate Gastrosurgical School, which is under the astute direction of Joy Goedkoop.

Finally, I should make it clear that it would be impossible to do what I do at the Academic Medical Center without my secretary, Marion van Haaster. Although there are many days in the week in which I do not even find 5 minutes to go through the work I have asked her to prepare, she keeps on showing a big smile to me and to everyone else. Furthermore she sets a fantastic example of hospitality to our guests, even when I forget to inform her of their arrival. She is an indispensable help in arranging my daily work.

Paul Fockens, M.D.

Dedication
For Chris, Grant and Taylor
For Marischka, Matthijs and Kiki

BASICS OF EUS

Principles of Ultrasound

Joo Ha Hwang and Michael B. Kimmey

KEY POINTS

- Ultrasound is mechanical energy in the form of vibrations that propagate through a medium such as tissue.

- Ultrasound interacts with tissue by undergoing absorption, reflection, refraction, and scattering, and produces an image representative of tissue structure.

- Imaging artifacts can be recognized and understood based on a knowledge of the principles of ultrasound.

INTRODUCTION

A basic understanding of the principles of ultrasound is requisite for an endosonographer's understanding of how to obtain and accurately interpret ultrasound images. In this chapter, the basic principles of ultrasound physics and instrumentation are presented, followed by illustrations of how these principles are applied to ultrasound imaging and Doppler ultrasound, and to explain some common artifacts seen with endosonography. Knowledge of the basic principles of ultrasound will help the endosonographer to understand the capabilities of ultrasound imaging – and also its limitations.

BASIC ULTRASOUND PHYSICS

Sound is mechanical energy in the form of vibrations that propagate through a medium such as air, water, or tissue.[1] The frequency of audible sound ranges from 20 to 20 000 Hz (cycles per second). Ultrasound involves a frequency spectrum that is greater than 20 000 Hz, with medical applications utilizing frequencies in the range of 1 000 000–50 000 000 Hz (1–50 MHz). The propagation of ultrasound results from the displacement and oscillation of molecules from their average position and the subsequent displacement and oscillations of molecules along the direction of propagation of the ultrasound wave.

Ultrasound waves can be described using the common properties of waves. Fig.1.1 is an illustration of a sinusoidal wave with the pressure amplitude along the *y*-axis and the time or distance along the *x*-axis. This figure will be referred to in the following sections to introduce the basic properties of waves.

Wavelength, frequency, and velocity

The wavelength is the distance in the propagating medium that includes one complete cycle (Fig. 1.1). The wavelength (λ) is dependent on the frequency (f) of the oscillations and the velocity (c) of propagation in the medium. The relationship between wavelength, frequency, and velocity is given in Eqn 1.1.

$$c = f\lambda \tag{1.1}$$

The frequency of a wave is the number of oscillations per unit of time. Typically in ultrasound this is stated in terms of cycles per second or Hertz (Hz) (1 cycle/s = 1 Hz). The period of a wave (τ) is the inverse of the frequency and represents the time required to complete one cycle. The relationship between frequency and period are given in Eqn 1.2.

$$f = \frac{1}{\tau} \tag{1.2}$$

The velocity of propagation is dependent on the physical properties of the medium in which the wave is propagating. The primary physical properties governing the velocity of propagation are the density and compressibility of the medium.

Density, compressibility, and bulk modulus

The density (ρ) of a medium is the mass per unit volume of that medium (kg/m³ in SI units). The compressibility (K) of a medium is a property that reflects the relationship between the fractional decrease in volume and the pressure applied to a medium. For example, air has a high compressibility (a small amount of pressure applied to a volume of air will result in a large fractional decrease in volume), whereas bone has a relatively low compressibility (a large amount of pressure applied to a volume of bone will result in a small fractional decrease in volume). Lastly, the bulk modulus (β), which is the inverse of the compressibility, is the negative ratio of pressure applied to a medium and the fractional change in volume of the medium and reflects the stiffness of the medium.

The acoustic velocity (c) of a medium can be determined once the density (ρ) and the compressibility (K), or bulk modulus (β), are known. Eqn 1.3 demonstrates the relationship between the three physical properties.

$$c = \frac{1}{\sqrt{K\rho}} = \frac{\sqrt{\beta}}{\sqrt{\rho}} \tag{1.3}$$

It is important to realize that the density, compressibility, and bulk modulus are not independent of one another. Typically, as density increases, the compressibility decreases and bulk modulus

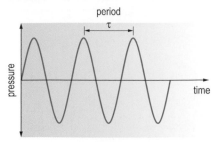

Fig. 1.1 Sinusoidal wave depicted on the time axis and distance axis. The time to complete one cycle is the period (τ). The distance to complete one cycle is the wavelength (λ).

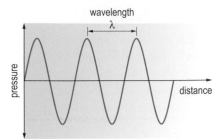

increases. However, the compressibility and bulk modulus typically vary more rapidly than the density and dominate in the above equation (Eqn 1.3).

The acoustic velocity in different media can be determined by applying the equations to practice. For example, water at 30°C has a density of 996 kg/m³ and a bulk modulus of 2.27×10^9 newtons/m².[2] Inserting these values into Eqn 1.3 yields an acoustic velocity of 1509 m/s in water. Values for density and bulk modulus have been characterized extensively and can be found in the literature.[2] A summary of relevant tissue properties are given in Table 1.1. Of note, the acoustic velocity is not dependent on the frequency of the propagating wave (i.e., acoustic waves of different frequencies all propagate with the same acoustic velocity within the same medium).[3]

Ultrasound interactions in tissue

Ultrasound imaging of tissue is achieved by transmitting short pulses of ultrasound energy into tissue and receiving reflected signals. The reflected signals that return to the transducer represent the interactions of a propagating ultrasound wave with tissue. A propagating ultrasound wave can interact with tissue resulting in *reflection, refraction, scattering,* and *absorption.*

Reflection

Specular reflections of ultrasound occur at relative large interfaces (greater than one wavelength) between two media of differing acoustical impedances. At this point it is important to introduce the concept of *acoustic impedance.* The acoustic impedance (Z) of a medium represents the resistance to sound propagating through the medium and is the product of the *density* (ρ) and the *velocity* (c):

$$Z = \rho c \qquad (1.4)$$

Sound will continue to propagate through a medium until an interface is reached where the acoustic impedance of the medium in which the sound is propagating differs from the medium that it encounters. At an interface where an acoustic impedance difference is encountered, a proportion of the ultrasound wave will be reflected back towards the transducer and the rest will be transmitted into the second medium. The simplest case of reflection and transmission occurs when the propagating ultrasound wave is perpendicular (90°) to the interface (Fig. 1.2). In this case the percentage of the incident beam that is reflected is:

$$\% \; reflected \; = \left(\frac{Z_2 - Z_1}{Z_2 + Z_1} \right)^2 \times 100 \qquad (1.5)$$

The percentage of the incident beam that is transmitted is:

$$\% \; transmitted = 100 - \% \; reflected \qquad (1.6)$$

Refraction

When the incident beam arrives at the interface at an angle other than 90°, the transmitted beam path diverges from the incident beam path due to refraction (Fig. 1.3). The angle at which the transmitted beam propagates is determined by Snell's law:

$$\frac{\sin \phi_1}{\sin \phi_2} \; = \; \frac{c_1}{c_2} \qquad (1.7)$$

The angle of refraction is determined by the *acoustic velocities* in the incident (c_1) and transmitted (c_2) media. There are three possible scenarios for a refracted beam, depending on the

PHYSICAL PROPERTIES OF TISSUE[2]			
Tissue or fluid	Density (kg/m³)	Bulk modulus ($\times 10^9$ N/m²)	Acoustic velocity (m/s)
Water (30°C)	996	2.27	1509
Blood	1050–1075	2.65	1590
Pancreas (pig)	1040–1050	2.63	1591
Liver	1050–1070	2.62	1578
Bone, cortical	1963–2017	28.13	3760

Table 1.1 Physical properties of tissue[2]

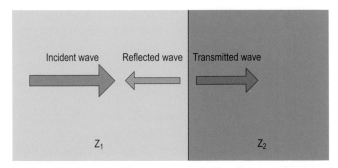

Fig. 1.2 Reflection of an ultrasound wave at normal incidence to an interface between two media with different acoustic impedances (Z).

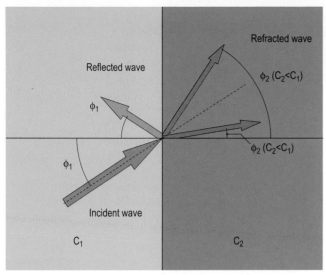

Fig. 1.3   Refraction and reflection of an incident wave that is not normal to the interface between media with different acoustic velocities (c). The angle of reflection is identical to the angle of incidence. The angle of the refracted wave is dependent on the acoustic velocities of the two media and can be determined by applying Snell's law (see text).

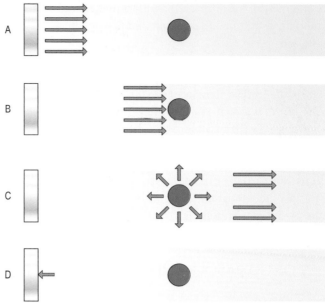

Fig. 1.4   Schematic representation of single scattering. Scattering occurs from an interface that is smaller than the wavelength of the propagating ultrasound signal. The transducer is responsible for sending and receiving the signal. I_b is the backscattered intensity that will propagate back to the transducer. **A,** The ultrasound signal transmitted by transducer and propagates toward the scatterer. **B,** The pulse reaches the scatterer. **C,** The incident acoustic intensity is scattered in different directions. **D,** The back-scattered energy received by the transducer is only a small fraction of the incident acoustic intensity that is scattered.

relative speeds of sound between the two media: (1) if $c_1 > c_2$, the angle of refraction will be bent toward normal ($\phi_1 > \phi_2$); (2) if $c_1 = c_2$, the angle of refraction will be identical to the angle of incidence and the beam will continue to propagate without diverging from its path; (3) if $c_1 < c_2$, the angle of refraction will be bent away from normal ($\phi_1 < \phi_2$).

Scattering

Scattering, also termed *non-specular reflection*, occurs when a propagating ultrasound wave interacts with different components in tissue that are smaller than the wavelength and have different impedance values than the propagating medium.[4] Examples of scatterers in tissue include individual cells, fat globules, and collagen. When an ultrasound wave interacts with a scatterer, only a small portion of the acoustic intensity that reflects off of the scatterer is reflected back to the transducer (Fig. 1.4). In addition, a signal that has undergone scattering by a single scatterer will usually undergo multiple scattering events before returning to the transducer. Scattering occurs in heterogeneous media, such as tissue, and is responsible for the different echotextures of organs such as the liver, pancreas, and spleen. Tissue containing fat or collagen scatters ultrasound to a greater degree than other tissues, which is why lipomas and the submucosal layer of the gastrointestinal tract appear hyperechoic (bright) on ultrasound imaging.[4]

Multiple reflections from non-specular reflectors within the tissue returning to the transducer result in a characteristic acoustic speckle pattern, or echotexture, for that tissue.[4] As speckle originates from multiple reflections and does not represent the actual location of a structure, moving the transducer will change the location of the speckle echoes while maintaining a similar speckle pattern. In addition, the noise resulting from acoustic speckle increases with increasing depth due to a greater number of signals that have undergone multiple reflections from non-specular reflectors returning to the transducer.

Absorption

Ultrasound energy that propagates through a medium can be absorbed, resulting in the generation of heat. The absorption of ultrasound energy depends on tissue properties and is highly frequency dependent. Higher frequencies cause more tissue vibration, resulting in greater absorption of the ultrasound energy and more heat generation.

Ultrasound intensity

The intensity of the ultrasound signal is a parameter that describes the power of the ultrasound signal over a cross-sectional area. As ultrasound waves propagate through tissue, the intensity of the wave becomes attenuated. Attenuation is due to effects of both scattering and absorption of the ultrasound wave.[1] The attenuation coefficient (a) is a function of frequency that can be determined experimentally, and increases with increasing frequency. The frequency of the ultrasound pulse impacts both the depth of penetration of the pulse and the obtainable resolution. In general, as the frequency is increased, the depth of penetration decreases owing to attenuation of the ultrasound intensity, and axial resolution improves, as discussed later in this chapter.

The intensity of the propagating ultrasound energy decreases exponentially as a function of depth and is given by the following equation:

$$I_x = I_o e^{-2ax} \qquad (1.8)$$

where I_o is the initial intensity of the ultrasound pulse, I_x is the intensity of the ultrasound pulse after it has passed a distance x through tissue with an attenuation coefficient a in Neper/cm (Np/cm). As the attenuation coefficient increases with frequency, intensity also decreases exponentially as frequency increases. This equation partially explains the limitation on the depth of imaging, as the returning ultrasound pulse from the tissue must be of sufficient intensity to be detected by the ultrasound transducer.

BASICS OF ULTRASOUND INSTRUMENTATION

The key component of an ultrasound system is the transducer. A transducer is a device that converts one form of energy to another. In the case of ultrasound transducers, electrical energy is converted to mechanical energy, resulting in the transmission of an ultrasound pulse. When an ultrasound signal is then received by the ultrasound transducer, the received mechanical signal is converted back to an electrical signal that is then processed and digitized by the ultrasound processor to yield a real-time image of the tissue being interrogated by the ultrasound transducer (Fig. 1.5).

Transducers

The active element of an ultrasound transducer, responsible for generating and receiving acoustic signals, is made typically from a piezoelectric ceramic. Piezoelectric ceramics are composed of polar crystals that are aligned in a particular orientation such that when an electric field is applied the material changes shape.[3] Therefore, if an alternating electrical field is applied to the material at a particular frequency, the material will vibrate mechanically at that frequency, similar to an audio speaker. In addition, if the piezoelectric material is deformed by sufficient mechanical pressure (e.g., a reflected ultrasound

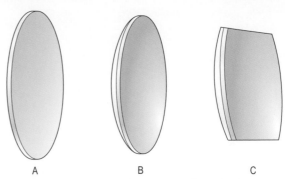

Fig. 1.6   Potential configurations of single element transducers. **A,** Flat circular disk. **B,** Spherically curved disk. **C,** Truncated, spherically curved disk.

wave), a detectable voltage can be measured across the material with a magnitude that is proportional to the applied pressure. The magnitude of the voltage then determines how bright that signal is represented in B-mode imaging (this is explained in the section on B-mode imaging, below).

Single-element transducers

The single-element transducer represents the most basic form of ultrasound transducer and is the easiest to understand owing to its geometric symmetry; therefore, single-element disk transducers will be explained in some detail to illustrate the basic principles of ultrasound transducers. Single-element transducers can be of any shape or size, and can be focused or unfocused. Fig. 1.6 illustrates variations of a single-element disk transducer.

The beam width originating from a flat circular disk transducer in a non-attenuating medium is shown in Fig. 1.7. The beam width is an important concept to understand, because this parameter determines the lateral resolution (further discussed in the section on imaging principles, below). There are two distinct regions of the ultrasound field, termed the *near-field* and *far-field*. The near-field to far-field transition is the location where the flat circular disk transducer has a natural focus, with the focal diameter equal to one-half of the diameter

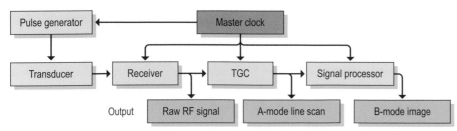

Fig. 1.5   Ultrasound instrumentation schematic. The overall system is synchronized by a master clock. A pulse generator sends an electrical signal to the transducer resulting in a transmitted ultrasound pulse. The transducer then receives the back-reflected signal resulting from the transmitted pulse. This signal is then passed on to the receiver, which amplifies the entire signal. The output from the receiver is the raw radiofrequency (RF) signal. The signal can then undergo time gain compensation (TGC) and the subsequent output will be the A-mode line scan. After TGC the signal is further processed, including demodulation and registration, to yield a B-mode image.

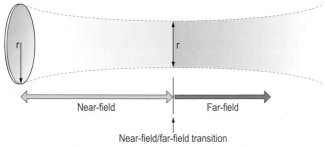

Fig. 1.7   Single-element unfocused disk transducer. In a non-attenuating medium, an unfocused transducer has a self-focusing effect with the diameter of the ultrasound beam at the focus qual to the radius of the transducer (*r*). The location of the beam waist occurs at the near-field/far-field transition.

(or equal to the radius) of the transducer. The distance from the transducer at which this occurs is given by the following equation:

$$D = \frac{r^2}{\lambda} \tag{1.9}$$

where D is the near-field to far-field transition distance or focal length, r is the radius of the transducer, and λ is the wavelength of ultrasound in the propagating medium. Eqn 1.9 demonstrates that, as the radius of the transducer decreases, the focal length is reduced if the frequency remains constant. In adddition, for a constant radius, increasing the wavelength (i.e., decreasing the frequency) also reduces the focal length. However, in attenuating media such as tissue, this self-focusing effect is not seen and the beam width in the near-field is approximately equal to the diameter of the transducer (Fig. 1.8). The beam width then rapidly diverges in the far field.

Focusing

A single-element transducer can be focused by fabricating the transducer with a concave curvature (spherically curved) or by

placing a lens over a flat disk transducer. Focusing is used to improve the lateral resolution and results in a narrow beam width at the focal length (distance from the transducer to the location of the beam width that is most narrow). However, the degree of focusing impacts the depth of focus (the range where the image is in focus) and the focal length. For weak focusing, the focal length is long, as is the depth of focus. Conversely, for a beam that is highly focused the focal length is short, as is the depth of focus (Fig. 1.9).

Arrays

Multiple single-element transducers can be combined in several different configurations. The linear array configuration is the most widely employed clinically. The array is composed of multiple identical crystals that are controlled electronically (Fig. 1.10). They can be fired individually in sequence or in groups depending on the imaging algorithm. This configuration allows for electronic focusing at different depths based on the timing of the excitation of the individual transducer crystals.

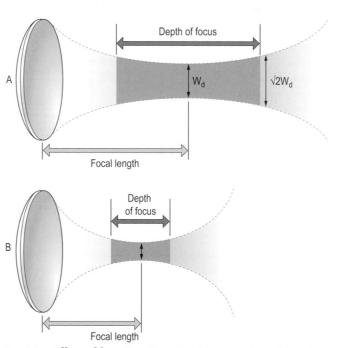

Fig. 1.9   Effect of focusing. Focusing increases lateral resolution by decreasing the beam waist in the focal region (highlighted in blue). The depth of focus is the distance between where the diameter of the beam is equal to $\sqrt{2}w_d$, where w_d is the diameter of the beam at the waist or focus. The degree of focusing influences the focal length as well as the depth of focus. This figure compares two transducers of equal diameters with different degrees of focusing. The transducer in (**A**) exhibits weak focusing, whereas that in (**B**) exhibits strong focusing. The diameter of the waist at the focus is narrower with strong focusing, leading to improved lateral resolution in the focal region. However, the trade-off for this is a decrease in the depth of focus with rapid divergence of the beam beyond the focus. In addition, the focal length is much shorter (i.e., the focus is closer to the transducer) for the highly focused transducer.

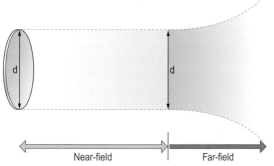

Fig. 1.8   Single-element unfocused disk transducer. In an attenuating medium, the beam width of an unfocused transducer is approximately equal to the diameter of the transducer (*d*) until the near-field/far-field transition. The beam then rapidly diverges in the far-field.

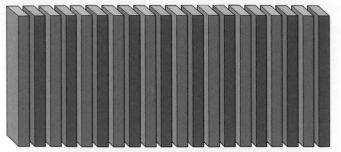

Fig. 1.10   Configuration of a linear array transducer. This configuration consists of several individual rectangular elements, which are controlled individually. The sequence and timing of excitation of each individual element dictates the beam pattern that is transmitted from the array.

Processors

Fig. 1.5 is a block diagram of the components of an ultrasound imaging system. The main components are the ultrasound transducer, processor, and display. Within the processor are electronic components that are responsible for controlling the excitation of the transducer, amplification of the received signal, time gain compensation (TGC), and signal processing resulting in an output signal to the display.

Transmit/receive

As described above, the ultrasound transducer is responsible for transmitting the ultrasound pulse and receiving reflected pulses. The time interval between the transmission of a pulse and the detection of the reflected pulse gives information as to the distance from the interface or non-specular reflector where the reflection occurred. The distance, or depth, of the interface from the transducer is given by:

$$D = \frac{v \times t}{2} \qquad (1.10)$$

where D is the distance from the transducer, v is the velocity of ultrasound in tissue (assumed to be uniform [1540 m/s] by most ultrasound processors), and t is the time between the transmitted and received pulses. The product of v and t is divided by 2 because the pulse travels twice the distance (to the reflector and back). In addition, the strength of the received signal gives information regarding the impedance mismatch at the interface where the reflection occurred.

System gain and time gain compensation

The amplification of the output can be adjusted by the operator in two ways. One is to increase the overall gain of the system, which uniformly increases the amplitude of all echoes received by the transducer. This can improve the detection of weak echoes; however, it generally comes at the expense of overall resolution.

Time gain compensation (TGC) is used to compensate for the decreased intensity of echoes that originate from structures further from the transducer. As described above, the intensity of the ultrasound signal diminishes exponentially with distance (Eqn 1.8); therefore, reflections from interfaces further from the transducer have significantly decreased intensities. The TGC function of ultrasound processors allows selective amplification of echoes from deeper structures. Current EUS processors allow the operator to vary the gain by depth.

Signal processor

After time gain compensation of the signal has occurred, additional signal processing is performed. The algorithms for signal processing performed differ between ultrasound processors and are closely held proprietary information. In general, some form of demodulation of the radiofrequency (RF) signal is performed to obtain an envelope of the RF signal, which is used to produce a B-mode image. In addition, processing can include threshold suppression to eliminate signals that are below an operator-specified threshold. Leading edge detection, peak detection, and differentiation are additional methods that can be employed by processors to improve the image quality.[1]

IMAGING PRINCIPLES

Now that the basic principles of ultrasound physics and instrumentation have been introduced, an overview of imaging principles can be described.

Resolution

In ultrasound imaging, three different aspects of resolution must be considered: axial, lateral, and elevation or azimuthal resolution.

Axial resolution

Axial resolution refers to the smallest separation distance between two objects along the beam path that can be detected by the imaging system. Axial resolution is determined by the ultrasound frequency and the spatial pulse length (SPL) of the transmitted ultrasound pulse.[5] The SPL can be determined by the following equation:

$$SPL = \frac{c}{f} \times n \qquad (1.11)$$

where c is the speed of sound in tissue, f is the center frequency of the transmitted ultrasound pulse, and n is the number of cycles per pulse (typically 4–7 cycles). The limit of axial resolution is equal to SPL/2. This equation demonstrates why using higher frequencies results in greater axial resolution (assuming pulses have the same number of cycles per pulse). To illustrate this concept two different ultrasound pulses with qualitatively different center frequencies and SPL are shown (Fig. 1.11). Axial resolution is the most important property in imaging the layered structures of the gastrointestinal tract wall.

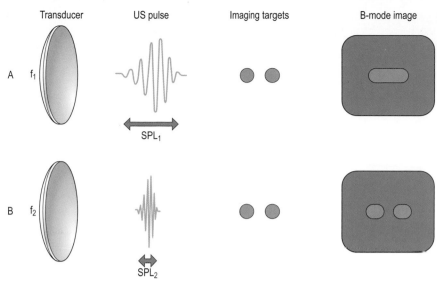

Fig. 1.11   Concept of axial resolution. The axial resolution is limited by the spatial pulse length (SPL). This figure compares the axial resolution of two different ultrasound pulses with different frequencies ($f_1 < f_2$) and identical pulse lengths; therefore, $SPL_1 > SPL_2$. In (**A**), the distance between the imaging targets is less than $SPL_1/2$, resulting in a B-mode image that is not able to resolve the two discrete targets. In (**B**), the distance between the imaging targets is greater than $SPL_2/2$, resulting in the ability to resolve the two discrete targets.

Lateral resolution

The lateral resolution of an imaging system represents the ability to discriminate between two points that are in a plane perpendicular to the ultrasound beam. The beam width of the transducer determines the achievable lateral resolution and is a function of the transducer size, shape, frequency, and focusing. Fig. 1.12 illustrates the concept of lateral resolution.

Elevation resolution

Elevation, or azimuthal, resolution relates to the fact that, although the image displayed is two dimensional, the actual interrogated plane has a thickness associated with it. The factors governing elevation resolution are similar to those for lateral resolution. In fact, the elevation resolution for a focused, circular disk transducer (as incorporated in the Olympus GF-UM series) is the same as for lateral resolution because of its circular symmetry. For the linear array transducers, the elevation resolution is determined by the beam width characteristics along the plane of imaging.

A-mode scanning

A-mode, or amplitude mode, scanning is obtained by the transmit/receive process described previously with an output yielding a radiofrequency (RF) line scan of the echoes detected along the axis of a stationary transducer after a pulse of ultrasound has been transmitted. The received signal by the transducer is amplified, yielding the A-mode signal (Fig. 1.13). This form of scanning is rarely used by the clinician, but is the basis for all other modes of scanning including B-mode scanning. In addition, RF signal analysis is an important aspect of research in the area of advanced imaging techniques.

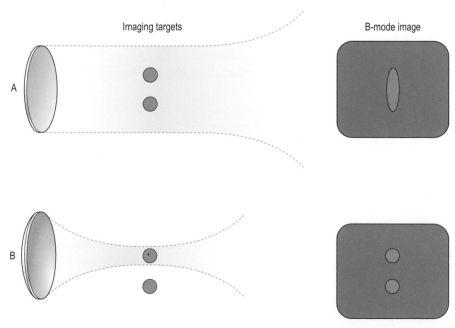

Fig. 1.12   Concept of lateral resolution. The lateral resolution is determined by the ultrasound beam width. This figure compares the lateral resolution of an unfocused (**A**) and focused (**B**) transducer with apertures of the same diameter. The beam width of the unfocused transducer in (**A**) cannot resolve the two imaging targets; therefore, the two targets are displayed as one target on B-mode imaging. The beam width of the focused transducer in (**B**) is sufficiently narrow to resolve the two imaging targets. Note that if the imaging targets were beyond the focus of the transducer in (**B**), the broadened beam width would not be able to resolve the two objects and the B-mode image would be similar to that in (**A**).

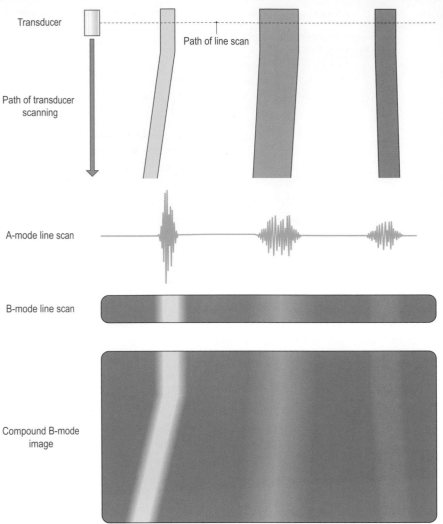

Transducer

Path of line scan

Path of transducer scanning

A-mode line scan

B-mode line scan

Compound B-mode image

Fig. 1.13   Conceptual representation of how A-mode line scans, B-mode line scans, and compound B-mode images are obtained. The transducer output is directed into the tissue determining the path of the line scan. An A-mode line scan is obtained after amplification of the received signals by the transducer. The B-mode line scan is obtained after demodulation and additional signal processing of the A-mode signal. The compound B-mode image is produced by obtaining multiple line scans by translating the path of the line scan. This can be accomplished either by mechanically scanning the transducer or by electronically steering a linear array transducer.

B-mode imaging

B-mode, or brightness mode, scanning results in additional signal processing and movement of the transducer either mechanically or electronically. A B-mode image is created by processing a series of A-mode signals (Fig. 1.13). For each line in the B-mode image (corresponding to a single A-mode line scan), the digitized RF signal is demodulated, yielding an envelope of the RF signal. The amplitude of the demodulated signal is then used to determine the brightness of the dot corresponding to its location in the B-mode image. As the axis of the transducer output is translated (either mechanically or electronically), additional A-mode signals are obtained and processed, eventually yielding a compound B-mode image (Fig. 1.13). EUS imaging systems generate a compound B-mode image.

DOPPLER

The Doppler effect is used in ultrasound applications to identify objects that are in motion relative to the transducer. In biologic applications, the reflective objects in motion are red blood cells. Doppler ultrasound is used in EUS examinations to identify blood flow in vessels. The fundamental basis for the Doppler effect in ultrasound is that an object in motion relative to the source transducer will reflect an ultrasound wave at a different frequency relative to the frequency transmitted by the source transducer; this is termed the *Doppler shift*. The difference between the transmitted frequency and the 'shifted' frequency is dictated by the velocity (v) of the object in motion relative to the transducer. The Doppler shift can be determined by the following equation:

$$f_D = \frac{2vf_t \cos \theta}{c} \tag{1.12}$$

where f_D is the Doppler shift frequency, which is the difference between the transmitted and reflected frequencies; v is the velocity of the object in motion (red blood cells); f_t is the transmitted frequency; θ is the angle at which the object in motion is traveling relative to the direction of the source beam (Fig. 1.14); and c is the speed of sound in tissue (1540 m/s). This equation illustrates why a Doppler shift is not detected if the transducer is aimed perpendicular (90°) to a blood vessel. At an angle of 90°, Eqn 1.12 demonstrates that $f_D=0$, as cos 90°=0. Therefore, interrogation of a blood vessel should be at an angle

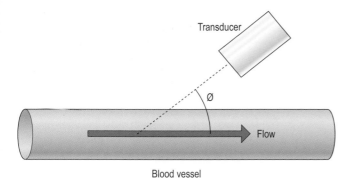

Fig. 1.14   Conceptual image of Doppler measurements. The angle θ determines the strength of the Doppler signal. If θ is 90° then no Doppler signal can be detected.

other than 90°, with the greatest Doppler shift detected when the object in motion is moving along the axis of the transmitted ultrasound wave (cos 0°=1 and cos 180°=−1).

There are different implementations of Doppler ultrasound, including continuous-wave, pulsed-wave, color, and power Doppler.

Continuous-wave Doppler

Continuous-wave Doppler represents the simplest configuration of Doppler ultrasound and requires two different transducers: a transmitting and a receiving transducer. The transmitting transducer produces a continuous output of ultrasound at a fixed frequency. The receiving transducer then receives the continuous signal. The transmitted and received signals are added, resulting in a waveform that contains a beat frequency that is equivalent to the Doppler shift frequency. Continuous-wave Doppler does not give any information regarding the depth at which the motion causing the Doppler shift is occurring.

Pulsed-wave Doppler

Pulsed-wave Doppler was developed to obtain depth information regarding where the motion causing the Doppler shift was occurring. In addition, a pulsed-wave Doppler system requires only a single transducer to transmit and receive ultrasound signals. The pulse length used for pulsed-wave Doppler is substantially longer than pulses used for imaging. Using electronic gating to time the interval between transmitting and receiving a pulse, this method allows the operator to interrogate a specific location along the axis of the transmitted ultrasound beam for motion. The output from pulsed-wave Doppler is usually in the form of an audible signal. The combination of pulsed-wave Doppler with B-mode imaging is termed *duplex scanning* and allows the operator to interrogate a specific location within a B-mode image.

Color Doppler

Color Doppler is a method of visually detecting motion or blood flow using a color map that is incorporated into a standard B-mode image. The principles of color Doppler are similar to those of pulsed-wave Doppler; however, a larger region can be interrogated and detected blood flow is assigned a color, typically blue or red depending on whether the flow is moving toward or away from the transducer. Frequency shifts are estimated at each point at which motion is detected within an interrogated region, yielding information on direction of motion and velocity. Shades of blue or red are used to reflect the relative velocities of the blood flow. All stationary objects are represented on a gray-scale, as in B-mode imaging. The benefits of color Doppler are that information on the direction and relative velocity of blood flow can be obtained. The limitation of color Doppler is its dependence on the relative angle of the transducer to the blood flow.

Power Doppler

Power Doppler is the most sensitive Doppler method for detecting blood flow. Again, the basis for power Doppler is similar to that for pulsed-wave and color Doppler; however, in processing the Doppler signal, instead of estimating the frequency shift as in color Doppler, the integral of the power spectrum of the Doppler signal is estimated. This method essentially determines the strength of the Doppler signal and discards any information on velocity or direction of motion. This method is the most sensitive for detecting blood flow and should be used to identify blood vessels when information on direction of flow and velocity is not needed.

IMAGING ARTIFACTS

Image artifacts are findings on ultrasound imaging that do not accurately represent the tissue being interrogated. An understanding of the principles of ultrasound can be used to explain image artifacts. It is important to identify and to understand the basis for image artifacts in order to interpret ultrasound images correctly. Some common ultrasound imaging artifacts are discussed.

Reverberation

Reverberations occur when a single transmitted pulse undergoes multiple reflections from a strong reflector over the time of a single line scan. The transmitted pulse first gets reflected by the reflector back to the transducer. The reflected pulse then is reflected off the transducer back toward the reflector. This sequence is repeated, and each time a reflection returns to the transducer a signal is generated, until the signal has been attenuated to the point where it is not detected by the transducer or the line scan has been completed (Fig. 1.15). The duration of the line scan is dependent on the depth of imaging. A reverberation artifact can be identified by the equal spacing between hyperechoic (bright) bands, with decreasing intensity as the distance from the transducer increases. Reverberation artifact from a mechanical radial scanning ultrasound probe is demonstrated in Fig. 1.16. This particular reverberation artifact is also called the *ring artifact*.[6] The reflections are from

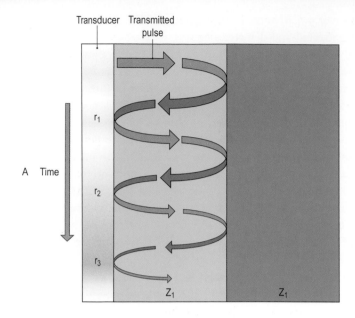

A Time

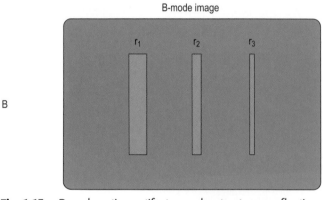

B-mode image

B

Fig. 1.15 Reverberation artifacts are due to strong reflections of a transmitted pulse from an interface with a large impedance mismatch (e.g., air–water interface). **A,** Depiction of how a transmitted signal is reflected by an interface with a large impedance mismatch. The reflected signal is detected by the transducer and redirected back into the medium. This sequence can be repeated multiple times, depending on the depth of imaging. The reflected signal is progressively attenuated. **B,** The corresponding B-mode image from the reverberation depicted in (**A**). The reflected signals (r_1, r_2, and r_3) are spaced equally.

the housing of the ultrasound transducer. Reverberation artifacts are also seen with air–water interfaces, such as bubbles (Fig. 1.17).

Reflection (mirror image)

The reflection, or mirror image, artifact occurs when imaging near an air–water interface such as a lumen filled partially with water.[7] In this scenario, transmitted ultrasound pulses reflect off the air–water interface (due to the significant impedance mismatch) resulting in multiple reflections that are eventually received by the transducer, leading to a mirror image being produced opposite the air–water interface (Figs 1.18 & 1.19). This artifact is easily identified and can be avoided by removing air and adding more water into the lumen.

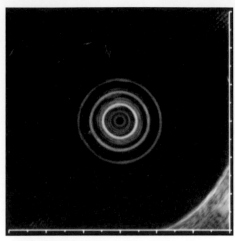

Fig. 1.16 EUS image of reverberation artifact due to multiple reflections from the transducer housing. The concentric rings are equally spaced, with the intensity of the rings decreasing as the distance from the transducer increases.

Acoustic shadowing

Acoustic shadowing is a form of a reflection artifact that occurs when a large impedance mismatch is encountered. When such a mismatch is encountered, a majority of the transmitted pulse is reflected with minimal transmission. This results in a hyperechoic signal at the interface and no echo signal detected beyond the interface, resulting in a 'shadow' effect. This finding is useful in diagnosing calcifications in the pancreas (Fig. 1.20) and gallstones in the gallbladder (Fig. 1.21).

Acoustic shadowing can also occur due to refraction occurring at a boundary between tissues with different acoustic velocities, especially if the boundary is curved (e.g., tumor or cyst). As discussed above, refraction of an ultrasound beam occurs when the angle of incidence is not normal to the boundary between tissues with different acoustic velocities, resulting in bending of the ultrasound beam. As the ultrasound beam is

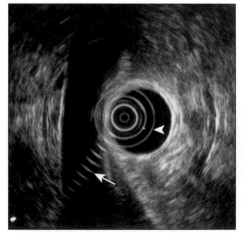

Fig. 1.17 EUS image of reverberation artifact (arrow) due to multiple reflections from an air bubble in the water-filled balloon. Note that the intensity of the artifact does not decrease as rapidly as the reverberation artifact (arrowhead) from the transducer housing, because the impedance mismatch of the air–water interface is much greater than the transducer housing interface, resulting in reflected signals with greater intensity.

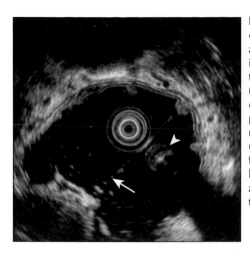

Fig. 1.18 Reflection or mirror image artifact. A mirror image of the transducer (arrowhead) and gastric wall is produced by the reflection of the ultrasound signal from the interface between water and air (arrow) within the gastric lumen.

goes less attenuation as it propagates through the cyst and as the reflected signal returns to the transducer. This finding is useful in diagnosing fluid-filled structures such as a cyst or blood vessel (Fig. 1.23).

Tangential scanning

If the thickness of a structure is being measured, it is important that the ultrasound beam is perpendicular to the structure. If the transducer is at an angle other than 90° to the structure, the thickness will be overestimated.[9] This is particularly important when assessing the thickness of the layers of the gastrointestinal (GI) tract wall and in staging tumors of the GI tract. On radial scanning examination of the GI tract, this artifact can be identified because the thicknesses of the wall layers will not be uniform throughout the image (Fig. 1.24). When staging tumors involving the GI tract wall, tangential imaging can result in overstaging of the tumor. To avoid this artifact the endoscope tip should be maneuvered to maintain the proper orientation such that the plane of imaging is normal (at 90°) to the structure being imaged.

redirected at this boundary, there are regions of the tissue that do not get interrogated by the ultrasound beam, resulting in an acoustic shadow (Fig. 1.22).[8]

Through transmission

Through transmission is the enhancement of a structure beyond a fluid-filled structure such as a cyst. The structure beyond a fluid-filled structure demonstrates increased enhancement because the intensity of transmitted ultrasound under-

Side lobe artifacts

Side lobes are off-axis secondary projections of the ultrasound beam (Fig. 1.25).[3] The side lobes have reduced intensities compared with the main on-axis projection; however, they can

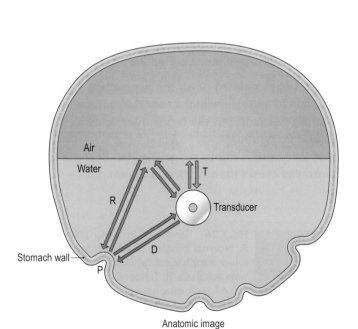

Anatomic image

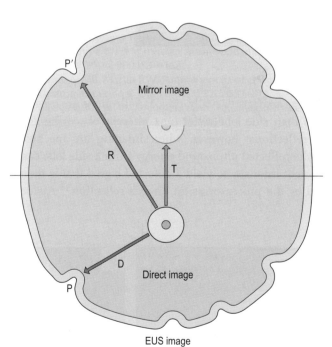

EUS image

Fig. 1.19 Reflection from an air–water interface produces a mirror image artifact. Due to the large impedance mismatch between water and air, an ultrasound signal that interacts with an air–water interface will be reflected almost completely. The figure on the left is an illustration of an ultrasound probe imaging the gastric wall with an air–water interface. The path denoted by D is the path that directly images location P along the gastric wall. The path denoted by R is the path that images location P due to a reflection from the air–water interface. The path T is the path that images the transducer due to a reflection from the air–water interface. The figure on the right is an illustration of the resulting ultrasound *image*. The ultrasound processor registers the location of the image by the direction of the transmitted pulse and the time it receives the reflected signal. The processor accurately registers point P, resulting from the reflected signal from path D; however, the signal from path R is incorrectly registered as point P′, resulting in the appearance of a mirror image. Also note that the reflected signal from path T results in shadowing artifact in the mirror image.

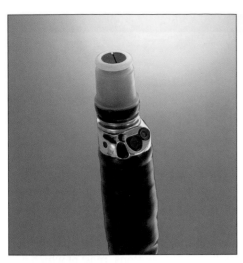

Fig. 2.1 The distal, mechanical transducer of the Olympus GF-UM2000/160 echoendoscope.

in these scopes capable of taking 'bronchoscopy'-sized mucosal biopsies; an elevator lifts the forceps into view.

Although robust and capable of a long clinical life, the dual requirement for a drive shaft and an exposed oil-bath housing might be perceived to be inherent weaknesses. In practice, the mechanical nature of these scopes does not carry any greater susceptibility to breakdown. Care must be exercised, however, when placing or removing the balloon, that the oil bath is not crushed or dislocated – a potentially significant problem in units with many trainees. The development of a bubble and resulting diffuse degradation in the quality of the ultrasound image is a sign that the oil bath requires topping up; this may occur once or twice a year.

Pentax was the first company to market an electronic radial instrument (Pentax/Hitachi EG-3630UR) (Fig. 2.2A). This forward-viewing instrument relies on solid-state electronics, a slightly bulbous band-like transducer placed just proximal to the scope tip. Being a modified curvilinear array instrument with multiple crystal transducers, a large part of the scope shaft is taken up with hard-wiring. This technical sophistication is offset by a narrowing of EUS view to 270°. The 90° wedge deficit occupies the upper quadrant of the screen but does not compromise EUS views, except when staging circumferential

luminal cancers. Although the distal tip of this scope was originally blunt, the leading edge has now been rounded. This scope is to be supplanted by a 360°-viewing model (Pentax/Hitachi EG-3670URK), which will connect to the Pentax endoscopic EPK-1000 color chip processor.

The Pentax EG-3630UR scans at 5, 7.5, and 10 MHz, and has forward endoscopic views (120°). This apparent advantage over oblique-viewing instruments is somewhat offset by the bulkiness and distal stiffness common to all echoendoscopes. Such lack of plasticity raises the question of whether formal endoscopy ought to be performed with one of these instruments; if a full endoscopic examination is important, a standard gastroscope must be used.

Olympus has developed an electronic radial echoendoscope with a near 360° field of examination (Olympus GF-UE260/160) (Fig. 2.2B). In build, this scope is of similar appearance to current mechanical models, the ultrasound transducer again lying distal to the endoscopic lens.

LINEAR SCOPES

The Pentax FG-32, launched in 1991, was the standard linear echoendoscope for many years. The EUS transducer sited distal to the viewing lens is gently curved, similar in shape to those used for transabdominal studies, and gives a 120° field of ultrasonic view. The range has been expanded, offering wider-bore channels and the presence of an elevator. Biopsy channels range in size from 2.0 to 3.8 mm (fiberoptic models: FG-34UX [2-mm channel] and FG-38UX [3.2 mm]; video models: EG-3630U [2.4 mm] and EG-3830UT [3.8 mm]). The smaller channel format is designed for the passage of fine-needle aspiration (FNA) needles alone, the larger-bore scope permitting placement of a 10-Fr stent (under ideal circumstances with a straight scope). As with all Pentax instruments, an extra control knob on the handle redirects the suction controls to either lumen or balloon. The introduction of the Pentax color chip endoscope processor (EPK-1000) is matched by the introduction of a further linear echoendoscope model (EG-3870UTK).

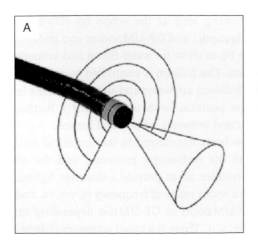

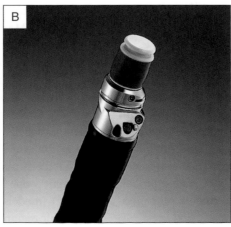

Fig. 2.2 **A,** The forward-viewing Pentax/Hitachi electronic radial echoendoscope (270° plane of ultrasound scanning; EG-3630UR). The Pentax/Hitachi model EG-3670URK has a 360° plane of view. **B,** The Olympus electronic 360°-viewing radial echoendoscope (GF-UE260/160).

The Olympus linear echoendoscope has a pea-like tip transducer allowing for a 180° scanning plane. There are two models (Fig. 2.3A), differentiated by accessory channel size: 2.8 mm (GF-UC240P/140P-AL5) and 3.7 mm (GF-UCT240/140-AL5). Both scopes have elevators to assist needle guidance. The latter scope is said to be capable of deploying a 10-Fr stent; however, any angulation of the scope tip required to obtain appropriate views lessens the functional diameter of the accessory channel, making passage of large-bore stents difficult. It might be conjectured that performing FNA with the larger-channel scope might be more problematic due to the needle wobbling within the channel, but in practice this does not occur.

The Toshiba PEF-708FA linear echoendoscope handles well and allows views through a wide range of frequencies from 3 to 13 MHz. The lower frequency would allow for greater depth of view when inspecting the liver. It is promoted as having the advantage of not requiring a balloon. It is a moot point, however, whether a balloon is required with any linear scope, on account of the constant pressure apposing the scope tip with the mucosa.

Fujinon has developed an electronic linear echoendoscope with a 130° ultrasound view and a 2.3-mm accessory channel, complete with elevator, that will accept 22- and 19-G FNA needles.

All of the scopes mentioned above are electronic in format. The Olympus mechanical 'linear' echoendoscope (GUMP) represents a clever variation on the mechanical radial scope. If the problem with the radial scope is that the plane of view is perpendicular to the scope tip, then why not adjust the mirror so that it rotates in another plane, allowing for a linear-type view? The resulting 'GUMP' echoendoscope (GF-UMD240/140P; Fig. 3.3B) is certainly clever, and does yield an impressive, though largely redundant, 270° linear view. It can be plugged into the same Olympus processor as the mechanical models. However, the scope tip is bulbous and concerns have been raised about depth of view. There is no facility for Doppler.

EUS PROCESSORS

There is little to separate the various scope offerings available from the major companies. This can also be said of the processors

required to drive these instruments. Compatibility between radial and linear systems, however, is not universal.

Radial systems

The current high-end Olympus radial processor (models EU-M2000 or EU-M60, depending on geographic area) is a very fine unit, replacing the workhorse EU-M20 that has been around for many years. The new processor allows for a greater range of available frequencies (5–20 MHz), greater focus (to a range of 1 cm), greater image manipulation including instant video replay and, with appropriate software, mini-probe 3D rendering. It will not, however, drive a linear scope. The Olympus EU-M30 is a current, compact, radial processor model that is similar in capability to the old EU-M20.

The Olympus electronic radial echoendoscope (GF-UE 260/160) is driven by the aloka 5000 platform common to their electronic linear offering.

The processor for Pentax's electronic radial scope is the Hitachi 5000, 6000, or 8000 range. This is significant for two reasons: first, the same processor is used for both Pentax radial and electronic echoendoscopes and, second, it brings to EUS the capabilities of mainstream ultrasonography.

Linear systems

Both Pentax electronic and radial echoendoscopes run from a common Hitachi processor described above. The linear scopes alone may also be run from the older Hitachi platforms EUB405plus and EUB2000 (both lower-end 'compromise' processors), or the mid-range EUB525.

Scopes in the Olympus linear GF-UC 240/140 range, however, require a separate processor from their mechanical radial cousins, either from Aloka (SSD4000PHD and SSD-5000PHD range) or from Philips (North America and continental Europe). The Olympus EU-C2000 (or EU-C60, depending on geographic region; Fig. 2.4) is a very mobile, diminutive processor, measuring only 313 mm in width and 93 mm in height. Its small size means that it can be attached to a radial processor trolley, allowing for some improvement in user convenience. Although cheaper, considerably smaller, and more mobile than standard ultrasound

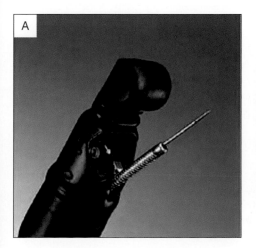

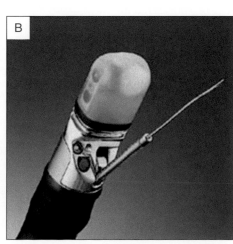

Fig. 2.3 Linear echoendoscopes. **A,** Olympus GF-UC240/140P-AL5 (electronic). **B,** Olympus GF-UMD240/140P (mechanical 'GUMP' scope).

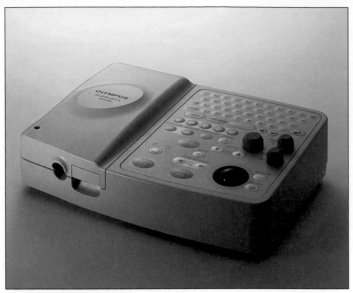

Fig. 2.4 The diminutive Olympus EU-C60/C2000 processor for Olympus electronic linear and endobronchial echoendoscopes.

processors, compromise comes at a price. Screen images are the result of 'averaging' factors such as frequency (7.5 MHz), depth of focus, and field of view (150° as opposed to 180° for the standard scope, an unimportant operating characteristic). It is also important to mention that the linear scopes run by the C2000/C60 have a modified connecting box, so they cannot be switched between Aloka/Philips platforms and the mini-processor. On the credit side of the equation, this processor is compatible not only with the Olympus gastrointestinal EUS linear scopes, but also with the endobronchial 'EBUS' scope.

Toshiba's PEF-708FA runs off a wide range of their processors including the PowerVision 6000, Nemio, CoreVision Pro, and Eccocee CX. The Fujinon linear scope, too, is operated through the Toshiba Nemio console. A feature of this latter scope is to permit on-screen marking of needle trajectory to aid with FNA.

SPECIALTY PROBES

A variety of probes is available for specific clinical situations. Although such instruments may be used only relatively infrequently, the advantages of their use must be considered in planning for departmental needs.

Esophagus and stomach

The Olympus MH908 slim probe is perhaps the unsung hero of the EUS world, and its value needs to be considered seriously in units that undertake a large volume of esophageal cancer staging.

The MH908 is a mechanical radial probe (7.5 MHz) that is driven by the same range of processors as all other Olympus mechanical scopes. It is a 'blind', cone-tipped scope that is passed over a standard endoscopic retrograde cholangiopancreatography (ERCP) wire, placed at endoscopy. The diameter of the scope is 8.5 mm, allowing for passage through the majority of esophageal strictures without the need for dilatation. The short length of

the insertion tube allows for proximal, but not distal, gastric tumors to be staged.

Concerns have been raised about the ability of the MH908 to inspect the celiac axis adequately (downward tip angulation being only 90° versus 130° for standard Olympus echoendoscopes). This difficulty has probably been overstated, as good regional views can be obtained. The advantages of using the MH908, obviating the need for dilatation, are obviously lessened in units where universal nodal FNA is the routine.

The facility to add an unplanned EUS examination to a gastroscopy is an ever-present aspiration. The Fujinon PL-2226B-7.5 is a torpedo-shaped, mechanical radial probe (7.5 MHz; head diameter 7.3 mm; Fig. 2.5) that may be back-loaded through a large-channel gastroscope in a fashion analogous to the loading of a variceal band cartridge. This cleverness in design is offset by a resultant diminishment in endoscopic luminal view, problematic with strictures. The probe is driven by the SP-711 UA processor through the TL-1A connector ('translator'). This processor also permits easy switching between radial and linear formats ('bi-planar' ultrasound) when using Fujinon mini-probes.

Mini-probes

Catheter probes range in size from 2 to 2.6 mm, are mostly mechanical radial, and require an additional small motor-drive unit intervening between the probe and the ultrasound processor. In length, all probes will reach to the duodenum and terminal ileum. They are usually of high frequency (12–30 MHz, most 20 MHz and above) with a shallow depth of view and a resultant reduction in useful application. Although such probes are particularly good at inspecting small mucosal or subepithelial lesions, and for intraductal use, they are not good for the regular staging of esophageal tumors or larger colonic polyps.

Another drawback with catheter probes is the difficulty of excluding air from the site of mucosal contact. Proprietary balloon

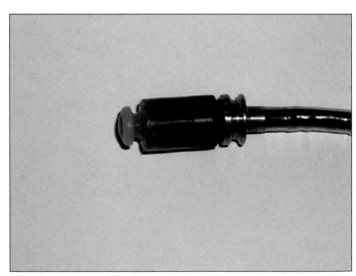

Fig. 2.5 Fujinon PL-2226B-7.5 mini-probe. This 7.5-MHz probe, of diameter 7.3 mm, is back-loaded through a large-channel gastroscope.

sheaths are available, but these require the use of scopes with large-caliber accessory channels. There have been many reports of other methods to provide a water interface, including use of (non-lubricated) condoms and water-flooding of the esophagus with prior cuffed intubation.

Mini-probes are said to have a useful life of 50 to 100 procedures. With care, the longevity of catheter probes can be extended considerably beyond this. In particular, storing probes in a hanging position, rather than coiled flat, prolongs lifespan. In use, the transducer should never be rotated when passing or withdrawing the probe through the scope, and the elevator should never, ever, be touched when the probe is in place.

Both Olympus and Fujinon offer a wide range of mini-probes. The probes from Olympus fall into two broad categories: those for general use (UM-2R [12 MHz], UM-3R [20 MHz], and UM-S30-25R [ultra-slim, 30 MHz]) and those for intraductal studies (wire-guided UM-G20-29R [20 MHz]; Fig. 2.6). The newer 'spiralling' UM-DP12-25R, UM-DP-20-25R, and UM-DP-29R probes (Fig. 2.7) offer the added capacity to permit dual-plane ('3D') rendering when used off the EU-M2000/EU-M60 processor, provided the appropriate software has been loaded. The UM-BS20-26R is a 20-MHz probe with a diameter of 2.6 mm and an inbuilt balloon. Such a balloon adds further

potential for shortened lifespan. The MAJ-935 unit (Fig. 2.8) is required to drive these probes as they do not plug directly into the ultrasound console.

Fujinon provides a broad range of catheter probes, ranging in frequency from 12 to 20 MHz (PL-2220-12, PL-2220-15, and PL-2220-20, all 2 mm in diameter, and PL-2226-12, PL-2226-15, and PL-2226-20, all 2.6 mm in diameter). These probes will run from a standard Hitachi radial/linear platform or from the Fujinon SP-711UA processor and TL-1A translator. This processor allows for dual-plane scanning (linear and radial).

Colon and anorectum

At first thought, the idea of a dedicated echocolonoscope seems attractive, standard scopes being difficult to maneuver safely beyond the rectosigmoid junction. The Olympus CF-UMQ230 answers this call, but its availability is restricted to certain regions (UK, Japan, and parts of Asia). The combination of standard colonoscope and mini-probe suffices, however, for most needs.

For many who have practiced endoanal ultrasonography in isolation, the probes from B-Kmedical have been the market leaders. Hitachi, however, has a range of both mono-plane and bi-plane probes (EUP range). The EUP-R54AW (5–10 MHz; working lengths 19 and 33 cm; Fig. 2.9) is the first electronic 360° radial anorectal probe. It might be conjectured that the small diameter of this probe (10 mm) would yield superior images to standard instruments on account of much decreased local compression. These instruments have the advantage of being run from the same platform as that used for both the Pentax/Hitachi linear and electronic radial echoendoscopes.

As with their longstanding radial echoendoscopes, Olympus offers the mechanical probes RU-75M-R1 and RU-12M-R1 operating at 7.5 and 12 MHz respectively. These rectal probes work from the EU-2000/EU-M60 processor, allowing compatibility across mechanical radial EUS scopes, mini-probes, and rectal probes, but not linear scopes. A probe driving unit (MAJ-935) is a further item of equipment needed to enable this. The EU-

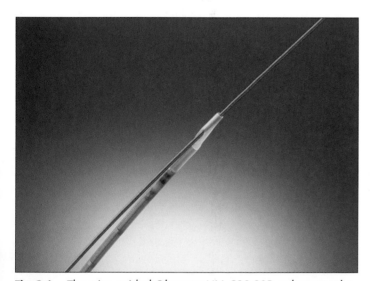

Fig. 2.6 The wire-guided Olympus UM-G20-29R catheter probe (20 MHz) is for intraductal use and may be passed over a short wire system at ERCP.

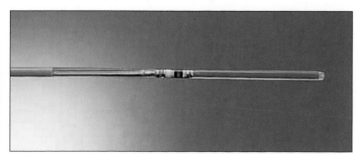

Fig. 2.7 The Olympus UM-DP range of mechanical probes 'spiral' within the catheter to yield dual-plane, or 3D, images.

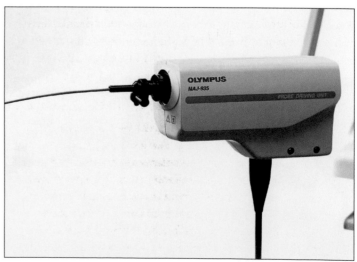

Fig. 2.8 Catheter probes require a motor drive (or translator) for use. The Olympus MAJ-935 Probe Driving Unit.

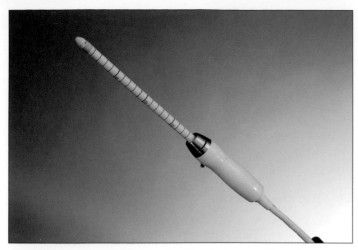

Fig. 2.9 Pentax/Hitachi, small-caliber (diameter 10 mm), electronic, 360°, radial electronic rectal probe.

M30S processor allows for more restricted funtionality between mini-probes and rectal probes. Of increasing interest with the advent of the Olympus electronic radial echoendoscope, is the Aloka ASU-67 dual-frequency (7.5 and 10 MHz) rectal probe, which is driven by the Aloka SSD5000PHD processor. This allows the SSD5000 to play 'mother hen' to a full clutch of echoendoscopes: electronic radial, linear, and endoanal, thereby matching the versatility provided by Pentax/Hitachi.

Endobronchial probes

Olympus offers a diminutive bronchial linear probe (outer diameter 6.9 mm, operating length 600 mm) with a FNA capability (BF-UC260/160F-OL8) (Fig. 2.10). The 2-mm accessory channel allows for passage of a dedicated transbronchial needle (NA-201SX-4022). In use, this scope is somewhat different to a gastrointestinal echoendoscope, as mucosal contact and thus ultrasound view are very easily lost. The probe is run through the C2000/C60 processor.

ACCESSORIES

Needles for FNA

Needles for FNA remain expensive and less than ideal, but have come a long way from simply being modifications of those used for variceal injection. The range of needle sizes has been extended to allow for a needle more suited to lymph node sampling. Additionally, specialized needles for specific tasks, such as pancreatic sampling, celiac axis neurolysis, core biopsy, and pancreatic cyst drainage, have been introduced. There have been refinements to the attached suction syringes, permitting variable degrees of negative pressure to suit a specific clinical situation. The tips of all needles are specially treated to allow for good EUS visualization.

Much tedious work has been performed in an attempt to define the best needle size and appropriate amount of negative pressure for a given task. These factors are covered elsewhere in this book but, in general, the basic principle is that the larger the needle, the more bloody the sample and the less happy the cytopathologist. A 22-G needle can be used in most situations, applying suction for the pancreas but not for lymph nodes. A 25-G needle may be better in the latter situation. A capacity to fix the syringe plunger in different positions, and so vary the degree of negative pressure, is an advantage.

The larger, stiffer, and more awkward 19-G needle is often required to drain larger cysts, as it allows for a quicker procedure, the aspiration of viscous contents, and, where needed, the passage of an 0.035-inch guidewire. Core samples of nodes and lesions such as gastrointestinal stromal tumors may be obtained with this large needle, without resorting to the Tru-Cut model.

Wilson-Cook

Cook produces a broad multipurpose range of fully disposable EUS-FNA needles (Echotip; 19, 22, and 25 G). The original build of these needles was not completely reliable as there were too many connecting joints, a relatively thin handle, and a poorly shaped luer-lock hub for the suction syringe. All of these issues have been addressed with the introduction of a one-piece sturdy handle, easily adaptable to the length of scope. Furthermore, the green-sheathed, slippery coated EUSN-3 22-G needle can be passed with great ease, even under conditions of marked scope torque. The 19-G needle (Fig. 2.11) still retains the older, less slippery, EUSN-1 blue sheath, and is considerably

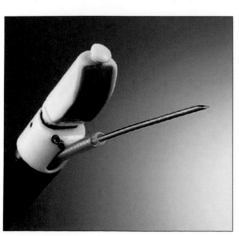

Fig. 2.10 Olympus electronic linear endobronchial echoendoscope (BF-UC260/160F-OL8) with a scope-specific FNA needle (NA-201SX-4022).

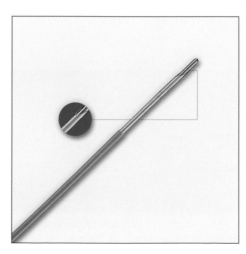

Fig. 2.11 Cook 19-G needle with a ball-tipped protruding stylet.

less easy to advance when the scope is beyond the pylorus. These needles come with a two-step, double-trigger (5 ml/10 ml) suction syringe.

Needles in the EUSN-1 range come with a stylet whose tip is beveled to the needle tip, whereas a protruding ball-tip stylet accompanies the EUSN-3 needles. The ball-tip version might protect the scope channel should the needle be deployed accidentally. In general use, the ball-tip stylet must be withdrawn by about 1 cm before puncture in order to 'sharpen' the needle. Following puncture, the stylet is pushed in to extrude any plugs of extraneous tissue. The 19-G needle cannot be used with Pentax echoendoscope models FG-32UA or FG-34UA owing to accessory channel size.

A 19-G Tru-Cut needle (Fig. 2.12) will yield core samples. The Cook 'Quick-Core' needle, however, is often neither quick to use nor does it always produce a core. The stiffness inherent to 19-G needles lessens the effectiveness of this instrument. Although it can be deployed successfully in the mediastinum and stomach, transduodenal sampling is often impossible.

Both 19- and 22-G needles can be used for celiac axis neurolysis. A specially styled 20-G 'spray' needle is available for this task from Cook (EUSN-20-CPN, available only in certain geographic regions) (Fig. 2.13). The needle has a solid, sharp, cone-tip with proximal side-holes, in order to allow for a bilateral spray effect.

Pancreatic pseudocyst drainage with placement of a transgastric or duodenal stent is achieved using a combination of 19-G needle, guidewire, biliary dilatation balloon, and biliary

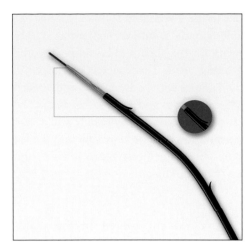

Fig. 2.14 Giovannini stent system for pancreatic pseudocyst drainage. An 8.5-Fr stent is loaded onto a needle-knife catheter (Cook NWOA-8.5; not available in all geographic regions).

endoprosthesis. Cook, however, produces a single-step, 8.5-Fr, stent-loaded needle-wire for this purpose (Giovannini needle wire; NWOA-8.5; certain geographic regions only) (Fig. 2.14). A 10-Fr cystotome delivering a 5-Fr catheter with 0.038-inch needle knife is also available (Cook CST-10; certain geographic regions only).

Cystic, potentially neoplastic, lesions of the pancreas present a specific problem for obtaining representative epithelial cell samples; standard aspirates are generally acellular. To address this difficulty, a dedicated EUS cytologic (nylon) brush has been marketed (EchoBrush).

Olympus

Olympus produces both disposable and partially disposable FNA needles, as well as a spring-loaded device designed for hard lesions.

The single-sized (22 G), fully disposable FNA needle (EZ-Shot; NA-200H-8022) comes with a 20-ml suction syringe that will allow for variable degrees of negative pressure by twisting and locking the plunger in place. The brown-colored needle sheath is not as slippery as that of the Cook 22-G needle, making it slightly more difficult to deploy in the duodenum. Olympus also produces a reusable handle/sheath apparatus with a disposable needle-piece (NA-10J-1).

The Olympus 'Power-Shot' apparatus is a reusable, spring-loaded device that fires a disposable needle (22 G) into a lesion, to a defined depth (NA-11J-1). This instrument has been designed with pancreatic tumors in mind. It must be pointed out, however, that the majority of such tumors are in fact quite soft and that the sensation of 'hardness' comes from poor scope positioning or the needle being gripped by the scope's elevator.

The NA-201SX-4022 needle is for use specifically with the Olympus EUS-bronchoscope (BF-UC260/160OF-OL8).

GIP/Mediglobe

These were perhaps the first dedicated EUS-FNA needles to be developed. Two formats are available: one with a reusable, autoclavable, aluminum piston handle, the other format being

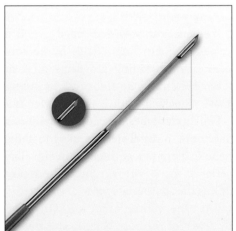

Fig. 2.12 Cook 19-G Tru-Cut needle ('Quick-Core').

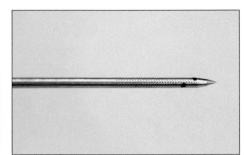

Fig. 2.13 This Cook needle is tailor-made for celiac axis neurolysis. The needle tip is solid with proximal side-holes permitting a bilateral 'spray' effect (Cook Echotip EUSN-20-CPN; not available in all geographic regions).

fully disposable. Needles in the disposable Sonotip II range (22 and 19 G) have a 'double' handle structure, somewhat akin to those from Cook, allowing for the sheath to be simply tailored to the make of scope being used. The stylet is of Nitinol (a nickel–titanium alloy), and comes with both rounded and beveled tips (22G: models GUS-01-18-022 and GUS-01-27-022). The 19-G needle (GUS-01-21-019), beveled-tip stylet only, will accept a 0.039-inch wire. The aspiration syringe allows for only a fixed negative-pressure volume. These needles are available through Medi-globe, or, in some regions, Hitachi.

Balloons

Proprietary balloons are obviously offered by the major echoendoscope manufacturers but usually at exorbitant prices. International Medical Products (Zutphen, The Netherlands) offers very cheap and reliable balloons for the Olympus mechanical radial EUS scopes. Where regulatory concerns allow such generic substitution, it is always worthwhile asking colleagues from other centers whether such products can be sourced in that region.

All EUS balloons contain latex, and so standard echoendo-scopes ought not to be used in patients with latex sensitivity. It may be possible, depending on the pathology in question, to use a mini-probe (those from Olympus are latex free) or a linear scope with no balloon.

Water pump

The UWS-1 water-instilling pump is available from Olympus in certain geographic regions. This pump permits the rapid instillation of water into the bowel lumen to allow for improved imaging of small epithelial lesions. Care must be exercised when water is used in the esophagus without prior cuffed intubation. Furthermore, it is important to change the connecting tube between each patient. It is always worth considering that sterile 50-ml syringes are universally available and cheap.

Reporting systems

There is no good, universally available, reporting system. Modules are offered by several sources including Endosoft, Fujinon (ADAM), and Olympus (EndoWorks, USA; EndoBase, continental Europe). The major drawback with these and other programs is that they require a tremendous amount of work to 'bed' them in for local use.

Archiving

Modern 'full size' processors from all the major manufacturers have inbuilt image/video capture units involving either local hard disks, magneto-optical drives, or DVD burners. The potential to store images in a Digital Imaging and Communications in Medicine (DICOM) format to digital archives (as in radiology departments) is common to current mid/upper range ultrasound processors such as the Aloka SSD5000/5500 and Hitachi 6000/8000 ranges. However, such software options may not be included in the 'package' offered to EUS users, and so must be discussed at the time of tender.

Lengthy paper streamers of photographs from a simple 'hot' black-and-white printer are always satisfying to see after an examination (although they may be a sign of uncertainty). Such images are a good option for most cases and will not fade even after many years, although folded paper may stick together. Hard transparent copies to a laser printer is another, albeit more expensive, option.

Hard-copy photographs can be scanned easily. If there is ever a chance that they might be used for publication, it is worthwhile scanning them as gray-scale images at a resolution of at least 300 dpi, but preferably 500 dpi (most scanners have a default setting of 200 dpi).

Video image capture is a mainstay of EUS teaching. Although high-specification digital recorders are available, these are expensive options. Any digital video camera may be hooked up to an EUS processor, either through an internally fixed video-out cable or from the monitor. Another option is to attach the camera to the line-out connector of the printer. There seems to be little degradation in the quality of image using these two latter simple solutions.

Editing of captured video is simple using generally available programs such as those from Pinnacle. High-specification, very expensive, video-editing software (Adobe, etc.) is not necessary. The type of connection between the video camera and the computer is important, as the system relies on rapid data transfer. For this reason, use a video camera with either a USB-2 or 'Firewire' socket. If using other types of video camera, including VHS, special connection adaptors, such as those from Dazzle, are available relatively cheaply.

Downloaded videos are usually in a format called .avi. The images from this file type are of very high quality but, consequently, of very large size. Video-editing programs offer to convert the snippets of movie into a range of formats including MPEG1, MPEG2, and .avi. Choosing MPEG1-type movies is a compromise in terms of quality, but they are widely playable on most computers. Furthermore, most projectors used to show such videos cannot handle file types of higher quality. The MPEG2 format is superior to that of MPEG1 but will not play on many computers, unless the appropriate piece of software (a 'codec') has been installed. One minute of an MPEG1 movie will take approximately 11 MB of memory. Single, still frames can be captured from downloaded videos using Pinnacle, but the quality does not compare with that of 'true' single-shot images taken at the time of the procedure.

When the EUS examination has been recorded, downloaded, edited, and put into a movie format, the next problem is how to show it. The easiest way is to double-click on the icon and allow a universal program such as Windows Media Player (WMP) to show it. This approach gives the advantage of control. The buttons of WMP allow freezing, fast-forwarding, etc. Another approach is to 'insert' the movie into PowerPoint. This will permit annotation and the incorporation of stills. PowerPoint, however, is not very good at handling video, and MPEG2 files are particularly problematic. Current PDA/hand-held computers are capable of storing large amounts of video and displaying them with good fidelity, even when placed on the platform of a video-type X-ray-viewing box/projector.

Patient confidentiality is a problem with videos, as masking names with a black box will not work in PowerPoint; this program automatically puts any video in front of anything else on that page. Video-editing programs will allow a mask to be placed, but it can be tedious to work out how to do this. In general, it is much easier not to put the patient's name or details on the EUS screen at all.

CHOOSING EQUIPMENT

The equipment for endoscopic ultrasonography is expensive and the choices are wide but not uniform; compromise is an ever-present shadow looming over purchase. Establishing an EUS service is considered elsewhere in this book (see Ch. 3), but it is worth stating several points that ought to be addressed when drafting a call for tenders.

The single most important question to be answered is: what is the equipment for? It is too easy to find a need for every type of equipment, but such loose thinking makes for an unfocused business plan.

Small lesions, celiac neurolysis, and pancreatic pseudocyst drainage are niche areas. The cornerstone of most EUS practice is cancer staging, supported possibly by benign work to extend equipment usage further, for example the substitution of EUS for magnetic resonance imaging in the investigation of possible choledocholithiasis. Another consideration is that not all centers will manage all types of cancer.

If the staging of non-small cell lung cancer will be a significant source of referrals, a linear system capable of FNA is an absolute requirement, the information yielded by radial EUS being vestigial. The situation is less clear for both esophageal and pancreatic cancer staging, and is heavily influenced by local practice.

In the UK, the majority of patients with operable esophageal cancer undergo neoadjuvant chemotherapy, and consequently linear EUS is not an absolute requirement for initial staging. The clinical significance of involved local nodes postchemotherapy (surgery or further chemotherapy) is unknown.

Pancreatic cancer can present an equally opaque decision process. If the lesion is operable, what is the role of FNA – does it add any useful information? If the lesion is inoperable, can a percutaneous biopsy not be performed? Perhaps a radial scan is all that is required?

The point of these few preceding paragraphs is to highlight the importance of detailing exactly how EUS is to be used and where it might fit in a local care pathway algorithm. This will help to prioritize the equipment needed.

Once the decision has been made about what the equipment is for, the next thorny issue to tackle is which system to buy.

Taking linear systems, is there a difference in the performance characteristics between the linear echoendoscopes? Could the shape of the different transducers translate into better or worse endosonographic views? In essence, the answers are 'no' and 'no'.

And radial equipment? Mechanical and electronic systems have their own champions and proponents but, once again, there is little to distinguish them in terms of performance. Consequently, in many ways the choice of processor and compatibility between linear and radial instruments has become the main battleground for EUS equipment (Table 2.1).

Outside regions where non-radiologists routinely perform transabdominal ultrasonography, discussions with radiologic colleagues will often yield preferences for one manufacturer over another, whether it be Hitachi, Toshiba, Aloka, Philips, etc., but it must be borne in mind that a significant amount of the capability of these processors is redundant to EUS. There is little advantage in buying a top-end processor over a more modest one, provided the quality of the screen image is adequate. Most processors are ergonomically similar to use.

The case for a high-specification processor might come from sharing the unit between radiology and endoscopy. If this is the case, it should be borne in mind that moving a complex electronic machine around an institution exposes it to risk, not to mention the inevitable aggravation of both parties needing it at the same time.

Compatibility between radial and electronic systems brings the discussion of purchase close to the thorny issue of cost. Why pay for two separate processors when one will do? Indeed, why have two bulky processors taking up limited endoscopy room space when one will do? The introduction of the Olympus electronic radial echoendoscope, driven by an Aloka processor common to linear Olympus scopes, will obviously level the playing field with Pentax/Hitachi, which have offered this facility for some time. Other considerations, however, remain; the Olympus slim probe may be indispensable for an esophageal cancer unit or, the compact Olympus C2000/C60 linear processor unit may be an acceptable compromise if cost is a consideration. Endoanal ultrasonography often falls under the remit of a unit different to that performing EUS. For this reason, probe compatibility with an EUS processor may not be of paramount importance. When considering the purchase of mini-probes, factor in the costs of a drive/translator unit and also the costs of a replacement catheter.

Cost, like beauty, is very much in the eye of the beholder. There are regional differences between how companies compete. In some areas, cost is the paramount issue, whereas in others a perception of quality carries a premium. The final price will be a balance between how much the unit is willing to pay and how much the company needs the business or the badge of a recognized 'trophy' name.

In choosing EUS equipment, the costs go beyond those of the initial set-up alone. This equipment is delicate, and pressure to train fellows exposes it to significant wear and tear. Support

COMPATIBILITY OF VARIOUS TYPES OF ECHOENDOSCOPE ACROSS AVAILABLE ULTRASOUND PROCESSOR PLATFORMS					
	Olympus EU-M2000/60	Olympus EU-C2000/C60	Olympus/Aloka	Pentax/Hitachi	Toshiba
Radial					
Mechanical	✓				
Electronic			✓	✓	
'Slim probe'	✓				
Linear					
Electronic		✓	✓	✓	✓
Mechanical	✓				
Mini-probes[a]	✓			✓	
Rectal probes					
Mechanical	✓				
Electronic			✓	✓	
EBUS		✓			

Table 2.1 Compatibility of various types of echoendoscope across available ultrasound processor platforms
[a]Fujinon mini-probes require a dedicated processor.
EBUS, endobronchial ultrasound.

packages, including the availability of replacement echoendo-scopes, are of great importance. The devil here is in the detail, as cheaper scopes may come with very expensive and/or weak service support. In a survey of 56 institutions performing EUS, mechanical radial-scanning echoendoscopes tended to break, on average, after 68 procedures, whereas curved linear-array echo-endoscopes failed after an average of 107 procedures.[1] Institutions paid an average of $10 534 over 12 months for echo-endoscope repairs. The average repair cost per procedure was $41. These data may serve as guidance when setting up a service.

REFERENCES

1 Schembre D, Lin O. Frequency and costs of echo endoscope repairs: results of a survey of endosonographers. Endoscopy 2004; 36:982–986.

Setting up an EUS Service

Ann Marie Joyce and Michael L. Kochman

KEY POINTS

- When establishing an EUS service, it is important to educate the principal referral sources (oncologists, surgeons, and gastroenterologists) as to the indications and utility of endoscopic ultrasonography with or without fine-needle aspiration.

- The keys to establishing and developing a vibrant EUS service include providing a timely service, performing careful quality examinations, and excellent communication with the patient and referral physician.

- In most cases, 60 minutes should be set aside for each EUS examination, and 'block' scheduling is by far the most efficient method for organizing EUS cases.

- It is highly recommended that a dedicated room and dedicated nursing staff be formed to provide an EUS service.

INTRODUCTION

Endoscopic ultrasonography (EUS) was first introduced in the late 1980s. The initial studies were focused on determining the reproducibility of the examinations and the operating parameters of the investigation, and defining the clinical applications of EUS. Over the past several years, the focus of research has been centered on the clinical utility and cost-effectiveness of EUS, and EUS with fine-needle aspiration (FNA), as it has now become standard of care in the staging of gastrointestinal malignancies when there are questions concerning the treatment plans. With the increased utilization of EUS, there is an increase in demand for EUS programs to provide these services. Initially this was limited to academic centers, but EUS programs can now be found in larger community hospitals and private practices.

There are several factors that are intrinsic to starting up an effective endoscopic ultrasound unit and program. This chapter discusses the referral sources for EUS, methods for documentation and communication, design of the EUS room, and staffing of the endoscopy unit. It also reviews the current literature regarding the clinical utility and cost-effectiveness of EUS.

BACKGROUND

EUS has been in clinical use for nearly two decades for the evaluation of lesions both within and outside the gastrointestinal tract. The unique capabilities of this technology enable the endoscopist to perform an endoscopy as well as to evaluate the wall layer pattern of the gastrointestinal tract by utilizing high-frequency ultrasound. Over the past 10 years, FNA has been introduced to enable tissue diagnosis in extraluminal areas such as the pancreas and mediastinum. Its primary use has been in the staging of gastrointestinal malignancies, but the indications are expanding for benign indications and non-gastrointestinal indications (i.e., evaluation of lung cancer, submucosal masses, chronic pancreatitis, and choledocholithiasis).

SETTING UP AN ENDOSCOPIC ULTRASOUND UNIT

EUS has become an integral component of the algorithms for staging of malignancies. There is an increasing demand for this service, due both to aging of the population and to the increasing availability of treatment options, many of which are less invasive than previous options. EUS was initially limited to large academic centers, but has moved into community hospitals and private practices as the availability of trained physicians increases concurrent with the demand for the investigation. Demand for the examinations and the availability of trained personnel are the two main factors to consider when setting up an EUS program and unit.[1]

Many gastroenterology fellows are exposed to EUS during their training, and some choose to proceed with more specialized training. The American Society for Gastrointestinal Endoscopy (ASGE) recommends a dedicated year of training in advanced procedures during a fourth year.[2] These fourth year positions have become quite competitive over the last several years, and there are relatively few training programs available throughout the United States. During this specialty year there should be training in the cognitive as well as technical components of the procedure: indications, complications, and follow-up care of the patient. In order to facilitate excellence in training there should be one, and preferably more, mentors with excellent endoscopic skills who are experienced, in order to assist the fellow in developing their own skills as well as encouraging clinical research and scholarly projects. This training typically occurs in an academic setting, as academic centers typically have a high volume of procedures and experienced endoscopists. Experience plays an important role in the interpretation and performance of the examinations. The ASGE Competency Guidelines and the American Gastroenterological Association (AGA) GI Fellowship core curriculum have recommended that a minimum of 100 luminal cases, 150 pancreaticobiliary cases, and at least 75 EUS examinations with FNA should be performed.[3] There are some programs emerging to help gastroenterologists who are already in practice. This training includes observation of procedures, a hands-on intensive course, and computer-based learning. These tools are recommended only for highly motivated gastroenterologists, and are only part of the training required. At this point in time, self-teaching is to be discouraged for a number of reasons.

DEMAND FOR ENDOSONOGRAPHIC INVESTIGATIONS

The need for EUS is dependent on the number of patients in the area who require EUS and the recognition of the clinical utility of EUS by the referral base. Referrals are typically from three main sources; oncologists, surgeons, and other gastroenterologists. It is important that these practitioners are aware of the indications and capabilities of EUS, and are easily able to request and schedule an examination for one of their patients. A survey was carried out among gastroenterologists and non-gastroenterologists in a large multispecialty academic practice to determine the knowledge of indications for EUS.[4] This study demonstrated that internists, non-gastroenterologist specialists, and surgeons had moderate knowledge of the indications and utility of EUS. The knowledge of this group of physicians was poor in the use of EUS in hepatopancreatobiliary and colorectal applications. Given these findings, it is prudent to educate the referring doctors. This education should encompass how the procedure is performed, the indications for examination, data to support the use of EUS, and a discussion concerning how to interpret and utilize the data provided by the EUS examination. This may be accomplished as both an educational and promotional experience, for example in the form of medical, surgical, or cancer center grand rounds, if EUS is new to the area.

Gastroenterologists who have not been trained in EUS typically refer patients for staging of a gastrointestinal malignancy and for evaluation of submucosal lesions found on routine endoscopy. Oncologists and surgeons tend to refer patients for further staging of gastrointestinal, mediastinal, or pulmonary malignancy prior to treatment selection or after chemotherapy and radiation to examine for progression or new lymphadenopathy. It is important that the referring doctor be aware of the indications for and limitations of EUS, as described by individual insurance carriers and gastrointestinal organizations to aid in preventing insurance approval delays and expediting pre-certification when necessary. In addition, some basic knowledge regarding the examination technique is needed, so that the patient can be educated about the procedure to help decrease the anxiety with testing.

The effective referral program will attempt to establish itself in the minds of the local medical community in order to garner primary referrals. This may be accomplished by a number of methods, but first and foremost is the provision of timely effective service; scheduling itself is discussed in the following section. Effective communication with the referral sources is paramount, and can be facilitated by having a patient coordinator or scheduling secretary as the point person, such that all calls are accommodated for scheduling purposes. A personal phone call to the referral source prior to the procedure may help in assuring that the information sought by the referring physician is reasonably attained by the examination, and it allows the endosonographer the opportunity to review the potential findings and change in management plans that may ensue.

Making the local physician community aware of the presence of your EUS program is multifaceted. First, it is best to ensure that the kinks of scheduling are worked out on a local basis prior to attempting to gather referrals from outside physicians. Internal referrals, and later external referrals, can be aided by attending and speaking at tumor boards, cancer center conferences, and various grand rounds. Many private institutions have 'Gut Clubs' where interesting and complex cases are discussed; either presenting your cases or discussing what EUS may have to add to an individual case may be of benefit. In most circumstances it is also helpful to perform clinical research and to publish the findings, even if not involved with an academic program. The use of an outreach liaison, who may be playing multiple roles, is helpful, as are personal visits to referral practices.

SCHEDULING AN EXAMINATION

In developing and maintaining a referral base, communication and the provision of a reliable efficient service are key. When a patient has been diagnosed with a malignancy, follow-up care must be carried out in a timely fashion so that the cancer can be dealt with expeditiously to minimize the anxiety of the patient. The patient may be seen by the endoscopist in an outpatient clinic or, with increasing frequency, may be directly referred for the endoscopy. If the patient is seen in clinic by the performing endoscopist, the EUS appointment should be arranged that day. Endosonography procedures are usually longer procedures and have longer recovery times than standard endoscopic procedures, and this must be taken into consideration when schedules are being prepared.

On average at least 60 minutes should be set aside, especially if there is the potential for FNA. We have found that the performance of an FNA adds at least 35 minutes to the base procedures, and not uncommonly adds close to 45 minutes. Most of this time is due to the travel time of the on-site cytopathology team, and the remainder is involved with slide preparation and interpretation. A great deal of data now exists indicating that the performance of FNA is augmented in diagnostic accuracy by the presence of on-site cytopathologists.

The patient should be given information regarding the examination (such as that published by the ASGE and modified for local use), the pre-procedure preparation, and instructions for arrival on the day of the procedure. Because office consultations can potentially delay treatment and are not always approved by insurance companies, direct referrals for endoscopy are becoming more common. The referring physician's office should contact the endoscopist's office for the initial exchange of information. A standardized form can be devised that would include all of the necessary information for the secretary or nurse to complete for scheduling purposes, with the clinical information to follow. It is the practice of some groups to require the provision of the clinical records at the time of the initial scheduling contact. This appears to have no deleterious effect on referrals, and indeed is time saving – only one contact with the referring physician's office is needed. The process of obtaining insurance approval should begin at this time. Once the appropriate clinical information has been gathered and reviewed by the performing endoscopist, direct contact with the referring physician may be needed. It is essential that the patient's relevant records and imaging studies be available to the endoscopist prior to the procedure, with the patient made part of the data-gathering process. We have found it imperative to remind patients verbally and in writing (in the brochure that is sent to them) that they need to bring the radiologic studies with them on the day of the procedure. Most do not understand that referring physicians typically forward only reports of the radiologic studies and not the studies themselves.

To provide an efficient service, endoscopists should be flexible in their schedule in order to add on urgent cases, or dedicated 'block' times should be allocated for these procedures. Some endoscopists have an endoscopy session on a weekly or biweekly basis that is able to accommodate these additional procedures. This allocated time period should be well known by the referring physicians; in some institutions it may be the same day as a multidisciplinary gastrointestinal cancer clinic. Busy referral practices may find that demand quickly escalates and that two or three physicians are needed to accommodate the patient flow in a timely fashion, and to provide a seamless service when one is away for vacation or meetings.

POSTPROCEDURE FOLLOW-UP

Good communication with the referring physician improves patient care and helps to strengthen your relationship with the doctor and their practice. Good communication begins with sending a complete endoscopy report with representative images and making phone contact with the referring physician on the day of the procedure. It is not unusual for patients to be confused or angry with the data that you provide: you may have found evidence that 'curative' surgery will not be possible, or you may make a cancer diagnosis that the patient was not aware was in the differential diagnosis. Often these patients will call the referring physician the same day, frequently from the car on their way home. A discussion with the referring physician and synthesis of a treatment plan, so that they are aware of the findings and the implications of the findings, will aid in garnering future referrals.

Computer-based procedure notes are usually adequate for upper endoscopies and colonoscopies, but without modification may not be appropriate for EUS. The endoscopy report should include the relevant findings, pertinent negatives, tumor node metastasis (TNM) staging, initial cytology result, representative images, and impression. If time allows, communication with the referring physician should be made, as decisions regarding malignancy are usually made expeditiously. Any important recommendations, such as further imaging or appropriate referrals, can be also noted on the report, including whether or not communication with the referring physicians has already taken place. The EUS examination can be recorded on videotape, computer hard-drives, PACS systems, or DVD.

STAFF REQUIREMENTS

A knowledgable and enthusiastic support staff is needed to make EUS more efficient. EUS is usually a relatively long procedure compared with esophagogastroduodenoscopy or colonoscopy, such that more time should be allocated for the procedure, with concomitant increases in sedation requirements. The nurse or anesthesiologist should be aware that higher doses of medications are routinely used for these procedures. In some endoscopy units, propofol may be the preferred choice for all advanced or complicated procedures.

A major role in the procedure is played by the technician. The technician should be aware of the equipment being used; a brief conversation with the technician prior to the patient being brought into the room will allow for a stress-free procedure, performed in an orderly and efficient manner. It is not unusual, for example, that in some procedures a standard gastroscope may be used, biopsies taken, and then a radial EUS device utilized, subsequently followed by a curvilinear device with an FNA being performed. The technician should be familiar with the use of all of the various needles that are kept in stock. There should be careful handling of the EUS scope because of the relatively fragile ultrasound tip and motor. Careful training and instruction in endoscope preparation, intraprocedure handling, and cleaning are key to the maintenance of the instrument pool and in keeping repair costs down.

Typically the technician is responsible for loading the balloon on the endoscope tip. The balloon should be properly placed on the ultrasound probe to avoid having it come off during the procedure and to prevent any leaks of water or air. Various techniques for loading the balloon are used by technicians; it would behoove the endoscopist to observe the technicians and train them in the loading of the balloon to ensure that it is performed appropriately. Once the endoscopy has started, the technician should be able to assist in recording selected images via digital capture devices or still pictures. This documentation may also be facilitated by the endoscopist with the use of foot pedals. The technician is responsible for proper labeling and filing of the images.

Once the procedure is complete, the echoendoscope should be cleaned and disinfected by a trained technician. It takes a minimum of 20 minutes to reprocess an endoscope, dependent upon the protocols used, so this should be taken into consideration when scheduling. The number of rooms that may run concurrently, the number of ultrasound processors available for use, and the number of echoendoscopes need to be assessed carefully in order to maximize efficiency. Redundancy of echoendoscopes is necessary for most units: loaners are hard to come by and, in order to protect your referral practice, you will not want to reschedule patients or delay scheduling while awaiting the return of an endoscope from repair.

ROOM SET-UP

This section focuses on the room and materials needed to perform EUS successfully. The first important aspect is the room and physical layout. The examining room will be where you spend most of your time (if you are performing six to ten examinations per day), so it is important that it is set up in the most comfortable and efficient fashion. The design of the room should encompass a team approach (i.e., architects, endoscopists, nursing staff, and technicians). There is a great deal of equipment needed for EUS that needs to be readily accessible and moved during the procedure, so this room may need to be the largest one in the endoscopic unit. On average, the room should measure 300 square feet, to allow space for the necessary equipment, and potentially for an anesthesiologist. In the room, a workstation should optimally be provided to allow for review of the electronic records of the patient. This workstation area should include an X-ray viewing box to review the patient's films if they are on hard copy. There should be at least two video monitors in the room, because of the different positions that the endoscopist may use successfully to obtain the best images and best needle tracks for FNA. The monitors should be placed on both sides of the patient. Additional monitors in the room will aid the nurse and technician during the procedure, and are also useful for teaching purposes.

The ultrasound console or tower should be within reach of the endoscopist so that imaging adjustments can be made easily. In some cases, both the radial and linear scopes are used, so these should be easily accessible to the endoscopist, whether on the same tower or with separate mobile towers. The complex wiring and cabling will require the close integration of the manufacturer and your hospital-based specialists to insure an ergonomic routing of the cables so that they are not damaged during the procedure or after hours by the janitorial staff.

Additional thought in the planning stage as to the in-room, or central location of the cytopathology team, will aid in the workflow and also make the team more comfortable during their time in your unit. The cytopathologist may have his or her own traveling microscope and table (which should fit comfortably into the room), or a specific workstation with fixed microscope for the cytopathologist should be installed within the examining room or endoscopy unit, potentially with electronic linkage to the cytopathology reading room.

ENDOSCOPIC ULTRASOUND EQUIPMENT

It is not the intention of this chapter to review in detail the various different endoscopes and ultrasound consoles on the market, nor is it to contrast the relative advantages and disadvantages or each one: rather it is to make the gastroenterologist aware of the factors that are in play when outfitting an endoscopy unit.[5] Specific details concerning the echoendoscopes, consoles, and needles are reviewed in Chapter 2. Two basic designs of echoendoscope are available: radial and curvilinear. The choice of echoendoscope is dependent on the area being examined and the endoscopist's preferences, as influenced by experience and training. Radial echoendoscopes are currently available in both mechanical and electronic versions, whereas all currently available curvilinear echoendoscopes are electronic. Electronic echoendoscopes have the ability to integrate Doppler into the feature set. Curvilinear echoendoscopes are the design of choice for needle biopsy, injection, and drainage procedures.[6] In addition, there are commercially available through-the-scope ultrasound mini-probes that appear to have utility in the biliary and pancreatic ducts and in the evaluation of superficial mucosal abnormalities.

A wide variety of ultrasound consoles is available commercially. The least expensive consoles are relatively limited in their utility; for example, they may only be able to drive mini-probes or contain a limited feature set that allows for a small, portable, fine-needle biopsy set-up. The larger (and more expensive) dedicated ultrasound consoles usually contain an expanded feature set, which may include digital capture capabilities, Doppler, and upgraded electronics that allow for better image quality.

A study by Gress et al.[7] compared the accuracy of the linear versus the radial endoscope for the staging of pancreatic cancer. Thirty-three patients were randomized and the findings detected by EUS were compared with those found at surgery. The results were equivalent, but the linear echoendoscope was preferred by the authors due to the advantage of being able to perform FNA without switching echoendoscopes. The radial echoendoscopes can image with a 270–360° field of view, dependent upon manufacture and design. These may be used for the initial examination, or the endoscopist may choose a curvilinear echoendoscope if FNA is anticipated as the primary indication for the procedure. The curvilinear echoendoscopes typically have a 120–180° field of view. The advantage of the curvilinear device is that FNA is performed under direct ultrasonographic control. The aspiration needle of the endoscopist's choice is advanced through the accessory channel and observed to enter into the target lesion. The needle is visualized on the monitor and its trajectory adjusted by use of an elevator on the endoscope coupled with fine movements of the endoscope head itself.

The endoscopy suite should have more than one echoendoscope available to facilitate flow and for the occasions when one is sent out for repair. Echoendoscopes may be purchased or leased from the suppliers under a variety of programs. The initial equipment investment may be capital intensive, so it may not be unreasonable to start with a leasing plan while the endosonographic program is in its initial stages. About 80% of academic institutions and large tertiary hospitals own their equipment. Along with the negotiation of equipment contracts, the repair contracts are equally important. Repairs cost the unit potential income because procedures may have to be postponed or cancelled, and due to the cost of the repair itself. According to the 2001 EUS repair survey, the average institution paid about $10 000 for three repairs in 2000.[8] On average, repairs added about $41 to each EUS procedure.

CYTOPATHOLOGY

An on-site cytopathologist can help to improve the results of FNA.[9] Klapman et al.[10] demonstrated that the presence of an on-site cytopathologist directly impacts the diagnostic yield of EUS-guided FNA. In this study, one endoscopist performed a total of 243 FNAs. At center 1,130 FNAs were done with the cytopathologist present. Malignancy was most commonly diagnosed at center 1 (58% versus 42%, $P=0.006$). In contrast, center 2 (without an on-site cytopathologist) had a much higher percentage of results reported as unsatisfactory (20% versus 9%, $P=0.035$) or as suspicious for malignancy (16% versus 3%, $P=0.024$). Two other studies by Chang et al.[11,12] also showed improved results with the presence of an on-site cytopathologist, and as a result one of the participating centers changed its policy.

The presence of a cytopathologist is not routine in all centers; this appears most likely to be related to inadequate reimbursement. Layfield et al.[13] demonstrated this in a cost and compensation analysis of on-site FNA techniques, including EUS-guided FNA, compared with routine surgical pathology sign-out. The cytopathologist spent an average of 56 minutes on-site at a cost of $83 per patient, which was $40–50 more than what was compensated. This was in comparison to $638 per hour for signing out surgical pathology cases. Another study demonstrated a cost savings by reducing the number of repeat procedures. Nasuti et al.[14] showed that non-diagnostic specimens occurred at a rate of 0.98%. It was determined mathematically that this would increase to 20% when there was no on-site evaluation. In this study, on-site evaluation resulted in a cost benefit with savings of $404 000 per year to their institution by reducing the need for repeat procedures.

CLINICAL UTILITY AND COST-EFFECTIVENESS

Recent studies have been undertaken to determine the role and clinical impact of EUS on daily practice.[15] Quantification of the impact on patient care and outcomes is not always easy to determine, as the studies are difficult to design with changing operating characteristics of the competitive and complementary imaging techniques, and with the ever-changing combinations of chemotherapy and radiotherapy. What is certain is that the ability of EUS to determine that a disease process is either early stage or advanced (with evidence for lymphadenopathy or vascular involvement that precludes curative resection) is clinically relevant; what was missing, but is now becoming clear in the literature, is that EUS is also cost-effective.

ESOPHAGEAL CARCINOMA

Esophageal carcinoma is one of the leading causes of death in men. The prognosis and treatment of esophageal carcinoma is dependent upon the stage of the disease at the time of diagnosis. The first imaging study performed is typically computed tomography (CT) to determine whether there are any distant metastases that would make surgical cure unlikely. If CT does not show any distant metastases then EUS is performed. EUS is better at determining the T stage and examining the celiac axis for lymphadenopathy compared with other imaging modalities. This more accurate staging identifies patients with advanced locoregional disease who would benefit most from preoperative neoadjuvant chemoradiation therapy.[16,17]

There have been a number of studies performed demonstrating the clinical impact of EUS on esophageal carcinoma. The surgical findings and the morbidity and mortality of patients have been examined to show a benefit with the use of EUS.[18] Hiele et al.[19] analyzed the survival data of 86 patients who underwent EUS for staging of tumors of the esophagus or esophagogastric junction. Surgical resection was then performed in 73 patients. Survival of patients was significantly dependent upon EUS T staging ($P=0.05$), EUS N staging ($P=0.02$), and the presence of stenosis ($P=0.02$). The worst prognosis was for patients with celiac lymph node metastasis ($P=0.003$). Harewood and Kumar[20] compared the outcome of patients diagnosed with esophageal cancer in 1998 (i.e., pre-EUS) with that of patients diagnosed in 2000. EUS was not available for the group diagnosed in 1998. Tumor recurrence and survival were better in the EUS-selected group. These authors demonstrated that EUS more accurately identified patients who benefited from preoperative neoadjuvant therapy. In this study, there were five patients with T1 disease who had endocopic mucosal resection performed and therefore did not require surgery. There are now a number of studies that suggest preoperative chemoradiation provides the best results for patients with stage II and III esophageal cancer. In this regard, it is important to identify these patients so that they receive the most appropriate care; EUS can provide the necessary information and therefore improve patient outcome.

It is important when a new modality is introduced that it is not only beneficial to the patient but also cost-effective. Three recent studies have shown that preoperative EUS in patients with esophageal cancer is cost-effective. Shumaker et al.[21] performed a retrospective review of the Clinical Outcomes Research Initiative (CORI) database to identify patients who had preoperative EUS for esophageal carcinoma. Cost analysis was performed for a cohort of 188 procedures. It was assumed that patients with stage I disease would go directly to surgery, whereas patients with stage IV disease would not have combined modality therapy. In this study, 26% of patients were spared the combined modality therapy, resulting in a cost savings. A prospective case series by Chang et al.[22] demonstrated similar findings. In this study, there was decreased cost of care by $12 340 per patient. This was achieved by reducing the number of thoracotomies as a result of improved staging. Harewood and Wiersema[23] used a computer model to determine the cost of EUS in the staging of esophageal cancer. EUS-FNA provided the least costly approach to patients with celiac lymph node involvement compared with CT-FNA or surgery. These data are dependent upon a prevalence of celiac lymph nodes of 16%, which is not unreasonable in some patient populations. Taken together, these three studies demonstrate cost savings for patients who have EUS, because appropriate treatment is provided to the patient as a result of more accurate staging.

EUS has also been used in restaging esophageal carcinoma after chemoradiation in an attempt to determine whether the patient has responded appropriately to the treatment. Multiple studies have been performed, with varying results. When the TNM classification is used in restaging, the majority of tumors are overstaged after chemoradiation. Kalha et al.[24] showed that T stage was assessed correctly by EUS in only 22 patients (29%). In evaluating the N stage, the sensitivity was 48% for N0 disease and 52% for N1 disease. In a pilot study, EUS with FNA was performed on enlarged lymph nodes and the accuracy of identifying malignant cells was 87.5%.[25] One promising method post-therapy appears to be the direct measurement of the size and cross-sectional area of the tumor. Isenberg et al.[26] demonstrated that measurement of the maximal cross-sectional area of the tumor was more useful than the TNM classification in the post-treatment cohort. In a small group of patients there was a statistically significant decrease in this measurement in patients who responded to chemotherapy. Larger studies are needed for further evaluation of the predictive power that the maximal cross-sectional area of the tumor has on patient survival.

SUBMUCOSAL TUMOR

Endoscopy is inaccurate in the evaluation of submucosal tumors of the gastrointestinal tract. With the introduction of EUS, the gastrointestinal wall can be clearly imaged and therefore the origin of the submucosal tumor (SMT) can be further defined.[27] There are certain sonographic characteristics that are suggestive of malignancy; EUS with FNA can further differentiate these lesions. With the use of immunohistochemical analysis along with histopathology, one group showed an accuracy rate of 80%.[28] Further analysis is needed to determine the malignant potential of SMTs and the impact that EUS-FNA has in defining SMTs as gastrointestinal stromal tumors – which may be of uncertain malignant potential and clinical course.[29]

PANCREATIC CARCINOMA

Pancreatic carcinoma has a poor overall prognosis; most patients unfortunately present with advanced disease. In appropriately selected patients, surgery can offer the only possibility of cure. CT, magnetic resonance imaging (MRI), and/or endoscopic retrograde cholangiopancreatoagraphy (ERCP) are currently used to evaluate patients with possible pancreatic carcinoma. The yield of tissue sampling with ERCP has been poor and should be discouraged.[30] EUS can effectively evaluate the pancreas and peripancreatic area. FNA may help to differentiate between other various benign and neoplastic processes, including lymphoma and neuroendocrine tumors.

EUS plays a major role in the staging and diagnosis of pancreatic carcinoma.[31] Chang et al.[32] demonstrated the safety, accuracy, and clinical utility of EUS-FNA in diagnosing and staging pancreatic carcinoma. In a study of 44 patients, EUS-FNA had a sensitivity of 92%, specificity of 100%, and diagnostic accuracy of 95%. EUS-FNA played an important role in decisions regarding surgery and further diagnostic testing. There was a cost saving of approximately $3300 per patient, because surgery was avoided for inappropriate candidates. Erickson et al.[33] compared the findings in patients diagnosed with CT-FNA with those diagnosed with EUS-FNA. There was a 62% increase in the number of pancreatic carcinomas diagnosed during the EUS-FNA period. This may be related to the better yield with EUS compared with CT, and a referral bias may have developed after the introduction of EUS. A cost savings was detected in the EUS era, mostly due to a 75% decrease in the number of purely diagnostic operations. Eighteen operations were avoided in the EUS group, resulting in a saving of approximately $360 000. These two studies demonstrate that EUS with FNA plays an important cost-effective role in the staging and diagnosis of pancreatic carcinoma. The cost saving in algorithms utilizing EUS was also demonstrated by a computer model cost analysis.[34] EUS-FNA proved to be more cost-effective when it was assumed that the frequency of lymphadenopathy was greater than 4%. False-negative examinations occur in the setting of chronic pancreatitis, prominent ventral anlagen of the pancreas, diffusely infiltrating neoplastic disease, and recent acute pancreatitis.[35]

NEUROENDOCRINE TUMORS OF THE PANCREAS

Neuroendocrine tumors (NETs) of the pancreas are also an area of great utility for EUS. These tumors are extremely rare, with a prevalence of approximately 10 per million persons; insulinomas and gastrinomas are encountered most commonly. About 50% of malignant NETs are slow growing. It is important to detect these tumors at an early stage, when they are often missed by traditional cross-sectional imaging. Preoperative localization typically has included CT, angiography, and somatostatin receptor scintigraphy. The latter test has been quite effective in detecting NETs, but it can be difficult to determine whether the test is positive in the parenchyma of the pancreas or in the peri-pancreatic lymph nodes. About 20% of all NETs do not have somatostatin receptors, so that other means of localization and diagnosis are critical. In the largest single-center experience, the sensitivity and accuracy of EUS was 93% for detecting pancreatic NETs.[36] Additional recent data indicate that there are significant cost savings associated with the preoperative use of EUS for the localization of NETs. The cost savings are multifaceted: a reduction in the use of angiographic studies and decreased operating room time are the main effects of EUS identification of NET location during preoperative evaluation.

RECTAL CARCINOMA

The prognosis and treatment of rectal carcinoma is stage dependent and well accepted. Rectal carcinoma has an increased tendency towards local recurrence, with 30–50% of patients developing local recurrence, which may also be found at the time of distant failure. EUS provides more accurate staging and thereby enables more appropriate initial treatment planning for patients. A cohort of patients in the pre-EUS staging era was compared with a group for which EUS was the routine local standard of care for the staging of rectal carcinoma.[37] More patients in the EUS group received preoperative chemoradiation ($P<0.0001$). Tumor recurrence was 21.9% in the EUS group, compared with 47.1% in the non-EUS group ($P=0.03$). The 5-year mortality rate was 6.9% in the EUS group and 19.1% in the non-EUS group ($P=0.76$). In this study there was a clinical benefit associated with EUS-FNA on recurrence rates of rectal carcinoma; interestingly, this was likely due to the more accurate T staging demonstrated on EUS compared with CT. Similar results were obtained in a study that evaluated retrospectively the records of 60 patients with rectal carcinoma.[38] Some 48 patients had undergone CT followed by EUS. EUS changed management in 38% of the patients by detecting lymph nodes not seen on CT. A total of 21 EUS-FNAs were performed on lymph nodes and suspicious lesions for recurrence. EUS-FNA changed the management of 3 of the 16 patients with lymph nodes. Importantly, in this study 78% of lymph nodes less than 5 mm in diameter were found to be malignant. All four patients who had suspicious lesions for recurrence had positive FNA. This paper, along with others, suggests that for patients with advanced pathology at the time of surgery there may be a role for EUS as part of postoperative surveillance, due to its high detection rate of recurrent disease.

After completion of chemoradiation therapy, it can be difficult to determine the response of the tumor prior to surgical resection. EUS has been used, but the results were disappointing. EUS cannot differentiate between tumor and radiation-induced inflammation and fibrosis of the rectal wall. In a study by Vanagunas et al.[39] this benign disruption of the wall resulted in overstaging of 45% of patients who demonstrated clear endoscopic evidence of substantial reduction of tumor. The accuracy rate of EUS in patients who received neoadjuvant chemoradiation was only 63%. The authors concluded that EUS-FNA is better suited to patients with rectal carcinoma who have a negative finding on CT and who have not undergone neoadjuvant chemoradiation.

SUMMARY

EUS is an important and integral component in the diagnosis of gastrointestinal and non-gastrointestinal diseases. There is relative underutilization of the technology. It has been demonstrated that EUS with or without FNA has a clinical impact in the management of these disease processes and that FNA is cost-effective in the staging of malignancy.

REFERENCES

1 Parada KS, Peng R, Erickson RA, et al. A resource utilization projection study of EUS. Gastrointest Endosc 2002; 55:328–334.

2 American Society for Gastrointestinal Endoscopy. Guidelines for advanced endoscopic training. Gastrointest Endosc 2001; 53:846–848.

3 Eisen GM, Dominitz JA, Faigel DO, et al. American Society for Gastrointestinal Endoscopy. Guidelines for credentialing and granting privileges for endoscopic ultrasound. Gastrointest Endosc 2001; 54:811–814.

4 Yusuf TE, Harewood GC, Clain JE, et al. Knowledge of indications for EUS among gastroenterologists and non-gastroenterologists. Gastrointest Endosc 2004; 60:575–579.

5 Ahmad N, Kochman ML. EUS instrumentation and accessories: a primer. Gastrointest Endosc 2000; 52:S2–S5.

6 Gress FG, Hawes RH, Savides TJ, et al. Endoscopic ultrasound-guided fine-needle aspiration biopsy using linear array and radial scanning endosonography. Gastrointest Endosc 1997; 45:243–250.

7 Gress F, Savides T, Cummings O, et al. Radial scanning and linear array endosonography for staging pancreatic cancer: a prospective randomized comparison. Gastrointest Endosc 1997; 45:138–142.

8 Schembre D. Potential and pitfalls of EUS in private practice. Digestive Disease Week meeting, May 2004. Online. Available: http://www.asge.org/pages/practice/sigs/eus.cfm [19 April 2005].

9 Chang KJ, Wiersema MJ. Endoscopic ultrasound-guided fine-needle aspiration biopsy and interventional endoscopic ultrasonography. Emerging technologies. Gastrointest Endosc Clin North Am 1997; 7:221–235.

10 Klapman JB, Logrono R, Dye CE, et al. Clinical impact of on-site cytopathology interpretation on endoscopic ultrasound-guided fine needle aspiration. Am J Gastroenterol 2003; 98:1289–1294.

11 Chang KJ, Katz KD, Durbin TE, et al. Endoscopic ultrasound-guided fine-needle aspiration. Gastrointest Endosc 1994; 40:694–699.

12 Wiersema MJ, Vilmann P, Giovannini M, et al. Endosonography-guided fine-needle aspiration biopsy: diagnostic accuracy and complication assessment. Gastroenterology 1997; 112:1087–1095.

13 Layfield LJ, Bentz JS, Gopez EV. Immediate on-site interpretation of fine-needle aspiration smears: a cost and compensation analysis. Cancer Cytopathol 2001; 93:319–322.

14 Nasuti JF, Gupta PK, Baloch ZW, et al. Diagnostic value and cost-effectiveness of on-site evaluation of fine-needle aspiration specimens: review of 5688 cases. Diagn Cytopathol 2002; 27:1–4.

15 Shah JN, Ahmad NA, Beilstein MC, et al. Clinical impact of endoscopic ultrasonography on the management of malignancies. Clin Gastroenterol Hepatol 2004; 2:1069–1073.

16 Pfau PR, Kochman ML. Pretreatment staging by endoscopic ultrasonography does not predict complete response to neoadjuvant chemoradiation in patients with esophageal carcinoma. Gastrointest Endosc 2000; 52:583–586.

17 Lerut T, Coosemans W, De Leyn P, et al. Optimizing treatment of carcinoma of the esophagus and gastroesophageal junction. Surg Oncol Clin N Am 2001; 10:863–884.

18 Pfau PR, Ginsberg GG, Lew RJ, et al. EUS predictors of long-term survival in esophageal carcinoma. Gastrointest Endosc 2001; 53:463–469.

19 Hiele M, De Leyn P, Schurmans P, et al. Relation between endoscopic ultrasound findings and outcome of patients with tumors of the esophagus or esophagogastric junction. Gastrointest Endosc 1997; 45:381–386.

20 Harewood GC, Kumar KS. Assessment of clinical impact of endoscopic ultrasound on esophageal cancer. J Gastroenterol Hepatol 2004; 19:433–439.

21 Shumaker DA, de Garmo P, Faigel DO. Potential impact of preoperative EUS on esophageal cancer management and cost. Gastrointest Endosc 2002; 56:391–396.

22 Chang KJ, Soetikno RM, Bastas D, et al. Impact of endoscopic ultrasound combined with fine-needle aspiration biopsy in the management of esophageal cancer. Endoscopy 2003; 35:962–965.

23 Harewood GC, Wiersema MJ. A cost analysis of endoscopic ultrasound in the evaluation of esophageal cancer. Am J Gastroenterol 2002; 97:452–458.

24 Kalha I, Kaw M, Fukami N, et al. The accuracy of endoscopic ultrasound for restaging esophageal carcinoma after chemoradiation therapy. Cancer 2004; 101:940–947.

25 Agarwal B, Swisher S, Ajani J, et al. Endoscopic ultrasound after preoperative chemoradiation can help identify patients who benefit maximally after surgical esophageal resection. Am J Gastroenterol 2004; 99:1258–1266.

26 Isenberg G, Chak A, Canto MI, et al. Endoscopic ultrasound in restaging of esophageal cancer after neoadjuvant chemoradiation. Gastrointest Endosc 1998; 48:158–163.

27 Kochman ML, Hawes RH. Endoscopic evaluation of submucosal lesions of the gastrointestinal tract. In: Barkin JS, O'Phelan A, eds. Advanced therapeutic endoscopy, 2nd edn. New York: Raven Press; 1994:133–145.

28 Arantes V, Logrono R, Faruqi S, et al. Endoscopic sonographically guided fine-needle aspiration yield in submucosal tumors of the gastrointestinal tract. J Ultrasound Med. 2004; 23:1141–1150.

29 Corless CL, Fletcher JA, Heinrich MC. Biology of gastrointestinal stromal tumors. J Clin Oncol 2004; 22:3813–3825.

30 NIH state-of-the-science statement on endoscopic retrograde cholangiopancreatography (ERCP) for diagnosis and therapy. NIH Consens State Sci Statements. 2002; 19:1–23.

31 Faigel DO, Ginsberg GG, Bentz JS, et al. Endoscopic ultrasound-guided real-time fine-needle aspiration biopsy of the pancreas in cancer patients with pancreatic lesions. J Clin Oncol 1997; 15:1439–1443.

32 Chang KJ, Nguyen P, Erickson RA, et al. The clinical utility of endoscopic ultrasound-guided fine-needle aspiration in the diagnosis and staging of pancreatic carcinoma. Gastrointest Endosc 1997; 45:387–393.

33 Erickson RA, Garza AA. Impact of endoscopic ultrasound on the management and outcome of pancreatic carcinoma. Am J Gastroenterol 2000; 95:2248–2254.

34 Harewood GC, Wiersema MJ. A cost analysis of endoscopic ultrasound in the evaluation of pancreatic head adenocarcinoma. Am J Gastroenterol 2001; 96:2651–2656.

35 Bhutani MS, Gress FG, Giovannini M, et al. The no endosonographic detection of tumor (NEST) study: a case series of pancreatic cancers missed on endoscopic ultrasonography. Endoscopy 2004; 36:385–389.

36 Anderson MA, Carpenter S, Thompson NW, et al. Endoscopic ultrasound is highly accurate and directs management in patients with neuroendocrine tumors of the pancreas. Am J Gastroenterol 2000; 95:2271–2277.

37 Harewood GC. Assessment of clinical impact of endoscopic ultrasound on rectal cancer. Am J Gastroenterol 2004; 99:623–627.

38 Shami VM, Parmar KS, Waxman I. Clinical impact of endoscopic ultrasound and endoscopic ultrasound-guided fine-needle aspiration in the management of rectal carcinoma. Dis Colon Rectum 2004; 47:59–65.

39 Vanagunas A, Lin DE, Stryker SJ. Accuracy of endoscopic ultrasound for restaging rectal cancer following neoadjuvant chemoradiation therapy. Am J Gastroenterol 2004; 99:109–112.

Chapter

4

Training and Simulators

Michael K. Sanders and Douglas O. Faigel

KEY POINTS

- EUS is an advanced endoscopic procedure that requires a level of training exceeding that of general endoscopy. Acquisition of the skills necessary to perform EUS competently often requires training beyond the scope of a traditional gastroenterology fellowship program.

- Competence in routine endoscopic procedures should be documented as it provides a vital foundation for EUS training.

- Competence in EUS requires both cognitive and technical skills, including an understanding of the appropriate indications for EUS, conducting appropriate pre- and post-procedure evaluations, and managing procedure-related complications.

- Upon successful completion of EUS training, the trainee must be able to integrate EUS into the overall clinical evaluation of the patient.

- A general consensus of expert endosonographers suggests that luminal endosonography requires at least 3–6 months of intensive training to establish competency, and that pancreatobiliary EUS and fine-needle aspiration (FNA) may require up to 1 year.

- Each program teaching EUS should have the ability to provide sufficient numbers of procedures that will substantially surpass those required for minimal competence.

- The threshold number of EUS-FNA cases needed to achieve competence has not been studied; however, it is generally agreed that FNA of pancreatic lesions carries a higher complexity and risk than that at other anatomic sites.

INTRODUCTION

Over the past decade endoscopic ultrasound (EUS) has emerged as a valuable endoscopic resource for the diagnosis and treatment of a variety of gastrointestinal disorders including, but not limited to, pancreatic cysts, mucosal and submucosal tumors, chronic pancreatitis, and various gastrointestinal malignancies. The diagnosis, staging, and treatment of gastrointestinal cancers have evolved into a multidisciplinary approach often utilizing endosonography as an initial tool for both diagnosis and staging. Multiple studies have demonstrated the superiority of EUS compared with conventional abdominal computed tomography (CT) in the staging of esophageal, gastric, and pancreatic cancers.[1–4] Furthermore, the advent of EUS-guided fine-needle aspiration (FNA) has provided an alternative approach to traditional percutaneous biopsies obtained under CT guidance. Moreover, compared with other modalities, the results of EUS-FNA from pancreatic masses are superior, with a sensitivity of 85–90% and a specificity of 100%.[5,6] Recently, EUS has been employed in the treatment of pancreatic adenocarcinoma with ultrasound-guided fine-needle injection of tumor-suppressing agents,[7] further expanding the future potential for therapeutic endosonography. Clearly, the introduction of EUS into clinical practice has revolutionized the field of gastroenterology, in particular gastrointestinal oncology, with potential applications continuing to evolve.

As the applications for EUS have become increasingly recognized by other clinical practitioners, the demand for well trained endosonographers has increased.[8] The limited availability of EUS is largely due to a lack of skilled endosonographers. Further barriers include equipment cost, ease of use, and reimbursement costs. A relative lack of training centers, combined with the extensive commitment required by the trainee, has limited the growth of EUS and its availability in community practices. Assuring adequate training of practicing endosonographers has become a priority for the American Society for Gastrointestinal Endoscopy (ASGE), evidenced by guidelines set forth on advanced training in EUS.[9] EUS is an advanced endoscopic procedure that requires a level of training exceeding that of general endoscopy. Acquisition of the skills necessary for conducting and understanding EUS often requires training beyond the scope of a traditional gastroenterology fellowship program. Additional training often involves a 1-year fellowship following completion of an accredited gastroenterology fellowship program. Although a minority of gastroenterology training programs may provide adequate exposure to EUS during a traditional 3-year fellowship, the provision of only a brief exposure to EUS and allowing independent practice by inadequately trained fellows are unacceptable. Although clinical workshops with hands-on training may provide an understanding of the indications and complications of EUS, they are not a substitute for formal fellowship training. This chapter covers the guidelines for individual trainees, training programs, and credentialing in EUS. Computer-based training simulators are in their infancy in the field of endosonography, but they represent an exciting adjunct to formal training and are also discussed.

GUIDELINES FOR TRAINING

Guidelines for training in advanced endoscopy have been published previously by the American Society for Gastrointestinal Endoscopy (ASGE).[10] Although many gastroenterology training programs have incorporated advanced endoscopy training into the second and third year curriculum, the majority of programs now require an additional fourth year of training for advanced procedures (endoscopic retrograde cholangiopancreatography [ERCP] and EUS). EUS training is available at relatively few academic centers in the USA. Currently, there are 29 recognized programs in the United States and one in Canada offering a fourth-year fellowship in EUS (ASGE website: http://www.asge.org/pages/education/training/eus.cfm). These programs may vary in the design of their training experience, but two critical components of a qualified training program include a large patient volume and recognized faculty expertise.

In certain unusual circumstances, a trainee may acquire the necessary skills for EUS in a standard 3-year fellowship, provided that an adequate patient volume is available and the trainee can demonstrate the necessary aptitude and skills required for advanced endoscopy. However, given the complexity of these procedures and necessary volume of cases required to achieve competency, it seems less likely that an individual would be adequately trained in a traditional 3-year program.

Competency is defined as the minimum level of skill, knowledge, and/or expertise acquired through training and experience, required to perform a task or procedure safely and proficiently.[11] Unfortunately, there have been few published reports regarding the training of individuals in EUS or the number of procedures required to attain competence.[12–14] A common goal for all gastroenterology training programs is the production of knowledgable, experienced, and competent endoscopists. Recognizing this goal for advanced endoscopy training and understanding the limitations of a 3-year curriculum has been a major impetus for establishing fourth-year fellowships in EUS.

Although the demand for qualified endosonographers is increasing, not all trainees should pursue such advanced training due to both variations in individual skill level and regional staffing needs. Similarly, not all training programs should offer EUS training owing to restraints on patient volume and faculty interests. Individuals wishing to pursue further training in EUS must have completed at least 24 months of a standard GI fellowship or demonstrate equivalent training. Moreover, competence in routine endoscopic procedures should be documented as it provides a vital foundation for advanced endoscopic training. Obviously, trainees in endoscopy develop skills at widely varying rates that can be evaluated objectively by experienced endoscopists. However, the use of an absolute or threshold number of procedures may be misleading and should therefore be employed with caution in the evaluation of individual trainees. The minimum number of procedures required to achieve competency in EUS will vary based on the individual's skill level, understanding of ultrasound principles, and quality of the training experience. Performing an arbitrary number of procedures does not necessarily guarantee competency. Although the Standards of Practice Committee of the ASGE has published a minimum number of procedures necessary before competency can be assessed (Table 4.1), these numbers simply represent a minimum requirement and should serve only as a guide in evaluating individual trainees. These numbers are derived from studies on training in EUS, published expert opinion, and the consensus of the Ad Hoc EUS and Standards of Practice committees of the ASGE. Ideally, competency should be gauged on objective criteria and direct observation by an experienced endosonographer.

Competence in EUS requires both cognitive and technical skills,[15] including an understanding of the appropriate indications for EUS, conducting appropriate pre- and post-procedure evaluations, and managing procedure-related complications. Trainees must be able to perform the procedure in a safe and efficient manner while also recognizing and understanding the ultrasound images. Furthermore, understanding the implications for EUS in staging gastrointestinal malignancies must be appreciated for integration of the endosonographic findings into the treatment plan for each patient (i.e., surgical versus medical and/or radiation oncology referrals). Formal supervised EUS training should also include reviews of cross-sectional anatomy, atlases of endoscopic or abdominal ultrasonography, videotaped teaching cases, and didactic courses in EUS. A combination of well supervised EUS procedures and didactic teaching will aid in assuring an adequate training experience as well as an overall understanding of EUS.

MINIMUM NUMBER OF EUS PROCEDURES REQUIRED BEFORE COMPETENCY CAN BE ASSESSED[18]	
Site or lesion	No. of cases required
Mucosal tumors (cancer of the esophagus, stomach, and rectum)	75
Submucosal abnormalities	40
Pancreaticobiliary	75
EUS-guided FNA	
Non-pancreatic	25
Pancreatic	25
Comprehensive competence	150[a]

Table 4.1 Minimum number of EUS procedures required before competency can be assessed[18]
[a]Including at least 75 pancreaticobiliary and 50 fine-needle aspiration procedures.

A crucial component to any EUS training program is focused on gastrointestinal tumor staging. When available, EUS has become the standard of care in staging several gastrointestinal malignancies including esophageal, gastric, rectal, and pancreatic cancers. Determining the accuracy of tumor staging by a trainee is an important aspect of training, allowing differentiation between potentially curable early-stage tumors and irresectable late-stage tumors. Studies in endosonographic staging of esophageal cancer suggested that at least 75 to 100 procedures were required before an acceptable level of accuracy was achieved.[13,14] Ideally, the accuracy of EUS staging should be compared to a gold standard such as surgical histopathology; however, surgical specimens are not always readily available and patients may have received preoperative radiation and chemotherapy, which may affect staging. In these circumstances, staging by a trainee should be compared to that of a skilled and competent endosonographer. Appropriate documentation of all EUS procedures in a training log, along with review of surgical pathology results, will further assist in determining both the quantity and accuracy of tumor staging cases.

Upon successful completion of EUS training, the trainee must be able to integrate EUS into the overall clinical evaluation of the patient. A thorough understanding of the indications, contraindications, individual risk factors, and benefit–risk considerations for individual patients must be demonstrated. Being able to describe the procedure clearly and accurately, and obtain informed consent, is a necessary requirement. A knowledge of the gastrointestinal anatomy and surrounding anatomic structures as imaged by EUS, and of the technical features of the equipment, workstation, and accessories, is vital for future independent practice. The trainee must be able safely to intubate the esophagus, pylorus, and duodenum to acquire the necessary images. Moreover, accurately identifying and interpreting the EUS images and recognizing normal and abnormal findings must be demonstrated and assessed by the mentor. The trainee must be able to demonstrate an accuracy in tumor staging comparable to that in the medical literature (Table 4.2).[9] Lastly, the trainee must be able to document and communicate the EUS findings with referring physicians, and understand the implications of these findings in formulating treatment plans for patient care. Adhering to these training requirements for EUS will further assist in assuring the production of skilled endosonographers.

TRAINING PROGRAM REQUIREMENTS

Although several institutions across the USA, Canada, and Europe offer brief training courses in EUS, these programs provide only limited exposure and arguably do not adequately train individuals as independent endosonographers. Formal, supervised training is the most accepted mode of training, but experience may be gained in other settings, such as hands-on short courses, use of animal models, EUS teaching videotapes, and computer-based training simulators. These teaching methods represent useful adjuncts to training and should not be used in lieu of a more formal supervised training experience. A general consensus by expert endonographers suggests that luminal endonography requires at least 3–6 months of intensive training to establish competency, whereas pancreaticobiliary EUS and FNA may require up to 1 year.[16] Short courses and computer-based learning without direct supervision may result in inadequate understanding and appreciation of the technical challenges and complexity of EUS.

When considering advanced training in EUS, a trainee should investigate all aspects of the training program. Arguably, the most important aspect of a program is the reputation and expertise of the endosonographer. Programs should have a minimum of one skilled endosonographer who is acknowledged as an expert by his/her peers and is committed to teaching EUS. Unfortunately, the majority of EUS programs across the USA have limited, if any, extramural funding and additional clinical responsibilities may be required to help support the trainee's salary. While understanding the financial limitations of most institutions, training programs should strive to limit the clinical responsibilities unrelated to EUS when developing the core curriculum. Ideally, programs should provide protected time and the necessary facilities for academic pursuits including designing research protocols, preparing manuscripts, writing grant proposals, and attending courses in EUS. Creating an environment that emphasizes endoscopic research and clinical investigation should be a fundamental goal for each training program. Trainees should be provided with the protected time and necessary funds to attend at least one scientific meeting during the course of training, preferably one related to endosonography. A common goal for all committed trainees should be the presentation of their endoscopic research at national or international meetings. Exposure to endoscopy unit management, including scheduling, staffing, equipment maintenance, and management skills, is also a valuable asset to any training program. Many of the trainees in EUS may pursue future academic positions, and these are invaluable skills to acquire early in an academic career. Although a common goal

REPORTED ACCURACY OF EUS COMPARED WITH HISTOPATHOLOGY FOR THE LOCAL STAGING OF ESOPHAGEAL CARCINOMA, GASTRIC CANCER, AMPULLARY CARCINOMA, AND RECTAL CANCER[9]			
Indication	No. of procedures	T stage	N stage
Esophageal cancer	739	85%	79%
Gastric cancer	1163	78%	73%
Pancreatic cancer	155	90%	–
Ampullary carcinoma	94	86%	72%
Rectal cancer	19	84%	84%

Table 4.2 Reported accuracy of EUS compared with histopathology for the local staging of esophageal carcinoma, gastric cancer, ampullary carcinoma, and rectal cancer[9]

for most training programs is the development of future academic endosonographers, some trainees may express different career interests that may conflict with the ideals of the training program. Understanding and recognizing the program's expectations and the trainee's career interests are crucial to an enjoyable and successful training experience.

Each program in EUS should have the ability to provide sufficient numbers of procedures that will substantially surpass those required for minimal competence (see Table 4.1). Although a large procedure volume does not necessarily guarantee competence, it is highly unlikely that a low volume of cases will provide sufficient exposure to these highly complicated and technically challenging procedures to allow adequate assessment of competency. Requiring a large volume of cases is not an elitist attempt by tertiary centers to exclude others from potential training opportunities, but rather an attempt to guarantee the delivery of skilled endosonographers into the workforce and to meet the demand for EUS. For these reasons, training in EUS has largely been limited to academic tertiary centers with highly skilled endosonographers conducting a large volume of cases, thus ensuring retainment of the skills necessary to train individuals interested in learning EUS.

CREDENTIALING IN EUS

Credentialing is the process of assessing and validating the qualifications of a licensed independent practitioner to provide patient care. Determining qualifications for credentialing is based upon an assessment of the individual's current medical license, knowledge base, training and/or experience, current competence, and ability to perform independently the procedure or patient care requested. The ASGE has provided guidelines for credentialing and granting hospital privileges to perform routine gastrointestinal endoscopy.[17] Furthermore, the ASGE has established guidelines for credentialing and granting privileges in advanced endoscopic procedures, including EUS.[18] Credentialing for EUS should be determined separately from other endoscopic procedures such as sigmoidoscopy, colonoscopy, esophagogastroduodenoscopy (EGD), ERCP, or any other endoscopic procedure. Determining competency and qualifications for credentialing can be somewhat challenging, as trained individuals possess varying degrees of skill in EUS along with recognized limitations. Nevertheless, providing a minimum number of procedures necessary prior to assessing competency (see Table 4.1) creates objective criteria for assessment in the credentialing process. As with credentialing in general gastrointestinal endoscopy, competency is ultimately assessed by the training director or other independent proctor.

EUS is performed in a variety of anatomic locations for various indications.[19] These locations include evaluation and staging of mucosally based neoplasms (esophagus, stomach, colon, and rectum), evaluation of subepithelial abnormalities, assessment of the pancreaticobiliary ducts, and performance of EUS-guided FNA. Endoscopists may be competent in one or more of these areas depending on their level of training and interest. Privileging in one or more of these areas may be considered separately, but training must be considered adequate in the areas for which privileging is requested.

MUCOSAL TUMORS

Safe intubation of the esophagus, pylorus, and duodenum is essential when evaluating mucosal tumors in the esophagus, stomach, and duodenum. Accurate imaging of the lesion and recognition of surrounding lymphadenopathy, in particular the celiac axis region for upper tract cancers, is critical to the diagnosis and correct staging of mucosally based tumors. Evaluation of rectal cancers should include intubation of the sigmoid colon and identification of the iliac vessels. A prospective study reported that competent intubation of the esophagus, stomach, and duodenum was achieved in 1 to 23 procedures (median 1–2), with visualization of the gastric or esophageal wall in 1 to 47 procedures (median 10–15).[12] Adequate evaluation of the celiac axis region required 8 to 36 procedures (median 10–15). Unfortunately, there are limited studies that have addressed the learning curve for evaluating mucosal tumors of the gastrointestinal tract. Only two studies have looked at the learning curve in staging esophageal cancers. Fockens et al.[13] reported that adequate staging accuracy was achieved only after 100 examinations, whereas Schlick et al.[14] reported an 89.5% T-stage accuracy after a minimum of 75 cases. A survey of the American Endosonography Club in 1995 suggested an average of 43 cases for esophageal imaging, 44 for gastric and 37 for the rectum.[20] Once competence is achieved in one anatomic location, the threshold number of procedures for other anatomic locations may be reduced, depending on the skill and training of the endosonographer. The ASGE currently recommends a minimum of 75 supervised cases, at least two-thirds in the upper gastrointestinal tract, before competency for evaluating mucosal tumors can be assessed.[18]

SUBEPITHELIAL ABNORMALITIES

Evaluation of subepithelial lesions has become a common indication for EUS. Discriminating between neoplasms, varices, enlarged gastric folds, and extrinsic compression from extramural masses can be performed with traditional echoendoscopes or catheter-based ultrasound probes. With the advent of the catheter-based probes, some practitioners have developed competency in subepithelial abnormalities without achieving competence in other indications for EUS. Although no studies are available for determining the threshold number of cases required for accurate assessment of subepithelial abnormalities, the ASGE Standards or Practice Committee currently recommends a minimum of 40 to 50 supervised cases.[21]

PANCREATICOBILIARY IMAGING

Most endosonographers will agree that accurate imaging and interpretation of images of the pancreaticobiliary system including the gallbladder, bile duct, pancreatic duct, and ampulla is more technically challenging than evaluating mucosal and submucosal lesions. For this reason, a larger volume of supervised pancreaticobiliary cases is required before competence can be assessed adequately. A multicenter, 3-year prospective study reported that adequate imaging of the pancreatic and bile ducts required 13 to 135 cases (median 55), whereas imaging of the pancreatic parenchyma required 15 to 74 cases (median 34).[12] Adequate assessment of the ampulla required 13 to 134 cases (median 54). Although technical competence in pancreaticobiliary imaging may be achieved in fewer than 100 cases, a survey from the American Endosonography Club suggests that interpretive competence of pancreatic images may require additional procedures (120 cases).[20] Other expert opinion suggests a higher threshold of 150 cases before assessing interpretative competence.[15] Currently, the ASGE Standards of Practice Committee recommends a minimum of 75 pancreaticobiliary cases before competence can be assessed.[18]

EUS-GUIDED FNA

EUS-guided FNA has emerged as an important diagnostic tool for obtaining tissue from intramural lesions, perigastrointestinal adenopathy, and pancreatic lesions.[22] Training in EUS-guided FNA requires knowledge of basic EUS principles along with acquisition of the skills necessary to obtain and interpret EUS images. Understanding and appreciating the complexity and risk that EUS-guided FNA adds to the procedure is critical for successful training. Unfortunately, the threshold number of FNA cases needed to achieve competence has not been studied. However, it is generally agreed that EUS-guided FNA of pancreatic lesions carries a higher complexity and risk for potential complications than that at other anatomic sites. Therefore, the number required for FNA of pancreatic lesions is considered separately from that for other anatomic locations. For nonpancreatic lesions (i.e., intramural lesions, lymph nodes, ascites), it is recommended that a trainee be competent in non-pancreatic EUS and conduct at least 25 supervised FNA cases before competence can be assessed.[18] Competence in EUS-guided FNA of pancreatic lesions requires demonstration of competence in pancreaticobiliary EUS (at least 75 cases) in addition to 25 supervised FNA procedures of pancreatic lesions.[18] Owing to the absence of literature supporting a threshold number for EUS-guided FNA, these threshold numbers were adopted from the guidelines set forth for therapeutic ERCP, requiring a minimum of 25 supervised cases in addition to 75 diagnostic cases.[21] The similarities between EUS and ERCP, such as side-viewing instruments and combined endoscopic and radiologic imaging, led to these recommendations. Clinical studies addressing this question for EUS-guided FNA of pancreatic and nonpancreatic lesions are needed for further assessment of the validity of these recommendations.

COMPREHENSIVE EUS COMPETENCE

Some practitioners may be interested in acquiring competence in only one or two areas of EUS, and can therefore focus their efforts on specific anatomic locations as outlined above. However, for practitioners interested in achieving competence in multiple areas of EUS, training must include exposure to a variety of procedures with differing clinical pathology. It is generally recognized that, once competence in one area of EUS has been established, the number of cases required to achieve confidence in other areas may be reduced. For trainees interested in only mucosal and submucosal lesions, it is generally recommended that a minimum of 100 supervised cases be performed. Consideration for comprehensive EUS competence, including pancreaticobiliary imaging and FNA, requires a minimum of 150 cases, including 50 EUS-guided FNAs and at least 75 pancreaticobiliary cases.[18]

RECREDENTIALING AND RENEWAL OF EUS PRIVILEGES

Over the course of time, physicians who have received appropriate privileges to perform EUS may change the scope of their clinical practice and subsequently reduce the frequency of performing one or more EUS procedures. It has been suggested that ongoing experience in advanced endoscopy is necessary to retain the technical skills required to perform these technically challenging procedures safely and adequately.[23,24] The goal of recredentialing is to assure continued clinical competence while promoting continuous quality improvement and maintaining patient safety. If ongoing experience is not maintained at some objective level, the quality of care provided to the patient may diminish, potentially leading to adverse events.

The ASGE has provided useful guidelines for renewing endoscopic privileges and assuring continued clinical competence in EUS.[25] However, it is the responsibility of each institution to develop and maintain individual guidelines for granting and renewing privileges. The threshold number of procedures necessary for recredentialing may vary between institutions; however, this threshold must be commensurate with the technical and cognitive skills required for advanced procedures such as EUS. Individual institutions must establish a frequency for the renewal process along with contingency plans when minimal competence cannot be assured. The Joint Commission on Accreditation of Healthcare Organizations (JCAHO) has mandated that renewal of clinical endoscopic privileges be made for a period of no more than 2 years.[26] Endosonographers seeking renewal of privileges must document an adequate caseload over a set period of time in order to maintain the necessary skills required for EUS. This documentation may include procedure log books or patient records, and should focus on objective measures such as number of cases, success rates, and complications. Continued cognitive training through participation in educational activities should also be a prerequisite for the recredentialing process. New EUS procedures and clinical applications continue to emerge, requiring a commitment to continued medical education within this specialized field.

SIMULATORS IN EUS

Endoscopic simulators have been developed for training in flexible sigmoidoscopy, EGD, colonoscopy, ERCP, and most recently EUS.[27] Since development of the first endoscopic mannequin simulator in the late 1960s,[28] considerable technologic advances have been made in the development of endoscopic simulators. A variety of simulators is available today, ranging from animal-based simulators (Erlangen Endo-Trainer; Erlangen Germany) to the computer-based simulators manufactured by Immersion Medical Corporation (Accutouch Endoscopy Simulator; Gaithersburg, MD), and Simbionix Corporation (GI Mentor II; Cleveland, OH).[29] Validation studies and small prospective clinical trials assessing the utility of endoscopic simulators have been conducted for upper endoscopy, flexible sigmoidoscopy, and colonoscopy;[30-34] however, the benefits of simulator training have not been clearly demonstrated, emphasizing the need for further investigation in large prospective trials. Nevertheless, this technology represents an exciting and potentially useful adjunct to formal endoscopic training.

Simbionix Corporation (http://www.simbionix.com) has recently developed the first and only EUS module providing a platform for hands-on training and practice of EUS procedures (Fig. 4.1).[29] The computer-based simulator generates ultrasound images in real-time from three-dimensional anatomic models constructed from CT and magnetic resonance images from real patients. The trainee inserts a customized echoendoscope into the specially designed GI Mentor mannequin and simultaneously receives visual feedback from the monitor along with tactile sensation from scope maneuvering during the procedure. A highly sensitive tracking system translates the position and direction of the camera into realistic computer-generated images. The EUS module allows the trainee to switch from endoscopic to ultrasound images in real time, and also provides training in both radial and linear ultrasound probes. Split-screen capability provides ultrasound images alongside three-dimensional anatomic maps, further assisting in the interpretation and understanding of generated EUS images. The module also allows trainees to practice keyboard functions such as labeling of organs, magnifying images, changing frequencies, and measuring with calipers. After completion of the examination, the computer software permits performance evaluation by reviewing all saved images (up to 50 frozen images per procedure) and indicating anatomy and landmarks that were incorrectly identified by the user.

Although the Simbionix GI-Mentor II EUS training module presents an exciting approach to training in EUS, there are currently no published validation studies or clinical trials assessing EUS simulators. Moreover, these simulators represent an adjunct, not a substitution, to formal supervised training. They may also serve as useful tools for skilled endosonographers interested in practicing new techniques. Unfortunately, these simulators are not readily available at most training institutions owing to cost restraints and regional needs. However, at select institutions (i.e., Mayo Clinic, Jacksonville), there are 1–2-week workshops in EUS utilizing these simulators and thus allowing exposure to this technology.

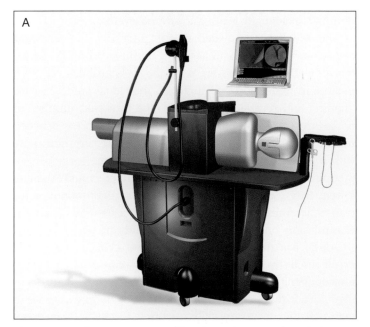
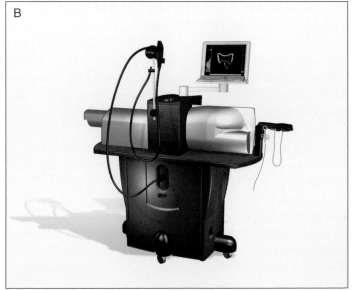

Fig. 4.1   Simbionix GI-Mentor Simulator. **A,** Front view. **B,** Rear view. (Courtesy of Simbionix Corporation, USA.)

SUMMARY

EUS has become an important imaging method for the evaluation of a variety of gastrointestinal diseases. It is a challenging endoscopic procedure requiring both cognitive and technical skills beyond the general scope of traditional gastroenterology fellowship training. As the demand for skilled endosonographers continues to increase, the guidelines for training must be critically analyzed to assure the production of well trained and competent future endosographers. Although guidelines have been established for credentialing and granting privileges in EUS, additional studies of threshold numbers necessary to achieve competence are needed to fill existing gaps in the current literature. Endoscopists interested in learning EUS must recognize and appreciate the complexity of these procedures and risks for potential complications. Clearly, a 1–2-week course in EUS is considered inadequate training and may potentially expose patients to increased risk and a diminished quality of care. For those truly interested in acquiring the skills required for EUS, a formal supervised training program is far superior to hands-on workshops, teaching videotapes, simulators, and inadequate exposure during a standard GI fellowship.

Simulators for training in EUS represent an exciting and useful adjunct to supervised instruction. Although clinical trials investigating the efficacy of simulators in EUS training are lacking, the potential applications for this technology are promising. Further studies are necessary to determine the role of endoscopic simulators in EUS training.

REFERENCES

1 Botet JF, Lightdale CJ, Zauber AG, et al. Preoperative staging of esophageal cancer: comparison of endoscopic US and dynamic CT. Radiology 1991; 181:419–425.

2 Ziegler K, Sanft C, Friedrich M, et al. Evaluation of computed tomography, endosonography, and intraoperative assessment in TN staging of gastric carcinoma. Gut 1993; 34:604–610.

3 Palazzo L, Roseau G, Gayet B, et al. Endoscopic ultrasonography in the diagnosis and staging of pancreatic adenocarcinoma: results of a prospective study with comparison to ultrasonography and CT scan. Endoscopy 1993; 25:143–150.

4 Muller MF, Meyenberger C, Bertschinger P, et al. Pancreatic tumors: evaluation with endoscopic US, CT and MR imaging. Radiology 1994; 190:745–751.

5 Wiersema MJ, Vilmann P, Giovannini M, et al. Endosonography-guided fine needle aspiration biopsy: diagnostic accuracy and complication assessment. Gastroenterology 1997; 112:1087–1095.

6 Gress FG, Hawes RH, Savides TJ, et al. Endoscopic ultrasound-guided fine-needle aspiration biopsy using linear array and radial scanning endosonography. Gastrointest Endosc 1997; 45:243–250.

7 Senzer N, Hanna N, Chung T, et al. Completion of dose escalation component of phase II study of TNFerade combined with chemoradiation in the treatment of locally advanced pancreatic cancer. American Society of Clinical Oncology Gastrointestinal Cancers Symposium 2005 (Abstract).

8 Parada KS, Peng R, Erickson RA, et al. A resource utilization projection study of EUS. Gastrointest Endosc 2002; 55:328–334.

9 ASGE. Guidelines for training in endoscopic ultrasound. Gastrointest Endosc 1999; 49:829–833.

10 ASGE. Guidelines for advanced endoscopic training. Gastrointest Endosc 2001;53:846–848.

11 ASGE. Methods of granting hospital privileges to perform gastrointestinal endoscopy. Gastrointest Endosc 2002; 55:780–783.

12 Hoffman B, Wallace MB, Eloubeidi MA, et al. How many supervised procedures does it take to become competent in EUS? Results of a multicenter three year study. Gastrointest Endosc 2000; 51:AB139.

13 Fockens P, Van den Brande JHM, van Dullemen HM, et al. Endosonographic T-staging of esophageal carcinoma: a learning curve. Gastrointest Endosc 1996; 44:58–62.

14 Schlick T, Heintz A, Junginger T. The examiner's learning effect and its influence on the quality of endoscopic ultrasonography in carcinoma of the esophagus and gastric cardia. Surg Endosc 1999; 13:894–898.

15 Boyce HW. Training in endoscopic ultrasonography. Gastrointest Endosc 1996; 43:S12–S15.

16 ASGE. Role of endoscopic ultrasonography. Gastrointest Endosc 2000; 52:852–859.

17 ASGE. Guidelines for credentialing and granting privileges for gastrointestinal endoscopy. Gastrointest Endosc 1998; 48:679–682.

18 ASGE. Guidelines for credentialing and granting privileges for endoscopic ultrasound. Gastrointest Endosc 2001; 54:811–814.

19 Chak A, Cooper GS. Procedure-specific outcomes assessment for endoscopic ultrasonography. Gastrointest Endosc Clin North Am 1999; 9:649–656.

20 Hoffman BJ, Hawes RH. Endoscopic ultrasound and clinical competence. Gastrointest Endosc Clin North Am 1995; 5:879–884.

21 ASGE. Principles of training in gastrointestinal endoscopy. Gastrointest Endosc 1999; 49:845–850.

22 ASGE. Tissue sampling during endosonography. Gastrointest Endosc 1998; 47:576–578.

23 Cass OW. Objective evalutation of competence: technical skills in gastrointestinal endoscopy. Endoscopy 1995; 27:86–89.

24 Jowell PS. Quantitative assessment of procedural competence: a prospective study of training in ERCP. Ann Intern Med 1996; 125:937–939.

25 ASGE. Renewal of endoscopic privileges. Gastrointest Endosc 1999; 49:823–825.

26 Joint Commission on Accreditation of Healthcare Organizations. Joint Commission comprehensive accreditation manual for hospital. Oakbrook, IL: JCAHO; 1997.

27 ASGE. Endoscopy simulators. Gastrointest Endosc 2000; 51:790–792.

28 Markman HD. A new system for teaching proctosigmoidoscopic morphology. Am J Gastroenterol 1969; 52:65–69.

29 Gerson LB, Van Dam J. Technology review: the use of simulators for training in GI endoscopy. Gastrointest Endosc 2004; 60:992–1001.

30 Moorthy K, Munz Y, Jiwanji M, et al. Validity and reliability of a virtual reality upper gastrointestinal simulator and cross validation using structured assessment of individual performance with video playback. Surg Endosc 2004; 18:328–333.

31 Datta V, Mandalia M, Mackay S, et al. The PreOp flexible sigmoidoscopy trainer. Validation and early evaluation of a virtual reality based system. Surg Endosc 2002; 16:1459–1463.

32 MacDonald J, Ketchum J, Williams RG, et al. A lay person versus a trained endoscopist: can the preop endoscopy simulator detect a difference? Surg Endosc 2003; 17:896–898.

33 Sedlack RE, Kolars JC, Alexander JA. Computer simulation training enhances patient discomfort during endoscopy. Clin Gastroenterol Hepatol 2004; 2:348–352.

34 Sedlack RE, Kolars JC. Colonsocpy curriculum development and performance-based criteria on a computer-based endoscopy simulator. Acad Med 2002; 77:750–751.

Chapter

5

Indications, Preparation, Risks, and Complications

Michael J. Levy and Mark Topazian

KEY POINTS

- The primary indications for EUS are cancer staging when there is potential additive value after computed tomography or magnetic resonance imaging has been performed, assessment (usually combined with EUS fine-needle aspiration [FNA]) of lymph node status, and evaluation of pancreatic disease and submucosal tumors.

- Antibiotics are recommended for prophylactic use with EUS-FNA of a cystic lesion.

- There are no reliable data regarding EUS-FNA in patients with increased risk of bleeding. In the absence of data, reasonable rules to follow include:
  International normalized ratio (INR) <1.5
  Platelet count >50 000
  Use a 22–25-gauge needle
  Make as few passes as possible (cytopathologist in room).

- The risk of perforation for EUS is higher than for standard endoscopy. Caution should be exercised when intubating the patient, traversing stenotic tumors, and passing the instrument past the apex of the duodenal bulb; these are all areas where the long rigid tip increases the difficulty of passing the instrument.

INDICATIONS

Endoscopic ultrasound (EUS) should be performed only when it has the potential to affect patient management,[1] as when establishing a diagnosis, performing locoregional tumor staging, or providing therapeutic intervention. As has occurred since its introduction in 1980, the indications and role for EUS will change as EUS and other diagnostic and therapeutic modalities continue to evolve. This discussion of the indications for EUS is limited to general comments, recognizing the inevitable changes that future technologic advances will bring. A detailed discussion of specific indications can be found in relevant chapters throughout this book.

Diagnostic imaging

The endosonographic appearance alone may provide a confident diagnosis for certain lesions including gut duplication cysts, lipomas, bile duct stones, and some branch duct intraductal papillary mucinous neoplasias (IPMNs). In none of these situations, however, does a 'classic' EUS image provide 100% diagnostic accuracy. As a result, EUS-guided biopsy is often indicated to allow histologic diagnosis. Follow-up imaging is often performed when EUS demonstrates a benign-appearing lesion, to identify interval growth or other signs suggestive of malignancy.

Tumor staging

Initial evaluation of patients with gastrointestinal (GI) cancers includes assessment of operative risk and determination of tumor stage. Accurate staging is necessary to determine prognosis, to guide administration of chemoradiation, and to select the ideal means and extent of resection, when appropriate. Staging usually begins with non-invasive imaging such as computed tomography (CT), magnetic resonance imaging (MRI), or positron emission tomography (PET), which are generally superior to EUS for excluding distant metastases. In the absence of metastasis, EUS is often subsequently performed for tumor (T) and node (N) staging, because it provides an accuracy of about 85% for GI luminal cancers.[2–5] Prior radiation therapy substantially decreases the accuracy of EUS. Although EUS currently offers a clear advantage over non-invasive imaging modalities for locoregional staging of luminal cancers, its value in pancreatic cancer staging has been questioned. In particular, recent studies have questioned its accuracy for diagnosis of vascular invasion by pancreatic cancer, and advances in CT and MRI have improved their pancreatic T-stage accuracy. At this point, EUS has maintained its advantage for nodal staging of pancreatic cancer and for the detection of small pancreatic mass lesions.

EUS provides important nodal staging information in patients with lung, esophageal, and rectal cancer. Use of sonographic features of lymph nodes is at best 75% accurate for predicting malignancy. The typical EUS characteristics of malignant lymph nodes are echo-poor appearance, round shape, a smooth border, and size greater than 1 cm in the short axis.[6–8] Overlap in appearance between benign and malignant lymph nodes makes nodal staging problematic. For instance, malignant perirectal lymph nodes secondary to rectal cancer are often 'benign appearing', according to the aforementioned criteria. Overstaging may occur due to enlarged reactive lymph nodes that mimic malignant lymphadenopathy. The addition of fine-needle aspiration (FNA) improves nodal staging accuracy. When biopsying lymph nodes, one should avoid traversing the primary tumor to minimize the risk of a false-positive cytologic finding and tumor seeding.

EUS has a limited role in establishing the presence or absence of distant metastasis (M stage). Occasionally a suspicious lesion is best approached for aspiration via EUS, or a previously unsuspected metastasis is diagnosed during EUS performed for local staging (for instance, a liver lesion in a patient with pancreatic cancer). In these cases EUS-FNA appears reasonably safe, at least with regard to the liver and adrenal glands.[9–12]

Tissue acquisition

Development of linear EUS technology in the early 1990s allowed ultrasound-guided FNA of lesions within and extrinsic to the GI tract wall. This has further enhanced diagnostic and staging accuracy. Indications for FNA include, but are not limited to, biopsy of locally advanced pancreatic cancer and nodal staging of esophageal, pancreatic, and rectal cancers. EUS often provides the least invasive and most successful route for obtaining tissue specimens.

Less invasive approaches for establishing a tissue diagnosis include transabdominal ultrasonography or CT-guided biopsy. The accuracy and safety of these methods are well established, and support their use for initial attempts at diagnosis when they are likely to provide the needed material (as in patients with liver metastases). However, these methods may be limited by their poor sensitivity in the diagnosis of small lesions, or by concern for potential tumor seeding of the biopsy needle track. EUS may be favored in these situations, as well as when EUS is indicated for other reasons such as for locoregional staging or celiac plexus neurolysis. In these settings, FNA can be performed during the same examination, offering a cost-effective approach and simplified patient care. This is in contrast to percutaneous approaches for biopsy that are routinely performed as a separate procedure. While the diagnostic accuracy of EUS-FNA for pancreatic cancer and nodal metastasis is generally over 85%, it is less accurate in other settings, including diagnosis of pancreatic cystic lesions, stromal tumors, and autoimmune pancreatitis, owing to limitations associated with cytologic evaluation. An EUS-guided Tru-Cut biopsy (TCB) device was designed to provide a core biopsy, thereby permiting assessment of tissue architecture. The ability of EUS-TCB safely to improve the diagnostic accuracy of EUS in selected settings is under investigation.[13]

Therapy

Linear echoendoscopes may also be used to deliver therapeutic intervention. The first to be developed was EUS-guided celiac plexus neurolysis (CPN) and celiac plexus block (CPB),[14,15] followed by EUS-guided pseudocyst drainage.[16] More recently, EUS fine-needle injection (EUS-FNI) has also been introduced as a means to deliver novel, potentially therapeutic, agents into solid pancreatic cancers[17] and for therapy of pancreatic cystic neoplasms with EUS-guided ethanol lavage. EUS-guided therapy may become an increasingly common indication in the future. However, limited data are available to judge the safety and efficacy of EUS-FNI for the management of solid and cystic GI neoplasms. Use of EUS for drug delivery has theoretical advantages over other approaches (percutaneous, systemic, or surgical) and may provide a treatment advantage. Further study is needed to establish clearly the safety, cost efficacy, and patient acceptance before EUS-FNI can be advocated.

CONTRAINDICATIONS

Absolute contraindications to EUS are few, and include unacceptable sedation risks. EUS-FNA is generally contraindicated in the presence of coagulopathy (INR >1.5), thrombocytopenia (platelet count <50 000), or the presence of intervening structures that prohibit biopsy. Relative contraindications to EUS include: (1) newly diagnosed cancer in a patient who has not undergone appropriate initial evaluation; (2) altered anatomy prohibiting access; and (3) mild coagulopathy or thrombocytopenia. EUS-FNA may be relatively contraindicated in patients with mild coagulopathy, but there are data (reported only in abstract form) suggesting that EUS-FNA is safe in patients taking antiplatelet agents. Likely of more concern than clinically significant bleeding is the tendency for bloody aspirates, thereby decreasing diagnostic sensitivity. Limited data suggest that EUS-FNA may be relatively safe in patients with portal hypertension.

PATIENT PREPARATION

General measures

Although EUS is typically undertaken in an ambulatory setting, it is also performed in hospitalized patients and practices are increasingly allowing open-access referrals. As a result, the setting of the pre-procedure evaluation can vary, as may the extent of the evaluation. At a minimum, an initial evaluation including a history, physical examination, and review of the medical records must be conducted to identify factors that influence the need, risks, benefits, alternatives, and timing of EUS, and to document acquisition of informed consent (Table 5.1).[18,19] As emergency EUS is uncommon, involved parties should generally have the necessary time for adequate evaluation, discussion of patient and family concerns, and for answering questions. A professional and unhurried demeanor facilitates open communication and helps patients and their families develop trust and a bond with the physician.

Initial planning and preparation for EUS of the upper and lower GI tract are similar to those for routine endoscopy and colonoscopy.[20,21] These efforts are undertaken to help assure a proficient and accurate EUS examination while maintaining patient comfort and safety. During pre-procedure consultation,

FACTORS THAT MAY AFFECT THE PERFORMANCE OF EUS
Severity and urgency of EUS examination
Prior endoscopic examinations (findings and complications)
Other imaging studies (findings and results of tissue sampling)
Administrations of chemoradiation (and timing relative to EUS)
Co-morbid illnesses
Cardiopulmonary
Hepatic disease
Hematologic disease
Bleeding diathesis
Altered anatomy
Medications
Antihypertensives
Anticoagulants
Antiepileptics
Aspirin and other non-steroidal anti-inflammatory agents
Cardiac
Hypoglycemic agents
Monoamine oxidase (MAO) inhibitors
Oral birth control pills
Pulmonary
Psychiatric
Drug allergies
Ability to give informed consent
Available transportation

Table 5.1 Factors that may affect the performance of EUS

patients are instructed as to their preparation responsibilities, use of other medications, and need to avoid alcohol and other sedatives. Patients are advised as to the use of conscious sedation and resulting restrictions on post-procedure activities and need for transportation. The potential signs and symptoms of adverse outcomes as well as contact persons and phone numbers are given in the event of procedure-related complications. These instructions are reviewed following the procedure with the patient and accompanying adult.

Heavier sedation may be required for EUS than for routine endoscopic procedures because of the often longer examination duration and need to minimize patient movement. As for all sedated endoscopic procedures, careful monitoring of pulse, blood pressure, and oxygen saturation is required throughout the procedure and recovery period. The authors administer supplemental oxygen to all patients receiving sedation. Although conscious sedation is routinely given for upper GI EUS, it is optional for rectal EUS.

Upper GI EUS is ideally performed after an overnight fast. At a minimum, patients should avoid solid foods for 6 h and liquids (except sips of water to ingest medications) for 4 h prior to procedure. When there is concern regarding incomplete gastric emptying due to dysmotility and/or obstruction, a 1–2-day diet of clear liquids may be advised. Retained gastric contents risk aspiration, may compromise acoustic coupling, produce image artifacts, and impair the overall examination quality.

Although some perform rectal EUS after administering enemas alone, we prefer a full colonic preparation to optimize acoustic coupling, minimize image artifacts, and potentially reduce infectious complications associated with FNA by decreasing intraluminal contents. More intense and/or prolonged efforts for cleansing may be required in patients with chronic constipation or recent barium study.

Laboratory studies

The need for, and benefit of, routine laboratory evaluation has never been formally studied in patients undergoing endoscopic procedures. Current recommendations are based on extrapolation of surgical data. Surgical series have consistently demonstrated lack of utility for routine preoperative studies such as hemoglobin level, blood cross-matching, routine chemistries, coagulation parameters, urinalysis, chest radiography, and electrocardiography for patients with no evidence of underlying pathology.[21–28] Routine preoperative testing in healthy patients rarely identifies abnormal findings and does not predict or correlate with patient outcomes.[25,28–30] Therefore, routine screening in asymptomatic patients is discouraged. Instead, endoscopists are advised to order pre-procedure testing selectively, based on clinical suspicion arising from the initial evaluation, including a history of bleeding diathesis.[24,28,31,32] This more focused approach greatly enhances the yield of preoperative testing without compromising patient outcomes.[26,33]

An exception may be women of childbearing age in whom pregnancy is possible. Although pregnancy is not a contraindication to endoscopic procedures or conscious sedation, there are situations in which it is important to know whether a woman is pregnant, because of the impact on certain procedural aspects. Such circumstances include administration of general anesthesia (in difficult to sedate patients) or use of fluoroscopy (when performing EUS as part of a rendezvous procedure following failed ERCP).[34] When possible, it is advisable to avoid or delay EUS until after delivery. When EUS cannot be delayed, appropriate measures must be undertaken to lessen the risk to the unborn child.

Medications

Daily medications

In the absence of controlled trials to guide management, we instruct patients to continue their cardiac, antihypertensive, pulmonary, antiepileptic, psychiatric drugs, and oral birth control pills. These medications are ingested with sips of water early on the day of the procedure. We advise diabetic patients to take half of their morning insulin dose at the usual time and the remaining dose with a post-procedure meal. Oral hypoglycemic agents are withheld on the morning of the procedure and until resumption of the patient's normal diet.

Prophylactic antibiotics

There is minimal risk (0–6%) of developing bacteremia after 'routine' endoscopies such as esophagogastroduodenoscopy (EGD), flexible sigmoidoscopy, and colonoscopy.[35,36] The risk of bacteremia is not increased as a result of mucosal biopsy, polypectomy, endoscopic mucosal resection, or sphincterotomy.[37] There is, however, an increased rate of bacteremia, or local infection, following other endoscopic procedures, including esophageal sclerotherapy,[38,39] esophageal stricture dilatation,[40,41] endoscopic retrograde cholangiopancreatography with biliary obstruction,[42,43] endoscopic drainage of a pancreatic pseudocyst,[44] and endoscopic placement of a feeding tube.[45] Although the risk of developing endocarditis or other infectious complication as a result of endoscopic procedures is low, the resulting morbidity and mortality rates are high. These findings have led the American Heart Association (AHA),[46] American Society for Gastrointestinal Endoscopy (ASGE),[38] and other societies and interest groups[47,48] to recommend antibiotic prophylaxis for high-risk patients undergoing high-risk procedures. There are few data regarding the risk of bacteremia following EUS-guided FNA, and hence some uncertainty regarding the need for antibiotics.

Risk of bacteremia and antibiotic recommendations for other endoscopic procedures

Bacterial endocarditis usually develops in patients with high-risk congenital or acquired cardiac lesions who develop bacteremia with microorganisms commonly associated with endocarditis.[46] Cardiac abnormalities are stratified as high, moderate, and low or negligible risk on the basis of the relative risk of developing endocarditis and the potential outcome if endocarditis develops (Table 5.2).[46] In most patients, with or without underlying risk factors, the resulting transient bacteremia is limited in duration (<15 min) and of no clinical significance.[41,49] Rarely, bacteria may lodge on damaged or abnormal heart valves and result in bacterial endocarditis.

Most cases of bacterial endocarditis (60–75%) develop in the absence of a procedure or intervention typically associated with bacteremia.[50] However, certain endoscopic procedures are associated with a high frequency of bacteremia caused by microorganisms commonly associated with endocarditis. The reported rate of bacteremia following particular endoscopic procedures varies greatly among studies. These are mostly small and uncontrolled trials. The discrepancy in results can be explained partly by widely varying differences in methodology. Studies vary in regard to technical aspects of the procedures and in the timing, number, and volume of blood cultured. However, there is general consensus that several endoscopic procedures place patients at higher risk for developing bacteremia. High-risk procedures include esophageal stricture dilatation[40,41] and variceal sclerotherapy,[39] which are associated with bacteremia in approximately 30% of patients. Other high-risk procedures include endoscopic retrograde cholangiography with biliary obstruction and endoscopic drainage of a pancreatic pseudocyst.[38] Although endocarditis rarely develops following these endoscopic

CARDIOVASCULAR RISK FACTORS[46]	
Risk	Condition
High	Prosthetic heart valve (bioprosthetic and homograft)
	History of bacterial endocarditis
	Complex cyanotic congenital heart conditions
	Single ventricle states:
	Transposition of the great arteries
	Tetralogy of Fallot
	Surgically constructed systemic–pulmonary shunt or conduits
	Synthetic vascular graft (less than 1 year old)
Moderate	Most other congenital cardiac malformations (other than those above or below)
	Acquired valve dysfunction (e.g., rheumatic heart disease)
	Hypertrophic cardiomyopathy (with latent or resting obstruction)
	Mitral valve prolapse with murmur and/or valve regurgitation and/or thickened leaflets and/or emergent need for procedure
Negligible[a]	Isolated secundum atrial septal defect
	Surgical repair of (without residua beyond 6 months):
	Atrial septal defect
	Ventricular septal defect
	Patent ductus arteriosus
	Coronary artery bypass graft (prior)
	Mitral valve prolapse (without valve regurgitation)
	Physiologic, functional, or innocent heart murmurs
	Prior Kawasaki disease (without valve dysfunction)
	Prior rheumatic heart disease (without valve dysfunction)
	Pacemaker (intravascular and epicardial)
	Implanted defibrillators

Table 5.2 Cardiovascular risk factors[46]
[a]Same risk as in general population.

procedures, antibiotic prophylaxis is recommended in properly selected patients, because of the high morbidity and mortality rates associated with endocarditis (Table 5.3).[51]

EUS studies

Data regarding the risk of infectious complications following EUS-FNA are limited (Table 5.4), and until recently there has been a notable absence of formal guidelines regarding the need for antibiotic prophylaxis. Several studies have addressed this issue. Van de Mierop and Bourgeois[52] prospectively evaluated the risk of bacteremia following EUS-FNA and published their data in abstract form. Fifteen patients underwent EUS-FNA of a total of 16 upper GI solid lesions. Transient bacteremia, excluding possible contaminates, was seen in three (19%) of 16 patients.

AMERICAN SOCIETY FOR GASTROINTESTINAL ENDOSCOPY RECOMMENDATIONS FOR ANTIBIOTIC PROPHYLAXIS

Patient condition	Procedure	Antibiotic prophylaxis
High-risk cardiac lesion	High risk	Yes
	Low risk	±
Moderate-risk cardiac lesion	High risk	±
	Low risk	No
Low-risk cardiac lesion	High risk	No
	Low risk	No
Cirrhosis (with acute GI bleed)	Any	Yes
Ascites, immunocompromised	High risk	±
Cirrhosis (without acute GI bleed)	Low risk	No
Biliary obstruction	ERCP	Yes
Pancreatic cystic lesion	ERCP	Yes
	EUS	Yes
All patients	PEG	Yes
Prosthetic joint	Any	No
Solid upper GI lesions	EUS	No
Solid lower GI lesions	EUS	Guidelines do not exist
Non-pancreatic cystic lesions	EUS	Guidelines do not exist

Table 5.3 American Society for Gastrointestinal Endoscopy recommendations for antibiotic prophylaxis

ERCP, endoscopic retrograde cholangiopancreatography; EUS, endoscopic ultrasound; GI, gastrointestinal.

±, Prophylaxis is optional for patients with moderate-risk lesions. There are insufficient data to make a firm recommendation and the physician should choose on patient-by-patient basis.

STUDIES EVALUATING THE RATE OF BACTEREMIA ASSOCIATED WITH EUS-FNA

Study	No. of patients enrolled	BACTEREMIA RATE (%) Before FNA	After FNA
Upper GI tract			
Barawi et al.[53] (2001)[a]	100	NA	0
Levy et al.[55] (2003)[b]	52	1.9	3.8
Janssen et al.[56] (2004)[c]	100	2.0	NA
	50	NA	4.0
Lower GI tract			
Levy et al. (2005)[d]	50	0	0

Table 5.4 Studies evaluating the rate of bacteremia associated with EUS-FNA
[a]Blood cultures (10 ml each) were collected 30 and 60 min after EUS-FNA.
[b]Blood cultures (20–30 ml each) were collected immediately before all endoscopic interventions. The second set of blood cultures was collected after EGD (if performed) and radial EUS examination (performed in all patients). A third set of blood cultures was obtained 15 min following EUS-FNA.
[c]100 patients underwent diagnostic linear EUS without FNA (group A) and another group of 50 patients underwent linear EUS with FNA (group B). None of the patients underwent radial EUS. Blood cultures (12 ml each) were collected immediately before EUS in group A and within 5 min after EUS-FNA in group B.
[d]Unpublished data from an ongoing study. Blood cultures (20–30 ml each) were collected immediately before all endoscopic interventions. The second set of blood cultures was collected after flexible sigmoidoscopy and radial EUS examination (performed in all patients). A third set of blood cultures was obtained 15 min after EUS-FNA.

NA, Data not available because blood cultures not performed during the given time period.

Barawi et al.[53] published a prospective study that evaluated the risk of bacteremia and other infectious complications associated with EUS-FNA. One hundred patients underwent EUS-FNA of a total of 107 lesions for a variety of upper GI indications. Other than contaminated blood cultures in six patients, none developed bacteremia or any infectious complication. The absence of true-positive bacteremia may be explained partly by the minimal quantity (10 ml) of blood collected and the delayed timing (30 min after EUS-FNA) of the first blood culture, both of which are associated with lower rates of positive blood cultures.[40,41,54]

We subsequently reported our findings in 52 patients who underwent EUS-FNA of 74 sites from solid lesions of the upper GI tract.[55] Patients underwent a mean of five needle passes. Coagulase-negative *Staphylococcus* grew in three patients (6%) and was considered a contaminant. Three patients (6%) developed bacteremia as the result of *viridans* group *Streptococcus* ($n=2$) and an unidentified Gram-negative bacillus ($n=1$). This rate is similar to that for routine endoscopy. None of the patients developed signs or symptoms of infection. It was concluded that EUS-FNA of solid upper GI tract lesions should be considered

a low-risk procedure for infectious complications and does not warrant antibiotic prophylaxis for bacterial endocarditis.

Janssen et al.[56] prospectively studied 100 patients undergoing diagnostic EUS, as well as 50 who underwent upper GI EUS-FNA. Excluding contaminants, bacteremia developed in four patients overall, two in each group. They concluded that the rate of bacteremia after EUS of upper GI tract lesions with and without FNA is low and that routine administration of antibiotics is not warranted.

Although the aforementioned studies address the risks of infectious complications following EUS-FNA, there are no controlled data concerning cystic lesions. However, based on limited data and anecdotal experience, FNA of cystic lesions is thought to be associated with a high risk of infectious complications.[57,58] In a subgroup analysis, Wiersema et al.[57] found that infectious complications developed in 9% of patients undergoing EUS-FNA of pancreatic cysts.

There are no data regarding the risk of infectious complications following EUS-FNA of rectal and perirectal lesions. In our preliminary experience, none of 50 patients had positive blood cultures and none developed immediate or delayed infectious complications after transrectal EUS-FNA. These data suggest that bacteremia is uncommon after EUS-FNA of rectal and perirectal GI lesions and that antibiotic prophylaxis for spontaneous bacterial endocarditis may not be warranted in patients with no specific indication for prophylaxis. However, these limited data do not allow firm conclusions to be made in this regard.

Summary recommendations regarding antibiotics

The results of these few studies have led the ASGE to recommend antibiotic prophylaxis for EUS-FNA of pancreatic cystic lesions while citing a lack of need for antibiotics with EUS-FNA of solid upper GI lesions.[59] The newly established ASGE guidelines do not address the need for antibiotics in patients undergoing EUS-FNA of non-pancreatic cystic lesions or solid rectal and perirectal lesions. Recognizing the lack of data, we routinely administer antibiotics prior to EUS-FNA of all cystic lesions, regardless of location. The decision to administer antibiotics prior to EUS-FNA of rectal and perirectal lesions seems less clear, and practice varies among centers and individual endosonographers. The same is true in our practice, where there is no standard of care regarding the administration of antibiotics in this setting.

Anticoagulants and antiplatelet agents

Anticoagulants are given to reduce the risk of stroke or systemic embolus in patients with atrial fibrillation, valvular heart disease, and mechanical heart valves.[60–62] In addition, they help to prevent deep vein thrombosis, thrombosis resulting from a hypercoagulable state, and occlusion of coronary artery stents.[60–62] Warfarin must often be discontinued at the time of surgery or endoscopy to minimize the risk of procedure-induced bleeding. However, this risks the development of thromboembolic events. In addition, thromboembolism may result from the transient hypercoaguability that develops following discontinuation of anticoagulation and from a prothrombic effect associated with surgical intervention.[63] Therefore, 'bridging therapy' with administration of unfractionated heparin (UFH) or low molecular weight heparin (LMWH) is often given to ameliorate the risk of thromboembolism.

ASGE recommendations

The ASGE classifies procedures as either high or low risk, depending on the likelihood of inducing bleeding[61] (Table 5.5). EUS without FNA is regarded as a low-risk procedure. Although patients undergoing EUS-FNA are not believed to be at increased risk of bleeding, EUS-FNA is considered a high-risk procedure because resulting bleeding is inaccessible or uncontrollable by endoscopic means. Also, patients' conditions are classified as high or low risk based on the likelihood of the patient developing a thromboembolic event[61] (Table 5.6). Based on both the procedural and condition risks, the ASGE has produced general guidelines for anticoagulation therapy in the peri-procedural period in patients receiving chronic warfarin therapy (Table 5.7). The ASGE is also in the process of formalizing recommendations for patients receiving chronic LMWH therapy (Table 5.8); this information was obtained from personal communication with the committee and is pending publication. As a result,

RISK OF BLEEDING BASED ON ENDOSCOPIC PROCEDURE	
High risk	Low risk
Increased risk of bleeding	**Diagnostic (with or without biopsy)**
Polypectomy	Esophagogastroduodenoscopy (EGD)
Gastric (4%)	Flexible sigmoidoscopy
Colonic (1–2.5%)	Colonoscopy
Laser ablation and coagulation (<6%)	Enteroscopy
Variceal therapy	EUS (without FNA)
Endoscopic sphincterotomy (2.5–5%)	ERCP (without sphincterotomy)
	Biliary/pancreatic stent (without sphincterotomy)
Inaccessible or uncontrollable endoscopically	
Dilatation (pneumatic, bougie)	
PEG/PEJ	
EUS-FNA	

Table 5.5 Risk of bleeding based on endoscopic procedure
ERCP, endoscopic retrograde cholangiopancreatography; PEG, percutaneous endoscopic gastrostomy; PEJ, percutaneous endoscopic jejunostomy.

RISK OF THROMBOEMBOLISM BASED ON UNDERLYING MEDICAL CONDITION	
High risk	Low risk
Atrial fibrillation (with valve disease)	Deep vein thrombosis
Mechanical valve (mitral)	Atrial fibrillation (no valve disease)
Mechanical valve (prior thromboembolic event)	Bioprosthetic valve
Mechanical valve (aortic)	

Table 5.6 Risk of thromboembolism based on underlying medical condition

these recommendations may be modified and the information provided in Table 5.8 should not be considered representative of the final report.

With regard to resuming anticoagulation following an endoscopic procedure, it is recommended that heparin be resumed 2–6 h after most procedures. For LMWH, the ASGE states only that resumption should be individualized, and makes no formal recommendation. The ASGE notes that coumadin can usually be resumed on the night of the procedure and that overlapping therapy is recommended for 4–5 days or until the INR is therapeutic for 2–3 days.

Despite the ASGE's recommendations, the ideal approach for managing anticoagulation in the perioperative period has not been established and is controversial.[60–69] Firm conclusions cannot be drawn concerning the efficacy and safety of different

RECOMMENDATIONS FOR ANTICOAGULATION THERAPY IN PATIENTS UNDERGOING ENDOSCOPIC PROCEDURES BASED ON THE RELATIVE RISKS OF THE PROCEDURE AND UNDERLYING CONDITION		
	CONDITION RISK FOR THROMBOEMBOLISM	
Procedure risk	High	Low
High	Stop warfarin 3–5 days before procedure	Stop warfarin 3–5 days before procedure
	Consider heparin while INR below therapeutic range	Reinstitute warfarin after procedure
Low	No change in anticoagulation	
	Elective procedures should be delayed while INR is in supratherapeutic range	

Table 5.7 Recommendations for anticoagulation therapy in patients undergoing endoscopic procedures based on the relative risks of the procedure and underlying condition
INR, international normalized ratio.

RECOMMENDATIONS FOR MANAGEMENT OF LMWH IN PATIENTS UNDERGOING ENDOSCOPIC PROCEDURES	
Procedure risk	High and/or low risk condition for thromboembolism
High	Consider stopping LMWH ≥8 h before procedure
	Decision to restart should be individualized
Low	No change in anticoagulation

Table 5.8 Recommendations for management of LMWH in patients undergoing endoscopic procedures
LMWH, low molecular weight heparin.

management strategies based on the current literature, owing to variations in patient populations, procedures, anticoagulation regimens, definitions of events, and duration of follow-up. The recommendations of the ASGE and most societies were based mostly on data from therapeutic regimens, treatment scenarios, and procedure that in many cases were quite dissimilar to endoscopic procedures. The need to stop coumadin and administer 'bridging therapy' is controversial and varies among societies. In general, firm recommendations are not given and many patient scenarios are not addressed. This is understandable, given the paucity of sound data. As for patient care in general, decisions regarding anticoagulation therapy must be made after careful consideration of the potential risks, benefits, and alternatives for an individual patient.

Although not addressed by the ASGE recommendations, and never formally studied, the use of anticoagulants may predispose to the development of bloody aspirates and may impair cytologic analysis. This should be considered when choosing the amount of negative pressure to apply during FNA, and may even alter the timing of EUS.

Anticoagulant administration (timing and technique)

Stopping coumadin When stopping coumadin, if the target INR is <1.5 and the initial INR is 2.0–3.0, then three to five doses of coumadin should be withheld.[63,64,70] If the initial INR

is >3.0, four to six doses should be withheld, especially in the elderly.[63,64,70] If the INR is not checked, the number of doses to withhold is based on the typical levels for a patient and the perceived risk of bleeding and thromboembolism.

Starting bridging therapy If bridging therapy is used, it should be started when the INR is expected to be at the lower limit of therapeutic range. As it is often impractical to check the INR daily, it is reasonable to start approximately 2 days after stopping coumadin.

Stopping bridging therapy UFH should be stopped 4–8 h prior to the procedure, and LMWH (when given as a single daily dose) should be stopped the morning before the procedure. When LMWH is given twice daily, it should be stopped the evening before the procedure.

Resuming anticoagulation Anticoagulants should generally be restarted without a bolus.[63,64,70] The timing, however, is greatly debated, with some favoring immediate administration with coumadin and either UFH or LMWH. Others favor waiting for 3 days after a procedure and administering coumadin alone (without UFH or LMWH). The approach is influenced by the occurrence of bleeding during the procedure, risk of thromboembolism, and clinical course.

Antiplatelet therapy

For antiplatelet agents there are virtually no data and what follows are the ASGE recommendations. For aspirin and other non-steroidal anti-inflammatory drugs, the recommendations state that, in the absence of a bleeding disorder, endoscopic procedures are safe. For clopidogrel (Plavix) and ticlopidine (Ticlid), low-risk procedures (regardless of the thromboembolic risk) require no change in anticoagulation. For high-risk procedures (regardless of the thromboembolic risk) the need to discontinue therapy is uncertain. The ASGE states that, if therapy is to be discontinued, this should be undertaken 7–10 days prior to the procedure. For dipyridamole, low-risk procedures (regardless of the thromboembolic risk) require no change in anticoagulation (unless there is an underlying bleeding disorder). Interestingly, for high-risk procedures (regardless of the thromboembolic risk) the need to discontinue therapy is uncertain, and no recommendation is given. Finally, for the glycoprotein IIb/IIIa inhibitors, these medications are given for acute coronary syndromes and are therefore not typically used prior to EUS. Although no guidelines are offered, the duration of action may help in guiding timing of the procedure, with abciximab having a duration of action of up to 24 h versus eptifibatide and tirofiban, with a duration of approximately 4 h.

RISKS AND COMPLICATIONS

EUS shares the risks and complications of other endoscopic procedures, including cardiovascular events, complications of conscious sedation, and allergic reactions to medications. This discussion focuses on adverse effects specifically associated with EUS. Some of these relate primarily to the unique features of echoendoscopes, whereas others are associated with the performance of FNA, TCB, or therapeutic interventions.

Perforation

The incidence of GI perforation during EUS ranges from 0%[71] to 0.4%[72] in prospective series enrolling over 300 patients. Although available data are limited, perforation is probably more common with upper GI EUS than with EGD.

The increased risk is partly accounted for by echoendoscope design, which combines oblique- or side-viewing optics with a relatively long rigid tip that extends well beyond the optical lens. The tip of the endoscope may cause luminal perforation during advancement, particularly in areas of angulation (oropharynx or apex of duodenal bulb), stenosis (esophageal cancer), or where a blind lumen exists (pharyngeal or esophageal diverticula). There is some evidence that perforation is more common early in an endosonographer'experience.[72] Risk may also be increased when experienced endosonographers use new equipment with different tip design, length, and deflection characteristics.

Approximately 15–40% of patients with esophageal cancer have a non-traversable obstructing esophageal tumor.[73-76] Some advocate dilatation, given the greater accuracy of EUS for T and N staging of traversable versus non-traversable tumors (81% versus 28%, and 86% versus 72%, respectively).[73,75,76] Others discourage routine dilatation given the risk and tendency for advanced disease (85–90% likelihood of T3 or T4 disease) in this setting.[74] However, distant lymphadenopathy (meriting M1a tumor staging) is diagnosed in 10–40% of patients requiring dilatation.[73,75,76]

Although initial studies reported perforation rates as high as 24% with esophageal dilatation followed by immediate EUS, more recent studies have found this practice quite safe.[73-76] There are several likely explanations for the apparent improvement in safety over time. Newer Olympus radial echoendoscopes introduced in the mid 1990s were of smaller diameter (13.2 mm for the GF-UM20), so dilatation was usually performed to 14 or 15 mm rather than 16–18 mm as in earlier studies. In addition, greater awareness of this potential complication has probably led to less aggressive dilatation practices.

Mini-probes passed through a stenotic esophageal cancer may improve the accuracy of T and N staging, but the limited depth of penetration does not allow a complete examination, particularly with regard to celiac axis nodes.[77] A small-caliber (7 mm) wire-guided echoendoscope without fiberoptic capability is available for staging stenotic tumors (Olympus MH-908). Use of this instrument in 130 patients allowed complete endoscopic staging in 90% (27 of 30), compared with 60% (60 of 100) in whom it was not used.[78]

For patients with circumferential stenosis, judicious stepwise dilatation is undertaken to a maximum of 15 mm. Two large studies reporting safety of dilatation[75,76] followed the 'rule of 3' (three stepwise 1-mm increases in dilator diameter above the diameter at which resistance was first encountered) and did not use 'unacceptable force' to dilate. Dilatation allowed immediate passage of an echoendoscope beyond the tumor in 75–85% of cases. We are particularly cautious when semi-circumferential infiltration is present, as the normal (and hence thinner) esophageal wall may be at increased risk of tearing in this setting, particularly if the proximal esophagus is dilated.

Bleeding

The risk of bleeding with EUS relates mainly to performance of FNA. The incidence of bleeding was 0%[71] to 0.4%[72] in two prospective studies enrolling over 300 patients, and 1.3% in a retrospective study.[79] FNA of pancreatic cystic lesions has been associated with a 6% rate of self-limiting bleeding.[80]

A small amount of luminal bleeding is often seen endoscopically at FNA puncture sites, but is generally without sequelae. Bleeding may also occur in the gut wall, adjacent tissue, or the target structure undergoing aspiration. Such bleeding may be detected sonographically as a hypoechoic expansion of soft tissue or enlargement of a node or mass. Alternatively echogenic material may be seen filling a previously anechoic cyst or duct lumen, or collecting in ascites. As blood clots, it increases in echogenicity and may thus become less apparent. When the bleeding is into a large potential space (such as the peritoneal cavity) the extent of blood loss may be difficult to assess due to pooling of blood outside the range of EUS imaging.

EUS-induced extraluminal bleeding is seldom associated with clinically important sequela such as the need for transfusion, angiography, or surgery. As most endosonographers avoid sonographically visible vessels when selecting a needle path for FNA, bleeding usually occurs from small vessels. Because the bleeding site is often extraintestinal, methods of endoscopic hemostasis are usually not applicable. In some cases it is possible to apply transmitted pressure to the bleeding site by deflecting the tip of the echoendoscope against the gut wall,[79] or to inject epinephrine.[81] The efficacy of these interventions is unknown.

Infection

Infectious complications have been reported in 0.3% of EUS-FNA procedures,[71,72] and may include those associated with the endoscopy itself (aspiration pneumonia) or from FNA (abscess or cholangitis).

Infection may develop secondary to aspiration of cystic lesions in the pancreas, mediastinum, and elsewhere.[82] A 9% rate of infection has been reported after EUS-FNA of cysts, the risk of which is markedly decreased by antibiotic administration prior to, and following, the examination.[72,80] The true incidence of cyst infection when antibiotics are given is unknown, but is likely to be low. Iatrogenic *Candida* infection of a cystic lesion has been reported after EUS-FNA performed with prophylactic antibiotics.[83] Technical issues may also affect the risk of cyst infection. Multiple needle passes into a cyst appear to increase the risk of infection, as does failure to aspirate completely all of the cyst fluid.

As reviewed in detail above, bacteremia after upper GI EUS-FNA is uncommon. Antibiotic prophylaxis for patients at increased risk of bacterial endocarditis is also discussed above.

Although little information is available regarding the risks of EUS-guided injection therapy, retroperitoneal abscess has been reported after EUS-guided celiac plexus block.

Pancreatitis

Pancreatitis may occur after EUS-FNA of both solid and cystic pancreatic lesions. In one pooled analysis of data from 19 American EUS centers, the incidence of pancreatitis after EUS-FNA of solid pancreatic lesions masses was 0.3%.[84] The incidence was higher (0.6%) at two centers with prospectively collected data, and was also 0.6% in another prospective study.[85] Aspiration of cystic lesions has been associated with pancreatitis in 1–2% of cases.[71] Pancreatitis following EUS-FNA is generally mild, but severe pancreatitis and fatal complications have been reported.[84]

The risk of pancreatitis may be ameliorated by limiting the number of needle passes, minimizing the amount of 'normal' pancreatic parenchyma that must be traversed, and avoiding the pancreatic duct during EUS-FNA procedures. In one small series, however, 12 patients with dilated pancreatic ducts underwent intentional EUS-guided aspiration of the duct without complications.[86] Cytologic yield on aspirated pancreatic duct fluid was 75%.

Other

There is a theoretical risk of tumor seeding along the needle track when performing EUS-FNA. We are aware of two cases with persuasive evidence of needle track seeding.[87] This is of minimal concern for pancreatic head lesions, due to inclusion of the needle track site within the field of resection during pancreaticoduodenectomy.

Bile peritonitis may result from traversal of the bile duct or gallbladder, especially in the presence of an obstructed biliary system.[88] If biliary puncture occurs, we favor administration of antibiotics in patients without biliary obstruction. In the presence of biliary obstruction, we also recommend biliary drainage.

REFERENCES

1 Hawes RH. Indications for EUS-directed FNA. Endoscopy 1998; 30:A155–A157.
2 Tio TL, den Hartog Jager FC, Tytgat GN. The role of endoscopic ultrasonography in assessing local resectability of oesophagogastric malignancies. Accuracy, pitfalls, and predictability. Scand J Gastroenterol Suppl 1986; 123:78–86.
3 Dittler HJ, Siewert JR. Role of endoscopic ultrasonography in esophageal carcinoma. Endoscopy 1993; 25:156–161.
4 Grimm H, Binmoeller KF, Hamper K, et al. Endosonography for preoperative locoregional staging of esophageal and gastric cancer. Endoscopy 1993; 25:224–230.
5 Rosch T. Endosonographic staging of esophageal cancer: a review of literature results. Gastrointest Endosc Clin North Am 1995; 5:537–547.
6 Bhutani MS, Hawes RH, Hoffman BJ. A comparison of the accuracy of echo features during endoscopic ultrasound (EUS) and EUS-guided fine needle aspiration for diagnosis of malignant lymph node invasion. Gastrointest Endosc 1996; 45:474–479.
7 Catalano MF, Sivak MV Jr, Rice T, et al. Endosonographic features predictive of lymph node metastasis. Gastrointest Endosc 1994; 40:442–446.
8 Grimm H, Hamper K, Binmoeller KF, et al. Enlarged lymph nodes: malignant or not? Endoscopy 1992; 24:320–323.
9 DeWitt J, LeBlanc J, McHenry L, et al. Endoscopic ultrasound-guided fine needle aspiration cytology of solid liver lesions: a large single-center experience. Am J Gastroenterol 2003; 98:1976–1981.

10 tenBerge J, Hoffman BJ, Hawes RH, et al. EUS-guided fine needle aspiration of the liver: indications, yield, and safety based on an international survey of 167 cases. Gastrointest Endosc 2002; 55:859–862.
11 Hollerbach S, Willert J, Topalidis T, et al. Endoscopic ultrasound-guided fine-needle aspiration biopsy of liver lesions: histological and cytological assessment. Endoscopy 2003; 35:743–749.
12 Jhala NC, Jhala D, Eloubeidi MA, et al. Endoscopic ultrasound-guided fine-needle aspiration biopsy of the adrenal glands: analysis of 24 patients. Cancer 2004; 102:308–314.
13 Levy MJ, Reddy RP, Wiersema MJ, et al. EUS-guided trucut biopsy in establishing autoimmune pancreatitis as the cause of obstructive jaundice. Gastrointest Endosc 2005; 61:467–473.
14 Gress F, Schmitt C, Sherman S, et al. Endoscopic ultrasound-guided celiac plexus block for managing abdominal pain associated with chronic pancreatitis: a prospective single center experience. Am J Gastroenterol 2001; 96:409–416.
15 Schmulewitz N, Hawes R. EUS-guided celiac plexus neurolysis – technique and indication. Endoscopy 2003; 35:S49–S53.
16 Seifert H, Dietrich C, Schmitt T, et al. Endoscopic ultrasound-guided one-step transmural drainage of cystic abdominal lesions with a large-channel echo endoscope. Endoscopy 2000; 32:255–259.
17 Chang KJ, Nguyen PT, Thompson JA, et al. Phase I clinical trial of allogeneic mixed lymphocyte culture (cytoimplant) delivered by endoscopic ultrasound-guided fine-needle injection in patients with advanced pancreatic carcinoma. Cancer 2000; 88:1325–1335.

18 Anonymous. Informed consent for gastrointestinal endoscopy. Gastrointest Endosc 1988; 34(Suppl):26S–27S.

19 Plumeri PA. Informed consent for gastrointestinal endoscopy in the '90s and beyond. Gastrointest Endosc 1994; 40:379.

20 Faigel DO, Eisen GM, Baron TH, et al for the Standards of Practice Committee, American Society for Gastrointestinal Endoscopy. Preparation of patients for GI endoscopy. Gastrointest Endosc 2003; 57:446–450.

21 Anonymous. ASGE guidelines for clinical application. Position statement on laboratory testing before ambulatory elective endoscopic procedures. American Society for Gastrointestinal Endoscopy. Gastrointest Endosc 1999; 50:906–909.

22 Rucker L, Frye EB, Staten MA. Usefulness of screening chest roentgenograms in preoperative patients. JAMA 1983; 250:3209–3211.

23 Smallwood JA. Use of blood in elective general surgery: an area of wasted resources. Br Med J Clin Res Ed 1983; 286:868–870.

24 Campbell IT, Gosling P. Preoperative biochemical screening. BMJ 1988; 297:803–804.

25 Kaplan EB, Sheiner LB, Boeckmann AJ, et al. The usefulness of preoperative laboratory screening. JAMA 1985; 253:3576–3581.

26 Blery C, Charpak Y, Szatan M, et al. Evaluation of a protocol for selective ordering of preoperative tests. Lancet 1986; i:139–141.

27 Rohrer MJ, Michelotti MC, Nahrwold DL. A prospective evaluation of the efficacy of preoperative coagulation testing. Ann Surg 1988; 208:554–557.

28 Turnbull JM, Buck C. The value of preoperative screening investigations in otherwise healthy individuals. Arch Intern Med 1987; 147:1101–1105.

29 Eika C, Havig O, Godal HC. The value of preoperative haemostatic screening. Scand J Haematol 1978; 21:349–354.

30 Suchman AL, Mushlin AI. How well does the activated partial thromboplastin time predict postoperative hemorrhage? JAMA 1986; 256:750–753.

31 Eisenberg JM, Goldfarb S. Clinical usefulness of measuring prothrombin time as a routine admission test. Clin Chem 1976; 22:1644–1647.

32 Robbins JA, Rose SD. Partial thromboplastin time as a screening test. Ann Intern Med 1979; 90:796–797.

33 Charpak Y, Blery C, Chastang C, et al. Usefulness of selectively ordered preoperative tests. Med Care 1988; 26:95–104.

34 Jamidar PA, Beck GJ, Hoffman BJ, et al. Endoscopic retrograde cholangiopancreatography in pregnancy. Am J Gastroenterol 1995; 90:1263–1267.

35 Botoman VA, Surawicz CM. Bacteremia with gastrointestinal endoscopic procedures. Gastrointest Endosc 1986; 32:342–346.

36 Low DE, Shoenut JP, Kennedy JK, et al. Prospective assessment of risk of bacteremia with colonoscopy and polypectomy. Dig Dis Sci 1987; 32:1239–1243.

37 Lee TH, Hsueh PR, Yeh WC, et al. Low frequency of bacteremia after endoscopic mucosal resection. Gastrointest Endosc 2000; 52:223–225.

38 Endoscopy ASfG. Antibiotic prophylaxis for gastrointestinal endoscopy. American Society for Gastrointestinal Endoscopy. Gastrointest Endosc 1995; 42:630–635.

39 Chen WC, Hou MC, Lin HC, et al. Bacteremia after endoscopic injection of N-butyl-2-cyanoacrylate for gastric variceal bleeding. Gastrointest Endosc 2001; 54:214–218.

40 Nelson DB, Sanderson SJ, Azar MM. Bacteremia with esophageal dilation. Gastrointest Endosc 1998; 48:563–567.

41 Zuccaro G Jr, Richter JE, Rice TW, et al. Viridans streptococcal bacteremia after esophageal stricture dilation. Gastrointest Endosc 1998; 48:568–573.

42 Motte S, Deviere J, Dumonceau JM, et al. Risk factors for septicemia following endoscopic biliary stenting. Gastroenterology 1991; 101:1374–1381.

43 Deviere J, Motte S, Dumonceau JM, et al. Septicemia after endoscopic retrograde cholangiopancreatography. Endoscopy 1990; 22:72–75.

44 Kolars JC, Allen MO, Ansel H, et al. Pancreatic pseudocysts: clinical and endoscopic experience. Am J Gastroenterol 1989; 84:259–264.

45 Sharma VK, Howden CW. Meta-analysis of randomized, controlled trials of antibiotic prophylaxis before percutaneous endoscopic gastrostomy. Am J Gastroenterol 2000; 95:3133–3136.

46 Dajani AS, Taubert KA, Wilson W, et al. Prevention of bacterial endocarditis: recommendations by the American Heart Association. Clin Infect Dis 1997; 25:1448–1458.

47 Simmons NA. Recommendations for endocarditis prophylaxis. The Endocarditis Working Party for Antimicrobial Chemotherapy. J Antimicrob Chemother 1993; 31:437–438.

48 Leport C, Horstkotte D, Burckhardt D. Antibiotic prophylaxis for infective endocarditis from an international group of experts towards a European consensus. Group of Experts of the International Society for Chemotherapy. Eur Heart J 1995; 16:126–131.

49 el-Baba M, Tolia V, Lin CH, et al. Absence of bacteremia after gastrointestinal procedures in children. Gastrointest Endosc 1996; 44:378–381.

50 Durack DT. Infective endocarditis. In: Alexander RW, Schlant RC, Fuster V, eds. Hurst's the heart, arteries and veins. New York: McGraw-Hill, 1998:2205–2239.

51 Watanakunakorn C, Burkert T. Infective endocarditis at a large community teaching hospital, 1980–1990. A review of 210 episodes. Medicine 1993; 72:90–102.

52 Van de Mierop F, Bourgeois S. Bacteremia after EUS guided puncture: a prospective analysis. Gastrointest Endosc 1999; 49:100A.

53 Barawi M, Gottlieb K, Cunha B, et al. A prospective evaluation of the incidence of bacteremia associated with EUS-guided fine-needle aspiration. Gastrointest Endosc 2001; 53:189–192.

54 Aronson MD, Bor DH. Blood cultures. Ann Intern Med 1987; 106:246–253.

55 Levy MJ, Norton ID, Wiersema MJ, et al. Prospective risk assessment of bacteremia and other infectious complications in patients undergoing EUS-guided FNA. Gastrointest Endosc 2003; 57:672–678.

56 Janssen J, Konig K, Knop-Hammad V, et al. Frequency of bacteremia after linear EUS of the upper GI tract with and without FNA. Gastrointest Endosc 2004; 59:339–344.

57 Wiersema MJ, Vilmann P, Giovannini M, et al. Endosonography-guided fine-needle aspiration biopsy: diagnostic accuracy and complication assessment. Gastroenterology 1997; 112:1087–1095.

58 Ryan AG, Zamvar V, Roberts SA. Iatrogenic candidal infection of a mediastinal foregut cyst following endoscopic ultrasound-guided fine-needle aspiration. Endoscopy 2002; 34:838–839.

59 Hirota WK, Petersen K, Baron TH, et al for the Standards of Practice Committee of the American Society for Gastrointestinal Endoscopy. Guidelines for antibiotic prophylaxis for GI endoscopy. Gastrointest Endosc 2003; 58:475–482.

60 Kearon C, Hirsh J. Management of anticoagulation before and after elective surgery. N Engl J Med 1997; 336:1506–1511.

61 Eisen GM, Baron TH, Dominitz JA, et al for the American Society for Gastrointestinal Endoscopy. Guideline on the management of anticoagulation and antiplatelet therapy for endoscopic procedures. Gastrointest Endosc 2002; 55:775–779.

62 Douketis JD, Johnson JA, Turpie AG. Low-molecular-weight heparin as bridging anticoagulation during interruption of warfarin: assessment of a standardized periprocedural anticoagulation regimen. Arch Intern Med 2004; 164:1319–1326.

63 Kearon C. Management of anticoagulation in patients who require invasive procedures. Semin Vasc Med 2003; 3:285–294.

64 Spandorfer J. The management of anticoagulation before and after procedures. Med Clin North Am 2001; 85:1109–1116.

65 Anonymous. Guideline on the management of anticoagulation and antiplatelet therapy for endoscopic procedures. American Society for Gastrointestinal Endoscopy. Gastrointest Endosc 1998; 48:672–675.

66 Ansell JE, Buttaro ML, Thomas OV, et al. Consensus guidelines for coordinated outpatient oral anticoagulation therapy management. Anticoagulation Guidelines Task Force. Ann Pharmacother 1997; 31:604–615.

67 Davis FB, Estruch MT, Samson-Corvera EB, et al. Management of anticoagulation in outpatients: experience with an anticoagulation service in a municipal hospital setting. Arch Intern Med 1977; 137:197–202.

68 Heit JA. Perioperative management of the chronically anticoagulated patient. J Thromb Thrombolysis 2001; 12:81–87.

69 Dunn AS, Turpie AG. Perioperative management of patients receiving oral anticoagulants: a systematic review. Arch Intern Med 2003; 163:901–908.

70 Douketis JD. Perioperative anticoagulation management in patients who are receiving oral anticoagulant therapy: a practical guide for clinicians. Thromb Res 2002; 108:3–13.

71 O'Toole D, Palazzo L, Arotcarena R, et al. Assessment of complications of EUS-guided fine-needle aspiration. Gastrointest Endosc 2001; 53:470–474.

72 Wiersema MJ, Vilmann P, Giovannini M, et al. Endosonography-guided fine-needle aspiration biopsy: diagnostic accuracy and complication assessment. Gastroenterology 1997; 112:1087–1095.

73 Kallimanis G, Gupta P, al-Kawas F, et al. Endoscopic ultrasound for staging esophageal cancer, with or without dilation, is clinically important and safe. Gastrointest Endosc 1995; 41:540–546.

74 Van Dam J, Rice T, Catalano M, et al. High-grade malignant stricture is predictive of esophageal tumor stage. Risk of endosonographic evaluation. Cancer 1993; 71:2910–2917.

75 Wallace MB, Hawes RH, Sahai AV, et al. Dilation of malignant esophageal stenosis to allow EUS guided fine-needle aspiration: safety and effect on patient management. Gastrointest Endosc 2000; 51:309–313.

76 Pfau PR, Ginsberg GG, Lew RJ, et al. Esophageal dilation for endosonographic evaluation of malignant esophageal strictures is safe and effective. Am J Gastroenterol 2000; 95:2813–2815.

77 Menzel J, Hoepffner N, Nottberg H, et al. Preoperative staging of esophageal carcinoma: miniprobe sonography versus conventional endoscopic ultrasound in a prospective histopathologically verified study. Endoscopy 1999; 31:291–297.

78 Mallery S, Van Dam J. Increased rate of complete EUS staging of patients with esophageal cancer using the nonoptical, wire-guided echoendoscope. Gastrointest Endosc 1999; 50:53–57.

79 Affi A, Vazquez-Sequeiros E, Norton ID, et al. Acute extraluminal hemorrhage associated with EUS-guided fine needle aspiration: frequency and clinical significance. Gastrointest Endosc 2001; 53:221–225.

80 Varadarajulu S, Eloubeidi MA. Frequency and significance of acute intracystic hemorrhage during EUS-FNA of cystic lesions of the pancreas. Gastrointest Endosc 2004; 60:631–635.

81 Varadarajulu S, Fraig M, Schmulewitz N, et al. Comparison of EUS-guided 19-gauge Trucut needle biopsy with EUS-guided fine-needle aspiration. Endoscopy 2004; 36:397–401.

82 Annema JT, Veselic M, Versteegh MIM, et al. Mediastinitis caused by EUS-FNA of a bronchogenic cyst. Endoscopy 2003; 35:791–793.

83 Ryan AG, Zamvar V, Roberts SA. Iatrogenic candidal infection of a mediastinal foregut cyst following endoscopic ultrasound-guided fine-needle aspiration. Endoscopy 2002; 34:838–839.

84 Eloubeidi MA, Gress FG, Savides TJ, et al. Acute pancreatitis after EUS-guided FNA of solid pancreatic masses: a pooled analysis from EUS centers in the United States. Gastrointest Endosc 2004; 60:385–389.

85 Eloubeidi MA, Chen VK, Eltoum IA, et al. Endoscopic ultrasound-guided fine needle aspiration biopsy of patients with suspected pancreatic cancer: diagnostic accuracy and acute and 30-day complications. Am J Gastroenterol 2003; 98:2663–2668.

86 Lai R, Stanley MW, Bardales R, et al. Endoscopic ultrasound-guided pancreatic duct aspiration: diagnostic yield and safety. Endoscopy 2002; 34:715–720.

87 Shah JN, Fraker D, Guerry D, et al. Melanoma seeding of an EUS-guided fine needle track. Gastrointest Endosc 2004; 59:923–924.

88 Chen H-Y, Lee C-H, Hsieh C-H. Bile peritonitis after EUS-guided fine-needle aspiration. Gastrointest Endosc 2002; 56:594–596.

Chapter
6

How to Perform EUS in the Esophagus and Mediastinum

Robert H. Hawes and Paul Fockens

ESOPHAGUS

Obtaining high-quality and high-resolution images of the esophageal wall is one of the more difficult techniques that an endosonographer will encounter. One has to deal with the 'catch 22' that pits adequate coupling of the ultrasound signal to the esophageal wall with wall compression; this can lead to missing lesions or inaccurate staging of malignancy. Numerous techniques have been employed to try to overcome these conflicting goals.

If one is dealing with a relatively large mass in the esophagus, either no or mild balloon inflation will be sufficient to couple the ultrasound image to the esophageal wall without causing compression. This technique is adequate for advanced esophageal cancers or for relatively large bulky mural tumors. This circumstance is one in which the electronic radial instrument has an advantage over mechanical radial because of the absence of ringdown artifact with the electronic array technology. Periesophageal structures (such as lymph nodes) are not affected by the degree of balloon inflation.

If it is important to avoid compression of the esophageal wall, there are multiple techniques that can be employed. The simplest is to instill water into the gut lumen by pressing on the air/water button to its first position. This will spray water across the endoscopic image lens. Interestingly, this does a very good job of filling the lumen with water without the risk of aspiration. This technique can be employed with the standard radial echoendoscope or when employing a high-frequency catheter probe in conjunction with a single- or dual-channel forward-viewing endoscope. The images generated, although of high quality, may not remain stationary for a long period of time and thus it is important to employ the cine review function, which continuously stores the last 100 images. High-resolution esophageal images can be obtained only when the esophagus is in its relaxed state, and this occurs only periodically. Agents normally used to paralyze the stomach, duodenum, and colon have little to no effect on esophageal contraction.

A second method that can be utilized with a radial scanning echoendoscope is to instill water through the biopsy channel. If this technique is employed, it is recommended that water be siphoned rather than actively instilled by pumping or vigorous syringe instillation. There is a very real risk of aspiration if high volumes are instilled over a short period of time, especially when topical pharyngeal anesthesia has also been applied.

Until the advent of electronic radial echoendoscopes, if one wanted to obtain precise images of the esophageal wall, the instrument of choice was a high-frequency ultrasound probe. However, the new electronic radial echoendoscopes have near-field imaging of very high quality, and allow high-resolution imaging of the esophageal wall layers without the need for significant balloon inflation. However, if one wishes to stage early esophageal cancer, that is, to determine whether the lesion penetrates through the muscularis mucosa, then high-frequency catheter probes are still the instrument of choice.

When using catheter probes for esophageal imaging, there are several techniques that can be employed. One, mentioned above, is to use a bare catheter and instill water via the air/water channel. A second method is to use a ultrasound catheter with an attachable balloon. This technique still risks compression of the wall layers with inflation of the balloon; however, the focal length of the catheter is such that only a small amount of balloon inflation is necessary, thereby minimizing this risk. Another technique that has been described is to affix a transparent, low-compliance condom onto the end of a two-channel endoscope. Approximately 2–3 cm of the condom protrudes beyond the tip of the endoscope. This redundant portion of the condom is folded across the imaging lens as the patient is intubated; during the intubation process, it is extremely important to avoid instilling air as this will inflate the condom and could compromise patient breathing. Once the esophagus is intubated, the instrument is passed into the stomach lumen and air is 'bled' from the condom tip. This is done by instilling water and then aspirating all of the contents. Once the condom has been bled, the endoscope is withdrawn to the level of the lesion and the condom is then filled with water. Because of the low compliance of the condom, it tends to elongate rather than compress the wall layers. The ultrasound catheter is then advanced into the lumen of the condom, and imaging proceeds. With this technique, the coupling of the ultrasound waves to the gut wall is virtually perfect, and with the transparent condom the lesion can be viewed endoscopically in real time, thus assuring that the catheter probe is positioned correctly. Because the water is completely contained within the condom, there is no risk of aspiration.

Whichever technique is employed, the risk of aspiration should be minimized while achieving good coupling of the

Chapter
7

EUS in Non-Small Cell Lung Cancer

Jouke T. Annema and Klaus F. Rabe

KEY POINTS

- Endoscopic ultrasound-guided fine-needle aspiration (EUS-FNA) is an accurate technique for the analysis of mediastinal lymph nodes located in the aorto pulmonary window and posterior mediastinum.

- EUS-FNA can diagnose intrapulmonary tumors adjacent to the esophagus directly and assess mediastinal tumor invasion (T4).

- In patients with non-small cell lung cancer, EUS-FNA can prevent surgical staging to a large extent by demonstrating lymph node metastases or tumor invasion.

- Incorporation of EUS-FNA in staging logarithms for non-small cell lung cancer reduces the number of mediastinoscopies and unnecessary thoracotomies, as well as costs.

INTRODUCTION

Transesophageal endoscopic ultrasound-guided fine-needle aspiration (EUS-FNA) is a novel technique for the diagnosis and staging of lung cancer. By demonstrating mediastinal lymph node metastases or tumor invasion, EUS-FNA provides a minimally invasive alternative to surgical staging.

Lung cancer has an annual worldwide incidence of more than one million cases, and presents with mediastinal metastasis in about one-third of those cases. Accurate diagnosis and staging is important for both prognostic and therapeutic reasons. Patients with mediastinal lymph node metastases or tumor invasion (stage III) are preferably treated with multimodality treatment, in contrast to patients without locally advanced disease who are treated primarily by surgery. Current staging of patients with non-small cell lung cancer (NSCLC) critically depends on surgical interventions, predominantly mediastinoscopy.

In this chapter, the role of EUS-FNA for the diagnosis and staging of lung cancer is evaluated, as well as the assessment of liver and adrenal metastases. Indications and limitations for EUS in the diagnosis and staging of lung cancer are discussed. The impact of EUS-FNA on patient management will be addressed, in particular its role in preventing surgical staging procedures as well as its position in non-small cell lung cancer staging algorithms.

DIAGNOSIS AND STAGING OF LUNG CANCER

Patients with suspected lung cancer primarily undergo bronchoscopy, which is non-diagnostic in up to 30% of cases.[1] As the next diagnostic procedure, several techniques are currently available, such as computed tomography (CT)-guided biopsy of the intrapulmonary tumor, mediastinoscopy in case of enlarged or positron emission tomography (PET)-positive mediastinal lymph nodes, video thoracoscopic surgery (VATS), or exploratory thoracotomy. EUS-FNA is a novel, minimally invasive, technique by which mediastinal lymph nodes or centrally located tumors can be analyzed.

Diagnosis and staging of intrapulmonary tumors

Biopsying intrapulmonary tumors

Intrapulmonary tumors that are located adjacent or near the esophagus can be visualized by EUS.[2,3] Once the primary tumor has been identified, a real-time EUS-guided biopsy of the intrapulmonary lesion is possible (Fig. 7.1A–C). Left upper lobe tumors located adjacent to the aorta are often detected by EUS but cannot be biopsied safely owing to the interposition of the aorta (Fig. 7.2). In a retrospective study of 18 patients with intrapulmonary tumors abutting the esophagus, EUS both identified intrapulmonary tumors and obtained a tissue diagnosis in all cases.[2] In a prospective study of 32 patients with suspected lung cancer and a primary tumor located adjacent to the esophagus, intrapulmonary masses were detected in all patients and the diagnosis of lung cancer was established in 97% of patients.[3]

T4 staging

Once the primary tumor has been identified, the presence or absence (Fig. 7.2) of mediastinal tumor invasion (T4) – invasion in the mediastinum, centrally located large vessels, or vertebrae – can be assessed. Patients with T4 lung tumors (stage IIIB) are not considered eligible for surgical resection. Currently, mediastinal tumor invasion is frequently assessed during surgery as CT has limited sensitivity and specificity (<75%) for mediastinal invasion[4] and PET has no value in detecting T4 tumors because of its limited anatomic resolution.[5] In a retrospective study that evaluated T4 staging in 308 patients, EUS had a sensitivity, specificity, and positive and negative predictive value of 88%, 98%, 70%, and 99% respectively.[6] In a cohort of 424 consecutive patients with (suspected)

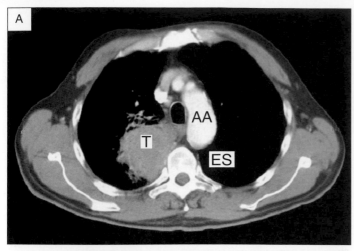

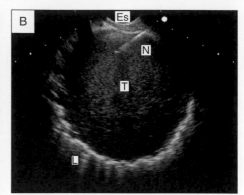

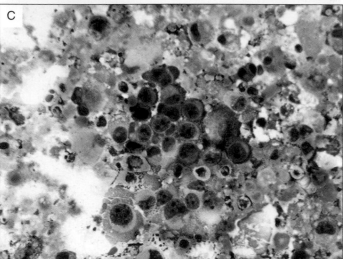

Fig. 7.1 A 53-year-old smoker with suspected lung cancer in whom bronchoscopy did not establish a diagnosis. **A,** CT of the chest demonstrating an intrapulmonary tumor (T) in the right upper lobe located adjacent to the esophagus (ES). AA, aortic arch. **B,** Corresponding EUS-FNA image. Notice the needle (N) located in the tumor (T). L, compromised lung tissue; Es, esophagus. **C,** Cytology of fine-needle aspirate demonstrating a squamous cell carcinoma.

lung cancer, EUS detected the primary tumor in 28%; 11% were staged as T4 based on tumor invasion in the mediastinum (8%) (Fig. 7.3A) or left atrium/centrally located vessels (3%) (Fig. 7.3B,C). In assessing T4 tumors, EUS had a sensitivity,

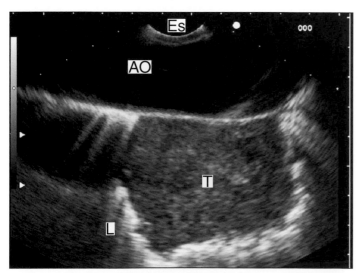

Fig. 7.2 Left upper lobe tumor (T) located adjacent to the aorta (AO). There are no signs of tumor invasion in the aorta (T4). ES, esophagus; L, compromised lung tissue.

specificity, positive predictive value, negative predictive value, and accuracy of 39%, 100%, 100%, 92%, and 92%, respectively.[7] Most cases of tumor invasion were assessed based on EUS images alone, and the authors of both of these studies agree that tumor invasion in large vessels or heart is easier to assess than invasion in the mediastinum, owing to the increased ultrasound contrasts between tumor and blood as well as the possibility of using a Doppler signal (Fig. 7.3C). It should be noted that in few patients surgical verification of EUS T4 findings occurred and that, therefore, the definitive value of EUS in T4 staging requires further investigation.

In conclusion, intrapulmonary tumors can be visualized and biopsied safely by EUS-FNA provided they are located adjacent to the esophagus. In addition to establishing a tissue diagnosis, EUS can detect mediastinal tumor invasion.

Mediastinal staging

Mediastinal staging is by far the most common indication for EUS-FNA in patients with (suspected) lung cancer. Accurate mediastinal staging is important as patients with locally advanced lung cancer are preferably treated with multimodality treatment, whereas those with no regional (and distant) metastases are preferably treated with surgery alone.[8] About one-

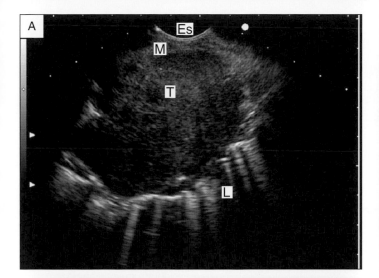

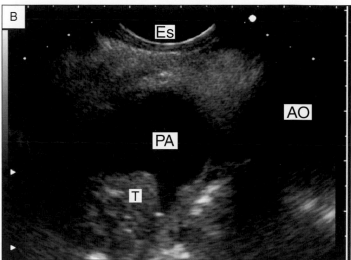

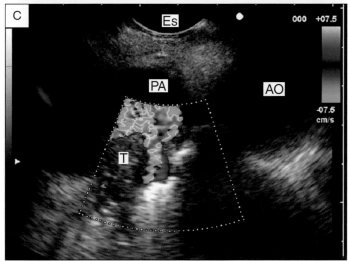

Fig. 7.3   A, Centrally located large cell carcinoma (T) invading the mediastinum (M). L, compromised lung tissue; Es, esophagus. **B & C,** Centrally located left-sided tumor (T) invading the pulmonary artery (PA), with (**C**) and without (**B**) color Doppler. AO, aorta.

third of patients with lung cancer present with mediastinal lymph node metastases.

EUS vs EUS-FNA

Specific ultrasonographic features of mediastinal lymph nodes – size >1 cm, a round shape, a homogeneous hypoechoic echo pattern, sharp distinctive borders – are associated with malignant involvement,[9,10] for which EUS has a sensitivity, specificity, and positive and negative predictive value of 78%, 71%, 75%, and 79% respectively.[11] EUS in combination with FNA is more accurate than imaging (EUS) alone,[9,11–13] and therefore FNA is always required before a lymph node can be designated as malignant. For this reason (curved) linear – not radial – ultrasound probes are required for mediastinal staging. The advised number of biopsies per lymph node depends on the presence or absence of on-site cytology. If on-site cytology is not available, three or five needle passes are recommended to obtain an optimal yield.[14,15] No benefit in diagnostic yield has been demonstrated regarding the position of the needle in the lymph node (central versus peripheral) or the application of suction.[14]

Diagnostic reach

Regional lymph nodes in NSCLC are classified using the tumor, node, metastasis (TNM) classification according to Mountain and Dresler.[16] Only lymph nodes that lie adjacent to the esophagus or centrally located vessels can be visualized by EUS. These lymph nodes are located in the following regions: low paratracheal on the left (station 4L; Fig. 7.4), in the aortopulmonary window (station 5; Fig. 7.5), para-aortal (station 6; Fig. 7.6), subcarinally (station 7; Figs 7.7 & 7.8), in the lower paraesophageal region (station 8), and the pulmonary ligamentum (station 9; Fig. 7.9) (Fig. 7.10[17]). Not all lymph nodes located in the aortopulmonary window or those located para-aortally can be biospied safely owing to the interposition of the pulmonary artery or aorta (see Fig. 7.6). EUS has limitations in its diagnostic reach as air in the trachea and main bronchi inhibits visualization of the upper paratracheal lymph node (stations 2) and the lower paratracheal station on the right (4R).

Procedure

Evaluation of the mediastinum by EUS should be performed in a standardized fashion in order to check all mediastinal lymph

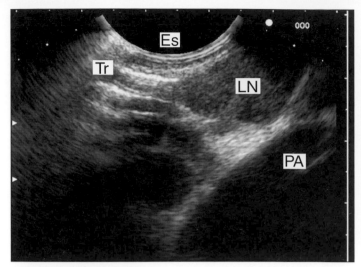

Fig. 7.4 Lower paratracheal lymph node (LN) on the left (station 4L) located between the esophagus (Es), trachea (Tr), and pulmonary artery (PA).

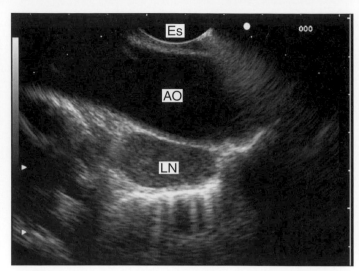

Fig. 7.6 Lymph node (LN) located adjacent to the descending aorta (AO) (station 6). Es, esophagus.

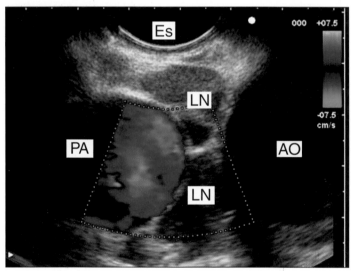

Fig. 7.5 Lymph node (LN) located in the aortopulmonary window (station 5), situated between the esophagus (Es), aorta (AO), and pulmonary artery (PA).

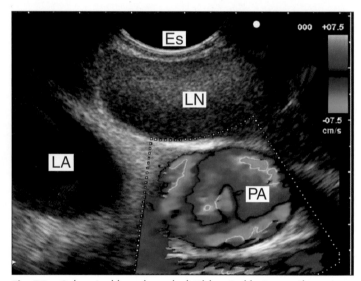

Fig. 7.7 Subcarinal lymph node (LN) located between the esophagus (Es), pulmonary artery (PA), with color Doppler signal, and left atrium (LA).

node stations (and, when indicated, the left liver lobe and left adrenal gland) that can be reached. After an initial orientation, (suspected) lymph nodes should be biopsied, starting with contralateral (N3) nodes before analyzing ipsilateral (N2) lymph node stations. A report should be made of each investigation with a description of the location of the lymph node in relation to anatomic landmarks, as well as the allocation of a number according to the Mountain and Dresler classification[16] (see Examination Checklist).

Accuracy of mediastinal staging

The operating characteristics of mediastinal staging by EUS-FNA, based on 1263 patients from 16 studies, are depicted in Table 7.1. These studies involved patients with (suspected) lung cancer (Fig. 7.11) or those with mediastinal masses suspect for malignancy (Fig. 7.12) who had subsequent analysis by EUS-FNA.[17–31] Although positive predictive values were reported in most studies, it should be noted that tumor-positive findings were verified by surgical–pathological staging in only one study.[28] Although false-positive EUS-FNA findings have seldom been reported, they are possible when the primary tumor is located immediately adjacent to a lymph node.[28] It should be noted that the majority of studies are performed in selected patients with enlarged (>1 cm) mediastinal lymph nodes at CT, and therefore the results apply only to patients in that category. One study reported a considerable proportion of patients with a normal mediastinum at CT,[28] and only two studies exclusively assessed the value of EUS in patients with a normal mediastinum[27,31] (Table 7.1).

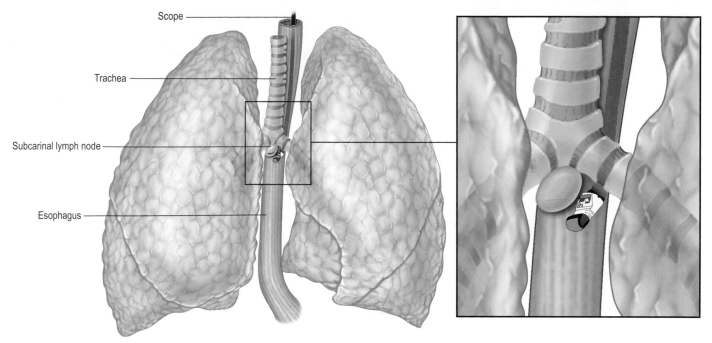

Scope
Trachea
Subcarinal lymph node
Esophagus

Fig. 7.8 Diagram showing a transesophageal ultrasound-guided FNA of a subcarinal lymph node.

Mediastinal restaging after induction chemotherapy is an increasing common indication for EUS-FNA. Accurate restaging is important in order to identify those patients who are successfully downstaged, as they benefit most from subsequent surgical resection.[32,33] The sensitivity (75%) of EUS-FNA in mediastinal restaging is slightly inferior compared with conventional staging, owing to the sampling error of small residual tumor metastases.[34]

Diagnostic yield

The diagnostic yield of EUS – expressed as the demonstration of lymph node metastases or mediastinal tumor invasion – obviously depends on the prevalence of mediastinal metastases

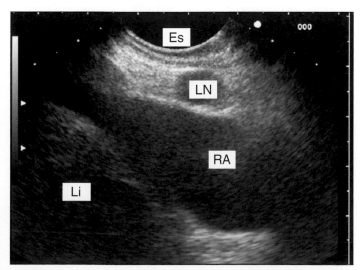

Fig. 7.9 Lymph node (LN) located in the pulmonary ligamentum (station 9). Es, esophagus; RA, right atrium; Li, liver.

and tumor invasion in the target population. In patients with a high pretest probability of locally advanced disease, for example those with enlarged or PET-positive mediastinal lymph nodes, a diagnostic yield of up to 70% has been reported.[17,29,35]

EUS compared with other techniques

How does EUS-FNA compare with other mediastinal staging techniques? It is important to distinguish between imaging techniques that provide information about lymph node size (CT of the chest) or metabolic activity (PET), and those staging techniques by which tissue is obtained (endobronchial ultrasound-guided transbronchial needle aspiration [EBUS-TBNA], EUS-FNA, video-assisted thoracoscopy [VATS], and mediastinoscopy).

In mediastinal staging, EUS-FNA is more sensitive (88% versus 57%) and specific (91% versus 82%) than CT.[11,12] EUS-FNA and PET have similar sensitivities (88% versus 84%) and specificities (91% versus 89%) in the analysis of mediastinal lymph nodes.[11,12] In a direct comparison study that had identification of inoperable patients as the outcome, EUS-FNA and PET had comparable sensitivities (63% versus 68%) and negative predictive values (68% versus 64%), but EUS was more specific (100% versus 72%).[36]

For accurate mediastinal staging, lymph node tissue is required, expect for small (<1 cm) nodes that are negative at FDG-PET. All available biopsy techniques have a different diagnostic reach and, unfortunately, none is able to sample all mediastinal N2–3 lymph node stations. For the various sampling techniques, sensitivity and specificity are regularly based on the specific area that can be reached by the technique under investigation, and not on the mediastinum as a whole. Real-time EUS-guided FNA is more accurate than 'blind' TBNA

ACCURACY OF EUS-FNA IN MEDIASTINAL STAGING OF PATIENTS WITH (SUSPECTED) LUNG CANCER OR MEDIASTINAL MASSES SUSPICIOUS FOR MALIGNANCY									
Reference	Year	No. of evaluable patients	Lymph node size[a]	Prevalence[b] (%)	Sensitivity (%)	Specificity (%)	PPV (%)	NPV (%)	Accuracy (%)
Silvestri et al.[18]	1996	27	<1>	67	89	100	100	82	93
Gress et al.[19]	1997	24	>1	63	93	100	100	90	96
Williams et al.[20]	1999	82	>1	73	87	100	100	73	90
Fritscher-Ravens et al.[21]	2000	153	>1	55	92	100	100	92	95
Wallace et al.[22]	2001	107	>1	79	87	100	100	68	90
Wiersema et al.[13]	2001	33	>1	76	100	88	96	100	97
Larsen et al.[23]	2002	79	>1	75	92	100	100	80	94
Fritscher-Ravens et al.[24]	2003	33	<1>	48	88	100	100	89	91
Annema et al.[17]	2004	36	<1>	78	93	100	100	80	94
Kramer et al.[25 c]	2004	81	<1>	85	72	100	100	39	77
Savides & Perricone[26]	2004	59	>1	42	96	100	100	97	98
Wallace et al.[27]	2004	69	<1	41	61	98	94	79	83
Annema et al.[28]	2005	100	<1>	36	76	97	92	91	91
Annema et al.[29]	2005	215	>1	71	91	100	100	74	93
Eloubeidi et al.[30 c]	2005	93	<1>	38	93	100	100	96	97
Leblanc et al.[31]	2005	72	<1	37	35	100	100	73	76
Total		1263		36–85	35–100	88–100	92–100	39–100	76–98

Table 7.1 Accuracy of EUS-FNA in mediastinal staging of patients with (suspected) lung cancer or mediastinal masses suspicious for malignancy
None of the studies, except for Annema et al.[28], included surgical–pathologic verification of tumor-positive EUS-FNA findings; therefore, positive predictive values cannot be determined.
[a]>1, Mediastinal lymph nodes >1 cm; <1, nodes <1 cm; <1>, both nodes <1 cm and >1 cm were included.
[b]Prevalence of mediastinal (N2–3) metastases.
[c]Also included upper retroperitoneal PET-positive lesions.

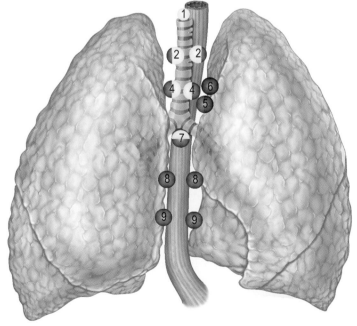
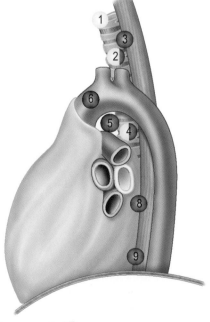

Fig. 7.10   Mediastinal staging techniques and their diagnostic reach. (Adapted from Annema et al.[17])

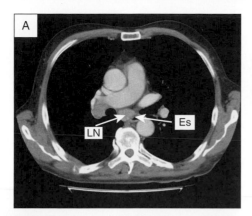

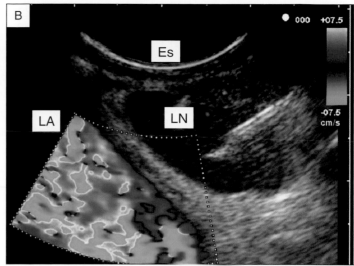

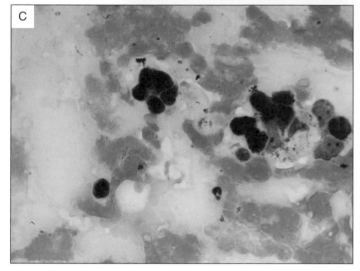

Fig. 7.11   A 54-year-old man with proven non-small cell lung cancer who was fit for surgical resection. **A,** CT of the chest demonstrating a centrally located non-small cell lung carcinoma of the right lung and an enlarged subcarinal lymph node (LN). Es, esophagus. **B,** Real-time EUS-guided aspiration of the subcarinal lymph node (LN) located between esophagus (Es), left atrium (LA). **C,** Cytologic appearance of a lymph node metastasis.

performed during bronchoscopy.[12,37] A comparison of EUS-FNA and real-time EBUS-TBNA is currently being investigated. EUS-FNA is complementary to mediastinoscopy, as mediastinoscopy provides access to the upper and lower paratracheal regions (stations 2 and 4) and the ventral part of the subcarinal station (region 7), and EUS provides access to the ventral as well as the dorsal part of station 7, the aorto pulmonary window (station 5), and the lower paraesophageal lymph nodes (station 8), as well as the nodes located in the pulmonary ligamentum (station 9) (see Fig. 7.10). In a comparison of EUS-FNA and mediastinoscopy, both techniques were found to have a comparable accuracy (91% versus 90%), but due to their complementary reach the combination of EUS-FNA and mediastinoscopy detected significantly more patients with lymph node metastases than either EUS-FNA or mediastinoscopy alone.[28]

Assessment of distant metastases

Unfortunately, most patients with lung cancer present with distant metastases and are therefore not a candidate for curative treatment. Lung tumors frequently metastasize to the liver, brain, bone, and adrenal glands. Of these predilection spots for distant metastasis, lesions located in the left liver lobe and left adrenal gland can be biopsied. In a study of patients (both with and without lung cancer) with enlarged left adrenal glands, EUS assessed malignant left adrenal involvement in 42% of

patients.[38] One case has been described in which a left adrenal metastasis was established by EUS-FNA in an adrenal gland that was not enlarged at CT.[39] Whether the left adrenal gland should be examined routinely during EUS in patients with lung cancer is the subject of debate.[39] Patients with disseminated lung cancer often present with liver metastases. The standard procedure for the detection of liver metastases is transabdominal ultrasonography. It has been reported that liver metastases can be assessed by EUS-FNA using a transgastric approach.[40–42] Whether EUS-FNA has additional benefits compared with transabdominal ultrasound-guided liver biopsy is not yet known.

IMPACT OF EUS-FNA ON PATIENT MANAGEMENT

The ultimate question is how does EUS-FNA influence the management of patients with lung cancer? By demonstrating ipsilateral (stage IIIA–N2) or contralateral (stage IIIB) lymph node metastases or mediastinal tumor invasion (stage IIIB), EUS can prevent unnecessary mediastinoscopies as well as exploratory thoracotomies. Patients with stage III lung cancer are preferably treated with multimodality therapy rather than surgery alone.[8] Various reports demonstrate that EUS-FNA prevents the need for surgical staging and reduces the number of futile thoracotomies (Table 7.2).

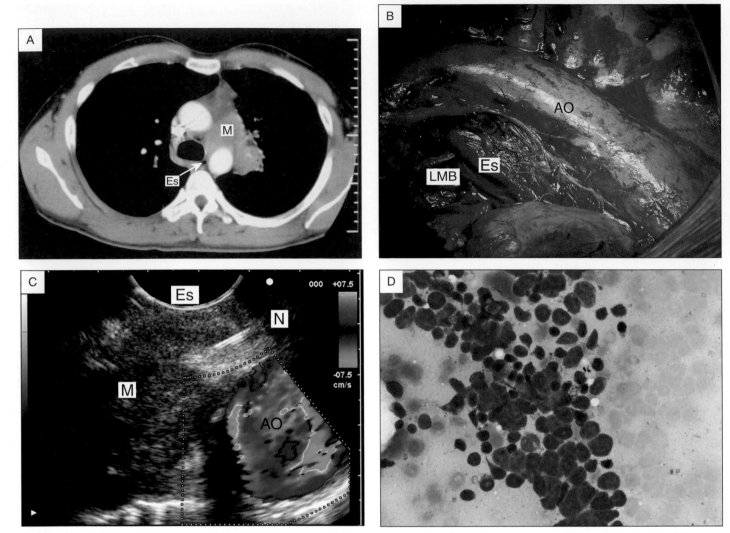

Fig. 7.12   A 66-year-old man, heavy smoker with suspected lung cancer, in whom bronchoscopy was non-diagnostic. **A,** CT of the chest demonstrating a mass (M) in the aortopulmonary window. Es, esophagus. **B,** Demonstrates another patient just after a left-sided pneumonectomy, showing the close relationship between the esophagus (ES) and the aortopulmonary window. AO, aorta; LMB, left main bronchus. **C,** Corresponding EUS image with fine-needle aspiration of the mass (M) located between esophagus (Es) and aorta (AO) (with color Doppler). N, needle. **D,** Cytologic appearance of small cell carcinoma.

IMPACT OF EUS-FNA ON THE MANAGEMENT OF PATIENTS WITH (SUSPECTED) NON-SMALL CELL LUNG CANCER				
Reference	Year	No. of patients	Outcome	Findings
Larsen et al.[23]	2002	41	Prevent mediastinoscopies	68%
		37	Prevent thoracoscopies/thoracotomies	49%
Fritscher-Ravens et al.[37]	2003	72	Identify inoperable patients	63%
Savides & Perricone[26]	2004	59	Prevent mediastinoscopies	39%
Annema et al.[28]	2005	100	Prevent mediastinoscopies/thoracotomies	16%
Annema et al.[29]	2005	242	Prevent surgical staging	70%
Larsen et al.[44]	2005	104	Prevent mediastinoscopies/thoracotomies	16%

Table 7.2 Impact of EUS-FNA on the management of patients with (suspected) non-small cell lung cancer

Preventing mediastinoscopies

In a prospective study of 84 patients with mediastinal masses suspected for malignancy, EUS prevented a thoracotomy or thoracoscopy in 48% and mediastinoscopy in 68% of patients by demonstrating lymph node metastases.[23] In a similar study population of 59 patients, all scheduled for mediastinoscpy, EUS-FNA proved mediastinal metastases in 39% of patients and a mediastinoscopy was eventually performed in only 22%.[26] In a prospective study of 242 patients with (suspected) NSCLC and enlarged mediastinal lymph nodes (all candidates for mediastinoscopy or mediastinotomy), EUS-FNA demonstrated lymph node metastases, tumor invasion, or an alternative diagnosis in 70% of patients, and therefore surgical interventions were prevented[29] (Table 7.2).

Identifying inoperable patients

In a prospective study of patients with NSCLC patients that identified 'inoperable patients' as the primary outcome, EUS had a similar sensitivity (63% versus 68%) and negative predictive value (68% versus 64%) as PET, but was more specific (100% versus 72%).[36]

Reducing unnecessary thoracotomies

In a prospective study of 108 patients with NSCLC, staging by EUS added to mediastinoscopy identified significantly more patients with either tumor invasion or lymph node metastasis (36%) compared with staging by mediastinoscopy alone (20%). Had EUS results been taken into account, one of six thoracotomies could have been prevented.[28] Additionally, in a randomized study of 104 patients, routine staging by EUS-FNA resulted in a 16% decrease in the number of futile thoracotomies compared with staging of selected patients by EUS.[43]

INDICATIONS FOR EUS-FNA IN THE DIAGNOSIS AND STAGING OF LUNG CANCER[7]
Suspected lung cancer, enlarged (>1 cm) mediastinal lymph nodes
Suspected lung cancer, primary tumor located adjacent to esophagus
Mediastinal staging of non-small cell lung cancer
Mediastinal involvement at FDG-PET in (suspected) lung cancer
Mediastinal restaging after induction chemotherapy
Assessment of tumor invasion (T4) in centrally located tumors

Table 7.3 Indications for EUS-FNA in the diagnosis and staging of lung cancer[7]

INDICATIONS AND POSITION OF EUS-FNA IN STAGING ALGORITHMS

Indications

Which patients with (suspected) non-small cell lung cancer (NSCLC) are candidates for EUS-FNA (Table 7.3)? EUS-FNA is indicated in the mediastinal (re)staging of patients with (suspected) lung cancer, especially in patients with enlarged or PET-positive mediastinal lymph nodes. Additionally EUS can diagnose and stage centrally located tumors, provided they are located adjacent to the esophagus (Fig. 7.13). EUS is also valuable in patients with NSCLC without mediastinal enlargement, as demonstrated in a study of 69 patients with NSCLC without enlarged lymph nodes at CT; EUS provided proof of advanced disease in 25% of patients.[27] Adding EUS to conventional staging in patients with (suspected) lung cancer reduced staging costs by 40%, predominantly by preventing surgical interventions.[25] A limitation of EUS is its inability to detect upper paratracheal lesions as well as those located paratracheally on the right (see

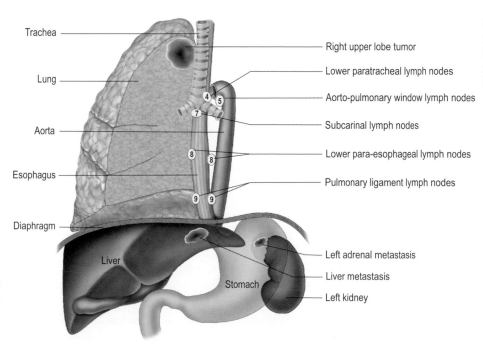

Trachea
Lung
Aorta
Esophagus
Diaphragm
Liver
Stomach

Right upper lobe tumor
Lower paratracheal lymph nodes
Aorto-pulmonary window lymph nodes
Subcarinal lymph nodes
Lower para-esophageal lymph nodes
Pulmonary ligament lymph nodes
Left adrenal metastasis
Liver metastasis
Left kidney

Fig. 7.13 EUS-FNA in NSCLC can biopsy intrapulmonary tumors and assess tumor invasion (T4), assess mediastinal lymph nodes, and assess distant metastasis located in the left liver lobe and left adrenal gland.

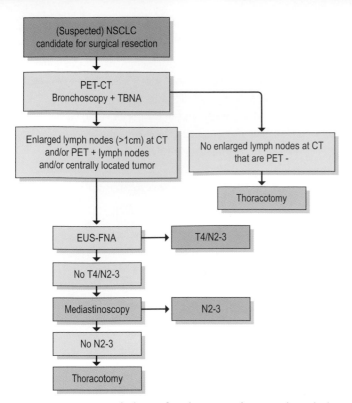

Fig. 7.14   Proposed place of endoscopic ultrasound-guided fine-needle aspiration (EUS-FNA) in the mediastinal staging of non-small cell lung cancer (NSCLC), including positron emission tomography (PET).[7] CT, computed tomography; TBNA, transbronchial needle aspiration.

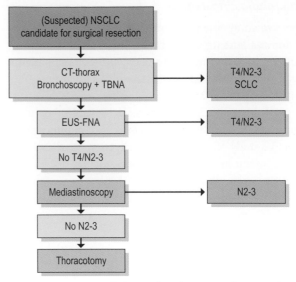

Fig. 7.15   Proposed place of endoscopic ultrasound-guided fine-needle aspiration (EUS-FNA) in the mediastinal staging of non-small cell lung cancer (NSCLC), excluding PET.[7] CT, computed tomography; SCLC, small cell lung cancer; TBNA, transbronchial needle aspiration.

Fig. 7.10), because of the interposition of air in the trachea by which the ultrasound waves are reflected.

Position of EUS in lung cancer staging algorithms

Where should EUS be positioned in staging algorithms for the diagnosis and staging of lung cancer? The strength of EUS is the assessment of mediastinal lymph node metastases or tumor invasion (to confirm advanced disease) in a minimally invasive way. EUS is complementary to PET, which has a high negative predictive value in excluding advanced disease.[11]

The authors advocate EUS early in staging algorithms for NSCLC, as EUS by itself can provide proof of tumor invasion or mediastinal metastases in at least 25% of patients with NSCLC regardless of CT findings (see Table 7.1).[27,31] The position of EUS-FNA in local staging algorithms depends on the availability of PET. In hospitals that have access to both EUS-FNA and PET, the following strategy is proposed for patients with (suspected) lung cancer who are candidates for surgical resection: PET-CT followed by bronchoscopy, including TBNA (Fig. 7.14[7]). In patients with either centrally located tumors, enlarged (>1 cm) or PET-positive mediastinal lymph nodes, further staging is required by EUS (first) and mediastinoscopy (when EUS does not indicate proof of mediastinal metastasis or tumor invasion). In patients with a peripherally located tumor without enlarged or PET-positive mediastinal lymph nodes, a thoracotomy can be performed directly, as the probability of mediastinal metastases is very low. In clinics with no access to PET, we advise staging patients by both EUS and mediastinoscopy (Fig. 7.15[7]), as combined staging significantly improves staging compared with EUS or mediastinoscopy alone.[28] In patients with stage IIIA–N2 disease with a radiologic response after induction chemotherapy, EUS-FNA should be considered for mediastinal restaging[34] in order to select patients who are downstaged to N0, as they will benefit most from subsequent surgical resection.[32,33]

FUTURE PERSPECTIVES

Reviewing the literature for non-small cell lung cancer, there is substantial evidence, in 2005, that EUS-FNA is a safe and accurate technique for lung cancer staging. By demonstrating mediastinal lymph node metastasis or tumor invasion, EUS provides a minimally invasive alternative for surgical staging and thus qualifies as the diagnostic technique of choice in many patients. At present, EUS-FNA is performed by a select group of dedicated chest physicians and gastroenterologists, and has only limited availability. Large-scale implementation of EUS-FNA in the diagnosis and staging of lung cancer is important, as EUS-FNA has a huge impact on patient managment. Dissemination of EUS from specialized academic institutions to large regional hospitals is needed in order to facilitate general availability. To achieve this goal, key professionals in lung cancer care – chest physicians and surgeons who perform lung surgery – should be aware of the indications of EUS and the alternative it provides for surgical staging. Furthermore, a group of specialists needs to be trained actually to perform

EUS. The fact that gasteroenterologists are in general not familiar with lung cancer staging, and chest physicians are not used to performing EUS, might be a barrier. Prospective studies of ultrasound-guided biopsies, comparing transesopheageal and transbronchial approaches, are needed. As the diagnostic reach of EUS-FNA and EBUS-TBNA in the mediastinum is complementary, complete mediastinal staging of NSCLC by combining these two endoluminal ultrasound techniques may be on the horizon.

EXAMINATION CHECKLIST

Celiac axis
Left adrenal gland
Left liver lobe (optional)
Periesophageal space below carina (area 8)
Subcarinal space (area 7)
Aortopulmonary window/pulmonary trunk (area 4L/5)
Paratracheal space (area 2R and 2L)
Pulmonary tumor visible? Mediastinal tumor invasion (T4)

REFERENCES

1 Mazzone P, Jain P, Arroliga AC, et al. Bronchoscopy and needle biopsy techniques for diagnosis and staging of lung cancer. Clin Chest Med 2002; 23:137–158, ix.

2 Varadarajulu S, Hoffman BJ, Hawes RH, et al. EUS-guided FNA of lung masses adjacent to or abutting the esophagus after unrevealing CT-guided biopsy or bronchoscopy. Gastrointest Endosc 2004; 60:293–297.

3 Annema JT, Veselic M, Rabe KF. EUS-guided FNA of centrally located lung tumours following a non-diagnostic bronchoscopy. Lung Cancer 2005; 48:357–361.

4 Venuta F, Rendina EA, Ciriaco P, et al. Computed tomography for preoperative assessment of T3 and T4 bronchogenic carcinoma. Eur J Cardiothorac Surg 1992; 6:238–241.

5 Pieterman RM, van Putten JW, Meuzelaar JJ, et al. Preoperative staging of non-small-cell lung cancer with positron-emission tomography. N Engl J Med 2000; 343:254–261.

6 Varadarajulu S, Schmulewitz N, Wildi SF, et al. Accuracy of EUS in staging of T4 lung cancer. Gastrointest Endosc 2004; 59:345–348.

7 Annema JT. Transoesophageal ultrasound guided fine needle aspiration in the diagnosis and staging of lung cancer and the assessment of sarcoidosis. PhD Thesis, Leiden; 2005.

8 Spira A, Ettinger DS. Multidisciplinary management of lung cancer. N Engl J Med 2004; 350:379–392.

9 Bhutani MS, Hawes RH, Hoffman BJ. A comparison of the accuracy of echo features during endoscopic ultrasound (EUS) and EUS-guided fine-needle aspiration for diagnosis of malignant lymph node invasion. Gastrointest Endosc 1997; 45:474–479.

10 Catalano MF, Sivak MV Jr, Rice T, et al. Endosonographic features predictive of lymph node metastasis. Gastrointest Endosc 1994; 40:442–446.

11 Toloza EM, Harpole L, McCrory DC. Noninvasive staging of non-small cell lung cancer: a review of the current evidence. Chest 2003; 123(Suppl):137S–146S.

12 Toloza EM, Harpole L, Detterbeck F, et al. Invasive staging of non-small cell lung cancer: a review of the current evidence. Chest 2003; 123(Suppl):157S–166S.

13 Wiersema MJ, Vazquez-Sequeiros E, Wiersema LM. Evaluation of mediastinal lymphadenopathy with endoscopic US-guided fine-needle aspiration biopsy. Radiology 2001; 219:252–257.

14 Wallace MB, Kennedy T, Durkalski V, et al. Randomized controlled trial of EUS-guided fine needle aspiration techniques for the detection of malignant lymphadenopathy. Gastrointest Endosc 2001; 54:441–447.

15 Leblanc JK, Ciaccia D, Al Assi MT, et al. Optimal number of EUS-guided fine needle passes needed to obtain a correct diagnosis. Gastrointest Endosc 2004; 59:475–481.

16 Mountain CF, Dresler CM. Regional lymph node classification for lung cancer staging. Chest 1997; 111:1718–1723.

17 Annema JT, Hoekstra OS, Smit EF, et al. Towards a minimally invasive staging strategy in NSCLC: analysis of PET positive mediastinal lesions by EUS-FNA. Lung Cancer 2004; 44:53–60.

18 Silvestri GA, Hoffman BJ, Bhutani MS, et al. Endoscopic ultrasound with fine-needle aspiration in the diagnosis and staging of lung cancer. Ann Thorac Surg 1996; 61:1441–1445.

19 Gress FG, Hawes RH, Savides TJ, et al. Endoscopic ultrasound-guided fine-needle aspiration biopsy using linear array and radial scanning endosonography. Gastrointest Endosc 1997; 45:243–250.

20 Williams DB, Sahai AV, Aabakken L, et al. Endoscopic ultrasound guided fine needle aspiration biopsy: a large single centre experience. Gut 1999; 44:720–726.

21 Fritscher-Ravens A, Sriram PV, Bobrowski C, et al. Mediastinal lymphadenopathy in patients with or without previous malignancy: EUS-FNA-based differential cytodiagnosis in 153 patients. Am J Gastroenterol 2000; 95:2278–2284.

22 Wallace MB, Silvestri GA, Sahai AV, et al. Endoscopic ultrasound-guided fine needle aspiration for staging patients with carcinoma of the lung. Ann Thorac Surg 2001; 72:1861–1867.

23 Larsen SS, Krasnik M, Vilmann P, et al. Endoscopic ultrasound guided biopsy of mediastinal lesions has a major impact on patient management. Thorax 2002; 57:98–103.

24 Fritscher-Ravens A, Bohuslavizki KH, Brandt L, et al. Mediastinal lymph node involvement in potentially resectable lung cancer: comparison of CT, positron emission tomography, and endoscopic ultrasonography with and without fine-needle aspiration. Chest 2003; 123:442–451.

25 Kramer H, van Putten JW, Post WJ, et al. Oesophageal endoscopic ultrasound with fine needle aspiration improves and simplifies the staging of lung cancer. Thorax 2004; 59:596–601.

26 Savides TJ, Perricone A. Impact of EUS-guided FNA of enlarged mediastinal lymph nodes on subsequent thoracic surgery rates. Gastrointest Endosc 2004; 60:340–346.

27 Wallace MB, Ravenel J, Block MI, et al. Endoscopic ultrasound in lung cancer patients with a normal mediastinum on computed tomography. Ann Thorac Surg 2004; 77:1763–1768.

28 Annema JT, Versteegh MI, Veselic M, et al. Endoscopic ultrasound added to mediastinoscopy for preoperative staging of patients with lung cancer. JAMA 2005; 294:931–936

29 Annema JT, Versteegh MI, Veselic M, et al. Endoscopic ultrasound guided FNA in the diagnosis and staging of lung cancer and its impact on surgical staging. J Clin Oncol 2005; Oct 11:[Epub ahead of print].

30 Eloubeidi MA, Cerfolio RJ, Chen VK, et al. Endoscopic ultrasound-guided fine needle aspiration of mediastinal lymph node in patients with suspected lung cancer after positron emission tomography and computed tomography scans. Ann Thorac Surg 2005; 79:263–268.

31 Leblanc JK, Devereaux BM, Imperiale TF, et al. Endoscopic ultrasound in non-small cell lung cancer and negative mediastinum on computed tomography. Am J Respir Crit Care Med 2005; 171:177–182.

32 Bueno R, Richards WG, Swanson SJ, et al. Nodal stage after induction therapy for stage IIIA lung cancer determines patient survival. Ann Thorac Surg 2000; 70:1826–1831.

33 Voltolini L, Luzzi L, Ghiribelli C, et al. Results of induction chemotherapy followed by surgical resection in patients with stage IIIA (N2) non-small cell lung cancer: the importance of the nodal down-staging after chemotherapy. Eur J Cardiothorac Surg 2001; 20:1106–1112.

34 Annema JT, Veselic M, Versteegh MI, et al. Mediastinal restaging: EUS-FNA offers a new perspective. Lung Cancer 2003; 42:311–318.

35 Fritscher-Ravens A, Soehendra N, Schirrow L, et al. Role of transesophageal endosonography-guided fine-needle aspiration in the diagnosis of lung cancer. Chest 2000; 117:339–345.

36 Fritscher-Ravens A, Davidson BL, Hauber HP, et al. Endoscopic ultrasound, positron emission tomography, and computerized tomography for lung cancer. Am J Respir Crit Care Med 2003; 168:1293–1297.

37 Annema JT, Veselic M, Rabe KF. Analysis of subcarinal lymph nodes in (suspected) non-small-cell lung cancer after a negative transbronchial needle aspiration – what's next? A preliminary report. Respiration 2004; 71:630–634.

38 Eloubeidi MA, Seewald S, Tamhane A, et al. EUS-guided FNA of the left adrenal gland in patients with thoracic or GI malignancies. Gastrointest Endosc 2004; 59:627–633.

39 Ringbaek TJ, Krasnik M, Clementsen P, et al. Transesophageal endoscopic ultrasound/fine-needle aspiration diagnosis of a malignant adrenal gland in a patient with non-small cell lung cancer and a negative CT scan. Lung Cancer 2005; 48:247–249.

40 Hollerbach S, Willert J, Topalidis T, et al. Endoscopic ultrasound-guided fine-needle aspiration biopsy of liver lesions: histological and cytological assessment. Endoscopy 2003; 35:743–749.

41 Nguyen P, Feng JC, Chang KJ. Endoscopic ultrasound (EUS) and EUS-guided fine-needle aspiration (FNA) of liver lesions. Gastrointest Endosc 1999; 50:357–361.

42 Prasad P, Schmulewitz N, Patel A, et al. Detection of occult liver metastases during EUS for staging of malignancies. Gastrointest Endosc 2004; 59:49–53.

43 Larsen SS, Vilmann P, Krasnik M, et al. Endoscopic ultrasound guided biopsy performed routinely in lung cancer staging spares futile thoracotomies: preliminary results from a randomised clinical trial. Lung Cancer 2005; 49:377–385.

EUS in Esophageal Cancer

Mohamad A. Eloubeidi

KEY POINTS

- Treatment and outcome in patients with esophageal cancer is stage dependent.

- One important role for endoscopic ultrasound (EUS) is the initial triage of patients to receive neoadjuvant therapy or to undergo immediate surgical resection or, in very early stages, endoscopic mucosal resection.

- EUS is superior to computed tomography and positron emission tomography in celiac and peritumoral lymph node detection.

- According to the American Joint Committee on Cancer (AJCC), the finding of a celiac lymph node is considered equivalent to metastatic disease, whether the tumor is in the distal (M1a) or proximal (M1b) esophagus.

- Application of EUS after administration of adjuvant chemoradiotherapy in esophageal cancer may provide a general idea of response but cannot accurately differentiate residual tumor from radiation effect. EUS-FNA can document persistent lymph nodes in celiac axis area that might preclude curative surgical resection.

INTRODUCTION

Treatment and outcome of patients with esophageal cancer is stage dependent. Since its introduction in the early 1980s, EUS has played a central and growing role in the staging of patients with esophageal cancer. The purpose of this chapter is to review data pertaining to accuracy of EUS in staging patients with esophageal cancer and to compare its operating characteristics with those of other staging modalities, such as positron emission tomography (PET) and computed tomography (CT). Data on the role of EUS in early and superficial esophageal cancer and Barrett's esophagus are reviewed. In addition, techniques of dilation of stricture to facilitate EUS, the use of alternative strategies, and the evaluation and staging of the celiac axis area are described. Data on restaging after chemotherapy and radiation therapy are reviewed. Finally, the vital role of EUS-guided fine-needle aspiration (EUS-FNA) in sampling celiac and peri-intestinal lymph nodes to complete the staging of patients with esophageal cancer is explored.

IMPORTANCE OF STAGING

Esophageal cancer is a leading health problem worldwide, but, fortunately, only about 14520 patients with this devastating condition are diagnosed each year in the USA, of whom 13750 will die from the disease.[1] Survival has improved slightly in patients with esophageal adenocarcinoma in the USA, but the overall 5-year survival rate remains dismal.[2] The treatment and outcome of patients with esophageal cancer is stage dependent.[2–5] EUS plays a vital role in the management and treatment planning of patients with esophageal cancer.

Perhaps the most important role for EUS is for initial triage of patients to receive neoadjuvant therapy or to undergo immediate surgical resection. Patients with any nodal involvement would typically receive preoperative therapy, whereas those with either T1 or T2 tumors (without nodal involvement) would go directly for surgical resection (Fig. 8.1 & Table 8.1). The second important role for EUS is restaging after the patient has received chemotherapy and radiation therapy. Although EUS is less accurate in determining the true stage in these patients, it helps to select those patients who are less likely to benefit from surgical resection or those who could potentially benefit from additional chemotherapy prior to surgical resection, such as patients with recalcitrant lymph nodes in the celiac axis area or persistent T4 disease.

EUS, CT, AND PET

Numerous studies to date have shown that EUS is superior to CT in the individual detection of tumor (T) stage in patients with esophageal cancer (Table 8.2).[6] Recent data also suggest that EUS retains its advantage in comparison with spiral CT.[7] This superiority of EUS stems from the fact that EUS can determine and examine esophageal wall layers with histologic correlates (Fig. 8.2).[8] In addition, EUS is superior to CT in the detection of peritumoral and celiac adenopathy (Tables 8.2 & 8.3).[6,9] When compared to PET, which relies on metabolic imaging, EUS can better delineate the wall layers, and hence has better operating characteristics than PET for tumor staging. In addition, EUS is superior to PET in the detection of peritumoral and celiac lymph nodes.[9] In a recent systematic review of the literature, FDG-PET showed moderate sensitivity and specificity in the detection of locoregional metastasis, and reasonable sensitivity and specificity in the detection of distant lymphatic and hematogenous metastases.[10] False-positive results

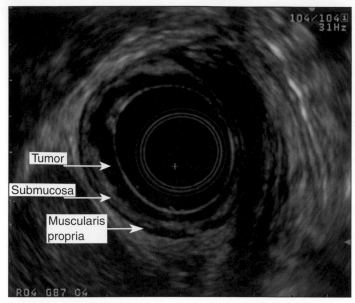

Fig. 8.1 EUS staging showed a tumor that invaded into but not through the submucosa, consistent with a T1 tumor. Findings were confirmed at surgery.

1997 AMERICAN JOINT COMMITTEE ON CANCER TNM CLASSIFICATION	
Stage	Description
Primary tumor (T)	
Tx	Tumor cannot be assessed
T0	No evidence of primary tumor
Tis	Carcinoma in situ
T1	Tumor invades lamina propria or submucosa
T2	Tumor invades muscularis propria
T3	Tumor invades adventitia
T4	Tumor invades adjacent structures
Regional lymph nodes (N)	
Nx	Regional lymph nodes cannot be assessed
N0	No regional lymph node metastasis
N1	Regional lymph node metastasis
Distant metastasis (M)	
Mx	Distant metastasis cannot be assessed
M0	No distant metastasis
M1	Distant metastasis
Tumors of the lower thoracic esophagus	
M1a	Metastasis in celiac lymph nodes
M1b	Other distant metastasis
Tumors of the mid-thoracic esophagus	
M1a	Not applicable
M1b	Non-regional lymph nodes and or other distant metastasis
Tumors of the upper thoracic esophagus	
M1a	Metastasis in cervical nodes
M1b	Other distant metastasis
AJCC stage groupings	
Stage 0	Tis, N0, M0
Stage I	T1, N0, M0
Stage IIA	T2, N0, M0
	T3, N0, M0
Stage IIB	T1, N1, M0
	T2, N1, M0
Stage III	T3, N1, M0
	T4, any N, M0
Stage IV	Any T, any N, M1
Stage IVA	Any T, any N, M1a
Stage IVB	Any T, nny N, M1b

Table 8.1 1997 American Joint Committee on Cancer TNM classification Esophagus. Used with permission of the American Joint Committee on Cancer (AJCC[7]), Chicago, Illinois. The original source of this material is the AJCC[7] Cancer Staging Manual, 5th edition (9), 65–68, 2000 (1977) published by Lipincott-Raven Publishers, Philadelphia, Pennsylvania.

were found in 13 of 86 patients (15%) in one study.[11] Proper interpretation of FDG-PET in staging esophageal cancer is impeded by false-positive results, so that positive FDG-PET findings still have to be confirmed by additional investigations.[11] EUS-FNA can be used in this setting to confirm positive findings on PET.[12] Although EUS is superior to PET and CT for locoregional recurrence, the latter modalities are better at detecting liver and lung metastasis.[9,10] Therefore, it is logical to perform EUS when CT and PET do not reveal distant metastasis, and thus help to triage the patient to surgery alone versus neoadjuvant therapy followed by surgery. Often, many investigations are needed in the same patient to complete staging. A recent study has shown that the combination of CT–PET–EUS reduces the number of unnecessary operations.[13] The number of unnecessary operations decreased from 44% when CT alone was used to 21% when the three modalities were incorporated in the preoperative staging protocol. Moreover, the presence of celiac axis metastasis during surgical exploration was significantly reduced in patients who underwent EUS (13%) or PET (7%), compared with CT (32%).[13] Finally, although not statistically significant, patients who underwent the trimodality staging had better survival than those who were staged with CT alone (48 versus 28 months).[13] The integration of PET-CT promises better resolution and hence better staging of patients with esophageal cancer.

MATERIALS AND METHODS

Echoendoscopes

A detailed description of equipment is given in Chapter 2. EUS equipment consists of radial (mechanical or electronic) and curved linear array (CLA; electronic) echoendoscopes with their respective processors. The radial mechanical echoendoscope is the most popular instrument used in the USA for the staging of esophageal cancer, whereas the curved linear echoendoscope is the most popular in Europe. The image created by the radial mechanical echoendoscope is in a 360° transverse plane per-

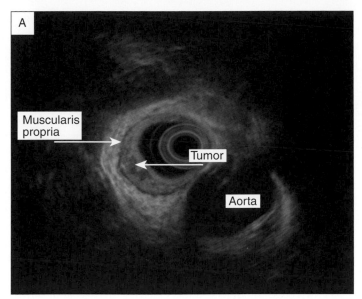

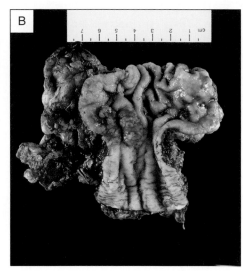

Fig. 8.2   A, EUS revealed a tumor limited to submucosa (muscularis propria is intact) with no lymph nodes observed (T1, N0). Surgery was recommended after EUS. **B,** Surgical resection confirmed no involvement of lymph nodes and disease that invaded submucosa consistent with T1 tumor.

pendicular to the long axis of the echoendoscope. Recent-generation mechanical radial echoendoscopes (GF-UM 130 series, 60 series) have broadband frequencies ranging from 5 to 20 MHz. The electronic radial instrument provides a 270° (Pentax) or 360° (Olympus) ultrasound field of view (a portion of the image is obscured by the fiberoptic bundle in forward-viewing instruments) via an electronic multi-element transducer. Image orientation is similar to that of radial mechanical instruments, but is augmented by the addition of pulsed, color and power Doppler. The electronic echoendoscope has adjustable frequencies from 5 to 12 MHz.

CLA instruments scan along the long axis of the endoscope, thereby permitting real-time visualization of a needle passed through the biopsy channel. Although both mechanical and electronic CLA systems exist, most users employ the electronic system because of its enhanced image quality and features associated with an advanced processor (e.g., Doppler, signal processing). The field of view of CLA echoendoscopes is narrower than that of radial echoendoscopes; this appears to lengthen the learning curve for CLA endosonography and makes luminal tumor staging more tedious.

Catheter probes

High-frequency transducers (12–30 MHz) can be incorporated into small catheters (2–3 mm in diameter). Currently, the best images are produced when the transducer is mechanically rotated 360°, as is done with radial endosonography. The most commonly used catheters in the USA are produced by Olympus (UM-2R, 20 MHz; UM-3R, 30 MHz). These catheters produce very high-resolution images of the gut wall and are important adjuncts to endoscopic mucosal resection (EMR) for early malignancies of the esophagus, stomach, and rectum. With the advent of the EUM-30S (a free-standing ultrasound unit), catheter probes are more accessible for use in general endoscopy units.

Blind probes

Passing standard echoendoscopes past a tight stricture can be quite problematic. Perforation of the esophagus has been reported, and can result from aggressive dilation or the applica-

COMPARISON OF ACCURACY OF CT AND EUS IN THE LOCOREGIONAL STAGING OF ESOPHAGEAL CANCER			
Technique	No. of patients	T accuracy (%)	N accuracy (%)
CT	1154	45 (40–50)	54 (48–71)
EUS	1035	85 (59–92)	77 (50–90)

Table 8.2 Comparison of accuracy of CT and EUS in the locoregional staging of esophageal cancer
Values in parentheses are ranges.
Data taken from Rosch.[6]

COMPARISON OF OPERATING CHARACTERISTICS OF CT, EUS, AND EUS-FNA IN PREOPERATIVE LYMPH NODE STAGING OF PATIENTS WITH ESOPHAGEAL CANCER			
Technique	Sensitivity (%)	Specificity (%)	Accuracy (%)
CT	29 (17–44)	89 (72–98)	51 (40–63)
EUS	71 (56–83)	79 (59–92)	74 (62–83)
EUS-FNA	83 (70–93)	93 (77–99)	87 (77–94)

Table 8.3 Comparison of operating characteristics of CT, EUS, and EUS-FNA in preoperative lymph node staging of patients with esophageal cancer
Values in parentheses are 95% confidence intervals.
Adapted from Vazquez-Sequeiros et al.[29]

tion of too much force when passing a malignant stricture. Characteristics that make use of the echoendoscope in esophageal strictures more difficult include the large diameter of the echoendoscope shaft, oblique optics, and a long rigid distal tip. The outer diameter of both radial and CLA echoendoscopes is approximately 13 mm, and the diameter of the lumen should be dilated to 45 Fr or greater to allow predictable passage of the echoendoscope.[14] Earlier studies reported an unacceptably high perforation rate in patients with esophageal cancer when dilation was performed in conjunction with endosonography.[15] Several studies since have confirmed that esophageal dilation prior to echoendoscopy is safe as long as the rules of sequential dilation are followed.[14,16,17] The use of a small-diameter non-optic probe that can be inserted over a guidewire provides an alternative to esophageal dilation.[18,19] The ultrasonic esophagoprobe (Olympus MH-908) has an Eden–Peustow-shaped metal tip and is passed over a guidewire in a 'mono-rail' fashion. The probe has an outer diameter of 7.9 mm and can usually be passed through an esophageal cancer without dilation.

TECHNIQUE

Patient preparation

Endoscopic evaluation is an important step in the evaluation of patients with dysphagia and esophageal strictures. By the time a patient is referred for endosonography for the staging of esophageal cancer, the diagnosis is usually established by the endoscopic image and mucosal biopsies. Review of the patient's prior barium swallow examination, recent endoscopy reports from referring colleagues, and assessment of the patient's degree of dysphagia will allow optimal planning for performing EUS. If the patient has difficulty swallowing soft (pureed) foods, it is predictable that dilation will be required to pass the echoendoscope. This information should be communicated to the staff so that dilation equipment and appropriate endoscopes can be prepared. An upper endoscopy is a must prior to endosonography, even in patients with no significant dysphagia, to assess the degree of stenosis and the distance of the stricture from the incisors, and to look for tortuosity within the stricture that might impact on the safety of EUS.

Radial endosonography

The patient is usually placed in the left lateral position. After administration of a topical anesthetic and conscious sedation, the radial echoendoscope is passed. Initial passage of the echoendoscope should be done carefully, gently, and slowly. Once in the esophagus, the instrument is advanced past the tumor by 'feel' rather than by direct visualization of the stenosed lumen. Once the echoendoscope is in position, ultrasound is switched on and imaging begins. In patients with esophageal cancer (see below), imaging actually begins in the duodenum and antrum of the stomach to examine the liver for possible metastasis. The area surrounding the fundus is scanned to look for perigastric and celiac axis lymphadenopathy. Once in the esophagus, attention is turned to the primary tumor, with particular attention to the wall layers. One must determine which layer of the esophagus has been invaded at the level of the deepest extent of tumor penetration (Fig. 8.3A). It is important to avoid tangential imaging, as this might lead

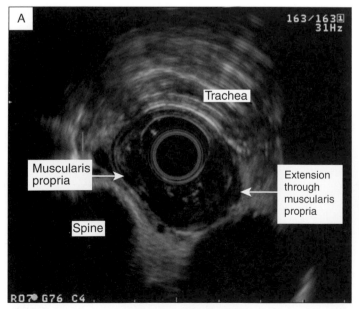

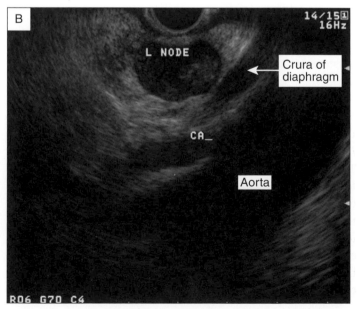

Fig. 8.3 **A,** EUS revealed a circumferential hypoechoic mass that invaded through the muscularis propria at the 3 o'clock position, although the muscularis propria was intact at the 9 o'clock position, consistent with T3 disease. **B,** Inspection of the celiac axis area revealed an enlarged, hypoechoic lymph node with sharp borders. Transgastric EUS-guided FNA confirmed the presence of malignant involvement. Neoadjuvant therapy was recommended after EUS.

to overstaging of the tumor. Imaging with 12 MHz (GF-UM 130) or 20 MHz (GF-UM Q 130) allows superior resolution of the esophageal wall layers. After adequate interrogation of the tumor, several passes are performed with 7.5 MHz to evaluate the celiac axis and the surrounding mediastinum, looking for lymph nodes (Fig. 8.3B & 8.4). Recent data suggest that staging patients with more advanced esophageal cancer can be performed equally well with the curvilinear echoendoscope alone.[20] Use of the CLA echoendoscope permits lymph node sampling without the need to switch to a second echoendoscope. The author uses the CLA echoendoscope first when prior imaging suggests enlarged lymph nodes and T staging becomes less important. However, the radial echoendoscope is more complete and less cumbersome for staging the primary tumor than the CLA echoendoscope.

Catheter probes

High-frequency catheter probes (CUS) provide high-resolution imaging of the gastrointestinal wall layers. They have proven to be indispensable in the staging of superficial esophageal cancer and in the selection of patients for EMR. Imaging of small superficial esophageal lesions with a radial echoendoscope is quite difficult, because achieving proper positioning is cumbersome and balloon inflation compresses the lesion, producing inaccuracies in staging. High-quality esophageal wall imaging depends on maintaining a water-filled lumen (despite esophageal peristalsis), positioning the transducer perpendicular to the lesion, and being able to adjust the distance between the probe and the lesion.

A few methods currently in use are able to achieve safe imaging of the esophageal wall with the high-frequency catheter probes: the free-floating catheter technique, the condom technique, and the most recently introduced balloon sheath.[21,22] The free technique does not rely on a sheath or condom to retain water in the esophagus. While achieving a column of water in the distal esophagus is possible for the expert endosonographer, this technique is limited by its short duration due to peristalsis washing the water down to the stomach. Occasionally, suctioning some of the air out from a hernia sac could bring the column of water back up into the esophagus. If the lesion cannot be demonstrated within a short period of time, repeated refilling of the distal esophagus is necessary. The most dreaded complication of this procedure is aspiration. Therefore, if attempted, the head of the bed should be elevated to at least 45° to minimize the risk of aspiration. In the author's experience, patients with Barrett's esophagus tend to tolerate this technique well. In addition, it is impossible to use this technique to image superficial lesions in the mid or upper esophagus. For these impractical reasons, alternative methods have been sought to image early esophageal lesions: the condom and the balloon sheath techniques.[21,22]

Fixing a condom to the end of a two-channel endoscope optimizes imaging by providing a contained column of water within the esophagus (that is not affected by peristalsis) and permits perpendicular imaging while being able to adjust the position of the catheter relative to the lesion.[22] Additionally, condoms are soft and very compliant, and thus do not compress esophageal wall layers. Adequate preparation is important in the success of this technique. A standard, non-lubricated, translucent latex condom is attached to a two-channel therapeutic endoscope. One inch of condom extends beyond the endoscope tip. The condom is fixed to the endoscope shaft at three locations with a rubber band, and then 2-cm wide strips of Tegaderm are wrapped full circle around the condom. As the condom is transparent, intubation can be performed under direct visualization but air insufflation *must* be avoided during intubation. The endoscope is passed into the stomach, the condom is filled with water, and then residual air and water are aspirated. The collapsed condom is then withdrawn into the esophagus and water is gently instilled. The lesion should be visible through the condom. Once in position, the ultrasound catheter is passed down the second channel and positioned against the lesion using visual contact. It is relatively easy to withdraw the scope, but if advancement is necessary it is best to aspirate some water first. The limitation of this technique is the formation of air pockets between the condom and the esophageal wall, resulting in image artifacts.

Another recently developed method is the balloon sheath technique.[21] The CUS probe is fitted with a sheath that has an acoustic coupling balloon at the distal end. The balloon can be filled with water and expanded by means of an adaptor at the proximal end outside the endoscope. With this device, standard endoscopy can be performed, and the CUS probe with balloon sheath can then be advanced through the accessory channel of the endoscope and placed in the area of interest. With the balloon filled with water and enhanced acoustic coupling, high-resolution images can be obtained.

ESOPHAGEAL DILATION AND ALTERNATIVES

Accurate staging directs the choice of therapy in patients with esophageal cancer. Up to one-third of patients with esophageal cancer present with marked luminal stenosis that does not permit passage of a 13 mm-tipped echoendoscope.[14] EUS examination from a position proximal to the tumor has been shown to result in inaccurate T staging and inadequate evaluation of the celiac axis. An earlier study using older echoendoscopes and dilation practices that did not adhere to the 'rule of 3s' reported an unacceptably high rate of esophageal perforation (24%) when dilation was employed before EUS.[15] Several studies have recently reported that dilation is safe and increases the yield of detection of celiac lymph node involvement.[14,17] Dilation to 45 Fr, or 15 mm, is usually needed to allow passage of the echoendoscope. Repeated dilation over a 2-day period should be employed if necessary.

In patients with inadequate dilation, and in situations where dilation is not preferred or is impractical, a narrow-caliber, tapered-tip, wire-guided echoendoscope can traverse high-grade malignant esophageal strictures with ease.[18,19] In addition, this probe has been shown to improve staging in this situation by evaluating both the primary tumor and the celiac axis. This esophagoprobe markedly reduced the occurrence of incomplete esophageal cancer staging and improved the detection of celiac disease in one study.[19] However, the celiac axis could not be identified in 10% of the patients with esophagoprobe due to either an extremely stenotic tumor or retained gastric air. Obviously, this instrument lacks the image orientation to permit EUS-guided FNA. In the case of T4 cancers (invasion into adjacent organ), FNA is not required. However, if celiac lymph nodes are seen, FNA is required to confirm that they are malignant. Finally, in patients with esophageal stenosis that cannot be overcome with dilation, or tumors with significant angulations, obtaining information from above the tumor (T3) can be sufficient to initiate chemotherapy and radiation therapy. In such situations, repeat EUS after neoadjuvant therapy might be appropriate to evaluate the presence of residual disease.

FINDING AND EVALUATING THE CELIAC AXIS

Celiac lymph node (CLN) metastasis carries a grave implication in patients with esophageal cancer.[4,23,24] Patients with esophageal cancer and CLN metastasis have worse survival than those without CLN involvement.[2] It is therefore crucial, when possible, both to identify and to inspect the celiac axis in all patients with esophageal cancer. To identify and evaluate the celiac axis with the radial instrument, the echoendoscope is usually placed at the gastroesophageal junction, and the aorta (anechoic and posterior) is located. Once identified, the aorta is placed at the 6 o'clock position on the screen and, as the echoendoscope is advanced forward, the aorta moves away from the echoendoscope towards the 5 o'clock position. With further advancement, the celiac axis emerges as a branching point from the descending aorta at the 7 o'clock position. Pushing 1–2 cm more will usually demonstrate the bifurcation of the celiac axis into the splenic artery and the common hepatic artery ('whale's tail sign'), and is typically seen at about 45 cm from the incisors. Sometimes it is not possible to locate the celiac axis by advancing the echoendoscope from the gastroesophageal junction (most commonly due to a hiatal hernia). In this case, beginning the examination in the gastric antrum and withdrawing slowly (while keeping the liver in the 11 o'clock position) will enable identification of the splenic–portal confluence and then, with an additional 2–3-cm withdrawal, the celiac axis can be seen.[25]

To identify the celiac axis with the CLA echoendoscope, the aorta is found at approximately 35 cm from the incisors (distal esophagus) as a long tubular structure. The endoscope is slowly advanced while maintaining the aorta in view. The first branching artery from the descending aorta is the celiac axis trunk (the superior mesenteric artery follows a few centimeters more distally). When in doubt, Doppler allows for proper identification and verification of the celiac axis trunk. Careful interrogation is performed to assess for lymphadenopathy.

Lymph node characteristics are helpful in differentiating benign from malignant lymph nodes. Malignant lymph nodes tend to be greater than 1 cm in diameter, round, sharply demarcated, and hypoechoic (Fig. 8.3B & 8.4).[26] Successively more criteria enhance the likelihood the lymph node is malignant.[27] In patients with esophageal cancer, the identification of CLNs is virtually synonymous with malignant involvement. Regardless of echo features and size, 90% of all detected CLNs were proven to be malignant in one study.[28] Moreover, 100% of lymph nodes greater than 1 cm in size were malignant. The clinical impact that malignant CLNs have on therapy leads to the performance of EUS-FNA, providing a means of documenting nodal involvement prior to neoadjuvant therapy.[28,29]

Once celiac lymph nodes have been identified and deemed suitable for biopsy, EUS-FNA is performed with a CLA echoendoscope.[25,28] The instrument is placed in the stomach lumen opposite the identified node. The FNA needle-sheath system is inserted through the biopsy channel of the echoendoscope and screwed into the Luer-Lok or the channel hub of the echoendoscope, and EUS-FNA is performed as described previously.[25] Some have suggested that suction during FNA of lymph nodes increases the bloodiness of the specimen but does not necessarily increase yield.[30] When this occurs, additional passes without suction are warranted. After 30–60 s, the needle is retracted. The aspirate is placed on a glass slide, processed with a Diff-Quick stain, and preferably reviewed immediately by an on-site cytologist or pathologist to ensure an adequate specimen. The availability of onsite interpretation is variable from center to center. A diagnosis of malignancy is usually obtained from the first two passes in the

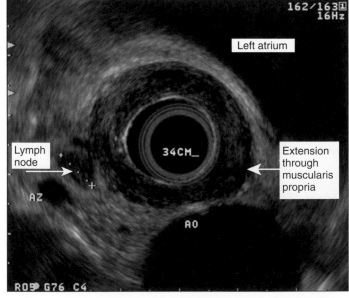

Fig. 8.4 EUS appearance of a tumor that invaded through the muscularis propria into the adventitia. A single peritumoral lymph node is seen and is consistent with malignant involvement (T3 N1). These lymph nodes are not amenable to EUS-FNA because the needle would have to traverse the tumor. AO, aorta. AZ, Azygous vein.

majority of malignant lymph nodes. We typically perform four passes in lymph nodes with benign EUS features to ensure that adequate sampling has been performed. The operating characteristics of EUS-FNA for assessing celiac lymph nodes are shown in Table 8.4.

EVALUATION OF THE LIVER

EUS can detect occult liver metastases in patients in whom non-invasive hepatic imaging studies are normal, although the frequency with which such lesions are detected is low. In addition, EUS-FNA can be performed to document liver metastatis.[31,32] The echoendoscope is usually placed in the antrum of the stomach to evaluate the parenchyma of the left lobe of the liver. Restricted by anatomic relations, not all segments of the liver can be viewed by endosonography. The latex balloon is inflated with water to allow better acoustic coupling and thus better imaging. Instillation of water in the stomach is not necessary. Imaging begins by pulling the endoscope slowly from the antrum. Metastases usually appear as discrete relatively hypoechoic areas in the liver. Once identified, EUS-FNA can be performed, yielding important diagnostic and prognostic information for the patient management.[31,32]

STAGING OF MALIGNANT STRICTURES

Accurate preoperative staging of esophageal cancer allows appropriate selection of therapy and prognostication. After dilation of the tumor (if necessary), staging is performed according to the tumor node metastasis (TNM) classification (see Table 8.1).[33] Inspection of the liver, celiac axis and gastrohepatic ligament areas are performed to determine the presence of liver metastasis and lymph nodes respectively. Attention is then turned to the primary tumor and the mediastinum to identify depth of tumor invasion and the presence of peritumoral and mediastinal adenopathy. The TNM system is based on the determination of depth of tumor invasion (T stage), the presence or absence of regional lymph node metastasis (N stage), and the presence or absence of distant metastasis (M stage). A global stage can be obtained by combining these components. There is an emerging body of data to suggest that EUS staging, similar to surgical staging, can predict long-term survival in patients with esophageal cancer.[4,34]

T stage

T stage is determined by the depth of tumor invasion and the involvement of esophageal wall layers. The earliest stage, Tis or carcinoma in situ is present when the cancer is limited to the epithelium and the lamina propria is intact. This stage is detected by biopsy and cannot be imaged by EUS. T1 tumors are defined when cancerous cells invade the lamina propria and submucosa. With the advent of high-frequency catheter probes, T1 tumors have been further classified into T1m (confined to mucosa) or T1sm (tumor invading submucosa). This classification becomes important in countries where esophageal cancer is detected at an early stage. These two tumors differ in their propensity to have early spread to lymph nodes through a dense network of esophageal lymphatics. This classification helps to identify appropriate therapy commensurate with the stage of disease. For example, EMR is appropriate treatment because there is rarely involvement with local lymph nodes. T1sm disease has a 15–30% rate of lymph node metastasis, and therefore surgery is the most appropriate treatment when lymph nodes are not detected. When the tumor invades the muscularis propria, the tumor is classified as T2. When the tumor progresses further to invade the adventitia, the tumor is classified as T3. Involvement of mediastinal structures, such as the aorta, pleura, azygous vein, or any adjacent structure, is classified as T4 disease. The accuracy of EUS and CT for various T stages is shown in Table 8.2.

N stage

Due to rich esophageal lymphatics, esophageal cancer has the propensity to spread early to local lymph nodes. It is clear that patients with N1 (nodal involvement) disease as classified by EUS have a poorer survival than those with N0 disease (no lymph node involvement).[4,35] Furthermore, the number of lymph nodes detected is an important predictor of survival.[3] The advantage of EUS is that these lymph nodes can be detected accurately before surgery. Lymph node characteristics are helpful in classifying benign from malignant lymph nodes.

OPERATING CHARACTERISTICS OF EUS-FNA IN CELIAC LYMPH NODES					
Reference	Year	No. of patients	Sensitivity (%)	Specificity (%)	Accuracy (%)
Giovannini et al.[44]	1995	26	100 (21/21)	–	81 (21/26)
Reed et al.[45]	1999	17	100 (15/15)	–	88 (15/17)
Williams et al.[46]	1999	27	96 (25/26)	100 (1/1)	96 (26/27)
Eloubeidi et al.[28]	2001	51	98 (45/46)	100 (5/5)	98 (50/51)

Table 8.4 Operating characteristics of EUS-FNA in celiac lymph nodes

Malignant lymph nodes tend to be greater than 1cm in diameter, round, sharply demarcated, and hypoechoic.[26] The higher the number of criteria a lymph node has acquired, the more likely it is to be malignant.[27] The location of the lymph node can help determine whether it contains cancer cells. For example, unlike the mediastinum, patients without upper abdominal pathology generally do not have CLNs detectable by EUS. In patients with esophageal cancer, the identification of CLNs is synonymous with malignant involvement.[28] Regardless of echo features and size, 90% of all detected CLNs were proven to be malignant in one study. Moreover, 100% of all lymph nodes greater than 1cm in diameter were malignant.[28] To eliminate or reduce uncertainty, EUS-FNA provides a means of documenting nodal involvement prior to neoadjuvant therapy.[28,29,36] A major limitation to EUS-FNA is the fact that intervening tumor does not allow sampling of these lymph nodes without the risk of contamination. The development of needle systems that allowed the sampling of peritumoral lymph nodes would clearly enhance further the role of EUS-FNA in this disease. The 1997 AJCC TNM classification takes into account the location of the primary tumor for classification of lymph nodes as local (N1) or metastatic (M1) disease.[33]

M stage

Involvement of sites distant from the primary tumor via hematogenous seeding of distant organs (liver, lung, bones) or distant lymph nodes is considered metastatic disease.[33] EUS provides excellent imaging of the medial two-thirds of the liver, but cannot exclude with certainty metastatic disease to all areas of the liver. Depending on the location of the tumor and the lymph nodes involved, metastasis to certain lymph nodes is classified as M1a or M1b disease. For example, for tumors of the lower and upper thoracic esophagus, metastasis to celiac and cervical lymph nodes is considered metastatic disease (M1a). M1b denotes metastasis to distant organs for tumors of the upper and lower thoracic esophagus, and metastasis to non-regional lymph nodes and/or other distant metastasis for tumors of the mid-thoracic esophagus.[33]

EUS IN SUPERFICIAL CANCER AND BARRETT'S ESOPHAGUS

With the advent of EMR and photodynamic therapy, accurate assessment of depth of tumor invasion is mandatory prior to their application. As the depth of tumor invasion correlates with lymph node metastasis, it is crucial to identify T stage prior to EMR. One study has shown that tumors limited to the epithelium and lamina propria (m1 and m2) have a 5% chance of metastasizing to lymph nodes. In contrast, tumors invading the muscularis mucosa or submucosa have a 12–27% chance of metastasizing to lymph nodes. Invasion of the deep submucosa reaching the proper muscle could lead to a 36–46% chance of lymph node metastasis.[37] The accuracy of the high-frequency catheter probe (HFCP) in distinguishing between mucosal cancer and cancer invading the submucosa is 81–100%.[38] The accuracy of EUS in patients with Barrett's esophagus and high-grade dysplasia or intramucosal carcinoma has been reported. The sensitivity, specificity, and negative predictive values of preoperative EUS for submucosa invasion were 100%, 94%, and 100%, and those for lymph node involvement were 100%, 81%, and 100%, respectively.[39] A nodule or stricture noted by endoscopy was associated with an increased likelihood of submucosal invasion.[39] Of note, this study used the regular echoendoscope and not the HFCP. With the exception of patients with Barrett's esophagus, early esophageal cancer is rarely seen in the USA and, therefore, the HFCP is less frequently used than in Japan.

EUS-GUIDED FNA BIOPSY OF CELIAC AND PERI-INTESTINAL LYMPH NODES

Prior to the advent of EUS-FNA, endosonographers relied on the echo features of lymph nodes to identify malignancy. These features included size greater than 1cm, sharp borders, round shape, and hypoechoic echo texture. Recent work suggests that EUS-FNA improves the accuracy of lymph node staging and is superior to EUS echo features.[27] EUS alone was only 33.3% accurate in differentiating between malignant and benign lymphadenopathy, whereas EUS-FNA had a significantly higher accuracy of 99.4%.[27] This study also found that lymph node echo features are particularly unreliable in the mediastinum. In patients with esophageal cancer, EUS-FNA was superior to helical CT and EUS for the preoperative staging of lymph nodes.[29] Owing to the small number of patients, EUS was equivalent to CT for the detection of CLNs. We have previously shown that EUS is superior to both CT and PET for the detection of CLNs.[9] The operating characteristics of EUS-FNA compared with CT and EUS, and the accuracy of EUS-FNA in sampling celiac lymph nodes, are shown in Tables 8.3 and 8.4 respectively.

EUS-FNA technique

Once lymph nodes have been identified and deemed suitable for biopsy, EUS-FNA is performed. EUS-FNA can be performed with either a CLA echoendoscope (FG-32-UA, Pentax Precision Instrument Company, Orangeburg, NY; or UC-30P, Olympus America Incorporated, Melville, NY) or the mechanical sector scanning biopsy echoendoscope (GF-UM 30 P, Olympus America Incorporated). Doppler ultrasound can be applied with CLA systems to ensure that there are no intervening vessels prior to EUS-FNA. The instrument is placed in the stomach lumen opposite the identified CLN. The FNA needle-sheath system, consisting of a 22- or 25-gauge needle, is inserted through the working channel of the endoscope. The needle is advanced from the sheath through the wall of the stomach and guided into the target site using real-time ultrasound. The stylet is removed and suction can be applied with a 10-ml syringe while the needle is manipulated back and forth within the target lesion. After 30–60 s, the suction is released and the needle retracted. The aspirate is placed on a glass slide, preserved with Diff-Quick stain, and reviewed immediately by an on-site pathologist to ensure an adequate specimen. If liver lesions are identified, these usually take priority in order of biopsy because they provide a higher stage that clearly precludes surgery. The CLA echoendoscope is usually placed in the stomach, and virtually the same technique is applied to liver lesions. It is prudent, however, to keep the patients on their right side for 3–4 h after EUS-FNA of a liver lesion to minimize the risk of bleeding.

EUS AND NEOADJUVANT THERAPY

Owing to its ability to image the gastrointestinal tract wall layers with accuracy and histologic correlates,[8] EUS is currently the best staging modality for locoregional disease in esophageal cancer. However, several studies have shown that standard EUS criteria are not accurate after neoadjuvant chemoradiation, as its performance is poor in differentiating tumor from necrosis or inflammatory reaction.[40,41] A recent study evaluated the utility of EUS after neoadjuvant therapy.[42] The authors studied 97 consecutive patients with esophageal cancer who were treated with preoperative chemoradiotherapy and a potentially curative surgical procedure. All patients had EUS examination prior to chemoradiotherapy, and 53 had a repeat EUS examination after treatment but before surgery. Surgical resection specimens were analyzed for the absence or presence of residual tumor and its location. Patients with residual tumor in the esophagus and those with no residual tumor had similar cumulative survival rates. Patients with residual cancer in lymph nodes showed a trend towards a shorter cumulative survival compared with patients with no residual tumor in lymph nodes. The actuarial survival rate in patients with involved lymph nodes was lower than that in patients with no lymph nodes at 1, 2, and 3 years. Patients with significant residual lymphadenopathy detected by EUS after therapy had a significantly worse postoperative survival than patients with no residual lymphadenopathy.[42] In eight patients, the authors reliably obtained cytologic specimens and were able to identify residual malignancy by EUS-FNA after chemoradiation therapy. The authors concluded that EUS and EUS-guided FNA can be helpful in identifying residual tumor in the lymph nodes after preoperative chemoradiotherapy to select patients who will benefit maximally from surgery. Another study[43] evaluated the accuracy of EUS in restaging 77 patients with esophageal adenocarcinoma after induction therapy. T classification was assessed correctly by EUS in 22 patients (29%). The proportion of individual T classifications by EUS that were correct were 0% for T0 tumors, 19% for T1 tumors, 27% for T2 tumors, 52% for T3 tumors, and 0% for T4 tumors when comparing results from the EUS restaging examination with the findings at surgical pathology. Nineteen of 77 patients (25%) were assigned the correct group stage by restaging EUS, 42 patients

(55%) were overstaged, and 15 (19%) were understaged. The accuracy of the restaging EUS examination for predicting the N classification of the tumor was 49%. The sensitivity of EUS for N classification was 48% for N0 disease and 52% for N1 disease. Interestingly, EUS-FNA was not performed routinely in this study to assess for residual disease. It is our current practice to sample lymph nodes after chemoradiotherapy; patients with residual disease, especially in the celiac axis, undergo more treatment prior to consideration of surgical resection. As neoadjuvant therapy was used initially to shrink and reduce the bulk of the tumor, perhaps it is more important to ask the question whether residual tumor is resectable so that the patient will undergo surgical resection. In addition, and more importantly, EUS-FNA has the ability to sample lymph nodes after chemotherapy and therefore can identify recalcitrant disease necessitating further chemotherapy. Many centers, including the author's own, do not offer surgical resection to patients with residual lymph nodes, especially in the celiac axis area, if they have persistent residual disease.

Another useful measure of tumor response is a reduction in the maximal cross-sectional area, as this offers better promise as a useful measure for assessing response to preoperative therapy.[40] In one study, responders (patients with a greater than 50% reduction in the maximal cross-sectional area) as assessed by EUS were more likely to survive than non-responders.[40] Moreover, it is apparent that responders with adenocarcinoma were more likely to survive than non-responders. However, this finding did not hold true for patients with squamous cell carcinoma of the esophagus. It is noteworthy that five of six patients in the R0 group were among the responders. None of the other clinical, endoscopic, or endosonographic variables studied was predictive of survival. This study was limited by small sample size. The lack of effect of known important variables on survival, such as T stage, N stage, the presence of celiac adenopathy, or overall AJCC stage, is probably due to a Type 2 error, that is, the study was underpowered to detect such a difference. The development of three-dimensional EUS that has the ability to measure the total volume of the tumor, rather than the cross-sectional area, might prove to be a superior modality in the assessment of response to multimodality therapy in patients with esophageal cancer.

SUMMARY

EUS is currently the only available modality that images the esophageal wall layers with histologic correlates. EUS is superior to CT and PET in the detection of peritumoral and celiac lymph nodes. EUS-FNA allows for documentation of locoregional and distant lymph node status prior to neoadjuvant therapy. EUS can select patients for surgical resection after neoadjuvant therapy. Future efforts should focus on implementing EUS as part of research protocols evaluating therapies for esophageal cancer.

EXAMINATION CHECKLIST

Liver

Celiac axis

Primary tumor

Periesophageal area above the aortic arch for lymph nodes

Note relationship of tumor to carina

For distal esophageal tumors, look for invasion into the
diaphragm

REFERENCES

1 Jemal A, Murray T, Ward E, et al. Cancer statistics, 2005. CA Cancer J Clin 2005; 55:10–30.

2 Eloubeidi MA, Mason AC, Desmond RA, et al. Temporal trends (1973–1997) in survival of patients with esophageal adenocarcinoma in the United States: a glimmer of hope? Am J Gastroenterol 2003; 98:1627–1633.

3 Eloubeidi MA, Desmond R, Arguedas MR, et al. Prognostic factors for the survival of patients with esophageal carcinoma in the US: the importance of tumor length and lymph node status. Cancer 2002; 95:1434–1443.

4 Eloubeidi MA, Wallace MB, Hoffman BJ, et al. Predictors of survival for esophageal cancer patients with and without celiac axis lymphadenopathy: impact of staging endosonography. Ann Thorac Surg 2001; 72:212–219.

5 Fockens P, Kisman K, Merkus MP, et al. The prognosis of esophageal carcinoma staged irresectable (T4) by endosonography. J Am Coll Surg 1998; 186:17–23.

6 Rosch T. Endosonographic staging of esophageal cancer: a review of literature results. Gastrointest Endosc Clin North Am 1995; 5:537–547.

7 Romagnuolo J, Scott J, Hawes RH, et al. Helical CT versus EUS with fine needle aspiration for celiac nodal assessment in patients with esophageal cancer. Gastrointest Endosc 1900; 55:648–654.

8 Kimmey MB, Martin RW, Haggitt RC, et al. Histologic correlates of gastrointestinal ultrasound images. Gastroenterology 1989; 96:433–441.

9 Akdamar M, Cerfolio R, Ojha B, et al. A prospective comparison of computerized tomography (CT), 18 fluoro-deoxyglucose positron emission tomography (FDG-PET) and endoscopic ultrasonography (EUS) in the preoperative evaluation of potentially operable esophageal cancer (ECA) patients. Am J Gastroenterol 2005; 98:s5.

10 van Westreenen HL, Westerterp M, Bossuyt PM, et al. Systematic review of the staging performance of ^{18}F-fluorodeoxyglucose positron emission tomography in esophageal cancer. J Clin Oncol 2004; 22:3805–3812.

11 van Westreenen HL, Heeren PA, Jager PL, et al. Pitfalls of positive findings in staging esophageal cancer with F-18-fluorodeoxyglucose positron emission tomography. Ann Surg Oncol 2003; 10:1100–1105.

12 Eloubeidi MA, Cerfolio RJ, Chen VK, et al. Endoscopic ultrasound-guided fine needle aspiration of mediastinal lymph node in patients with suspected lung cancer after positron emission tomography and computed tomography scans. Ann Thorac Surg 2005; 79:263–268.

13 van Westreenen HL, Heeren PA, van Dullemen HM, et al. Positron emission tomography with F-18-fluorodeoxyglucose in a combined staging strategy of esophageal cancer prevents unnecessary surgical explorations. J Gastrointest Surg 2005; 9:54–61.

14 Wallace MB, Hawes RH, Sahai AV, et al. Dilation of malignant esophageal stenosis to allow EUS guided fine-needle aspiration: safety and effect on patient managment. Gastrointest Endosc 2000; 51:309–313.

15 Van Dam J, Rice TW, Catalano MF, et al. High-grade malignant stricture is predictive of esophageal tumor stage. Risks of endosonographic evaluation. Cancer 1993; 71:2910–2917.

16 Kallimanis GE, Gupta PK, al-Kawas FH, et al. Endoscopic ultrasound for staging esophageal cancer, with or without dilation, is clinically important and safe. Gastrointest Endosc 1995; 41:540–546.

17 Pfau PR, Ginsberg GG, Lew RJ, et al. Esophageal dilation for endosonographic evaluation of malignant esophageal strictures is safe and effective. Am J Gastroenterol 2000; 95:2813–2815.

18 Binmoeller KF, Seifert H, Seitz U, et al. Ultrasonic esophagoprobe for TNM staging of highly stenosing esophageal carcinoma. Gastrointest Endosc 1995; 41:547–552.

19 Mallery S, Van Dam J. Increased rate of complete EUS staging of patients with esophageal cancer using the nonoptical, wire-guided echoendoscope. Gastrointest Endosc 1999; 50:53–57.

20 Siemsen M, Svendsen LB, Knigge U, et al. A prospective randomized comparison of curved array and radial echoendoscopy in patients with esophageal cancer. Gastrointest Endosc 2003; 58:671–676.

21 Vazquez-Sequeiros E, Wiersema MJ. High-frequency US catheter-based staging of early esophageal tumors. Gastrointest Endosc 2002; 55:95–99.

22 Wallace MB, Hoffman BJ, Sahai AS, et al. Imaging of esophageal tumors with a water-filled condom and a catheter US probe. Gastrointest Endosc 2000; 51:597–600.

23 Christie NA, Rice TW, DeCamp MM, et al. M1a/M1b esophageal carcinoma: clinical relevance. J Thorac Cardiovasc Surg 1999; 118:900–907.

24 Hiele M, De Leyn P, Schurmans P, et al. Relation between endoscopic ultrasound findings and outcome of patients with tumors of the esophagus or esophagogastric junction. Gastrointest Endosc 1997; 45:381–386.

25 Eloubeidi MA, Vilmann P, Wiersema MJ. Endoscopic ultrasound-guided fine-needle aspiration of celiac lymph nodes. Endoscopy 2004; 36:901–908.

26 Catalano MF, Sivak MVJ, Rice T, et al. Endosonographic features predictive of lymph node metastasis. Gastrointest Endosc 1994; 40:442–446.

27 Chen VK, Eloubeidi MA. Endoscopic ultrasound-guided fine needle aspiration is superior to lymph node echofeatures: a prospective evaluation of mediastinal and peri-intestinal lymphadenopathy. Am J Gastroenterol 2004; 99:628–633.

28 Eloubeidi MA, Wallace MB, Reed CE, et al. The utility of EUS and EUS-guided fine needle aspiration in detecting celiac lymph node metastasis in patients with esophageal cancer: a single-center experience. Gastrointest Endosc 2001; 54:714–719.

29 Vazquez-Sequeiros E, Wiersema MJ, Clain JE, et al. Impact of lymph node staging on therapy of esophageal carcinoma. Gastroenterology 2003; 125:1626–1635.

30 Wallace MB, Kennedy T, Durkalski V, et al. Randomized controlled trial of EUS-guided fine needle aspiration techniques for the detection of malignant lymphadenopathy. Gastrointest Endosc 2001; 54:441–447.

31 Prasad P, Schmulewitz N, Patel A, et al. Detection of occult liver metastases during EUS for staging of malignancies. Gastrointest Endosc 2004; 59:49–53.

32 tenBerge J, Hoffman BJ, Hawes RH, et al. EUS-guided fine needle aspiration of the liver: indications, yield, and safety based on an international survey of 167 cases. Gastrointest Endosc 2002; 55:859–862.

33 American Joint Committee on Cancer. Esophagus. In: AJCC cancer staging manual, 5th edn. Philadelphia: Lippincott-Raven; 2000:65–68.

34 Harewood GC, Kumar KS. Assessment of clinical impact of endoscopic ultrasound on esophageal cancer. J Gastroenterol Hepatol 2004; 19:433–439.

35 Pfau PR, Ginsberg GG, Lew RJ, et al. Endoscopic ultrasound predictors of long term survival in esophageal carcinoma. Gastrointest Endosc 2001; 53:463–469.

36 Penman ID, Williams DB, Sahai AV, et al. Ability of EUS with fine-needle aspiration to document nodal staging and response to neoadjuvant chemoradiotherapy in locally advanced esophageal cancer: a case report. Gastrointest Endosc 1999; 49:783–786.

37 Kodama M, Kakegawa T. Treatment of superficial cancer of the esophagus: a summary of responses to a questionnaire on superficial cancer of the esophagus in Japan. Surgery 1998; 123:432–439.

38 Murata Y, Napoleon B, Odegaard S. High-frequency endoscopic ultrasonography in the evaluation of superficial esophageal cancer. Endoscopy 2003; 35:429–435.

39 Scotiniotis IA, Kochman ML, Lewis JD, et al. Accuracy of EUS in the evaluation of Barrett's esophagus and high-grade dysplasia or intramucosal carcinoma. Gastrointest Endosc 2001; 54:689–696.

40 Chak A, Canto MI, Cooper GS, et al. Endosonographic assessment of multimodality therapy predicts survival of esophageal carcinoma patients. Cancer 2000; 88:1788–1795.

41 Isenberg G, Chak A, Canto MI, et al. Endoscopic ultrasound in restaging of esophageal cancer after neoadjuvant chemoradiation. Gastrointest Endosc 1998; 48:158–163.

42 Agarwal B, Swisher S, Ajani J, et al. Endoscopic ultrasound after preoperative chemoradiation can help identify patients who benefit maximally after surgical esophageal resection. Am J Gastroenterol 2004; 99:1258–1266.

43 Kalha I, Kaw M, Fukami N, et al. The accuracy of endoscopic ultrasound for restaging esophageal carcinoma after chemoradiation therapy. Cancer 2004, 101:940–947.

44 Giovannini M, Seitz JF, Monges G, et al. Fine-needle aspiration cytology guided by endoscopic ultrasonography: results in 141 patients. Endoscopy 1995; 27:171–177.

45 Reed CE, Mishra G, Sahai AV, et al. Esophageal cancer staging: improved accuracy by endoscopic ultrasound of celiac lymph nodes. Ann Thorac Surg 1999; 67:319–321.

46 Williams DB, Sahai AV, Aabakken L, et al. Endoscopic ultrasound guided fine needle aspiration biopsy: a large single centre experience. Gut 1999; 44:720–726.

Chapter

9

EUS Diagnosis of Posterior Mediastinal Masses, Lymph Nodes, and Cysts

Thomas J. Savides

KEY POINTS

- Criteria exist to differentiate benign from malignant mediastinal lymph nodes, but alone they are not sufficiently accurate and endoscopic ultrasound-guided fine-needle aspiration (EUS-FNA) is required to make sound clinical decisions.

- The overall accuracy for the diagnosis of posterior mediastinal malignancies with transesophageal EUS-FNA is greater than 90%.

- The diagnosis of lymphoma in the posterior mediastinum is made by cytology and flow cytometry studies on EUS-FNA specimens.

- EUS-FNA can be valuable in helping to establish a diagnosis of granulomatous disease involving the mediastinum (sarcoidosis, histoplasmosis, tuberculosis).

- Most mediastinal cysts are benign and, as the risk of infection is high, EUS-FNA should not be performed. If there is a high suspicion for malignancy, the cyst should undergo one puncture, be fully drained, and antibiotics should be administered.

INTRODUCTION

Transesophageal endoscopic ultrasound (EUS) with fine-needle aspiration (FNA) offers a unique ability to assess and biopsy posterior mediastinal lesions. Usually these lesions are first detected by computed tomography (CT), but occasionally they are seen during passage of the echoendoscope through the esophagus on the way to image gastrointestinal or pancreatic pathology. Transesophageal EUS is well suited to image the posterior mediastinum, but cannot visualize the middle or anterior mediastinum. This chapter focuses on EUS diagnosis of posterior mediastinal masses, lymph nodes, and cysts, while the role of EUS-FNA in lung cancer staging is discussed in Chapter 7.

EUS EVALUATION OF ENLARGED POSTERIOR MEDIASTINAL LYMPH NODES

EUS appearance of normal benign posterior mediastinal lymph nodes

Mediastinal lymph nodes are commonly encountered during EUS for non-thoracic indications. The most common EUS features of these benign nodes are triangular or crescent shape, with possibly an echogenic center (Fig. 9.1). The echogenic center represents the hilum of the lymph node. The prevalence of posterior mediastinal adenopathy in a study from Indianapolis evaluating patients undergoing EUS for non-thoracic indications was 86%, with an average of 3.6 periesophageal lymph nodes per patient.[1] These nodes had mean short- and long-axis diameters of 5 and 10 mm respectively. Because of the high rate of histoplasmosis exposure in Indiana, it is possible that the prevalence of benign posterior mediastinal lymph nodes in other geographic areas may be lower.

EUS appearance of malignant posterior mediastinal lymph nodes

EUS findings associated with malignant lymph nodes include round shape, short-axis diameter ≥10 mm, hypoechoic echotexture, and well demarcated borders (Fig. 9.2).[1,2] If all four features are present in a lymph node, the chance of malignancy is 80–100%.[2,3] However, all four features are seen in only 25% of malignant lymph nodes.[3] For this reason, tissue sampling is important to obtain diagnostic cytopathologic material of enlarged mediastinal lymph nodes.

Transesophageal EUS-FNA of mediastinal lymph nodes

The first report of EUS-assisted FNA of mediastinal lymph nodes was made in 1992 from the Indiana University Medical Center, where a diagnostic radial EUS scope was used to mark the site on the esophageal wall adjacent to a mass lesion, followed by FNA using a sclerotherapy needle through a standard forward-viewing endoscope.[4] The first use of a dedicated linear array echoendoscope to perform transesophageal EUS-FNA of posterior mediastinal lymph nodes was reported in 1993.[5] Table 9.1 shows the types of pathologic lesions that can be diagnosed with transesophageal EUS-FNA cytology.

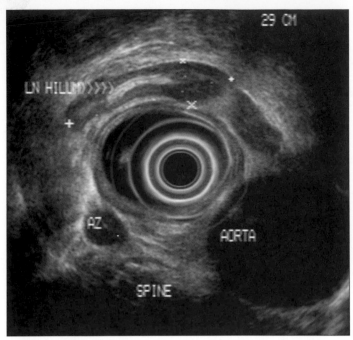

Fig. 9.1 Benign mediastinal lymph node. Note the triangular appearance with a central hyperechoic stripe.

Technique for EUS-FNA of posterior mediastinal lesions

Transesophageal EUS-FNA is generally performed as an outpatient procedure. Patients stop aspirin and non-steroidal anti-inflammatory drugs for 1 week prior to the procedure. Patients usually receive intravenous moderate sedation with meperidine and midazolam. EUS can be performed first using a radial echoendoscope to identify lesions, followed by a linear array echoendoscope to perform the FNA, or directly with the linear array scope to find and biopsy a lesion. The echoendoscope is passed through the patient's mouth into the stomach, and

ultrasound imaging is performed as the scope is withdrawn. The liver, celiac axis, left adrenal gland, and posterior mediastinum are evaluated for lesions. The location of each lesion is documented in terms of the distance (in centimeters) of the transducer tip from the incisors, anatomic location (subcarinal, left paraesophageal, right paratracheal, posterior aortopulmonic window, etc.), and size (short- and long-axis dimensions). For each lesion, the short- and long-axis diameters are measured. The shape is described as round, oval, or triangular. The echogenicity is described in terms of hypoechoic, hyperechoic, or anechoic.

Transesophageal EUS-FNA is performed using a linear array echoendoscope and usually a 22-gauge aspiration needle. Occasionally a 25-gauge or Tru-Cut needle may be used. If radial EUS is performed first, the linear array echoendoscope is then passed to the distance where the lesion was noted with the radial echoendoscope. If there is more than one possible lesion to biopsy, the lesion that is most likely to be malignant (i.e., rounder, larger, more demarcated) is chosen as the target.[6] If there is any question about whether the structure to be biopsied is vascular, color Doppler on the linear array scope can be used to assess for flow. Under constant ultrasound visualization, the needle is passed through the esophageal wall and into the lymph node. The internal stylet is then removed, and the needle is moved back and forth within the lesion using intermittent suction. The needle is then removed from the scope instrument channel, the stylet is slowly reintroduced into the needle, and the aspirate material is expressed onto a microscope slide, as well as into medium for cell block or flow cytometry.

In the USA, it is common that a cytotechnologist in the procedure room prepares the slides using a rapid staining procedure and then a cytopathologist immediately evaluates the slides under the microscope to determine whether there is adequate material for a preliminary diagnosis. If preliminary

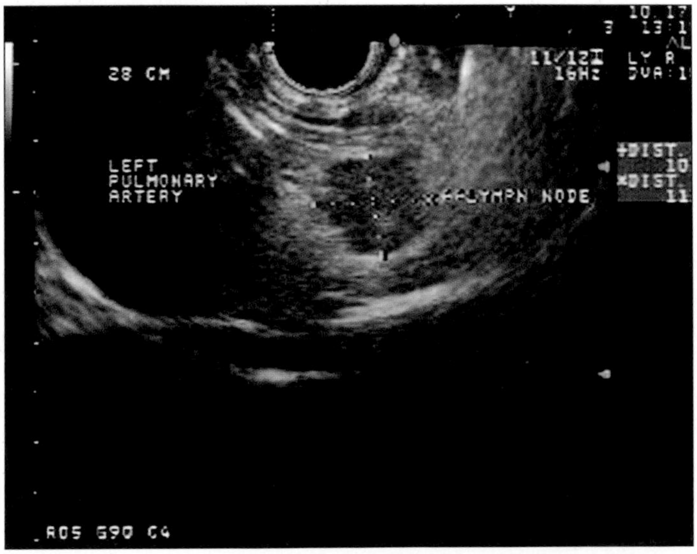

Fig. 9.2 Malignant appearing lymph node. Note the round shape, well demarcated border, hypoechoic echo pattern, and short-axis diameter ≥10 mm.

POSTERIOR MEDIASTINAL LESIONS THAT CAN BE DIAGNOSED WITH EUS-FNA
· Primary pulmonary cancer
Non-small cell lung cancer
Small cell lung cancer
· Metastatic cancer from extrathoracic malignancy
· Lymphoma
· Reactive lymph nodes
· Granulomatous disease
Sarcoid
Histoplasmosis
Tuberculosis
· Neurogenic tumors
· Duplication cysts
· Mediastinal abscess/mediastinitis

Table 9.1 Posterior mediastinal lesions that can be diagnosed with EUS-FNA

evaluation raises the possibility of lymphoma, additional passes may be obtained for flow cytometry. If preliminary evaluation is suspicious for infection, additional passes may be made for microbiologic studies. Final diagnosis is provided only once the pathologist has evaluated all processed specimen slides and cell-block material. Other possible approaches for evaluation of the cytologic material include having the endosonographer evaluate the cytologic material, a cytotechnician evaluate the material, the cytopathologist called only after several passes have been made, or the specimens delivered to a pathologist located in a part of the medical center distant from the EUS room.

Accuracy of EUS-FNA for diagnosing posterior mediastinal lesions

The overall accuracy rate for diagnosing posterior mediastinal malignancy with transesophageal EUS-FNA is approximately 93%.[6] Table 9.2 gives a summary of the accuracy rates for EUS-FNA for diagnosing malignancy in posterior mediastinal lesions. Several studies have shown that the diagnostic accuracy of malignant posterior mediastinal lymph nodes increases with the use of EUS-FNA cytology compared with the EUS appearance alone.[7–9]

EUS-FNA compared with other modalities for evaluating and biopsying posterior mediastinal lymph nodes or masses

The imaging modalities used to evaluate enlarged mediastinal lymph nodes are CT and positron emission tomography (PET).

These have been compared with EUS-FNA in the setting of suspected lung cancer. Both EUS alone and EUS-FNA have been shown to be more accurate than CT alone (using short-axis lymph node diameter >10 mm) for diagnosing malignant posterior mediastinal lymph nodes.[7,10]

PET detects increased uptake of the glucose analog ^{18}F-2-deoxy-D-glucose. Increased uptake can occur in both malignancy and inflammatory conditions. A meta-analysis comparing CT with PET in the evaluation of mediastinal adenopathy in patients with lung cancer revealed that when CT showed enlarged lymph nodes the sensitivity of PET was 100%, but the specificity was only 78%, in contrast to a sensitivity of 82% and a specificity of 93% when there were no CT findings of lymph node enlargement.[11] The low specificity of PET implies that 22% of patients with PET-positive enlarged mediastinal lymph nodes actually do not have malignancy (false-positive PET finding), and therefore these nodes should undergo tissue biopsy.[11] Several recent studies have confirmed the poor specificity of PET compared with EUS-FNA.[10,12,13] The largest and most recent study found that the EUS-FNA-positive predictive value of malignancy was 100%, compared with 40% for PET.[13] There has also been a report of EUS-FNA diagnosing malignancy in an enlarged posterior mediastinal lymph node that was falsely negative on PET.[14]

The other modalities for obtaining tissue samples from posterior mediastinal lesions are percutaneous CT-guided transthoracic FNA, bronchoscopy with transbronchial biopsy, transbronchial EUS-FNA, and mediastinoscopy. Percutaneous transthoracic FNA is generally not used to biopsy posterior mediastinal biopsies, because of the risk of pneumothorax

SUMMARY OF STUDIES EVALUATING THE OPERATING CHARACTERISTICS OF EUS-FNA FOR DIAGNOSING MALIGNANT MEDIASTINAL LESIONS							
Reference	Year	n	Sensitivity (%)	Specificity (%)	Accuracy (%)	PPV	NPV
Giovannini et al.[64]	1995	24	81	100	83	–	–
Silvestri et al.[65]	1996	27	89	100	–	–	–
Gress et al.[7]	1997	52	95	81	96	–	–
Hunerbein et al.[66]	1998	23	89	83	87	–	–
Serna et al.[67]	1998	21	86	100	–	–	–
Wiersema et al.[68]	2001	82	96	100	98	94	100
Fritscher-Ravens et al.[23]	2000	153	92	100	95	–	–
Wallace et al.[69]	2001	121	87	100	–	–	–
Devereaux et al.[24]	2002	49	–	–	94	–	–
Larsen et al.[41]	2002	79	92	100	94	100	80
Hernandez et al.[70]	2004	59	–	–	84	–	–
Savides & Perricone[21]	2004	59	96	100	98	100	97
Eloubeidi et al.[13]	2005	104	93	100	97	100	97
Overall			91	97	97	99	94

Table 9.2 Summary of studies evaluating the operating characteristics of EUS-FNA for diagnosing malignant mediastinal lesions
PPV, positive predictive value; NPV, negative predictive value.

or puncture of a major vessel. Transbronchial FNA can be performed into subcarinal lymph nodes, but this is a non-image-guided approach that also has risks of pneumothorax or bleeding. A comparative study, published only in abstract form, found EUS-FNA to be more accurate than bronchoscopy–FNA in the diagnosis of malignant enlarged mediastinal lymph nodes.[15,16] Additionally, the availability of bronchoscopy with transbronchial FNA may be limited, as a 1991 survey found that only 12% of bronchoscopists in the USA perform transbronchial FNA, which suggests this technique may not be widely available.[17] Transbronchial EUS-FNA is a newly described technique that has not been compared to transesophageal EUS-FNA for diagnosing mediastinal lesions.[18,19] Mediastinoscopy requires general anesthesia and has a 2% morbidity rate.[20] It also has difficulty reaching subcarinal and posterior aortopulmonic lymph nodes, which are easily accessible with EUS-FNA.

DIFFERENTIAL DIAGNOSIS OF ENLARGED POSTERIOR MEDIASTINAL LYMPH NODES

Enlarged mediastinal lymph nodes are usually defined by CT findings of lymph nodes ≥1 cm in diameter. In the setting of a peripheral lung mass and mediastinal lymph nodes, the main concern is that of primary lung cancer with metastatic disease. The finding of numerous posterior mediastinal and hilar lymph nodes raises the question as to whether the diagnosis is benign (sarcoid, histoplasmosis, tuberculosis, reactive) or malignant (especially lymphoma). Often the clinical history suggests the etiology, especially based on geographic location of the patient.

MALIGNANT POSTERIOR MEDIASTINAL LYMPH NODES

The rate of malignancy diagnosis in EUS-FNA of posterior mediastinal nodes of patients without a known diagnosis of cancer varies depending on prior bronchoscopic evaluation and local referral patterns, but is approximately 50%, with most cancers of pulmonary origin.[21–23] Table 9.2 shows the reported diagnostic operating characteristics of EUS-FNA for diagnosing malignancy in posterior mediastinal adenopathy. The overall sensitivity, specificity, and accuracy is greater than 90%.

Metastatic disease to the posterior mediastinum from primary pulmonary tumors

Lung cancer is generally divided into small cell and non-small cell lung cancer (NSCLC) pathologic types, with 80% of lung cancer due to NSCLC. EUS-FNA cytology can diagnose metastatic lung cancer to mediastinal lymph nodes from both small cell carcinoma and NSCLC. EUS-FNA is a very effective technique for diagnosing and staging lung cancer.[6,7] Further discussion of EUS-FNA in lung cancer staging is discussed in detail in Chapter 7.

Metastatic disease to the posterior mediastinum from extrathoracic malignancy

A variety of tumors result in metastases to the posterior mediastinum, appearing as either a lymph node or a mass (Fig. 9.3). Metastatic lymph nodes from breast, colonic, renal, testicular, laryngeal, pancreas, and esophageal cancer can be diagnosed by transthoracic EUS-FNA.[24–27]

Lymphoma

EUS-FNA can diagnose lymphoma in posterior mediastinal lymph nodes by obtaining material that can be evaluated by both cytology and flow cytometry.[28] If lymphoma is suspected, additional material should be sent for flow cytometry and immunocytochemistry stains. In one study the sensitivity of diagnosing lymphoma increased from 44% to 86% with the addition of flow cytometry and immunocytochemistry.[28] Lymphoma can be associated with granulomas on lymph node FNA cytology; therefore, if lymphoma is suspected, material should be sent for flow cytometry rather than concluding that the granulomas represent old infections or sarcoid. Sometimes it can be difficult to obtain sufficiently large quantities of adequate material on transesophageal EUS-FNA to diagnose lymphoma, and so more needle passes may be needed than for NSCLC. Tru-Cut needle biopsies may provide additional material for architectural evaluation of low-grade lymphomas.[29]

BENIGN POSTERIOR MEDIASTINAL LYMPH NODES

Reactive lymph nodes

Reactive lymph nodes are usually the result of previous pulmonary infections. They tend to be benign-appearing lymph

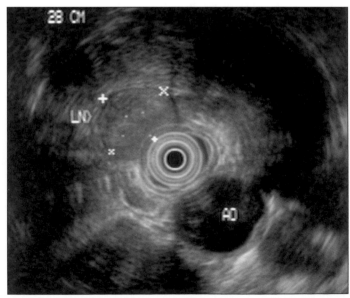

Fig. 9.3   EUS of metastatic renal cell carcinoma to the mediastinum.

nodes by EUS criteria. Cytologically, they appear as a mixture of lymphoid elements, with reactive and hyperplastic features.

Granulomatous lymph nodes

EUS-FNA cytology is able to demonstrate granulomatous disease in lymph nodes. The cytologic appearance is that of histiocytes in a swirling pattern. The differential diagnosis includes sarcoid, histoplasmosis, tuberculosis, and coccidiomycosis. Lymphoma can also be associated with granulomas. The presence or absence of caseating granulomas does not necessarily help with the diagnosis, as caseation can be seen in all of the above conditions. Sending EUS-FNA cytologic material for fungal stains and culture, acid-fast bacillus stain, and mycobacterial culture can help to determine whether there is an infectious etiology.

Sarcoid

Sarcoid is a multisystem granulomatous disease of unknown etiology. It typically involves mediastinal lymph nodes. The final diagnosis is made using clinical criteria, and by excluding other causes of granulomatous disease. There is no pathognomic laboratory or pathologic finding. Serum angiotensin-converting enzyme (ACE) levels may be raised to support this diagnosis. The diagnosis of non-caseating granulomas in a mediastinal lymph node supports the diagnosis of sarcoid.

The EUS appearance of mediastinal sarcoid lymph nodes is generally that of several enlarged lymph nodes (Fig. 9.4). EUS-FNA can obtain granulomatous material to support the diagnosis of sarcoid with high accuracy (Table 9.2).[30–32] One retrospective study found the sensitivity and specificity of EUS-FNA for diagnosing granulomas in suspected sarcoid to be 89% and 96% respectively.[33] Another study found that EUS-FNA demonstrated non-caseating granulomas in 41 of 50 patients (82%) with a final clinical diagnosis of sarcoidosis.[32]

Histoplasmosis

Histoplasmosis, caused by infection with *Histoplasma capsulatum*, is found worldwide. Within the USA, infection is most common in the mid-western states located in the Ohio and Mississippi River valleys. It is commonly associated with enlarged mediastinal adenopathy. The diagnosis is typically made by histopathology, serologic testing, and/or antigen testing.[34] Histoplasmosis is usually suspected because of either pulmonary symptoms or incidentally found mediastinal adenopathy.

EUS-FNA can diagnose granulomas in patients with suspected histoplasmosis.[35,36] Histoplasmosis should be suspected in patients with enlarged posterior mediastinal lymph nodes and EUS-FNA granulomas if they have spent time in areas endemic for *Histoplasma* infection.

Histoplasmosis can also cause dysphagia as a result of enlarged, fibrosing nodes compressing the esophagus (Fig. 9.5). The EUS appearance of mediastinal histoplasmosis causing dysphagia includes the finding of a large mass of matted lymph nodes that are adherent to a focally thickened esophageal wall.[36] The nodes can contain calcification, which is also suggestive of *Histoplasma* infection.

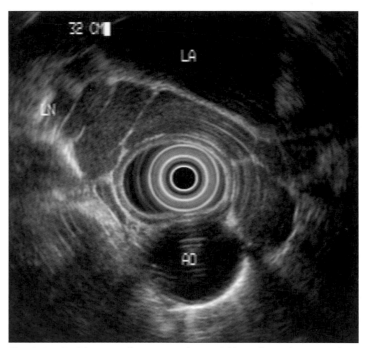

Fig. 9.4   EUS image of presumed sarcoid lymph node. Note that there are several lymph nodes adjacent to one another.

Tuberculosis

Mycobacterium tuberculosis can cause enlarged mediastinal lymph nodes, as well as a lymph node tuberculoma mass (Fig. 9.6). EUS-FNA can obtain material for *M. tuberculosis* culture.[23,31,37–39] Patients with granulomas identified on EUS-FNA should have material submitted for mycobacterial culture. The addition of polymerase chain reaction testing for *M. tuberculosis* in samples obtained by EUS-FNA has been reported to increase the diagnostic yield compared to cytology and culture in patients suspected of having tuberculosis.[40]

IMPACT OF EUS-FNA OF MEDIASTINAL LYMPH NODES ON SUBSEQUENT THORACIC SURGERY RATES

One study found that, of 59 patients with mediastinal adenopathy who were referred for surgical mediastinoscopy

DIAGNOSTIC ACCURACY OF EUS-FNA FOR SARCOIDOSIS				
Reference	Year	*n*	Sensitivity (%)	Specificity (%)
Fritscher-Ravens et al.[31]	2000	19	100	94
Wildi et al.[33]	2004	28	89	96
Annema et al.[32]	2005	50	82	–
Overall			90	95

Table 9.3   Diagnostic accuracy of EUS-FNA for sarcoidosis

Chapter 10

How to Perform EUS in the Stomach

Robert H. Hawes and Paul Fockens

There are two methods for examining the stomach: the balloon inflation and the water-filled stomach methods. The balloon inflation method is best for rapid screening of submucosal lesions and for examination of perigastric structures, whereas the water-filled method is best for examining the gastric wall layers and for careful and accurate examination of specific abnormalities. If one wishes to do a rapid screening of the gastric wall or a quick evaluation for perigastric structures, we recommend advancing the tip of the echoendoscope into the pre-pyloric antrum. The balloon is fully or overinflated and continuous suction is applied to remove air to the gastric lumen. With the gastric wall completely collapsed around the balloon, the scope is withdrawn slowly. The examiner's eyes should then be fixed on both the gastric wall and the perigastric structures, and then, when an abnormality is recognized, specific techniques can be applied to obtain detailed imaging.

With the water-filled method, the stomach is collapsed and 200–400 ml fluid is then usually instilled into the gastric lumen. High-quality imaging of the gastric wall requires attention to detail on two points: (1) to achieve perpendicular imaging to the gastric wall and (2) to position the gastric wall within the focal length of the transducer (see Ch. 2, Principles of ultrasound). To obtain superfine images with the water-filled method, one should consider using an agent to paralyze peristalsis, and instill water into the gastric lumen in a way that minimizes the production of micro-bubbles.

A significant challenge for imaging in the stomach arises from the fact that, in some areas, it may be difficult to obtain perpendicular imaging. This is particularly difficult in the antrum. It may be impossible to adjust the tip deflection in a way that allows the tip of the echoendoscope to lie perpendicular to an antral lesion while at the same time maintaining a 1–2-cm distance from the surface of the lesion. The consequence of an inability to achieve optimal orientation between the transducer and the surface of the stomach is tangential imaging. When the ultrasound waves cut across gastric surface lesions, it can be difficult to determine an accurate depth of penetration. For a large bulky tumor, where one is assessing T3 versus T4, this is less of an issue than with very superficial lesions in which you are trying to determine whether endoscopic mucosal resection is appropriate. In the antrum, it is sometimes easier to use a dual-channel endoscope and a high-frequency catheter probe to achieve good positioning. However, if the lesion is large, then depth of penetration of the catheter probe is insufficient for accurate staging.

Submucosal Lesions

Eun Young (Ann) Kim

KEY POINTS

- EUS can accurately differentiate a mural lesion from an extrinsic compression against the gut wall.

- Determination of the etiology of an intramural lesion is based on its layer of origin and internal echo characteristics.

- The finding of an intact submucosal layer running deep into a mural lesion indicates that the lesion can be removed safely by endomucosal resection.

- Carcinoid tumors can usually be diagnosed with standard mucosal biopsies because they emanate from the deep mucosal layer.

- Leiomyomas can be differentiated from gastrointestinal stromal tumors by immunohistochemical staining for the *c-kit* proto-oncogene protein (also known as CD117).

INTRODUCTION

The term submucosal lesion is used by endoscopists to describe any bulge covered with normal mucosa, usually found incidentally during gastrointestinal (GI) endoscopy or barium contrast radiography. Actually this lesion could be either an intramural subepithelial mass or an impression caused by extramural structures. The prevalence of suspected gastric submucosal lesions at routine endoscopy is not high, and has been reported as 0.36%.[1] To characterize the cause of protrusion, some non-invasive imaging methods, such as transabdominal ultrasonography, computed tomography (CT), and magnetic resonance imaging (MRI), have been used, but are often insufficient. However, endoscopic ultrasonography (EUS) has the ability to visualize clearly the structure of gut wall layers. Thus, EUS can not only differentiate subepithelial lesions from extraluminal structures, but also identify the layers of origin and endosonographic characteristics of the intraluminal lesions.[2–7] EUS is now accepted as the best modality for visualization of submucosal lesions with high precision.

The differential diagnosis of submucosal lesions includes a wide variety of benign and malignant subepithelial neoplasms, as well as non-neoplastic lesions. To evaluate submucosal lesions, the transition zone (the area where the tumor arises from normal gut wall layers) should be examined carefully to determine the layer of origin. Next, the size and echo pattern of the tumor, such as the smoothness of the border, internal features, echogenicity, and vascularity, should be observed. In addition, the presence of adjacent adenopathy provides valuable information. From the information gathered, a differential diagnosis of the submucosal tumor is possible with reasonable accuracy (Table 11.1).[7] Diagnostic information on the submucosal mass, including the origin of the wall layer provided by EUS, may also help in deciding whether a lesion should be removed or followed in situ.[8,9] Lesions confined to the mucosal or submucosal layers can be safely removed endoscopically. Surgical resection, if needed, is generally recommended for lesions located deep in muscularis propria, although several studies have shown no significant risk with endoscopic resection of lesions arising in the muscularis propria.[10]

COMPARISON OF ACCURACY BETWEEN EUS AND OTHER IMAGING MODALITIES

Differentiation of submucosal lesions is one of the main indications for EUS. Compared with endoscopy, barium contrast radiography, ultrasonography, CT, and MRI, EUS has a higher accuracy in detecting and assessing the size and location of subepithelial lesions (Table 11.2).[11]

When viewed endoscopically, the surface of submucosal lesions is usually smooth and has a similar color to the surrounding mucosa, without ulceration or erosion. Sometimes these lesions show a slight color change and morphologic characteristics, but it is often impossible to differentiate them with endoscopy.

Ultrasonography provides diagnostic information only for very large submucosal lesions. In a study of patients with endosonographically diagnosed gastric submucosal lesions, 82.5% of tumors were visualized and measured by ultrasonography after filling the stomach with water.[12] Uultrasonography can also provide useful information on perigastric structures, like CT and MRI. Using preoperative CT, large submucosal tumors previously identified by EUS could be visualized in only two-thirds of cases.[11] However, CT and MRI were able to diagnose large lipomas and malignant gastrointestinal stromal tumors (GISTs), especially those with metastatic spread.[13–15]

In addition to detection, EUS can establish the precise location of the lesion within the GI wall and give information

EUS CHARACTERISTICS OF VARIOUS SUBMUCOSAL TUMORS

Etiology	EUS layers	EUS appearance
Gastrointestinal stromal tumor	Fourth or second	Hypoechoic mass (irregular borders, echogenic foci, anechoic spaces suggest malignancy)
Aberrant pancreas	Second, third, and/or fourth	Hypoechoic or mixed echogenicity (anechoic ductal structure may be present)
Lipoma	Third	Hyperechoic
Carcinoids	Second and/or third	Mildly hypoechoic, homogeneous
Granular cell tumors	Second or third	Homogeneous mass with smooth borders
Cysts	Third	Anechoic, round or oval (3- or 5-layer walls suggestive of duplication cyst)
Varices	Third	Anechoic, tubular, serpiginous
Inflammatory fibroid polyp	Second and/or third	Hypoechoic, homogeneous or mixed echogenicity, indistinct margin
Glomus tumor	Third or fourth	Hypoechoic, smooth margin, internal heterogeneous echo mixed with high echoic spots
Metastatic deposits	Any or all	Hypoechoic, heterogeneous

Table 11.1 EUS characteristics of various submucosal tumors
Reproduced by permission of The American Society of Gastrointestinal Endoscopy.[7]

VISUALIZATION OF SUBMUCOSAL TUMORS BY EUS, UPPER GI SERIES, AND CT

Tumor localization[a]	EUS	Visualization by GI series	CT
Esophagus (n=14)	14/14	4/6	6/8
Stomach (n=20)	20/20	5/5	8/13
Duodenum (n=3)	3/3	2/2	2/3

Table 11.2 Visualization of submucosal tumors by EUS, upper GI series, and CT
[a] All tumors were previously diagnosed or suspected at upper GI endoscopy.
Reproduced by permission of Thomas Rösch.[11]

COMPARISON OF ACCURACY OF EUS WITH EXTRACORPOREAL ULTRASONOGRAPHY AND CT IN DIFFERENTIATING BETWEEN SUBMUCOSAL TUMOR AND EXTRALUMINAL COMPRESSIONS

	EUS	Ultrasonography	CT
No. of patients	68	68	39
Correct diagnosis	68	15	16
Misdiagnosis	0	53	24
Accuracy (%)	100	22	28

Table 11.3 Comparison of accuracy of EUS with extracorporeal ultrasonography and CT in differentiating between submucosal tumor and extraluminal compressions
Reproduced by permission of Q.-L. Zhang.[18]

on the sonographic characteristics of the submucosal tumor. The narrow differential diagnosis of subepithelial lesions afforded by the use of EUS enhances appropriate management decision-making. Based on EUS, the clinician can decide between observation with re-examination in patients with suspected benign lesions, or resection where the lesion is likely to be malignant.

In the differentiation between submucosal lesions and extraluminal compression, EUS also demonstrates higher accuracy than endoscopy, ultrasonography, and CT. Endoscopy was able to differentiate submucosal lesions from extraluminal compressions with a sensitivity and specificity of 87% and 29%, respectively, in a multicenter study.[16] In another study, [17] ultrasonography and CT established the diagnosis in only 16%, compared with 100% for EUS. Another comparison of ultrasonography, CT, and EUS reported an accuracy of 22%, 28%, and 100%, respectively, in differentiating submucosal tumors and extraluminal compressions (Table 11.3).[18]

EXTRALUMINAL LESIONS

EXAMINATION CHECKLIST

Check the integrity of the five wall layers between the lesion and the gut lumen

As EUS is able to visualize the gut wall layers in detail, it can readily differentiate the intramural and extramural nature of submucosal lesions. When EUS demonstrates the integrity of all gut wall layers between the gut lumen and the lesion, it is safe to say that the lesion is an impression caused by an extraluminal structure.

Extramural lesions may be adjacent to normal structures or pathologic masses. A normal spleen usually makes an impression in the gastric fundus and upper body (Fig. 11.1), and the gallbladder compresses the gastric antrum. Transient gastric impression is often caused by bowel loops. Other causes of gastric impression include vessels in the splenic hilum, the pancreatic tail, and the left lobe of the liver. Abnormal structures such as pancreatic pseudocysts, splenic artery aneurysm, aortic aneurysm, cystic tumor of the pancreas or liver, colonic tumors, and lymphoma may also produce endoscopically visible impressions on the gastric wall.

Adjacent structures, such as the aortic arch and vertebrae, can also press on the esophagus. Other potential causes of esophageal impression are vascular anomalies, such as a right descending aortic arch, anomalous branches of the aortic arch, aneurysms, and left atrial dilation. Enlarged mediastinal lymph nodes or mediastinal tumors, lung cancer, and lymphomas are also known to compress the esophagus.

Using EUS, the suspected area of gastric impression should be observed by the 'two-step' method. First, at a low frequency of 7.5 MHz, the examiner should survey the gross relation between the extramural structure and the gut wall. Then, at a higher frequency of 12 MHz, the outer hyperechoic serosal layer should be observed carefully to determine whether it is intact or disrupted. This method allows reliable differentiation between gastric wall impression and gastric wall infiltration caused by an extragastric tumor. In the esophagus, the endosonographer may encounter difficulties in this evaluation owing to interference from the air-filled bronchial system.

EVALUATION OF SUBMUCOSAL LESIONS

EXAMINATION CHECKLIST

Carefully examine the transition zone between the normal gut wall and the lesion to determine the layer of origin
Measure the size of the lesion and observe the echo pattern, for example echogenicity, internal features, vascularity, and smoothness of the border
Check the presence of adjacent lymphadenopathy

GASTROINTESTINAL STROMAL TUMOR

DIAGNOSTIC CHECKLIST

Origin in second or fourth gastric wall layer
Well circumscribed, hypoechoic, homogeneous mass
If malignant, features of heterogeneous echo texture with hyperechoic foci and/or anechoic necrotic zones, irregular extraluminal border, and adjacent malignant-looking lymphadenopathy are noticeable

GISTs are some of the most common mesenchymal tumors in the GI tract, and are also the most commonly identified intramural subepithelial mass in the upper GI tract. Previously, these tumors were classified as GI smooth muscle tumors, such as leiomyomas and leiomyosarcomas, owing to histologic findings of circular palisades of spindle cells with prominent nuclei and apparent origin in the muscularis propria layer of the gut wall. However, with the development of new molecular markers and an improved understanding of their biologic behavior, GISTs are now classified as a distinctive but heterogeneous group of mesenchymal tumors with varying differentiation. Interstitial cells of Cajal, also known as pacemaker cells of the GI tract, are now believed to be the precursor of GISTs. GISTs express *kit*, and show gain-of-function *kit* mutations. With immunohistochemical staining techniques, most GISTs are positive for c-*kit* (CD117) and CD34, but negative for desmin. However, leiomyomas express smooth muscle actin and desmin, and schwannomas produce S-100 protein and neuron-specific enolase.[19]

According to the recent classification, about 80% of GI mesenchymal tumors are GISTs. Approximately 10–30% of GISTs are malignant.[20] Leiomyomas are the most common mesenchymal tumors in the esophagus, but they rarely occur in the stomach and small bowel. In contrast, GISTs are rare in the esophagus, and are more common in the stomach (60–70%) and small bowel (20–25%).[21]

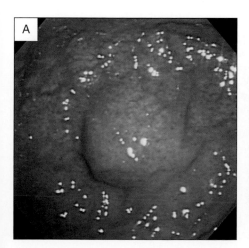
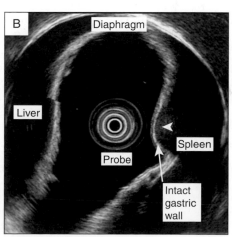

Fig. 11.1 Extraluminal compression. **A,** Endoscopic image of gastric wall compression by normal spleen. An ill defined, elevated area is seen at the gastric fundus. **B,** Endosonographic view of spleen (arrow) compressing the gastric wall.

The most common symptoms associated with GISTs are vague abdominal discomfort or pain, but most lesions are small (<2 cm) and asymptomatic. Larger lesions (>2 cm) may be ulcerated on top of the mass and present with bleeding or anemia. Occasionally GISTs cause intestinal obstruction.

In defining the prognosis of patients with GIST, it has been recommended that a 'grading as to the risk of aggressive behavior' be used instead of the term 'benign'. This means that no GIST can be definitively labeled as benign, and all are considered to have some malignant potential. Pathologists classify GISTs into 'very low risk', 'low risk', 'intermediate risk', and 'high risk' groups according to the size of the mass and the mitotic count of the resected specimen.[22]

Endosonographically, a GIST is typically a well circumscribed hypoechoic, homogeneous mass that can arise from either the second hypoechoic layer (muscularis mucosae) (Fig. 11.2) or the fourth hypoechoic layer (muscularis propria) (Fig. 11.3). GISTs, leiomyomas, and schwannomas cannot be differentiated with EUS without special immunohistochemical tissue staining. The sensitivity and accuracy of diagnosing GISTs has been reported as 95% and 87%, respectively.[23]

When malignant changes occur, GISTs show heterogeneous echo texture with hyperechoic deposits and/or anechoic necrotic zones inside large tumors (Fig. 11.4). According to one report,[24] EUS findings of tumor size greater than 4 cm, an irregular extraluminal border, echogenic foci, and anechoic spaces are good indicators of malignancy. The sensitivity ranged between 80% and 100% in detecting malignancy, when at least two out of four features were present.[24] Another study[25] found a correlation with malignancy when irregular extraluminal margins, cystic spaces, and lymph nodes were seen. The presence of two out of these three features had a positive predictive value of 100% for malignant or borderline malignant tumors.[25] Nonetheless, lack of defined risk factors cannot exclude a malignant potential. In addition to EUS, EUS-guided fine-needle aspiration (EUS-FNA) can be performed for immunohistochemical examination to achieve better diagnostic accuracy (Table 11.4).[23,26,27] EUS-FNA is discussed in greater detail below.

As small (<1 cm) asymptomatic mesenchymal tumors are rarely malignant, a policy of close follow-up with EUS may be justified, although an optimal surveillance strategy has not yet been established. Excision is advised when growth of the lesion, a change in the echo pattern, or necrosis is noted from yearly follow-up with EUS. Surgical treatment is indicated for lesions greater than 3 cm in diameter with features suggestive of malignancy. For lesions between 1 and 3 cm, EUS-FNA can

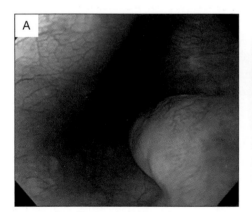
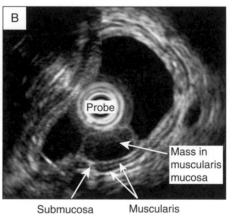

Fig. 11.2 Esophageal leiomyoma. **A,** Endoscopic image shows an elongated submucosal lesion visible in the mid esophagus. **B,** Endosonographic view using a 20-MHz catheter probe. The lesion is homogeneous, hypoechoic, and associated with muscularis mucosae.

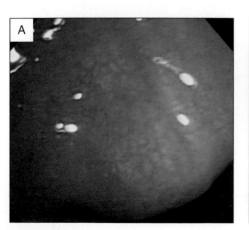
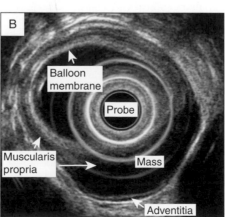

Fig. 11.3 Esophageal benign GIST. **A,** Endoscopic finding of histologically proven esophageal benign GIST. **B,** Radial scanning EUS image showing a homogeneous, hypoechoic mass arising from the fourth sonographic layer, corresponding to the muscularis propria.

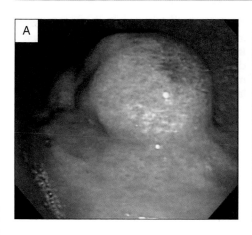

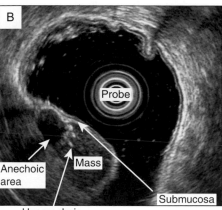

Fig. 11.4 Malignant GIST of the stomach. **A,.** Endoscopy shows a submucosal mass in the body of the stomach. **B,** Radial scanning EUS image of histologically proven malignant GIST showing hyperechoic spots and an anechoic area. The mass is contiguous with the fourth sonographic layer.

be recommended. When the lesion is confirmed to be a GIST, the risk of malignant transformation needs to be discussed with the patient; more careful follow-up or early resection should be considered.

ABERRANT PANCREAS

DIAGNOSTIC CHECKLIST

Origin in the second, third, and/or fourth layers
Hypoechoic or mixed echogenicity with internal anechoic ductal structure

The term aberrant pancreas is used to describe ectopic pancreatic tissue lying outside its normal location with no anatomic or vascular connection to the pancreas proper. These lesions are also termed ectopic pancreas, pancreatic rest, and heterotopic pancreas. They are typically discovered incidentally during endoscopy, surgery, or autopsy. Aberrant pancreas is encountered in about 1 of every 500 operations performed in the upper abdomen, and the incidence in autopsy series has been estimated as between 0.6% and 13.7%.[28] Aberrant pancreas is usually located in the stomach wall (frequently along the greater curvature of the antrum), duodenum, small intestine, or anywhere in the GI tract. Patients with aberrant pancreas are usually asymptomatic, but rare complications are pancreatitis, cyst formation, ulceration, bleeding, gastric outlet obstruction, obstructive jaundice, and malignancy.[29]

On endoscopy, an aberrant pancreas appears as a submucosal nodule, usually small, with a characteristic central umbilication that corresponds to a draining duct. The characteristic EUS features of aberrant pancreas are heterogeneous lesions, mainly hypoechoic or intermediate echogenic masses accompanied by scattered small hyperechoic areas, with indistinctive margins within the gut wall (Fig. 11.5). Generally, anechoic area and fourth layer thickening accompany the lesions. Anechoic cystic or tubular structures within the lesion correlate with ductal structures. They commonly arise from the third and fourth layers.[30] However, lesions may develop in one of the two layers, with varying location from mucosal to serosal.

The management of aberrant pancreas remains controversial. It should be guided by symptoms and the possibility of malignancy. Asymptomatic lesions do not necessarily require resection, and can be followed expectantly. If needed, endo-

DIAGNOSTIC ACCURACY OF EUS AND EUS-FNA FOR GASTROINTESTINAL STROMAL TUMORS (GISTS)					
Reference	No. of patients	Sensitivity (%)	Specificity (%)	Accuracy (%)	Diagnostic method
Okubo et al.[26] (2004)	14	40	100	79	EUS-FNA[a]
Brand et al.[23] (2002)	44	95	72	87	EUS[b]
Ando et al.[27] (2002)	23	83	77	78	EUS[c]
Ando et al.[27] (2002)	23	67	100	91	EUS-FNA[c]

Table 11.4 Diagnostic accuracy of EUS and EUS-FNA for gastrointestinal stromal tumors (GISTs)
EUS-FNA, endoscopic ultrasound-guided fine-needle aspiration.
[a] For differentiating between low- and high-grade malignancy of GISTs.
[b] For diagnosis of GISTs.
[c] For differentiating between benign and malignant GISTs.

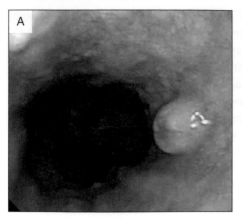

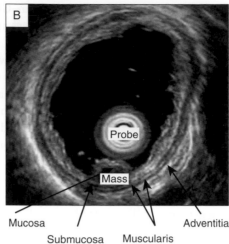

Fig. 11.8 Granular cell tumor of the esophagus. **A,** Small, round, molar tooth-like, polypoid lesion in the esophagus. **B,** Endosonographic image acquired with a 20-MHz mini-probe shows the nine-layered structure of the esophageal wall. A homogeneous, hypoechoic lesion with smooth margins is noted within the fourth layer.

myogenic tumors with advanced cystic degeneration, and gastric tuberculomas.

Gastric cyst is a rare clinical entity and is usually asymptomatic. It may result from a resolved inflammatory process. Endosonographically, the cysts appear in the submucosal layer of the gastric wall as sharply demarcated anechoic, rounded or ovoid structures with dorsal acoustic accentuation (Fig. 11.9). The inflammatory cyst always shows a single hyperechoic wall layer.

In adults, foregut cysts usually are asymptomatic and discovered incidentally during radiographic or endoscopic examination. Foregut cysts are categorized on the basis of their anomalous embryonic origin into bronchogenic and neuroenteric cysts. Bronchogenic cysts represent 50%–60% of all mediastinal cysts.[43] They can be diagnosed easily with EUS. Duplication cysts may involve the entire GI tract, with the ileum the most common site. The stomach is the least common site for GI duplication cysts. When examined endoscopically, duplication cysts may have a slightly transparent appearance. Endosonographic findings of duplication cysts are usually anechoic, homogeneous lesions with regular margins

arising from the third layer or extrinsic to the GI wall. The walls of duplication cysts may be shown as three- or five-layer structures because of the presence of submucosa or muscle layer.[44,45] Duplication cysts are believed to have a low malignant potential, but case reports have described malignant transformation. Complications are rare, and may include dysphagia, abdominal pain, bleeding, and pancreatitis when located near the ampulla of Vater.

VARICES

DIAGNOSTIC CHECKLIST

Origin in third layer
Anechoic, tubular, serpiginous mass

Patients with portal hypertension may have varices. Endoscopically, gastric varices can be misdiagnosed as submucosal tumors or thickened gastric folds. When found incidentally

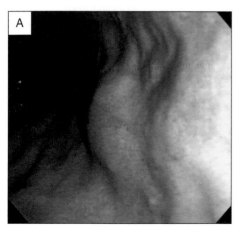

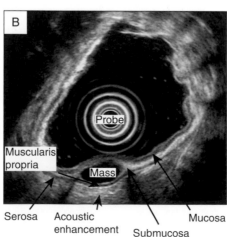

Fig. 11.9 Gastric cyst. **A,** Endoscopic view of a smooth bulge in the body of the stomach. **B.** EUS revealed a sharply demarcated, anechoic, ovoid structure within the third gastric wall layer.

during endoscopy in a patient with no relevant information, it is highly inappropriate and potentially hazardous to take a biopsy from such a lesion without EUS examination. On EUS, fundic varices appear as small, round to oval, and anechoic structures within the submucosa. They can be differentiated from submucosal cysts, which usually occur as solitary lesions, from their shape and easy compressibility by the ultrasound balloon. When gastric varices get larger, they appear as anechoic, serpentine, tubular structures with smooth margins, accompanied by perigastric collateral vessels (Fig. 11.10). In severe portal hypertension, cross-sections of multiple fundic varices may show a 'Swiss cheese pattern'.[46]

In portal hypertensive gastropathy, EUS findings are often normal and endosonographic intramural vessel changes are not normally observed. However, dilation of the azygos vein and thoracic duct, and thickening of gastric mucosa and submucosa, have also been reported.[47] In comparative studies, EUS was inferior to endoscopy for detecting and grading esophageal varices, but was able to detect fundic varices earlier and more often than endoscopy in patients with portal hyper-

tension.[48] EUS could be used in the treatment of varices, making it possible to inject sclerosing agent into perforating veins.[49]

INFLAMMATORY FIBROID POLYPS

DIAGNOSTIC CHECKLIST

Origin in second and/or third layer
Hypoechoic, homogeneous lesion with indistinct margins

Inflammatory fibroid polyp (IFP) is a rare benign polypoid lesion, usually found in the stomach, occasionally in the small bowel, and rarely in the esophagus or large bowel.[50] The lesion is located in the second and/or third sonographic layer of the gastric wall, with an intact fourth layer. The usual echo-endoscopic features of IFP are indistinct margin, hypoechoic, and homogeneous echo pattern (Fig. 11.11). These findings

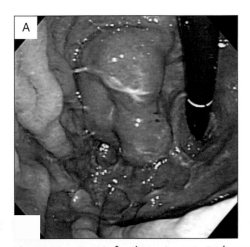
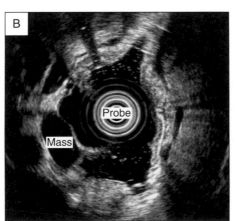
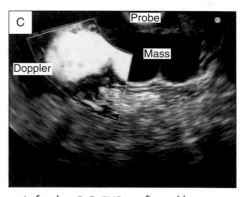

Fig. 11.10   Gastric fundic varices. **A,** Endoscopic view of a large bulging mass lesion at the gastric fundus. **B,C,** EUS confirmed large, anechoic, tubular, submucosal vessels with multiple extramural collateral vascular structures.

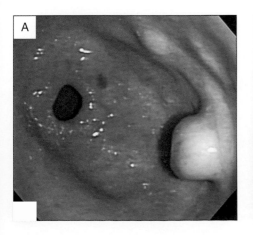
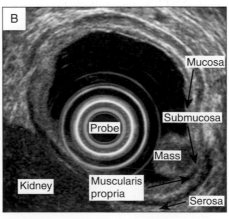

Fig. 11.11   Inflammatory fibroid polyp. **A,** Endoscopic image of a small, round, polypoid lesion at the gastric antrum. **B,** Gastric EUS demonstrates a homogeneous hypoechoic lesion with indistinct margins located deep in the mucosal layer.

correlate well with the histologic findings of proliferated, non-encapsulated fibrous tissue with vascular elements and eosinophilic infiltration, located in deep mucosal and submucosal layers. Sometimes, the internal echo is heterogeneous or hyperechoic. In that case, the inner hyperechoic area and bright echos correspond to the presence of many small blood vessels.[51]

The EUS patterns of leiomyomas originating from the muscularis mucosae and carcinoid tumors may be similar to that of IFP. However, these tumors have a distinctive margin.

RARE LESIONS

Many uncommon lesions have been reported in the endosonographic literature. The number of lesions is too small for their appearance on EUS to be described as characteristic. Some examples are given below.

The glomus tumor of the stomach presents as a circumscribed, low echoic mass in the third or fourth layer; it has an internal heterogeneous echo mixed with high echoic spots.[52] Glandular cysts present as small nodular to polypoid lesions in the body of the stomach. They create a uniform, relatively hyperechoic, internal echo pattern in the upper mucosa, but do not disrupt the normal layer pattern of the gastric wall.[46]

Distant metastases may also develop into submucosal masses in the GI tract. They appear as hypoechoic heterogeneous masses, and may involve any or all of the sonographic layers. Extrinsic malignant tumors directly infiltrating the gut wall and presenting as submucosal lesions can also be visualized by EUS.

TISSUE SAMPLING FOR HISTOLOGIC ASSESSMENT OF SUBEPITHELIAL LESIONS

During endoscopic examination of submucosal lesion, biopsies of the mucosa overlying the lesion are recommended to confirm the intact epithelium. Nevertheless, when the lesion appears cystic or vascular, biopsy should not be attempted before EUS.

Some subepithelial masses arising from the lamina propria or muscularis mucosae may be diagnosed on standard endoscopic forceps biopsy. However, for most submucosal lesions, mucosal biopsy is inconclusive. Conventional EUS does not provide a histologic diagnosis of subepithelial lesions. Recently, EUS-FNA was introduced to obtain specimens for cytologic examination. However, the sensitivity, specificity, and accuracy of cytologic evaluation of intramural lesions are lower than those for lymph nodes or organs adjacent to the GI tract. In one study, the sensitivity of EUS-FNA was 88% for mediastinal masses, 81% for mediastinal lymph nodes, 80% for celiac lymph nodes, 75% for pancreatic tumors, and 60% for submucosal tumors.[53] To overcome some limitations of EUS-FNA, EUS-guided core-needle biopsy has been introduced. Using a needle with a guillotine tip, adequate tissue was obtained in

more cases and no major complications occurred.[54,55] The average reported accuracy of EUS-FNA in the diagnosis of submucosal lesions is about 80% (Table 11.5).[36,55-59] EUS-FNA with histologic and immunohistochemical analysis has a high accuracy in the differential diagnosis of mesenchymal tumors of the GI tract.[23,26,27] However, any form of needle biopsy carries the possibility of sampling error, and a negative finding does not exclude malignancy in GISTs.

SUMMARY

Subepithelial lesions involving the GI tract are difficult to diagnose definitively by conventional imaging methods such as gastrointestinal radiography, ultrasonography, CT, and MRI. Endoscopic views are limited and standard biopsy techniques have a low yield. EUS is an essential modality in the evaluation of these lesions. Any subepithelial lesion that appears to be larger than 1 cm on endoscopic examination, and is not regarded as a lipoma, should be referred for EUS evaluation.[61] With the unique ability of EUS to visualize the layers of the GI tract wall, identification of the layer of origin, assessment of size, extent, and sonographic characteristics of subepithelial lesions can be made.

A characteristic endosonographic appearance has been described for some submucosal lesions, including GISTs, aberrant pancreas, lipomas, carcinoid tumors, granular cell tumors, cysts, varices, and inflammatory fibroid polyps. However, EUS cannot reliably distinguish benign from malignant lesions, especially in terms of the malignant potential of GISTs. Addition of EUS-FNA can be helpful to obtain histologic or cytologic samples from submucosal lesions. However, the accuracy is relatively low compared with that for other targets, such as lymph nodes or pancreatic masses.

EUS is helpful in the selection of patients for endoscopic resection as it can help determine the depth and originating

DIAGNOSTIC ACCURACY OF EUS AND EUS-FNA FOR GASTROINTESTINAL SUBMUCOSAL LESIONS			
Reference	No. of patients	Accuracy (%)	Diagnostic method
Kwon et al.[60] (2005)	58	79.3	EUS
Arantes et al.[56] (2004)	10	80	EUS-FNA
Levy et al.[55] (2003)	5	80	EUS-FNB
Kojima et al.[36] (1999)	54	74	EUS
Matsui et al.[57] (1998)	15	93	EUS-FNA
Matsui et al.[57] (1998)	15	60	EUS
Gress et al.[58] (1997)	27	81	EUS-FNA
Wiersema et al.[59] (1997)	12	50	EUS-FNA

Table 11.5 Diagnostic accuracy of EUS and EUS-FNA for gastrointestinal submucosal lesions
EUS-FNA, endoscopic ultrasound-guided fine-needle aspiration; EUS-FNB, endoscopic ultrasound-guided fine-needle biopsy using a TruCut needle.

wall layer of the lesion. EUS can also be used in the follow-up of submucosal tumors left in situ. The follow-up interval depends on the index of suspicion of the examiner, and is usually 1 year. When the characteristics of the lesion do not change for two consecutive follow-up examinations with EUS, a longer follow-up interval would be justified. Further research is necessary to determine appropriate long-term surveillance guidelines.

EXAMINATION CHECKLIST

Transition zone – perpendicular imaging at the edge of the lesion produces an image that shows where the normal gut wall layers are merging into the lesion

Overlying layers – perpendicular imaging with the transducer positioned on top of the lesion (but not touching it) demonstrates which layer(s) overlie the lesion

REFERENCES

1 Hedenbro JL, Ekelund M, Wetterberg P. Endoscopic diagnosis of submucosal gastric lesions. The results after routine endoscopy. Surg Endosc 1991; 5:20–23.

2 Caletti G, Zani L, Bolondi L, et al. Endoscopic ultrasonography in the diagnosis of gastric submucosal tumor. Gastrointest Endosc 1989; 35:413–418.

3 Yasuda K, Nakajima M, Yoshida S, et al. The diagnosis of submucosal tumors of the stomach by endoscopic ultrasonography. Gastrointest Endosc 1989; 35:10–15.

4 Boyce GA, Sivak MV Jr, Rosch T, et al. Evaluation of submucosal upper gastrointestinal tract lesions by endoscopic ultrasound. Gastrointest Endosc 1991; 37:449–454.

5 Nesje LB, Laerum OD, Svanes K, et al. Subepithelial masses of the gastrointestinal tract evaluated by endoscopic ultrasonography. Eur J Ultrasound 2002; 15:45–54.

6 van Stolk RU. Subepithelial lesions. In: Van Dam J, Sivak MV, eds. Gastrointestinal Endosonography, 1st edn. Philadelphia: Saunders; 1999:153–165.

7 Chak A. EUS in submucosal tumors. Gastrointest Endosc 2002; 56(Suppl):S43–S48.

8 Shen EF, Arnott ID, Plevris J, et al. Endoscopic ultrasonography in the diagnosis and management of suspected upper gastrointestinal submucosal tumours. Br J Surg 2002; 89:231–235.

9 Nickl NJ, Bhutani MS, Catalano M, et al. Clinical implications of endoscopic ultrasound: the American Endosonography Club Study. Gastrointest Endosc 1996; 44:371–377.

10 Hyun JH, Jeen YT, Chun HJ, et al. Endoscopic resection of submucosal tumor of the esophagus: results in 62 patients. Endoscopy 1997; 29:165–170.

11 Rösch T, Lorenz R, Dancygier H, et al. Endosonographic diagnosis of submucosal upper gastrointestinal tract tumors. Scand J Gastroenterol 1992; 27:1–8.

12 Futagami K, Hata J, Haruma K, et al. Extracorporeal ultrasound is an effective diagnostic alternative to endoscopic ultrasound for gastric submucosal tumours. Scand J Gastroenterol 2001; 36:1222–1226.

13 Thompson WM, Kende AI, Levy AD. Imaging characteristics of gastric lipomas in 16 adult and pediatric patients. AJR Am J Roentgenol 2003; 181:981–985.

14 Hasegawa S, Semelka RC, Noone TC, et al. Gastric stromal sarcomas: correlation of MR imaging and histopathologic findings in nine patients. Radiology 1998; 208:591–595.

15 Scatarige JC, Fishman EK, Jones B, et al. Gastric leiomyosarcoma: CT observations. J Comput Assist Tomogr 1985; 9:320–327.

16 Rosch T, Kapfer B, Will U, et al. Accuracy of endoscopic ultrasonography in upper gastrointestinal submucosal lesions: a prospective multicenter study. Scand J Gastroenterol 2002; 37:856–862.

17 Motoo Y, Okai T, Ohta H, et al. Endoscopic ultrasonography in the diagnosis of extraluminal compressions mimicking gastric submucosal tumors. Endoscopy 1994; 26:239–242.

18 Zhang QL, Nian WD. Endoscopic ultrasonography diagnosis in submucosal tumor of stomach. Endoscopy 1998; 30(Suppl 1):A69–A71.

19 Miettinen M, Sobin LH, Lasota J. Gastrointestinal stromal tumors of the stomach: a clinicopathologic, immunohistochemical, and molecular genetic study of 1765 cases with long-term follow-up. Am J Surg Pathol 2005; 29:52–68.

20 Miettinen M, Sarlomo-Rikala M, Lasota J. Gastrointestinal tumors: recent advances in understanding of their biology. Hum Pathol 1999; 30:1213–1220.

21 Berman J, O'Leary TJ. Gastrointestinal stromal tumor workshop. Hum Pathol 2001; 32:578–582.

22 Fletcher CD, Berman JJ, Corless C, et al. Diagnosis of gastrointestinal stromal tumors: a consensus approach. Hum Pathol 2002; 33:459–465.

23 Brand B, Oesterhelweg L, Binmoeller KF, et al. Impact of endoscopic ultrasound for evaluation of submucosal lesions in gastrointestinal tract. Digest Liver Dis 2002; 34:290–297.

24 Chak A, Canto MI, Rosch T, et al. Endosonographic differentiation of benign and malignant stromal cell tumors. Gastrointest Endosc 1997; 45:468–473.

25 Palazzo L, Landi B, Cellier C, et al. Endosonographic features predictive of benign and malignant gastrointestinal stromal cell tumours. Gut 2000; 46:88–92.

26 Okubo K, Yamao K, Nakamura T, et al. Endoscopic ultrasound-guided fine-needle aspiration biopsy for the diagnosis of gastrointestinal stromal tumors in the stomach. J Gastroenterol 2004; 39:747–753.

27 Ando N, Goto H, Niwa Y, et al. The diagnosis of GI stromal tumors with EUS-guided fine needle aspiration with immunohistochemical analysis. Gastrointest Endosc 2002; 55:37–43.

28 Armstrong CP, King PM, Dixon JM, et al. The clinical significance of heterotopic pancreas in the gastrointestinal tract. Br J Surg 1981; 68:384–347.

29 Jovanovic I, Knezevic S, Micev M, et al. EUS mini probes in diagnosis of cystic dystrophy of duodenal wall in heterotopic pancreas: a case report. World J Gastroenterol 2004; 10:2609–2612.

30 Matsushita M, Hajiro K, Okazaki K, et al. Gastric aberrant pancreas: EUS analysis in comparison with the histology. Gastrointest Endosc 1999; 49:493–497.

31 Parmar JH, Lawrence R, Ridley NT. Submucous lipoma of the ileocaecal valve presenting as caecal volvulus. Int J Clin Pract 2004; 58:424–425.

32 Watanabe F, Honda S, Kubota H, et al. Preoperative diagnosis of ileal lipoma by endoscopic ultrasonography probe. J Clin Gastroenterol 2000; 31:245–247.

33 Zhou PH, Yao LQ, Zhong YS, et al. Role of endoscopic miniprobe ultrasonography in diagnosis of submucosal tumor of large intestine. World J Gastroenterol 2004; 10:2444–2446.

34 Garcia M, Buitrago E, Bejarano PA, et al. Large esophageal liposarcoma: a case report and review of the literature. Arch Pathol Lab Med 2004; 128:922–925.

35 Nakamura S, Iida M, Yao T, et al. Endoscopic features of gastric carcinoids. Gastrointest Endosc 1991; 37:535–538.

36 Kojima T, Takahashi H, Parra-Blanco A, et al. Diagnosis of submucosal tumor of the upper GI tract by endoscopic resection. Gastrointest Endosc 1999; 50:516–522.

37 Ichikawa J, Tanabe S, Koizumi W, et al. Endoscopic mucosal resection in the management of gastric carcinoid tumors. Endoscopy 2003; 35:203–206.

38 Matsumoto T, Iida M, Suekane H, et al. Endoscopic ultrasonography in rectal carcinoid tumors: contribution to selection of therapy. Gastrointest Endosc 1991; 37:539–542.

39 Nakachi A, Miyazato H, Oshiro T, et al. Granular cell tumor of the rectum: a case report and review of the literature. J Gastroenterol 2000; 35:631–634.

40 Love MH, Glaser M, Edmunds SE, et al. Granular cell tumour of the oesophagus: endoscopic ultrasound appearances. Australas Radiol 1999; 43:253–255.

41 Palazzo L, Landi B, Cellier C, et al. Endosonographic features of esophageal granular cell tumors. Endoscopy 1997; 29:850–853.

42 Hizawa K, Matsumoto T, Kouzuki T, et al. Cystic submucosal tumors in the gastrointestinal tract: endosonographic findings and endoscopic removal. Endoscopy 2000; 32:712–714.

43 Wildi SM, Hoda RS, Fickling W, et al. Diagnosis of benign cysts of the mediastinum: the role and risks of EUS and FNA. Gastrointest Endosc 2003; 58:362–368.

44 Geller A, Wang KK, DiMagno EP. Diagnosis of foregut duplication cysts by endoscopic ultrasonography. Gastroenterology 1995; 109:838–842.

45 Faigel DO, Burke A, Ginsberg GG, et al. The role of endoscopic ultrasound in the evaluation and management of foregut duplications. Gastrointest Endosc 1997; 45:99–103.

46 Dancygier H, Lightdale CJ. Endoscopic ultrasonography of the upper gastrointestinal tract and colon. In: Stevens PD (ed.) Endosonography in gastroenterology: principles, techniques, findings. New York: Thieme; 1999:76–89.

47 Faigel DO, Rosen HR, Sasaki A, et al. EUS in cirrhotic patients with and without prior variceal hemorrhage in comparison with noncirrhotic control subjects. Gastrointest Endosc 2000; 52:455–462.

48 Tio TL, Kimmings N, Rauws E, et al. Endosonography of gastroesophageal varices: evaluation and follow-up of 76 cases. Gastrointest Endosc 1995; 42:145–150.

49 Lahoti S, Catalano MF, Alcocer E, et al. Obliteration of esophageal varices using EUS-guided sclerotherapy with color Doppler. Gastrointest Endosc 2000; 51:331–333.

50 Matsushita M, Hajiro K, Okazaki K, et al. Endoscopic features of gastric inflammatory fibroid polyps. Am J Gastroenterol 1996; 91:1595–1598.

51 Matsushita M, Hajiro K, Okazaki K, et al. Gastric inflammatory fibroid polyps: endoscopic ultrasonographic analysis in comparison with the histology. Gastrointest Endosc 1997; 46:53–57.

52 Imamura A, Tochihara M, Natsui K, et al. 1: Glomus tumor of the stomach: endoscopic ultrasonographic findings. Am J Gastroenterol 1994; 89:271–272.

53 Giovannini M, Seitz JF, Monges G, et al. Fine-needle aspiration cytology guided by endoscopic ultrasonography: results in 141 patients. Endoscopy 1995; 27:171–177.

54 Varadarajulu S, Fraig M, Schmulewitz N, et al. Comparison of EUS-guided 19-gauge Trucut needle biopsy with EUS-guided fine-needle aspiration. Endoscopy 2004; 36:397–401.

55 Levy MJ, Jondal ML, Clain J, et al. Preliminary experience with an EUS-guided Trucut biopsy needle compared with EUS-guided FNA. Gastrointest Endosc 2003; 57:101–106.

56 Arantes V, Logrono R, Faruqi S, et al. Endoscopic sonographically guided fine-needle aspiration yield in submucosal tumors of the gastrointestinal tract. J Ultrasound Med 2004; 23:1141–1150.

57 Matsui M, Goto H, Niwa Y, et al. Preliminary results of fine needle aspiration biopsy histology in upper gastrointestinal submucosal tumors. Endoscopy 1998; 30:750–755.

58 Gress FG, Hawes RH, Savides TJ, et al. Endoscopic ultrasound-guided fine-needle aspiration biopsy using linear array and radial scanning endosonography. Gastrointest Endosc 1997; 45:243–250.

59 Wiersema MJ, Vilmann P, Giovannini M, et al. Endosonography-guided fine-needle aspiration biopsy: diagnostic accuracy and complication assessment. Gastroenterology 1997; 112:1087–1095.

60 Kwon JG, Kim EY, Kim YS, et al. Accuracy of endoscopic ultrasonographic impression compared with pathologic diagnosis in gastrointestinal submucosal tumors. Korean J Gastroenterol 2005; 45:88–96.

61 Hwang JH, Kimmey MB. The incidental upper gastrointestinal subepithelial mass. Gastroenterology 2004; 126:301–307.

Chapter

12

EUS in Gastric Cancer

Mitsuhiro Kida

KEY POINTS

- EUS is useful for staging gastric cancer but is an ineffective modality for screening.

- Two methods for imaging can be utilized: water-filled stomach and balloon contact.

- Endoscopic mucosal resection (EMR) can be applied to gastric cancer if the lesion is well differentiated and intramucosal (any size), or if ulcerative, with a diameter less than 3cm.

- If a gastric cancer extends into the superficial submucosal (<500μm), EMR can be performed if the diameter is less than 3cm.

INTRODUCTION

Endoscopic ultrasonography (EUS) has assumed an important role in the diagnosis and staging of malignant gastrointestinal and biliopancreas tumors since its development in 1980.[1,2] For malignant gastrointestinal tumors, an appropriate treatment such as endoscopic mucosal resection (EMR), surgical treatment, and chemotherapy can be chosen following EUS staging of the lesion. Endoscopy is usually performed prior to EUS to establish the diagnosis, which should be confirmed by histologic examination of biopsy specimen. Generally, ultrasonographic endoscopes with 360° radial sector scanners are used for local staging of tumors because of their maneuverability compared with ultrasonographic endoscopes with convex or linear scanners, which are used to perform EUS-guided fine-needle aspiration cytology/biopsy (EUS-FNAB).[3,4] However, EUS is not useful as a screening method as it takes considerable time to examine all of the upper gastrointestinal tract with this technique.

HOW TO VISUALIZE THE LESION

There are two scanning methods for diagnosing gastric lesions: the water-filling method and the balloon contact method. In general, the water-filling method is employed for small and flat lesions such as early gastric cancers, and the balloon contact method is used for large lesions such as advanced gastric cancer. It is difficult to detect early gastric cancer with conventional EUS, because early cancer is detected as an irregularity of the first layer and slightly thickened second and third layers of the stomach wall. Using the balloon contact method, therefore, it is sometimes problematic to identify the irregular first layer of flat lesions and the thickened stomach wall, which is compressed by the balloon. In this situation, an ultrasonic thin probe should be employed, as it is then easy to detect flat lesions with endoscopic guidance.

In the water-filling method, the stomach is washed with about 200ml of de-aerated water, which is aspirated again when mucus and food remnants are present. Generally 300–800ml de-aerated water is instilled into the stomach; the volume of water should be controlled by keeping the transectional stomach wall including the lesion circular. In practice, 300–500ml deareated water is used when there is a lesion in the body of the stomach, and 600–800ml in patients with a lesion of the antrum. However, lesions around the cardia, fornix, and pyloric ring are difficult to visualize by the water-filling method. When evaluable pictures cannot be obtained with the water-filling method, the balloon contact method should be tried.

To obtain a clear image, it is important to keep the transducer tip of ultrasonographic endoscope perpendicular to the lesion. As each transducer has its own focusing point, the distance between the ultrasonographic endoscope and the lesion should optimally be kept at 2–3cm for a 7.5-MHz transducer and 1–2cm for a 20-MHz transducer. The distance is controlled by manipulating with angle of scope, the volume of de-aerated water, changing the position of the patient from left lateral to prone or supine, and filling de-aerated water to the tip of the balloon, and so on.

INSTRUMENT

For staging gastric cancer, EUS with a radial scanning transducer is generally used because of the ease of manipulation and detection of lesions. There are two types of EUS: conventional EUS with normal endoscopy and an ultrasonic transducer, and an ultrasonic mini-probe (without endoscopic function). In addition, there are two scanning types of EUS: mechanical radial scanners (e.g., GF-UM2000; Olympus, Tokyo, Japan) and electronic radial scanners (e.g., GF-UE260; Olympus). With electronic scanning, it is possible to evaluate blood flow using the Doppler function.

Generally, conventional EUS is used for relatively large lesions such as advanced gastric cancer. The ultrasonic mini-probe is useful for small, flat lesions. As mentioned above, it is sometimes difficult to detect early gastric cancer with conventional EUS; in this situation an ultrasonic mini-probe should be employed, as it is easy to detect flat lesions with endoscopic guidance.

The first prototype scanner capable of performing three-dimensional EUS (3D-EUS) was developed in 1994, and the second generation of 3D-EUS scanners was commercialized in 1999,[5–7] although a 'home-built' 3D-EUS scanner was tried in 1991.[8] The 3D-EUS system consists of an image processor, an ultrasound unit, a probe driving unit, and two 3D-EUS scanning ultrasound probes (UM-DG20-25R (20 MHz) and UM-DG12-25R (12 MHz) (Fig. 12.1). While the 3D-EUS probe is pulled back in the sheath by the driving unit, its transducer carries out maximally 160 mechanical spiral scans, as in helical computed tomography (CT) (Fig. 12.2). Three-dimensional information is obtained from the area around the probe, and both a real-time radial image and a computer-reconstructed linear image are displayed simultaneously on the monitor. Images can be reviewed after scanning to select the optimal radial and linear images, and to adjust imaging conditions. Using 3D-EUS maximally, 160 consecutive radial images can be reviewed, so this method is expected to have a higher accuracy in determining the depth of gastric cancer invasion. With 3D-EUS, it is also possible to measure tumor volume.

INDICATIONS FOR EUS IN GASTRIC CANCER

Local staging

EUS is the most accurate method for local staging of gastric cancer.[9–18] The clinical utility of EUS depends on whether preoperative assessment of local tumor extent will affect the

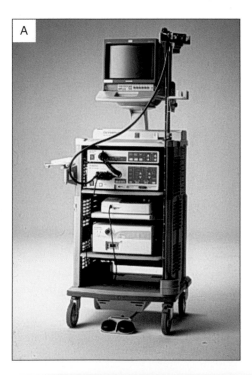

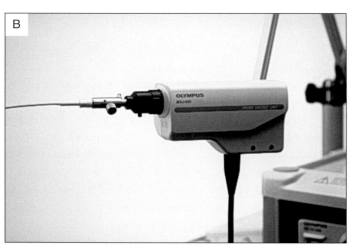

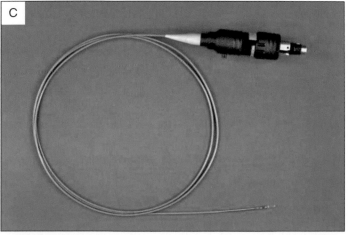

Fig. 12.1 A, Three-dimensional endoscopic ultrasonography (3D-EUS) system. **B,** Driving unit. **C,** 3D-EUS probe.

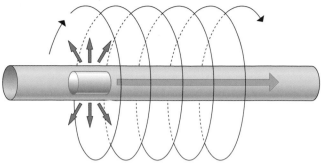

UM-DP20-25R: 20 MHz
UM-DP12-25R: 12 MHz
Scan: Mechanical spiral scan
Pitch: 1.0, 0.75, 0.5, 0.35, 0.25 mm
Range: 40, 30, 20, 15 mm
Maximum diameter: 2.5 mm

Fig. 12.2 Principle of three-dimensional endoscopic ultrasonography.

choice of therapeutic procedure. Several alternative procedures are currently available for the treatment of both early and advanced gastric cancer. Protocols with curative aim offer two possibilities. The first is a choice between conventional primary resection and local treatment such as EMR, laparoscopic resection, argon plasma coagulation (APC), photodynamic therapy, and laser treatment. According to the Japanese guidelines for gastric cancer,[19] the classic indication for EMR is intramural, well differentiated adenocarcinoma without ulceration or ulcer scar, and with a diameter of less than 2 cm. Furthermore, the indications for EMR have been widened recently:[19]

- Intramucosal, well differentiated adenocarcinoma without ulceration or ulcer scar, no size limitation
- Intramucosal, well differentiated adenocarcinoma with ulceration or ulcer scar, less than 3 cm in diameter
- sm1 (submucosal invasion less than 500 μm), well differentiated adenocarcinoma, less than 3 cm in diameter.

These cancers have no likelihood of distant metastasis, such as lymph node metastasis, and can therefore be treated curatively by endoscopic techniques.

The main role of EUS is to select candidates with the above indications. Therefore, m and sm1 tumors have to be differentiated from sm2 lesions (submucosal invasion more than 500 μm).

The second choice is between conventional primary resection and chemotherapy or radiation therapy. Secondary resection is proposed when there is a significant response to chemotherapy with tumor downstaging. If there is no response, treatment is shifted to palliation. Therefore, it is important to determine whether a stage T2 or T3 tumor is present, as these tumors are curable by surgical resection, and therefore primary resection is generally indicated. Patients with stage T4 tumors without distant metastasis will benefit from preoperative chemotherapy or radiation therapy. Secondary resection is proposed when there is a significant response to chemotherapy or radiation therapy (neoadjuvant therapy) with tumor

downstaging. If there is no response the treatment is shifted to palliation. EUS plays a role in this important decision. The overall accuracy of EUS is better than that of CT or magnetic resonance imaging (MRI), although it is still not completely satisfactory.

Differentiation and follow-up

It is sometimes difficult to diagnose scirrhous gastric cancer and malignant lymphoma by means of biopsy, even when endoscopic findings indicate a strong suspicion. In this situation, EUS may be important in differentiating these conditions from hyperplastic gastritis and Ménétrièr's disease.[20-22]

EUS is also employed to diagnose recurrence after surgery or local treatment such as APC, laser treatment, or photodynamic therapy, and chemotherapy.[11] Anastomotic recurrence of cancer is first diagnosed by forceps biopsy; however, EUS also has an important role in detecting recurrence of malignant tumor from benign tumorous lesions.[23] Using EUS, it is also possible to evaluate the efficacy of chemotherapy and endoscopic treatment in case of recurrence.

WALL STRUCTURE AND THE DIAGNOSIS OF GASTRIC CANCER INVASION

Normal gastric wall structure

Along the entire length of the digestive tract, the normal wall is visualized by EUS with 7.5–12-MHz transducers as a five-layered structure (Fig. 12.3).[24,25] From the digestive tract lumen inwards, the first hyperechoic and the second hypoechoic layers correspond to the mucosa, the third hyperechoic layer to the submucosa, the fourth hypoechoic layer to the muscularis propria, and the fifth hyperechoic layer to the subserosa and the serosa in the stomach.

Using high-frequency transducers (12–20 MHz, sometimes 30 MHz), the gastric wall is detected under optimal conditions as a nine-layer structure (Figs 12.3 & 12.4). In addition to the normal five layers, there is a border echo of the muscularis mucosae, a hypoechoic muscularis mucosae, a hypoechoic inner muscle, a border echo between inner and outer muscle, and a hypoechoic outer muscle.[26] However, with a high-frequency transducer, the gastric wall is usually visualized as a seven-layered structure without the components of the muscularis mucosae.

T staging

The tumor node metastasis (TNM) system is generally employed worldwide, but in Japan the Japanese classification is mainly used. According to the endoluminal shape of gastric tumors, protruded, flat, depressed, and ulcerated lesions can be visualized by EUS. The tumor mass itself may be classified as follows:

- T1 – thickening or tumor infiltration of the mucosal and submucosal layer, leaving the fourth layer (muscularis propria)

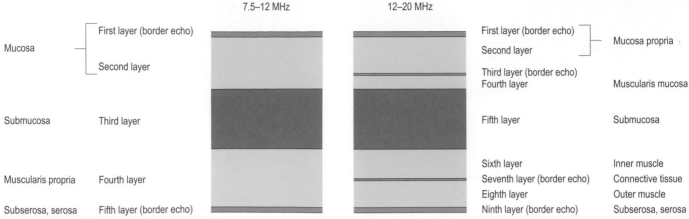

7.5–12 MHz   12–20 MHz

Mucosa — First layer (border echo) / Second layer

First layer (border echo) / Second layer — Mucosa propria

Third layer (border echo) / Fourth layer — Muscularis mucosa

Submucosa — Third layer

Fifth layer — Submucosa

Muscularis propria — Fourth layer

Sixth layer — Inner muscle
Seventh layer (border echo) — Connective tissue
Eighth layer — Outer muscle

Subserosa, serosa — Fifth layer (border echo)

Ninth layer (border echo) — Subserosa, serosa

Fig. 12.3 EUS of the normal stomach wall.

intact. Discrete flat or depressed early gastric cancer is detected as an irregularity of the first layer and a slightly thickened second layer. However, histologic examination of biopsy material should be undertaken to confirm a T1 diagnosis.

- T2 – tumor infiltration into the muscularis propria and subserosa. Pattern analysis is required to differentiate subserosal from serosal invasion (see below).
- T3 – tumor penetration through the serosa (visceral peritoneum) without invasion of adjacent organs or structures.
- T4 – tumor invasion of adjacent organs or structures.

To diagnose the depth of gastric cancer invasion, it is usually possible with EUS to detect the deepest layer that is damaged by tumor infiltration. However, it is sometimes difficult to diagnose depressed-type gastric tumors from peptic ulceration or fold convergence, as peptic ulcer fibrosis is seen as a hypoechoic area, similar to cancer invasion. Although early gastric cancer is not so frequent in Western countries, in Asian countries (especially Japan) some 50–70% of gastric tumors are classified as early gastric cancer. About 20–30% of early gastric cancers have ulcer fibrosis (type 0–IIc+III, or 0–IIc+ulcer scar). Therefore, a method of pattern analysis

capable of distinguishing between cancer invasion and ulcer fibrosis was introduced to evaluate depressed-type gastric cancer (Fig. 12.5),[27,28] and several studies with similar pattern analysis have been reported.[29,30]

To diagnose the extent of subserosal or serosal invasion, it is first necessary to differentiate between medullary and scirrhous growth, based on the internal pattern (Fig. 12.6). Generally, the medullary pattern has a well demarcated border and a homogeneous hypoechoic internal pattern; the scirrhous pattern, however, has an undefined border, a heterogeneous internal echo, and vestiges of the five-layered structure. In the medullary group, a hump on the outer border means that the cancer is still limited to the subserosa, and a serrated outer border indicates serosal invasion. In the scirrhous group, an indistinct hump on the outer border indicates serosal invasion, even if it is small, and a distinct hump of the outer border indicates cancer invasion limited to the subserosa.

N staging

After scanning of the primary lesion, lymph node metastasis is investigated around the primary lesion, lesser curvature, greater curvature, and celiac trunk. The ultrasonographic features of lymph nodes (homogeneous versus heterogeneous) are the most sensitive parameter for malignant involvement of nodes, followed by border demarcation (sharp versus fussy),

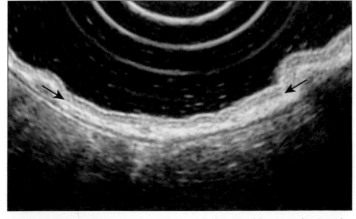

Fig. 12.4 Muscularis mucosae (arrows) detected by EUS (20 MHz).

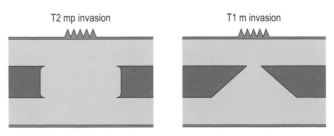

T2 mp invasion   T1 m invasion

Fig. 12.5 Differentiation of cancer invasion from ulcer fibrosis with EUS (basic principle).[26,27]

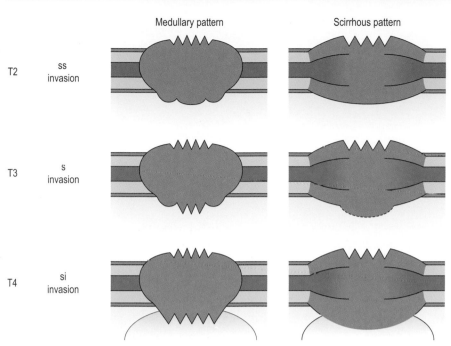

Medullary pattern　　　　Scirrhous pattern

T2　ss invasion

T3　s invasion

T4　si invasion

Fig. 12.6 Differentiation of T2 subserosa (ss), T3 serosa (s), and T4 (si) with EUS.

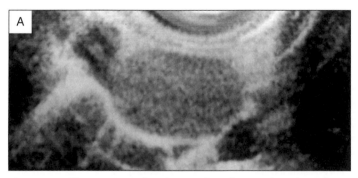
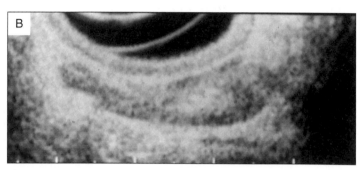

Fig. 12.7 Differentiation of malignant from benign lymph nodes. **A,** Malignant. **B,** Benign.

shape (round versus elliptical), and size (>10 mm versus <10 mm). If all four parameters are present, the positive predictive value is 100%, whereas central hyperecho is the pattern typical of benign lymph nodes (Fig. 12.7). However, all four of these features are present in only 25% of malignant lymp nodes, and a single feature can independently predict malignant involvement.[31,32]

CASE PRESENTATION

Case 1 – gastric cancer, mucosal invasion (Fig. 12.8)

There is a slightly depressed lesion, designated 0–IIc by the Japanese classification, on the anterior wall of angulus. EUS reveals this lesion as an irregularity of the first layer and slight thickening of the second layer. The third to fifth layers are intact. This lesion is thus diagnosed as intramural cancer. Histologic examination showed that cancer invasion was limited to the mucosa.

Case 2 – gastric cancer, submucosal cancer (Fig. 12.9)

There is a slightly depressed lesion, designated 0–IIc by the Japanese classification, in the posterior wall of the lower body. EUS shows this lesion as an irregularity and elevation of the first layer, a thickening of the second layer, and a narrowing of the third layer, corresponding to submucosal invasion. Histologic examination demonstrated that the tumor invaded deeper into the submucosa, designated sm2 by the Japanese classification.

Case 3 – gastric cancer, mucosal invasion (Fig. 12.10)

There is a slightly depressed lesion, designated 0–IIc + ulcer scar by the Japanese classification, in the lesser curvature of lower body. EUS reveals this lesion as an irregularity of the first layer, slight thickening of the second layer, and interruption or narrowing of the third layer. According to the usual diagnostic criteria, this lesion is diagnosed as invasion of the muscularis mucosa or submucosa. However, histologically this tumor was

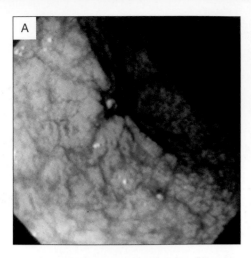

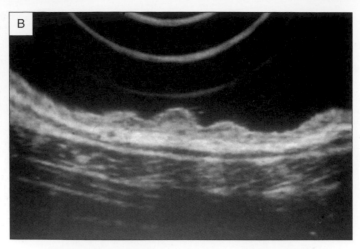

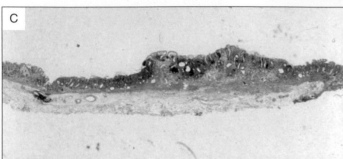

Fig. 12.8 Case 1, 0–IIc, mucosal invasion.

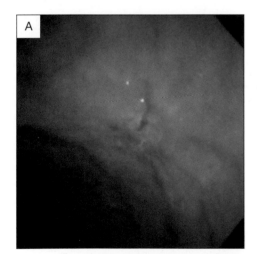

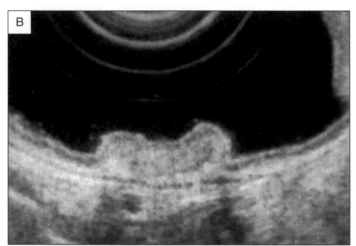

Fig. 12.9 Case 2, 0–IIc, submucosal invasion.

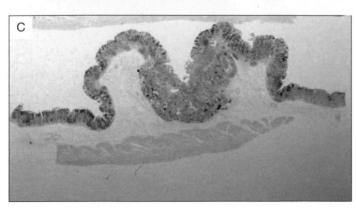

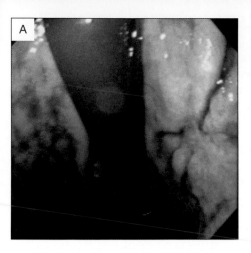

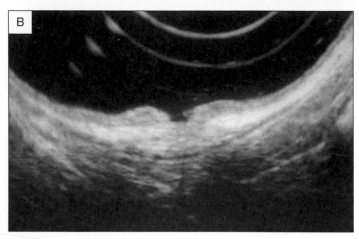

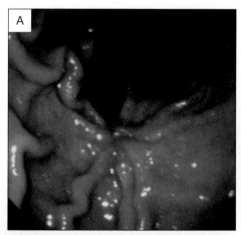

Fig. 12.10 Case 3, 0–IIc+III, mucosal invasion with ulcer fibrosis.

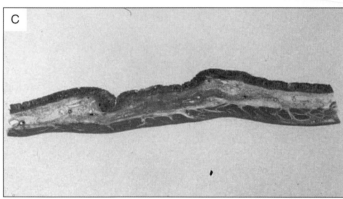

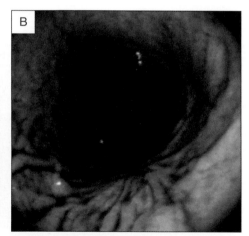

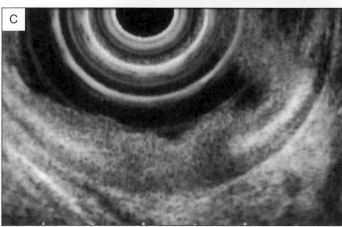

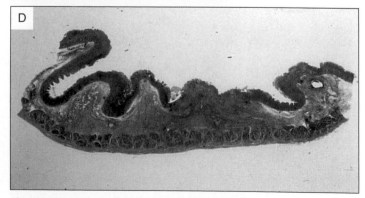

Fig. 12.11 Case 4, advanced cancer (IIc+III), muscularis propria invasion.

limited to the mucosa, and fan-shaped ulcer fibrosis was detected in the submucosa, causing interruption or narrowing of the third layer endosonographically. In this situation, pattern analysis was employed to differentiate ulcer fibrosis from cancer invasion (see Fig. 12.5).

Case 4 – gastric cancer, invasion of muscularis propria (Fig. 12.11)

There is a depressed lesion, which looks likes 0–IIc + III of the Japanese classification, in the posterior wall of the mid body. EUS reveals this lesion as an irregularity of the first layer, thickening of the gastric wall, and an arch-shaped interruption of the third layer on the right-hand side; however, a fan-shaped interruption of third layer is visible on the left-hand side. On pattern analysis, the arch-shaped interruption and gastric wall thickening indicates invasion of the muscularis musoca, although ulcer fibrosis remains in the third layer because a fan-shaped interruption is revealed on the left hand side. Finally, this lesion was diagnosed as invasion of the muscularis propria. Histologically, tumor invasion of the muscularis propria with ulcer fibrosis was confirmed.

Case 5 – gastric cancer, subserosal invasion (T2) (Fig. 12.12)

There is an irregular, ulcerated lesion, designated as Borrmann 3, in the lesser curvature of the body. EUS detected a hypoechoic tumor, homogeneous, well demarcated, and classified as having a medullary pattern. The tumor reaches the fifth layer, and shows the smooth hump sign. According to pattern analysis for differentiating subserosal from serosal invasion, this lesion was diagnosed as subserosal invasion. This diagnosis was confirmed histologically.

Case 6 – gastric cancer, serosal invasion (T3) and colonic invasion (T4) (Fig. 12.13)

There is an irregular ulcerated lesion, designated as Borrmann 3, in the lesser curvature of the antrum. EUS reveals a hypoechoic tumor, homogeneous, well demarcated, and classified as having a medullary pattern. The tumor invades the fifth layer, which demonstrates an irregular serrated outline, and loss of the border between the tumor and the colon (T4). According to pattern analysis for differentiating subserosal from serosal invasion, the irregular serrated outline indicates serosal invasion (T3) and disappearance of the border with

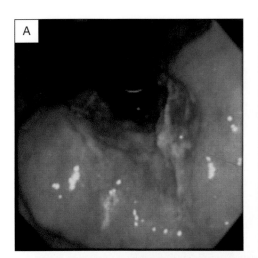

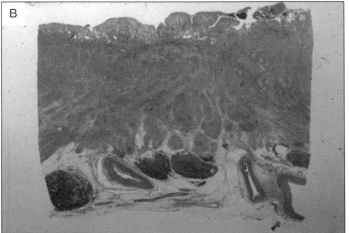

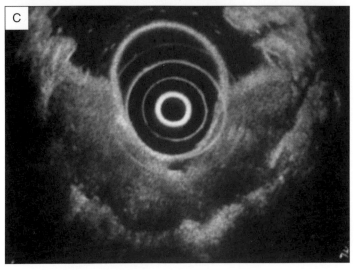

Fig. 12.12 Case 5, Borrmann 3, T2 ss invasion (medullary pattern).

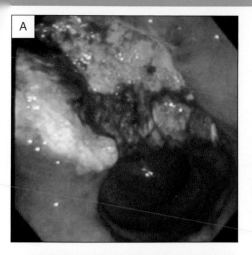

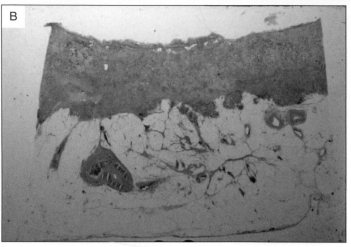

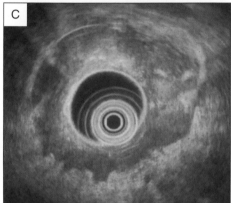

Fig. 12.13 Case 6, Borrmann 3, T3 s and T4 si to colon invasion (medullary pattern).

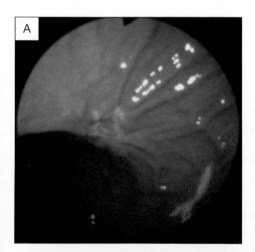

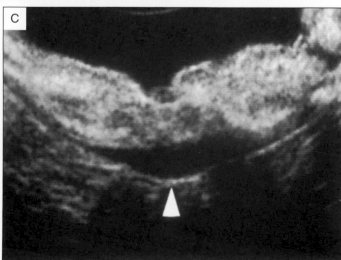

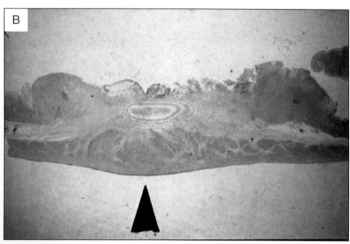

Fig. 12.14 Case 7, Borrmann 3, T2 ss invasion (scirrhous pattern).

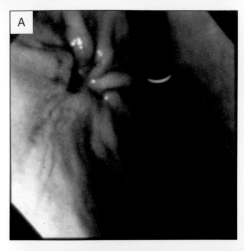

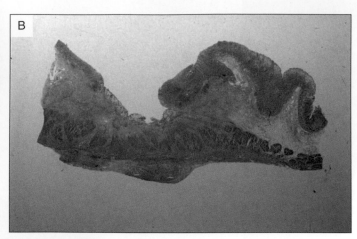

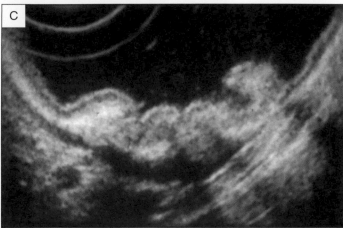

Fig. 12.15 Case 8, Borrmann 3, T3 s invasion (scirrhous pattern).

adjacent organ corresponds to a T4 lesion. This lesion is diagnosed as colonic invasion (T4), and was confirmed by histologic examination.

Case 7 – gastric cancer, subserosal invasion (T2)
(Fig. 12.14)

This is an irregular ulcerated lesion, which appears to be 0–IIc+III according to the Japanese classification, in the posterior wall of the lower body. EUS reveals a heterogeneous tumor that has vestiges of a five-layered structure, an obscure border, smooth hump of the fifth layer, and classified as having a scirrhous pattern. According to pattern analysis for differentiating subserosal from serosal invasion, the hump of the fifth layer indicates subserosal invasion, even though it is slight. Histologically, tumor invasion was seen to be limited to the subserosa.

Case 8 – gastric cancer, serosal invasion (T3)
(Fig. 12.15)

This is an irregular ulcerated lesion with fold convergence in the greater curvature of the lower body. EUS reveals a heterogeneous tumor with vestiges of a five-layered structure, an irregular hump of the fifth layer, an obscure border, and classified as having a scirrhous pattern. According to pattern

analysis for differentiating subserosal from serosal invasion, the irregular hump of the fifth layer indicates serosal invasion, even though slight. Histologically, this tumor was seen to invade into the serosa.

Case 9 – 3D-EUS: gastric cancer, 0–IIc, sm1
(Fig. 12.16)

There is a slightly depressed lesion in the anterior wall of the lower body. 3D-EUS provides radial (D) and linear (E) images at the same time; the arrow indicates a tiny narrowing of the submucosa. This lesion was thus diagnosed as submucosal invasion. Histologic examination revealed microinvasion (583 μm) to the submucosa. Using 3D-EUS, it is possible to review a maximum number of 160 consecutive images, so that tiny findings can be noticed.

ACCURACY OF EUS

T staging

After endoscopy, EUS is the most important diagnostic procedure for patients with gastric cancer. Numerous studies have investigated the accuracy of EUS in TNM staging of gastric cancer (Table 12.1). These vary with respect to instrumentation, scanning frequency, and location of the tumor

TNM STAGING WITH EUS				
Reference	Year	n	T staging (%)	N staging (%)
Aibe et al.[34]	1989	67	73	69
Tio et al.[35]	1989	72	84	68
Heintz & Junginger[36]	1991	19	79	72
Botet et al.[37]	1991	50	92	78
Akahoshi et al.[38]	1991	74	81	50
Cerizzi et al.[39]	1992	27	90	55
Roesch et al.[40]	1992	41	71	75
Caletti et al.[41]	1993	42	91	69
Nattermann et al.[42]	1993	50	82	78
Ziegler et al.[43]	1993	108	86	74
Grimm et al.[44]	1993	147	78	87
Dittler & Siewert[45]	1993	254	83	66
De Angelis et al.[46]	1994	86	80	75
Massari et al.[47]	1996	65	89	68
Wang et al.[48]	1998	119	70	65
Mancino et al.[49]	2000	79	76	67
Willis et al.[50]	2000	116	78	77
Xi et al.[51]	2003	32	80	69
Shimoyama et al.[52]	2004	45	71	80
Javaid et al.[53]	2004	112	83	64
Total		1605	83	69

Table 12.1 TNM staging with EUS

(cardia vs rest of the stomach). The accuracy of EUS in determination of the T stage of the primary tumor ranges from 71% to 92%, with an average of 83%. In general, EUS is least accurate (range 60–70%) for T2 lesions. This is because of the difficulty of differentiating between muscularis propria and subserosal (T2) or serosal (T3) invasion. Whereas findings of T2 invasion is small and limited histologically, T3 includes both small and far advanced invasion, and the stomach is not covered completely by the serosa. As proposed pattern analysis before, there are two types of infiltration (medullary and scirrhous), and it is necessary to diagnose the deeper invasion by tiny findings in the scirrhous group, compared with the medullary group. EUS can readily differentiate between T3 and T4 lesions; this is useful when deciding whether the treatment should be surgical or chemotherapeutic, and may also be helpful in reducing the number of unnecessary laparotomies.

When using EUS, it is important to differentiate intra-mucosal from submucosal cancer for EMR.[62] Numerous studies have investigated the accuracy of EUS in staging gastric cancer with the Japanese classification (Table 12.2). The

diagnostic accuracy of EUS is summarized as follows: mucosal cancer, 86% (n=1391); submucosal cancer, 68% (n=744); cancer of the muscularis propria, 65% (n=264); subserosal cancer, 80% (n=370); serosal cancer, 85% (n=227); si (infiltration of adjacent organ) cancer; 62% (n=61); and overall totally 79% (n=3442). EUS is least accurate for tumors extending into but not through the muscularis propria (T2). The data for T4si are not satisfactory, because they are based mainly on surgically resected cases.

Generally, reasons for incorrect diagnosis with EUS are microinvasion, peritumorous inflammation such as peptic ulcer fibrosis, macroscopic type such as a protruding lesion, and inadequate scanning. Microinvasion may result in understaging, as it is difficult to diagnose sm1 lesions (vertical invasion into submucosa <500 µm) with conventional EUS and an ultrasonic thin probe. If pattern analysis for depressed gastric cancer is not employed, ulcer fibrosis may result in overstaging, according to the depth of ulcer fibrosis. Even when pattern analysis is employed, it is almost impossible to differentiate microinvasion such as sm1 from ulcer fibrosis, although it is feasible to distinguish SM2 or more invasion from ulcer fibrosis. Protruding lesions introduce artifact, interrupting the layer structure, even when tumor invasion is not present, and the third layer (submucosa) under the lesion generally protrudes into the lesion. Consequently, it is also difficult to detect narrowing or real interruption due to cancer invasion. Inadequate scanning has been a problem since the beginning of EUS, as it is difficult in practice to maintain the scope in a vertical position in relatively small lesions around the cardia, greater curvature of upper body, lesser curvature of angle, and pyloric ring. In addition, there are many factors such as pulsation, breathing, air bubble, and mucus, that may cause artifact.

In order to perform endoscopic treatment such as EMR and endoscopic submucosal dissection (ESD), mucosal and sm1 tumors have to be diagnosed before surgery with high accuracy. As mentioned above, conventional EUS is not sufficiently accurate for clinical purposes. However, by using 3D-EUS it is possible to diagnose submucosal invasion of more than 500 µm with high accuracy. According to our data, the diagnostic accuracy of 3D-EUS for diagnosing the depth of gastric cancer invasion is 96% (n=243) in the mucosa, 75% (n=106) in the submucosa, 67% (n=12) in muscularis propria, 75% (n=16) in subserosa, 67% (n=12) in serosa, 0% (n=3) in si (invasion to adjacent organ), and 87% (n=392) overall.[54] In the submucosa, invasion to more than 500 µm can be detected with an accuracy greater than 80%, which is satisfactory for selecting candidates for EMR or ESD.

N staging

Assessment of lymph node metastasis is slightly less accurate than T staging, with a range of 50–87% (see Table 12.1). Although the criteria for TNM staging have changed recently,

JAPANESE STAGING SYSTEM (M, SM, PM, SS, S, SI) WITH EUS

Reference	Year	n	T1m	T1sm	T2pm	Advanced	T2ss	T3s	T3ss–T4si	T4si	Overall	Comment
Yamanaka et al.[55]	1985	50	87	83		84			100		86	
Yoshino et al.[56]	1987	41	88	77		82					83	
Kida et al.[27]	1989	171	95	71	67				94		86	
Yasuda et al.[57]	1992	500	80	78	53				81		79	
Yanai et al.[58]	1997	108	63	78		20					65	
Akahoshi et al.[59]	1998	78	70	46		75					67	USP
Nakamura et al.[60]	1999	325	74	71	66		98		100		81	
Kida et al.[61]	1999	1428	91	70	70		76	84		63	79	EUS
		352	92	61	39		67	71		50	79	USP
Fujino et al.[62]	1999	272	88	66	64		89		98		82	
Hizawa et al.[63]	2002	234	84	52							76	EGC
Total		3559	86	68	65	74	80	85	96	62	79	

Table 12.2 Japanese staging system (m, sm, pm, ss, s, si) with EUS
Values for stages are percentages.
EUS, conventional endoscopic ultrasonography; USP, ultrasonic probe; EGC, early gastric cancer.

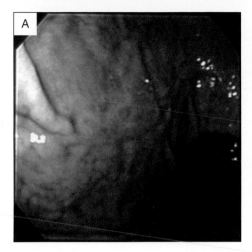

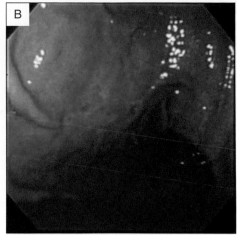

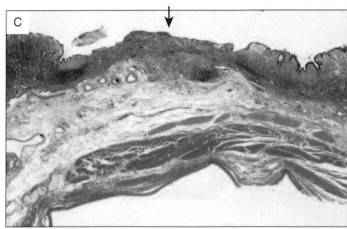

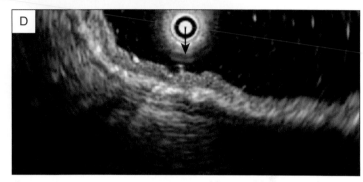

Fig. 12.16 Case 9, 0–IIc, sm1 invasion (detected by 3D-EUS).

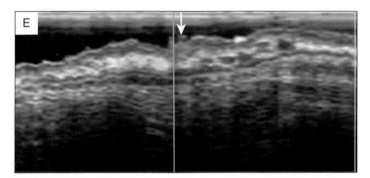

the overall accuracy for assessment of lymph node metastasis in 20 reports (1608 patients in total) was 69% in a study that compared EUS results with histopathologic diagnosis using TNM criteria (see Table 12.1). There is a strong correlation between increasing T stage and the presence of lymph node metastasis; therefore, concomitant T stage may be suitable for determing the probability of lymph node metastasis on EUS. If the study sample includes mainly T3 and T4 tumors, the accuracy and sensitivity of EUS for diagnosing lymph node metastasis is rather high. In contrast, it is difficult to detect lymph node metastasis in T1 cancer because, in general, a large proportion of T1m and about 15% of T1sm tumors have metastasis to only one or two lymph nodes. However, the reliable accuracy of EUS for lymph node diagnosis in T1 lesions is of critical importance in determining whether or not local endoscopic treatment of early gastric cancer is suitable. Therefore, in Japan, the suitability of local treatments such as EMR and ESD is decided mainly by T staging. In general, EUS can detect lymph node metastasis around the lesser curvature of the stomach more easily than that of the greater curvature or sites more than 3 cm from the primary lesion, such as the celiac trunk; this is because EUS has to follow a wide area along the greater curvature and has a maximum depth of penetration of approximately 5–7 cm, thus limiting its ability to detect lymph node metastasis around a greater or distant curvature.

As mentioned above, malignant lymph nodes can be difficult to distinguish from benign nodes. Even benign lymph nodes sometimes have one or two malignant findings. Therefore, EUS-guided fine-needle aspiration cytology and biopsy (EUS-FNAB) is often employed, when indicated.

COMPARISON WITH OTHER MODALITIES

CT has been the primary examination for staging of gastric cancer. EUS is superior to CT in its ability to reveal the structure of the gastric wall, but it is not accurate in the assessment of distant lymph node metastasis and other distant metastasis. The literature shows that, in terms of accuracy, EUS and CT are complementary rather than competitive: EUS is superior in diagnosing the depth of gastric cancer invasion (Table 12.3),

and CT is preferred for the diagnosis of distant metastases.[68] For N staging, EUS is superior to CT, although CT has become competitive as a result of recent advances in its application (Table 12.4).

EXAMINATION CHECKLIST

Primary lesion – depth of penetration and presence or absence of local lymph nodes
Celiac axis
Liver
Hilum of the spleen
Gastrohepatic ligament (between stomach and liver)

T STAGING WITH ENDOSCOPIC ULTRASONOGRAPHY (EUS), COMPUTED TOMOGRAPHY (CT), AND MAGNETIC RESONANCE IMAGING (MRI)						
Reference	Year	n	EUS (%)	CT (%)	MRI (%)	Comment
Botet et al.[37]	1991	50	92	42		
Grimm et al.[64]	1991	118	82	11		
Ziegler et al.[43]	1993	108	86	43		
Kuntz & Herfarth[65]	1999	82	73	51	48	
Polkowski et al.[66]	2004	88	63	44		Helical CT
Bhandari et al.[67]	2004	63	88	83		Multidetector row CT
Total		509	80 (393/494)	41 (200/489)	48 (32/67)	

Table 12.3 T staging with endoscopic ultrasonography (EUS), computed tomography (CT), and magnetic resonance imaging (MRI)

N STAGING WITH EUS, CT, AND MRI						
Reference	Year	n	EUS	CT	MRI	Comment
Botet et al.[37]	1991	50	78	48		
Grimm et al.[64]	1991	118	88	21		
Ziegler et al.[43]	1993	108	74	51		
Kuntz & Herfarth[65]	1999	82	87	65	69	
Polkowski et al.[66]	2004	60	30	47		Helical CT
Bhandari et al.[67]	2004	48	79	75		Multidetector row CT
Total		466	75	48	69	

Table 12.4 N staging with EUS, CT, and MRI

REFERENCES

1 DiMagno EP, Buxton JL, Regan PT, et al. Ultrasonic endoscope. Lancet 1980; i:629–631.

2 StrohmWD, Classen M. Anatomical aspects in ultrasonic endoscopy. Scand J Gastroenterol Suppl 1984; 94:21–33.

3 Vilmann P, Jacobsen GK, Henriksen FW, et al. Endoscopic ultrasonography with guided fine needle aspiration biopsy in pancreas disease. Gastrointest Endosc 1992; 38:172–173.

4 Grimm H, Binmoeller K, Soehendra N. Endosonography-guided drainage of a pancreas pseudocyst. Gastrointest Endosc 1992; 38:170–171.

5 Kida M, Watanabe M, Sugano A, et al. 3-Dimensional endoscopic ultrasonography (3D-EUS) for upper gastrointestinal diseases. Endoscopy 1996; 28(Suppl):S38.

6 Yoshino J, Nakazawa S, Inui K, et al. Volume measurement using tissue characterization of three-dimensional endoscopic ultrasonography. Endoscopy 2000; 32:624–629.

7 Watanabe M, Kida M, Yamada Y, et al. Measuring tumor volume with three-dimensional endoscopic ultrasonography: an experimental and clinical study. Endoscopy 2004; 36:976–981.

8 Hashimoto H. The capability of three dimensional display during endoscopic ultrasonography. Digest Endosc 1991; 3:194.

9 Roesch T, Classen M. Gastric carcinoma. In: Gastroenterologic endosonography. New York: Thieme Medical Publishers; 1992:71–80.

10 Roesch T. Endosonographic staging of gastric cancer: a review of literature results. Gastrointest Endosc Clin North Am 1995; 5:549–557.

11 Siewert JR, Sendler A, Dittler HJ, et al. Staging gastrointestinal cancer as a precondition for multimodal treatment. World J Surg 1995; 19:168–177.

12 Pollack BJ, Chak P, Sivak MV. Endoscopic ultrasonography. Semin Oncol 1996; 23:336–346.

13 Brugge WR. Endoscopic ultrasonography: the current status. Gastroenterology 1998; 115:1577–1583.

14 Bergman J, Fockens P. Endoscopic ultrasonography in patients with gastro-esophageal cancer. Eur J Ultrasound 1999; 10:127–138.

15 Lambert R, Caletti G, Cho E, et al. International workshop on the clinical impact of endoscopic ultrasound in gastroenterology. Endoscopy 2000; 32:549–584.

16 Standards of Practice Committee of ASGE. Role of endoscopic ultrasonography. Gastrointest Endosc 2000; 52:852–859.

17 Kida M. Endoscopic ultrasonography in Japan: present status and standardization. Digest Endosc 2002; 14(Suppl): S24–S29.

18 Fusaroli P, Caletti G. Endoscopic ultrasonography. Endoscopy 2003; 35:127–135.

19 Japan Gastric Cancer Association. Guideline of gastric cancer treatment. Tokyo: Kanehira; 2001.

20 Souquet JC, Valette PJ, Berger F, et al. Contribution of endosonography to the diagnosis of gastric linitis. Gastrointest Endosc 1988; 34:209 (abstract).

21 Andriulli A, Reccina S, De Angelis C, et al. Endoscopic ultrasonographic evaluation of patients with biopsy negative gastric linitis plastica. Gastrointest Endosc 1990; 36:611–615.

22 Caletti G, Ferrari A, Bocus P, et al. Endoscopic ultrasonography in gastric lymphoma. In: Sivak MV. ed. Tenth International Symposium on Endoscopic Ultrasonography, Cleveland, Ohio, October 1995:119–125.

23 Lightdale CJ, Botet JF, Kelsen DP, et al. Diagnosis of recurrent upper gastrointestinal cancer at the surgical anastomosis by endoscopic ultrasound. Gastrointest Endosc 1989; 35:407–412.

24 Aibe T, Fuji T, Okita K, et al. A fundamental study of normal layer structure of the gastrointestinal wall visualized by endoscopic ultrasonography. Scand J Gastroenterol 1986; 21(Suppl):34–40.

25 Kimmey MB, Martin RW, Haggitt RC, et al. Histologic correlates of gastrointestinal ultrasound images. Gastroenterology 1989; 96:433–441.

26 Yamanaka T. Endosonographic correlation with histology in a layered structure of the gastrointestinal wall. Gastroenterol Endosc 2001; 43:1091–1092.

27 Kida M, Saigenji K, Okabe H. Endoscopic ultrasonography in the diagnosis of the depth of gastric cancer invasion: differential diagnosis between cancerous invasion and fibrosis of the co-existing ulcer. Gastroenterol Endosc 1989; 31:1141–1155.

28 Kida M, Tanabe S, Kokutou M, et al. Staging of gastric cancer with endoscopic ultrasonography and endoscopic mucosal resection. Endoscopy 1998; 30(Suppl):A64–A68.

29 Ohashi S, Nakazawa S, Yoshino J. A study of the depth of invasion of depressed type of early gastric cancer by endoscopic ultrasonography. Gastroenterol Endosc 1989; 31:1471–1479.

30 Chonan A, Mochizuki F, Ikeda T, et al. Clinical evaluation of the endoscopic ultrasonography (EUS) on the diagnosis for depressed type early gastric cancer associated with ulceration. Gastroenterol Endosc 1990; 32:1081–1091.

31 Catalano MF, Sivak MVJ, Rice T, et al. Endosonographic features predictive of lymph node metastasis. Gastrointest Endosc 1994; 40:442–446.

32 Bhutani MS, Hawes RH, Hoffman BJ. A comparison of the accuracy of echo features during endoscopic ultrasound (EUS) and EUS-guided fine needle aspiration for diagnosis of malignant lymph node invasion. Gastrointest Endosc 1997; 45:474–479.

33 Ohashi S, Segawa K, Okamura S, et al. The utility of endoscopic ultrasonography and endoscopy in the endoscopic mucosal resection of early gastric cancer. Gut 1999; 45:599–604.

34 Aibe T, Fujimura H, Noguchi T, et al. Endosonographic detection and staging of early gastric cancer. In: Dancygier H, Classen M, eds. Fifth International symposium on EUS, Munich, Germany, 1989:71–78.

35 Tio TL, Schouwink MH, Cikot RJ, et al. Preoperative TNM classification of gastric carcinoma by endosonography in comparison with pathological TNM system: a prospective study of 72 cases. Hepatogastroenterology 1989; 36:51–56.

36 Heintz A, Junginger T. Endosonographisches staging von karzinomen in speiserohre und magen. Bildgebung (Imaging) 1991; 58:4–8.

37 Botet JF, Lightdale CJ, Zauber AG, et al. Preoperative staging of gastric cancer: comparison of endoscopic US and dynamic CT. Radiology 1991; 181:426–432.

38 Akahoshi K, Misawa T, Fujishima H, et al. Preoperative evaluation of gastric cancer by endoscopic ultrasound. Gut 1991; 32:479–482.

39 Cerizzi A, Botti F, Carrara A, et al. EUS in preoperative staging of gastric cancer. Endoscopy 1992; 24(Suppl):380 (abstract).

40 Roesch T, Lorenz R, Zenker K, et al. Local staging and assessment of respectability in carcinoma of the esophagus, stomach, and duodenum by endoscopic ultrasonography. Gastrointest Endosc 1992; 38:460–467.

41 Caletti G, Ferrari A, Brocchi E, et al. Accuracy of endoscopic ultrasonography in the diagnosis and staging of gastric cancer and lymphoma. Surgery 1993; 113:14–27.

42 Nattermann C, Galbenu-Grunwald R, Nier H. Endoskopischer ultraschall im TN-staging des magenkarzinims. Ein vergleich mit der computertomographie und der knoventionellen sonographie. Z Gesamte Inn Med 1993; 48:60–64.

43 Ziegler K, Sanft C, Zimmer T, et al. Comparison of computed tomography, endosonography, and intraoperative assessment in TN staging of gastric carcinoma. Gut 1993; 34:604–610.

44 Grimm H, Binmoeller KF, Hamper K, et al. Endosonography for preoperative locoregional staging of esophageal and gastric cancer. Endoscopy 1993; 25:224–230.

45 Dittler HJ, Siewert JR. Role of endoscopic ultrasonography in gastric carcinoma. Endoscopy 1993; 25:224–230.

46 De Angelis C, Gindro T, Recchia S, et al. Value and limitations of preoperative endoscopic ultrasonography in predicting stage and respectability of gastric cancer. Gastroenterology 1994; 106:380 (abstract).

47 Massari M, Cioffi U, De Simone M, et al. Endoscopic ultrasonography for preoperative staging of gastric carcinoma. Hepatogastroenterology 1996; 43:542–546.

48 Wang JY, Hsieh JS, Huang YS, et al. Endoscopic ultrasonography for preoperative locoregional staging and assessment of respectability in gastric cancer. Clin Imaging 1998; 22:355–359.

49 Mancino G, Bozzetti F, Schicci A, et al. Preoperative endoscopic ultrasonography inpatients with gastric cancer. Tumori 2000; 86:139–141.

50 Willis S, Truong S, Gribnitz S, et al. Endoscopic ultrasonography in the preoperative staging of gastric cancer. Surg Endosc 2000; 14:951–954.

51 Xi WD, Zhao C, Ren GS. Endoscopic ultrasonography in preoperative staging of gastric cancer: determination of tumor invasion depth, nodal involvement and surgical resectability. World J Gastroenterol 2003; 9:254–257.

52 Shimoyama S, Yasuda H, Hashimoto M, et al. Accuracy of linear-array EUS for preoperative staging of gastric cardia cancer. Gastrointest Endosc 2004; 60:50–55.

53 Javaid G, Shah O, Dar MA, et al. Role of endoscopic ultrasonography inpreoperative staging of gastric carcinoma. Aust N Z J Surg 2004; 74:108–111.

54 Kida M, Kikuchi H, Saigenji K. Three-dimensional endoscopic ultrasonography (in Japanense with English abstracts). Endoscopia Digestiva 2005; 17:828–835.

55 Yamanaka T, Yoshida Y, Ueno N, et al. Endoscopic ultrasonography in the diagnosis of the degree of vertical invasion of gastric cancer. Jpn J Gastroenterol 1985; 82:1865–1874.

56 Yoshino J, Nakazawa S, Nakamura T, et al. The depth of invasion in depressed gastric cancer estimated by roentgenography and endoscopic ultrasonography. Stomach Intestine 1987; 22:169–177.

57 Yasuda K, Uno K, Tanaka S, et al. Evaluation of the degree of gastric cancer invasion by endoscopic ultrasonography for endoscopic treatment. Stomach Intestine 1992; 27:1167–1174.

58 Yanai H, Matsumoto Y, Harada T, et al. Endoscopic ultrasonography and endoscopy for staging depth of invasion in early gastric cancer: a pilot study. Gastrointest Endosc 1997; 46:212–216.

59 Akahoshi K, Chijiwa Y, Hamada S, et al. Pretreatment staging of endoscopically early gastric cancer with a 15MHz ultrasound catheter probe. Gastrointest Endosc 1998; 48:470–476.

60 Nakamura T, Suzuki T, Matsuura A. Assessment of the depth of gastric carcinoma by endoscopic ultrasonography (EUS) focused on peptic ulcer. Stomach Intestine 1999; 34:1105–1117.

61 Kida M, Kokutou M, Watanabe M, et al. Accuracy of endoscopic ultrasonography for diagnosing the depth of early gastric cancer with or without ulcer. Stomach Intestine 1999; 34:1095–1103.

62 Fujino Y, Nagata Y, Ogino K, et al. Evaluation of endoscopic ultrasonography as an indicator for surgical treatment of gastric cancer. J Gastroenterol Hepatol 1999; 14:540–546.

63 Hizawa K, Iwai K, Esaki M, et al. Is endoscopic ultrasonography indispensable in assessing the appropriateness of endoscopic resection for gastric cancer. Endoscopy 2002; 34:973–978.

64 Grimm H, Hamper K, Maydeo A, et al. Accuracy of endoscopic ultrasonography (EUS) in determining local/regional spread of gastric cancer: results of a prospective controlled study. Gastrointest Endosc 1991; 37:279 (abstract).

65 Kuntz C, Herfarth C. Imaging diagnosis for staging of gastric cancer. Semin Surg Oncol 1999; 17:96–102.

66 Polkowski M, Palucki J, Waronska E, et al. Endosonography versus helical computed tomography for locoregional staging of gastric cancer. Endoscopy 2004; 36:617–623.

67 Bhandari S, Shim CS, Kim JH, et al. Usefulness of three-dimensional, multidetector row CT (virtual gastroscopy and multiplanar reconstruction) in the evaluation of gastric cancer: a comparison with conventional endoscopy, EUS, and histopathology. Gastrointest Endosc 2004; 59:619–626.

68 Kelly S, Harris KM, Berry E, et al. A systemic review of the staging performance of endoscopic ultrasound in gastro-oesophageal carcinoma. Gut 2001; 49:534–539.

Chapter
13

EUS in the Evaluation of Gastric Wall Layer Abnormalities – Non-Hodgkin Lymphoma and Other Causes

Pietro Fusaroli and Giancarlo Caletti

KEY POINTS

- In large gastric folds, endoscopic ultrasonography (EUS) can determine different levels of gastric wall involvement, allowing the clinician to narrow down the differential diagnosis.

- EUS is the most accurate imaging modality for evaluation and staging of infiltrative gastric lesions.

- The gastrointestinal tract is the most common extranodal site for non-Hodgkin lymphomas.

- The importance of EUS lies not only in its ability to stage mucosa-associated lymphoid tissue (MALT) lymphoma before treatment, but also in the follow-up, as EUS may determine response to therapy and detect relapse early.

INTRODUCTION

Non-Hodgkin lymphomas (NHLs) are composed of many histologically and biologically distinct lymphoid malignancies. It is estimated that approximately 54 000 persons are diagnosed with this disease every year in the USA, accounting for a proportion of 4% of all malignancies.[1] The overall incidence is about 50% higher for males than for females, the difference in incidence rate being more marked in younger than older individuals.

The majority of NHLs arise in lymph nodes, although primary extranodal disease accounts for 20–30% of all cases. The most frequent primary extranodal sites are the stomach, small intestine, skin, and brain. Etiologic factors that have been advocated include immunodeficiency, infectious organisms, familial predisposition, blood transfusion, pesticide exposure, lifestyle factors, and genetic susceptibility.

The gastrointestinal (GI) tract is the most commonly involved extranodal site for NHLs, gastric localization being by far the most common. The stomach can harbor a primary NHL or be involved secondarily by disseminated nodal disease.

This chapter focuses mainly on primary gastric NHL, as endoscopic ultrasonography (EUS) plays a central role in the diagnosis and staging of disease in this location. In contrast, secondary gastric NHL, which occurs in 20–60% of newly diagnosed cases, reflects disseminated disease that necessitates systemic diagnostic, staging, and treatment strategies. Studies analyzing the incidence of secondary gastric NHL have shown a large discrepancy between the frequency of diagnosis before treatment and in post-mortem findings.[2,3] These results reveal that the majority of cases of secondary gastric involvement by NHL may go undetected.

The difference between primary and secondary gastric lymphoma was studied by Kolve et al.,[4] who evaluated whether differences in the pathogenesis were associated with distinct clinical and endoscopic features. Of 205 patients enrolled, 176 presented with primary gastric NHL (65 low grade, 111 high grade) and 29 with secondary gastric NHL (19 low grade, 10 high grade). The analysis of various clinical symptoms and endoscopic findings revealed a relationship between primary disease and the occurrence of abdominal pain, vomiting, and unifocal growth pattern ($P < 0.001$). However, tumor localization in the gastric fundus was found predominantly in secondary gastric involvement ($P < 0.001$). Additionally, duodenal involvement was diagnosed more frequently in patients with secondary disease. However, the gastric body and antrum were the predominant sites of infiltration in both primary and secondary gastric NHL. As a result, an equation was generated to help predict primary or secondary gastric NHL with a very high accuracy. Knowledge of these differential features by the endoscopist is important, particularly when upper endoscopy is the first modality to diagnose the disease; in this case other investigative methods can be employed, according whether a primary or a secondary malignancy is suspected.

PRIMARY GASTRIC NHLs– THE MALT LYMPHOMA CONCEPT

Considering the special properties of the digestive tract, Isaacson and Spencer[5] introduced the mucosa-associated lymphoid tissue (MALT) concept, thus classifying primary gastric lymphoma as a distinct entity with particular histologic and biologic features.[6,7]

Marginal zone lymphomas are divided in nodal, primary splenic, and extranodal lymphomas; the latter derive from MALT and are the most frequent type, representing 20–30% of all NHLs. They are composed of small B lymphocytes with a centrocytic, immunocytic, or monocytoid appearance and varying degrees of plasmacellular differentiation. MALT lymphoma cells, like marginal zone B lymphocytes, are CD20+, CD21+, CD35+, IgM+, CD5−, CD10−, IgD− (Figs 13.1 & 13.2).[8]

The most common karyotypic abnormalities associated with MALT lymphomas are trisomy 3, trisomy 18, and breakpoints at 1q21 and 1p34–36. Translocations t(11;18)(q21;q21) and t(1;14)(p22;q32) have been demonstrated, but these lymphomas never show t(11;14)(q13;q32) or t(14;18)(q32;q21) translocations.[9]

MALT lymphomas were first differentiated from low-grade nodal B-cell lymphomas in 1983, by Isaacson and Wright,[10] who demonstrated that MALT lymphomas have different sites, clinical and histologic characteristics compared with nodal B-cell lymphomas. Some years later, the International Lymphoma Study Group accepted MALT lymphomas as an independent category in the REAL classification (Table 13.1).[11]

With the exception of intestinal Peyer's patches, this class of lymphoma arises in organs that are congenitally devoid of lymphoid tissue and subsequently acquire MALT secondary to an infection or autoimmune process.[12,13] The majority of these lesions arise in the GI tract, where they represent 3–5% of all primary GI malignancies.[14] Digestive MALT lymphomas grow particularly in the stomach, where up to 90% are related to the presence of *Helicobacter pylori*;[15] the antigens of this bacterium

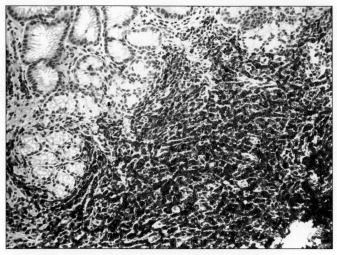

Fig. 13.1 Positivity at immunohistochemistry for the B cell-associated antigen CD20 (alkaline phosphatase–antialkaline phosphatase [APAAP] labeling technique, ×300).

seem to have a triggering and trophic action on MALT lymphoma cells, dependent on specific T-cell activation.[16–19] Histologic evidence of a lymphoid infiltration in endoscopic biopsies is obviously not sufficient for a definitive diagnosis of MALT lymphoma; the molecular evidence of B-cell monoclonality detected by polymerase chain reaction (PCR) is needed to distinguish chronic gastritis from lymphoma. Moreover, a correct differential diagnosis between MALT gastric lymphomas and other gastric small B-cell lymphomas, based on immunohistochemistry, is crucial for correct management of the malignancy: mantle cell gastric lymphomas do not demonstrate transformed blasts, but express CD5, IgD, and cyclin D1 in the nucleus; lymphocytic gastric lymphomas are CD5+, CD23+, and IgD+, but do not express nuclear cyclin D1; follicular gastric lymphomas are CD10+ and express BCL6 in the nucleus.

In the stomach, MALT lymphoma cells infiltrate gastric glands, forming the characteristic lymphoepithelial lesions

THE REAL CLASSIFICATION OF NON-HODGKIN LYMPHOMAS	
B-cell lymphomas	T-cell lymphomas
Precursor B-cell lymphomas	**Precursor T-cell lymphomas**
B-lymphoblastic	T-lymphoblastic
Mature B-cell lymphomas	**Mature T-cell lymphomas**
B-cell CLL/small lymphocytic	Mycosis fungoides/Sézary syndrome
Follicular	Peripheral T-cell (many subtypes)
Marginal zone nodal	Anaplastic large T-cell/null cell
Extranodal marginal zone (MALT)	Adult T-cell leukemia/lymphoma
Splenic marginal zone	
Lymphoplasmacytic	
Mantle cell	
Diffuse large B-cell	
Primary mediastinal large B-cell	
Burkitt-like	
Burkitt	

Table 13.1 The REAL classification of non-Hodgkin lymphomas
CLL, chronic lymphocytic leukemia; MALT, mucosa-associated lymphoid tissue.

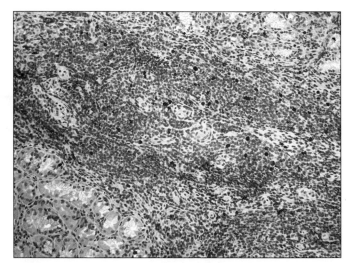

Fig. 13.2 Immunohistochemistry – a low proliferative index can be seen with Ki-67/MIB1 staining.

(Fig. 13.3); this tumoral involvement can sometimes be multifocal.[20] From the mucosa, MALT lymphoma gradually infiltrates the underlying submucosa, muscularis propria, and serosa (Figs 13.4–13.10); simultaneously, malignant cells can reach regional lymph nodes (Fig. 13.11), other parts of the GI tract or the spleen, reflecting the homing properties of MALT cells; metastases at bone marrow are rare. Moreover, low-grade MALT lymphomas can evolve into high-grade lymphomas, with a variable component of large cells, forming sheets or clusters; this transformation shows a more aggressive histologic and clinical behavior of the tumor.

The response of gastric MALT lymphomas to therapy depends on all of the above characteristics: presence of chromosome translocations, presence of large cell clusters, depth of gastric infiltration, presence of lymph node metastases, spleen or bone marrow involvement.[21]

Although the stomach is the most common site of MALT lymphoma, other intestinal and extraintestinal sites have been described, such as small and large bowel, esophagus, rectum, nasal mucosa, gingiva, tonsil, Waldeyer's ring, salivary gland, pharynx, larynx, thymus, liver, gallbladder, kidney, dura, and skin (Fig. 13.12).[22–26] Outside the stomach, the role of a yet unidentified infective agent is less clear, although healing of extragastric MALT lymphoma following administration of antibiotics has been reported.[27,28]

Other forms of gastric lymphoma are of non-MALT type, although many may initially have been MALT tumors (Table 13.2, Fig. 13.13). Rare tumors may be T cell in origin.

TREATMENT OF GASTRIC NHL

Surgery, chemotherapy, radiotherapy, and combined treatments represent the standard of gastric lymphoma therapy when *H. pylori* eradication fails or is not indicated.[29,30] *H. pylori* eradication therapy is addressed below in the specific EUS section.

Surgery

Surgery has been the mainstay of treatment for many years. However, the value of gastrectomy has recently been disputed,

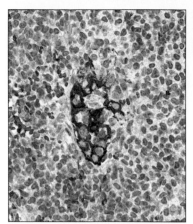

Fig. 13.3 Lymphoepithelial lesion highlighted by the anticytokeratin antibody (APAAP technique, ×400).

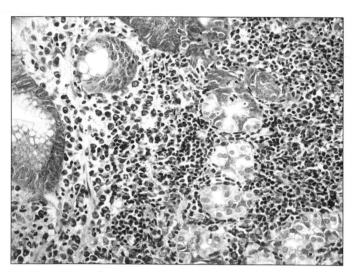

Fig. 13.4 Stomach – lymphoid infiltration in the lamina propria (Giemsa stain, ×100).

and considered unnecessary. Tissue collection for definitive staging, exploration of the abdomen, and reduction of tumor burden represent the advantages of surgery.

Many reports have shown a superior outcome when surgery is performed in the early stages of the disease, with a 5-year survival rate of up to 93%.[31,32] Fischbach et al.[33] reported one of

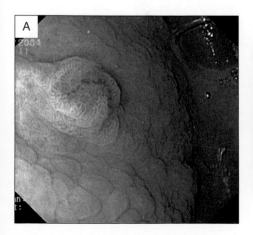

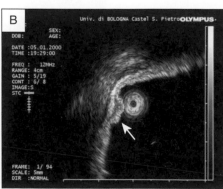

Fig. 13.5 A, Small sessile polypoid lesion in the gastric body. Histology revealed a low-grade MALT lymphoma. **B,** Scanning of the same lesion (arrow) with a 12-MHz miniprobe revealed the disease to be limited to the second layer (stage T1m N0).

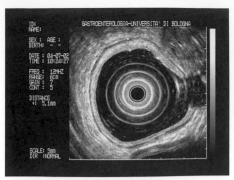

Fig. 13.6 Radial scanning of the gastric antrum at 12 MHz. The second and third layers are thickened, with no clear boundary in between; the fourth layer is preserved (stage T1sm N0).

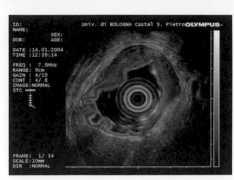

Fig. 13.7 Radial scanning of the gastric corpus at 7.5 MHz: the second, third, and fourth layers are thickened and fused together; only the fifth layer is preserved (stage T2 N0).

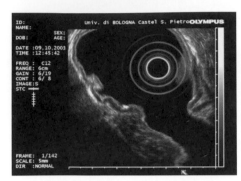

Fig. 13.8 Radial scanning of the gastric corpus at 12 MHz. The transition zone between normal and pathologic wall is displayed, showing progressive disruption of the second, third, and fourth layers (stage T2 N0). A careful assessment of the transition zone is always required for accurate staging.

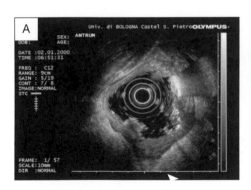

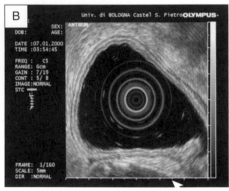

Fig. 13.9 A, Radial scanning of the gastric antrum at 12 MHz; all layers are thickened and disrupted. Solution of continuity of the fifth layer is visible (arrow), corresponding to lymphomatous penetration of the serosa without invasion of adjacent structures (stage T3 N0). **B,** Radial scanning of the gastric antrum in the same patient 6 months after finishing chemotherapy. Complete restoration of the gastric wall thickness and layering is shown.

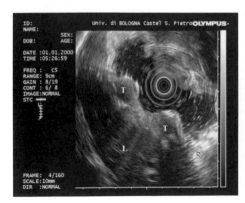

Fig. 13.10 High-grade gastric lymphoma infiltrating the anterior wall and lesser curvature of the gastric corpus and fundus. The tumor (T) has infiltrated all layers of the gastric wall and invaded the perigastric structures. In particular, no cleavage plane between the lesion and the left lobe of the liver (L) is visible (stage T4). This finding was confirmed at surgery.

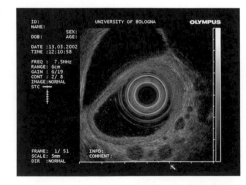

Fig. 13.11 Enlarged hypoechoic regional lymph nodes are clearly detected outside the stomach (stage T1sm N1).

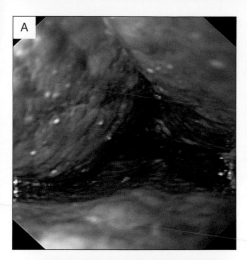

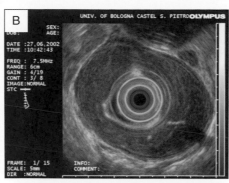

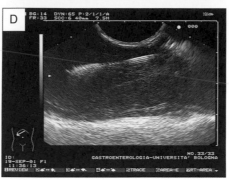

Fig. 13.12 A, Huge, elongated, vegetating masses are visible in the middle and distal esophagus, covered by irregular mucosa. Differential diagnosis with varices may be problematic. **B,** Radial scanning demonstrated a huge circumferential thickening of the esophageal wall by solid tissue, infiltrating the second, third, and fourth layers. A lymph node is also visible outside the wall. **C,** Curvilinear scanning with an electronic echoendoscope confirmed thickening and disruption of the layers. **D,** EUS-FNA was performed to obtain deep sampling of the lesion, allowing a diagnosis of low-grade esophageal MALT lymphoma (prior standard endoscopic biopsies had been unrevealing).

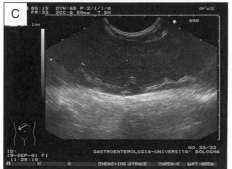

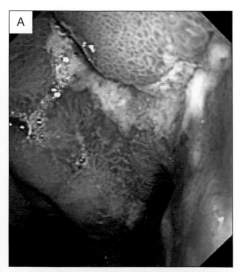

Fig. 13.13 A, Ulcerated vegetating lesion in the gastric fundus. Histology showed low-grade lymphoma with a high degree of plasmacellular differentiation. **B,** Radial scanning showed that the lesion is infiltrating the muscularis propria (stage T2).

HISTOLOGIC CLASSIFICATION OF GASTROINTESTINAL LYMPHOMAS
B-cell lymphomas

MALT-type (extranodal marginal zone lymphomas):
     Low grade
     High grade (with or without a low-grade component)

Immunoproliferative small intestinal disease (IPSID):
     Low grade
     High grade (with or without a low-grade component)

Lymphomatous polyposis (mantle cell lymphoma)
Burkitt and Burkitt-like
Other types of low- or high-grade lymphoma corresponding to lymph node equivalents
T-cell lymphomas
Enteropathy-associated T-cell lymphomas (EATCLs)
Other types not associated with enteropathy

Table 13.2 Histologic classification of gastrointestinal lymphomas

the largest experiences in this respect. They enrolled 266 patients with primary gastric B-cell lymphoma, 236 with stage IE or IIE. Non-responders to *H. pylori* eradication therapy and patients with stage IIE low-grade disease underwent gastric surgery. Depending on the residual tumor status and pre-defined risk factors, patients received either radiotherapy or no further treatment. Patients with high-grade disease underwent surgery and chemotherapy, complemented by radiation in those with incomplete resection. In this experience, surgical therapy was the treatment of choice in the majority of cases (Fig. 13.14). However, in view of the increasing tendency towards stomach-conserving therapy, the authors claimed the need for further studies to compare control of the disease and quality of life with surgical and conservative treatment.

Another prospective study[34] found that in stages IE and IIE the complete response rate, survival rate, and disease-free survival rate were similar among those who underwent complete resection, partial or no surgery prior to chemotherapy. A survival rate of 60% was reported with surgery alone, compared with 85% when adjuvant chemotherapy was given.

Surgical treatment has been almost abandoned owing to increased morbidity and mortality, often outweighing the benefits gained in terms of survival.[35] Moreover, gastric conservation may substantially contribute to the preservation of quality of life in these patients. Another large multicenter study,[36] conducted in 208 patients, failed to show any difference in therapeutic outcome between surgically or conservatively treated patients, again favoring the caution surrounding surgery as a treatment for gastric lymphoma.

Chemotherapy

The efficacy of chemotherapy as the sole treatment for gastric lymphoma is still under debate. Chemotherapy has been advocated to avoid the morbidity and mortality related to gastrectomy. Moreover, improved quality of life as a result of stomach

preservation is another factor that favors non-surgical treatment (Fig. 13.15).

A trial by Maor et al.[37] showed good results for chemotherapy, combined with radiotherapy, in a small group of patients with stage IE and IIE disease. Salvagno et al.[32] reported a survival rate of 71% in patients receiving chemotherapy. Another study[38] of patients with high-grade lymphoma found chemotherapy useful in inducing complete remission in 81% of patients, with fewer complications such as perforation or bleeding. No apparent difference in survival between surgery and chemotherapy was shown in these reports.

In patients with co-morbidities and at increased risk for surgery, chemotherapy offers at least an equally effective treatment.

In the past, the fear of complications such as bleeding and perforation was a discouragement to the initiation of chemotherapy. However, it was subsequently reported that the incidence of chemotherapy-related bleeding was very low (0–3%), and that of perforation was almost nil.[35,39] Since then, chemotherapy has become the treatment of choice. The most effective regimen for low-grade lymphomas combines cyclophosphamide, doxurubicin, vincristine, and prednisolone (CHOP). For high-grade lymphomas, regimens including doxurubicin, teniposide, cyclophosphamide, and prednisolone have been adopted. These pharmacologic regimens combined with surgical resection are associated with 80–100% survival rates.[40]

Radiotherapy and combined treatments

Radiotherapy is often employed as an adjuvant to surgery, chemotherapy, or both. Radiotherapy alone has been rarely studied; however, some authors maintain that it can be utilized as the primary treatment with a reasonable outcome. Schechter et al.[41] administered low-dose radiotherapy as an alternative to surgery in 17 patients with low-grade MALT lymphoma without evidence of *H. pylori* or with persistent disease after antibiotic therapy. The median total radiation dose was 30 Gy, delivered in

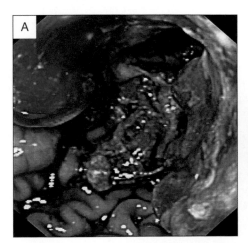
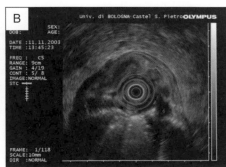
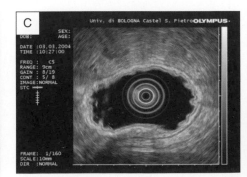

Fig. 13.14 A, A huge ulcerated lesion, spontaneously bleeding, infiltrating the whole gastric antrum. Biopsies revealed high-grade MALT lymphoma. **B,** Radial scanning revealed marked thickening of the gastric wall, with disruption of the layers and penetration of the serosa (stage T3). The patient was subsequently operated on due to bleeding that resulted in marked anemia. **C,** Postsurgical follow-up, showing no EUS sign of recurrence in the gastric remnant.

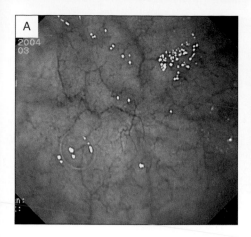

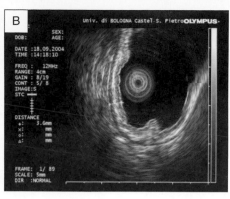

Fig. 13.15 A, Atrophic aspect of gastric fundal mucosa after chemotherapy administered for a T1sm N1 low-grade MALT lymphoma, not responsive to anti-*H. pylori* treatment. **B,** Radial scanning at the same level shows that the gastric wall thickness and layers have returned to normal.

1.5-Gy fractions within 4 weeks to the stomach and adjacent lymph nodes. All patients had a complete response. At a median of 27 months after completion of radiotherapy, the event-free survival rate was 100%. Treatment was well tolerated with few side-effects. Results from this and other trials suggest that radiotherapy can be a feasible, safe, and effective treatment in selected patients, allowing stomach preservation.

Finally, combined protocols including chemotherapy, radiotherapy, and eventually surgical resection have become the standard of care in many centers and now represent the mainstay of treatment of gastric lymphoma after *H. pylori* eradication failure, or when it is not indicated. This multimodal therapy has induced a significant improvement in the 5-year survival rate compared with single therapy.

ROLE OF EUS IN MALT LYMPHOMA

Diagnosis and staging

Differential diagnosis between gastric lymphoma and other forms of gastric wall infiltrative disease, usually encompassed under the term of large gastric folds (LGFs) (see below), is fundamental for therapeutic purposes, but may be challenging. Standard endoscopic mucosal biopsies are often unrevealing and have been shown to provide a limited diagnostic yield, as they contain only superficial mucosa. In some series of infiltrative malignancies of the stomach, traditional biopsies were positive in only 50% of cases.[42–45] Specimens obtained by large-valve biopsy forceps may increase diagnostic sensitivity by only a small amount; a diathermic snare can be used to obtain deeper

specimens, but at the cost of increased risk of hemorrhage and perforation.[46,47] For these reasons, even laparotomy has been advocated to obtain a surgical, full-thickness, gastric biopsy specimen. Other authors have suggested even more refined techniques, such as EUS-guided fine-needle aspiration (EUS-FNA) (Fig. 13.16) and the guillotine-needle biopsy.[48–50]

Nevertheless, LGFs may still escape the traditional combined endoscopic–histologic diagnostic approach. The advent of EUS has led to a marked improvement in diagnostic accuracy in this respect.[51]

Several studies of gastric cancer and lymphoma have demonstrated specific EUS features that allow correct diagnosis and staging of lymphoma in the majority of patients. Although infiltrative carcinoma tends to show a vertical growth in the gastric wall, with transmural involvement, lymphoma shows a mainly horizontal extension. At an early stage, lymphoma may be seen at EUS as a thickening of the second layer alone, or of the second and third layers, preserved as different layers (Figs 13.17–13.19). Interestingly, these alterations of the gastric wall may be found not only within and around the lesions observed at endoscopy, but also in areas where the mucosa appears normal.[52,53] At an advanced stage, lymphoma shows an ultrasonographic pattern of diffuse hypoechoic thickening with fusion of the layers (Figs 13.20–13.22).

At present, EUS is the most accurate imaging modality for the evaluation and staging of infiltrative gastric lesions. As additional evidence, the number of published papers considering EUS staging of gastric MALT lymphoma has increased progressively in recent years (Fig. 13.23).[54]

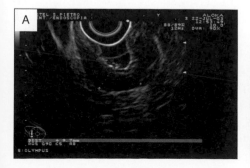

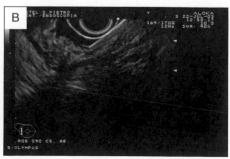

Fig. 13.16 A, Curvilinear scanning of the gastric wall showing deep infiltration of the layers involving the muscularis propria. Standard endoscopic biopsies were negative for malignancy. **B,** EUS-FNA was performed to obtain deep sampling of the gastric wall, thus allowing a positive cytologic diagnosis of lymphoma.

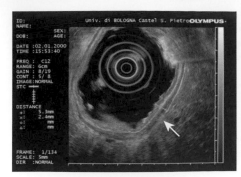

Fig. 13.17 Radial scanning showing a mild thickening of the stomach wall, limited to the second layer and circumscribed to a small portion of the gastric circumference (arrow). The rest of the gastric wall was normal. Subsequently, endoscopic biopsies were performed as directed by EUS findings, showing high-grade lymphoma (stage T1m N0).

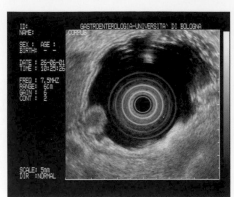

Fig. 13.18 Polypoid aspect of a gastric low-grade MALT lymphoma. Thickening of the second layer is visible; underlying layers are preserved (stage T1m N0).

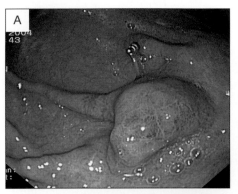

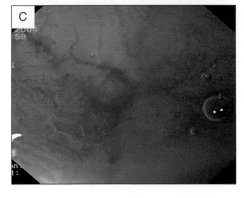

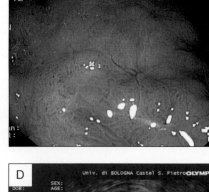

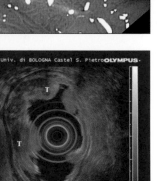

Fig. 13.19 A, Vegetating irregular lesion on the anterior face of the gastric corpus, creating retraction of the surrounding rugal folds. **B,** At a closer view, irregular mucosa and neoangiogenesis are visible on the surface of the lesion. **C,** High-magnification view with a zoom endoscope, showing a neoangiogenesis pattern in great detail (×100). **D,** Radial scanning at 12 MHz, showing a marked, hypoechoic, and irregular thickening of the second layer consistent with lymphomatous infiltration (T). The third layer is still identifiable but disrupted, demonstrating infiltration of the submucosa too. The fourth layer is preserved (stage T1sm N0).

Fig. 13.20 Marked thickening of the gastric antrum, viewed from the corpus. The second, third, and fourth layers are fused and no longer identifiable as single layers (stage T2 N0).

The great accuracy of EUS for staging gastric lymphoma, both before and after therapy, has been demonstrated by several authors.[55–59] In particular, the authors' group reported an 89% sensitivity, 97% specificity, and 95% overall accuracy for EUS evaluation of depth of lymphoma invasion.[60]

However, Fischbach et al.[61] recently raised a word of caution in this respect. They performed a multicenter study evaluating the accuracy of EUS in the staging of gastric lymphoma at 34 different centers. Data from preoperative EUS procedures were compared with the histopathologic stage of resection specimens in 70 patients with newly diagnosed primary

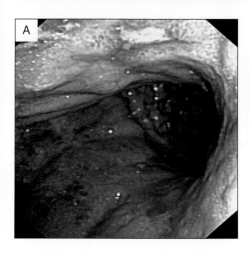

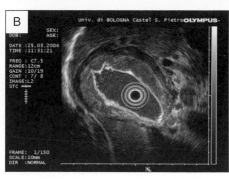

Fig. 13.21 A, Large gastric folds covered by ulcerated mucosa are visible in the fundus and corpus. **B,** Diffuse circumferential thickening of the second, third, and fourth layers, which are disrupted but still identifiable. The serosa is irregular but still preserved. Several perigastric enlarged lymph nodes are visible. At this stage, differential diagnosis with linitis plastica can be difficult. However, endoscopic biopsies provided the answer, demonstrating high-grade lymphoma (stage T2 N1).

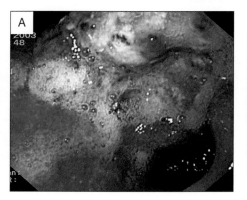

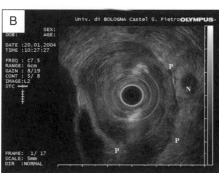

Fig. 13.22 A, Huge ulcerated lesion of the stomach with a large amount of necrotic debris inside. **B,** Radial scanning shows a circumferential thickening of the wall; all the layers are infiltrated by the lymphoma and are no longer identifiable as individual entities. The serosa shows minimal interruptions (pseudopodia, P) consistent with lymphomatous infiltration. A lymph node (N) is also visible (stage T3 N1). In this case, as opposed to that shown in Fig. 13.21, linitis plastica is less likely and differential diagnosis is somewhat easier.

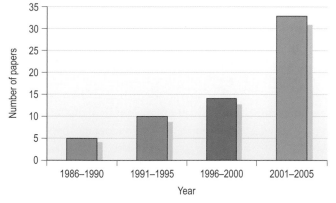

Fig. 13.23 Number of published papers dealing with EUS staging of gastric lymphoma.

gastric lymphoma; EUS classified the lymphoma correctly in only 37 (53%). the sensitivity of EUS was as follows: stage I1, 67%; stage I2, 83%; and stage II1, 71%. In conclusion, according to this study, it seems that the accuracy of EUS in the local staging of gastric lymphoma has to be improved if non-surgical treatment strategies are to be used. However, the authors themselves found an explanation of the relative lack of accuracy: a high number of participating centers were performing few EUS procedures. Nevertheless, this study underlines the importance of having highly experienced operators in large-volume EUS centers in order to maximize the accuracy and diagnostic yield of the technique.

Shimodaira et al.[62] were among the first to state that EUS assessment of the depth of lymphoma infiltration should be based on the tumor node metastasis (TNM) classification. According to the most recent update of the TNM classification,[63] EUS staging can be explained as follows: EUS-T1 is a hypoechoic tumor located in the mucosa or submucosa; EUS-T2 is a hypoechoic tumor located in the mucosa and submucosa extending into the muscularis propria or subserosa; EUS-T3 is a transmural hypoechoic tumor that penetrates into the serosa; and EUS-T4 is a transmural hypoechoic tumor that infiltrates into adjacent structures.

The present authors believe that the TNM rather than the modified Ann Arbor classification should be adopted to stage gastric lymphoma by EUS. The TNM classification allows a detailed assessment of lymphoproliferative disease as it differentiates the degree of mural involvement layer by layer, whereas the modified Ann Arbor classification contemplates only two stages of mural involvement.[64,65] For instance, modified Ann Arbor stage IE1 corresponds to T1m and T1sm, and modified Ann Arbor stage IE2 corresponds to multiple stages including T2, T3, and T4 (Tables 13.3 & 13.4). As shown below, an accurate EUS assessment of infiltration of every single layer is fundamental for predicting prognosis and establishing the appropriate therapy (Fig. 13.24).

ANN ARBOR CLASSIFICATION, MODIFIED BY MUSSHOFF AND SCHMIDT-VOLLMER[64]	
Grade	Description
IE	Lymphoma restricted to GI tract on one side of diaphragm
IE$_1$	Infiltration limited to mucosa and submucosa
IE$_2$	Lymphoma extending beyond submucosa
IIE	Lymphoma additionally infiltrating lymph nodes on same side of diaphragm
IIE$_1$	Infiltration of regional lymph nodes
IIE$_2$	Infiltration of lymph nodes beyond regional nodes
IIIE	Lymphoma infiltrating GI tract and/or lymph nodes on both sides of diaphragm
IVE	Localized infiltration of associated lymph nodes together with diffuse or disseminated involvement of extragastrointestinal organs

Table 13.3 Ann Arbor classification, modified by Musshoff and Schmidt-Vollmer[64]

COMPARISON OF MODIFIED ANN ARBOR AND TNM CLASSIFICATIONS		
Ann Arbor	TNM	Comment
IE$_1$	T1m–sm N0	
IE$_2$	T2–4 N0	
IIE$_1$	T1–4 N1	Perigastric lymph nodes
IIE$_2$	T1–4 N2	Regional lymph nodes
IIIE	T1–4 N3	Lymph nodes on both sides of diaphragm
IVE	T1–4 N0–3 M1	Visceral metastases or second extranodal site

Table 13.4 Comparison of modified Ann Arbor and TNM classifications

Another classification that should be cited for the sake of completeness, in addition to the modified Ann Arbor classification and the TNM staging system, is represented by the Lugano classification. The Lugano classification was constructed by Rohatiner et al.,[66] who introduced stage IIE for 'serosa penetration' without lymph node involvement into the Ann Arbor system. However, this classification is still intended mainly for clinical rather than EUS use (Table 13.5).

The same issue of inadequacy of the modified Ann Arbor and Lugano classifications to stage properly the different gastric levels of lymphomatous infiltration, resulting in very different prognoses, was also raised by Ruskoné-Fourmestraux et al.[67] These authors tend to agree with us regarding the use of the TNM system for EUS purposes of staging. However, as the TNM was created for staging carcinomas rather than lymphomas, they suggested a modified staging system, termed the Paris classification, that centered on the TNM system, but with some slight modifications. This new staging system adequately records the depth of tumor infiltration, extent of nodal involvement, and specific lymphoma spreading (Table 13.6). It is adjusted to the GI origin of the lymphoma, considering histopathologic characteristics of extranodal B- and T-cell lymphomas. According to the authors, the use of this system in future studies will permit accurate comparison of reported cohorts and should allow rapid accumulation of good data for proper stratification of patients for risk assessment and treatment options.

As far as lymph nodes are concerned, EUS can detect nodes as small as 3–4 mm in diameter. However, reliance on EUS features in the differential diagnosis of benign and malignant lymph nodes can be problematic. One of the most comprehensive series on this subject came from Catalano et al.,[68] who suggested that rounded, sharply demarcated, homogeneous, hypoechoic lymph nodes greater than 1 cm in diameter indicate malignancy, whereas elongated, heterogeneous, hyperechoic

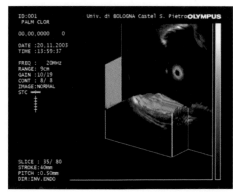

Fig. 13.24 Scanning of a gastric lymphoma at 20 MHz with a 3D-EUS mini-probe. 3D reconstruction and surface rendering are software functions that may help to enhance the accuracy of assessment of the level of lymphomatous infiltration. In this case it is nicely shown that only the second layer is thickened and that the underlying layers are preserved (stage T1m).

LUGANO STAGING OF GASTROINTESTINAL NON-HODGKIN LYMPHOMAS	
Stage	Description
I	Tumor confined to GI tract (single primary site or multiple non-contiguous sites)
II	Tumor extending into abdomen from primary GI site
II$_1$	Local nodal involvement
II$_2$	Distant nodal involvement
II$_E$	Penetration of serosa to involve adjacent organs or tissues
IV	Disseminated extranodal or supradiaphragmatic nodal involvement

Table 13.5 Lugano staging of gastrointestinal non-Hodgkin lymphomas

PARIS STAGING SYSTEM FOR PRIMARY GASTROINTESTINAL LYMPHOMAS[a]

Stage	Description
TX	Extent of lymphoma not specified
T0	No evidence of lymphoma
T1	Lymphoma confined to mucosa/submucosa
T1m	Lymphoma confined to mucosa
T1sm	Lymphoma confined to submucosa
T2	Lymphoma infiltrates muscularis propria or subserosa
T3	Lymphoma penetrates serosa (visceral peritoneum) without invasion of adjacent structures
T4	Lymphoma invades adjacent structures or organs
NX	Involvement of lymph nodes not assessed
N0	No evidence of lymph node involvement
N1[b]	Involvement of regional lymph nodes
N2	Involvement of intra-abdominal lymph nodes beyond the regional area
N3	Spread to extra-abdominal lymph nodes
MX	Dissemination of lymphoma not assessed
M0	No evidence of extranodal dissemination
M1	Non-continuous involvement of separate site in gastrointestinal tract (e.g., stomach and rectum)
M2	Non-continuous involvement of other tissues (e.g., peritoneum, pleura) or organs (e.g., tonsils, parotid gland, ocular adnexa, lung, liver, spleen, kidney, breast, etc.)
BX	Involvement of bone marrow not assessed
B0	No evidence of bone marrow involvement
B1	Lymphomatous infiltration of bone marrow
TNM	Clinical staging: status of tumor, node, metastasis, bone marrow
PTNMB	Histopathologic staging: status of tumor, node, metastasis, bone marrow
PN	The histologic examination ordinarily includes six or more lymph nodes

Table 13.6 Paris staging system for primary gastrointestinal lymphomas[a]

[a]Valid for lymphomas originating from the gastroesophageal junction to the anus (as defined by identical histomorphologic structure). In cases with more than one visible lesion synchronously originating in the gastrointestinal tract, give the characteristics of the more advanced lesion.

[b]Anatomic designation of lymph nodes as 'regional' according to site: (a) stomach – perigastric nodes and those located along the ramifications of the celiac artery (i.e., left gastric artery, common hepatic artery, splenic artery) in accordance with compartments I and II of the Japanese Research Society for Gastric Cancer (1995); (b) duodenum – pancreaticoduodenal, pyloric, hepatic, and superior mesenteric nodes; (c) jejunum/ileum – mesenteric nodes and, for the terminal ileum only, the ileocolic as well as the posterior cecal nodes; (d) colorectum – pericolic and perirectal nodes, and those located along the ileocolic, right, middle, and left colic, inferior mesenteric, superior rectal, and internal iliac arteries.

lymph nodes with indistinct borders are more likely to be benign. However, assessment of these features is highly operator-dependent and may be impossible in the presence of micrometastases. The issue of interobserver agreement in lymph node assessment is discussed below.

MÉNÉTRIÈR'S DISEASE AND OTHER LGFs: DIFFERENTIAL DIAGNOSIS WITH EUS

Diagnosis of LGFs is made when folds do not flatten at endoscopy, or when folds of 1.5 cm or more are seen at barium upper GI series or CT.[69,70] Ménétrièr was the first person to describe the presence of giant gastric folds in patients with hypertrophic gastritis, and Ménétrièr's disease has been the most commonly used eponym since then.[71]

The normal gastric wall thickness range at EUS is assessed as 0.8–3.6 mm.[72] Diagnosis of gastric wall thickening is generally established at EUS under routine clinical conditions when the overall thickness of the five layers is greater than 4 mm.[73,74] Nevertheless, the differential diagnosis can be very hard to make by means of endoscopic appearance, radiography, and even biopsy, because widening of the gastric folds is seen in a large number of benign and malignant conditions.

Some inflammatory and infectious diseases can be involved (Fig. 13.25), including *H. pylori* infection;[75–80] vascular and infiltrating diseases can sometimes be present, although these do not appear to play a major etiologic role;[81,82] and finally malignant diseases, such as carcinoma and lymphoma, must always be considered[83,84] (Table 13.7). All of these diseases causing LGFs show different levels of EUS infiltration of the gastric wall; thus the number of differential diagnostic possibilities can be somewhat limited (Table 13.8).

EUS differential diagnosis between early lymphoma and Ménétrièr's disease may be challenging. These lesions show a fairly similar echo pattern, which is displayed as an extended thickening of the second and sometimes the third layer, with preservation of the layers as distinctive structures. Nevertheless, as the distinction among these different pathologies is very important because of their different prognosis, it is possible to find some particular differences.

Ménétrièr's disease displays a more localized thickening, which is hyperechoic rather than hypoechoic, and involves mainly the second layer (Fig. 13.26).[85]

ETIOLOGY OF LARGE GASTRIC FOLDS

Malignancies	Adenocarcinoma, linitis plastica, lymphoma, metastases
Infections	Secondary syphilis, tuberculosis, cytomegalovirus, herpes simplex virus, histoplasmosis, cryptococcosis, aspergillosis, *H. pylori* infection, anisakiasis
Infiltrative diseases	Crohn's disease, sarcoidosis, amyloidosis, gastritis (eosinophilic, granulomatous, and lymphocytic)
Vascular diseases	Portal hypertensive gastropathy, gastric varices
Benign conditions	Ménétrièr's disease, Zollinger–Ellison syndrome, gastritis, hyper-rugosity, gastritis cystica profunda

Table 13.7 Etiology of large gastric folds

LAYERS PRINCIPALLY INVOLVED ACCORDING TO ETIOLOGY	
Disease	Layers
H. pylori infection	2, 2+3
Ménétrièr's disease	2
Gastritis, hyper-rugosity	2
Anisakiasis	3
Gastritis cystica profunda	3
Gastric varices	3
Adenocarcinoma, linitis plastica	2, 2+3, 2+3+4
Gastric lymphoma	2, 2+3, 2+3+4

Table 13.8 Layers principally involved according to etiology

The ability of EUS to examine patients with LGFs has been investigated by several authors. Mendis et al.[86] examined the utility of EUS in 28 patients with endoscopically or radiographically diagnosed LGFs, in most of whom endoscopic biopsies had been inconclusive for malignancy. EUS demonstrated gastric varices in four patients and biopsy specimens were not taken. In three patients, biopsy results were negative for malignancy. However, because of ultrasonographic findings of wall thickening involving layers three and four, the patients underwent laparotomy, which revealed primary gastric carcinoma. In the remaining 24 patients, large-forceps endoscopic biopsy revealed acute or chronic inflammation in 16 (67%), malignancy in 4 (17%), and Ménétrièr's disease in 1 (4%). Malignancy did not develop in any of the patients with gastric wall thickening limited to layer two and negative biopsy results during a mean follow-up of 35 months. The authors concluded that when EUS abnormalities involve only the mucosal layer, endoscopic biopsies are diagnostic. Abnormalities involving the muscularis propria in the absence of ulceration strongly suggest malignancy and should be investigated further if endoscopic biopsy findings are negative. Moreover, with EUS, potentially dangerous biopsies of gastric varices can be avoided.

Songur et al.[87] analyzed the EUS features of 35 patients with giant gastric folds describing some findings useful in

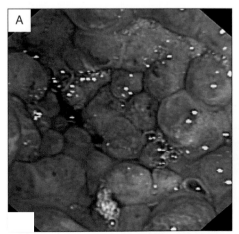
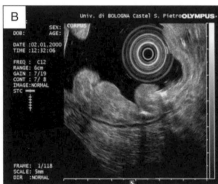
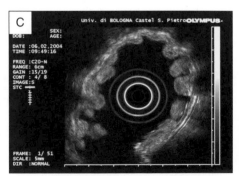
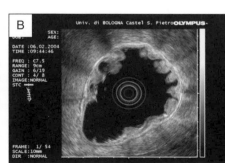
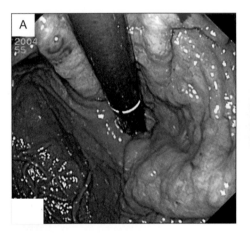

Fig. 13.25 A, Hypertrophic gastric folds are detected in the gastric fundus during upper endoscopy performed in a patient with a recent history of perforated duodenal ulcer. Differential diagnosis can be problematic on the basis of endoscopy, and biopsies should not be taken before ruling out the presence of fundal varices. **B,** Radial scanning at the same level, showing marked thickening of the second layer with a non-homogeneous echogenicity. In view of the clinical picture and other diagnostic investigative data, this finding was consistent with the diagnosis of Zollinger–Ellison syndrome.

Fig. 13.26 A, Large gastric folds covered by irregular mucosa. This woman had hypoalbuminemia, anemia, and diarrhea. **B,** General view of the gastric corpus by radial scanning at 7.5 MHz. A hyperechoic diffuse thickening of the second layer is visible. **C,** Closer view of the wall by radial scanning at 20 MHz. Isolated hyperechoic thickening of the second layer is clearly shown. Moreover, some small anechoic lacunae, compatible with cystic spaces, are present inside the second layer itself. This finding is highly suggestive of Ménétrièr's disease. After antibiotic treatment for *H. pylori*, the patient experienced a complete and stable normalization of her symptoms and signs.

characterizing each type of lesion. According to these authors, when the second layer alone is thickened, Ménétrièr's disease may be one of the possible pathologic entities, whereas when the third layer alone is abnormally enlarged, anisakiasis might be suspected. Most of the patients with scirrhous carcinoma showed an abnormally enlarged third and fourth layer. Thus, the second and third layers may be thickened in healthy subjects with simple hyperrugosity, but also in patients with gastric lymphoma. The fourth layer was significantly thickened only in malignant conditions. The authors concluded that EUS can visualize the structure of giant gastric folds and may facilitate the differentiation of benign from malignant etiologies.

Maunoury et al.[88] stated that endosonographic aspects may be helpful in distinguishing Ménétrièr's disease from lymphocytic gastritis, although biopsies are necessary for final confirmation of diagnosis because some overlapping endosonographic aspects may exist.

Okada et al.[89] described two patients suffering from gastritis cystica profunda, a rare condition in which multiple small cysts in the mucosa and submucosa of the stomach are encountered, presenting as giant gastric folds. In these cases the diagnosis was made based on findings from EUS and mucosectomy.

It must be always kept in mind that EUS is not a histologic technique. For this reason, it must be used always in combination with endoscopic biopsy. EUS can help in determining the site at which to take a biopsy in order to avoid false-negative results, and sometimes the need for a large-particle biopsy can be suggested. Conversely, contraindication to biopsies can result from an EUS examination at which gastric varices are depicted.

In conclusion, a final protocol based on EUS findings can be suggested for patients with gastric lymphoma or LGFs of different etiology. For an early diagnosis, when the EUS pattern is normal and endoscopic findings are inconclusive, an adequate number of standard endoscopic biopsies should be performed, and even repeated in multiple sessions. Large-valve forceps biopsy and snare biopsy must also be considered. When abnormalities involve layer two, endoscopic biopsies are diagnostic; when abnormalities involve layers two and three, large-particle biopsy should be considered; when abnormalities involve layer four, malignancy should be strongly suspected even if standard biopsies are negative; thus, FNA or guillotine-needle biopsy should be performed.

EUS FOR PREDICTING THERAPEUTIC RESPONSE

Several studies have shown that anti-*H. pylori* therapy may lead to regression of early-stage primary gastric MALT lymphoma. However, complete response figures are variable, ranging from zero to 100% in different case series. This striking disparity in response rate may be highly dependent on the accuracy of pretreatment staging of the MALT lesions. On average, regression of gastric MALT lymphoma after eradication of *H. pylori* with antibiotics has been reported in approximately 50–60% of treated patients (Table 13.9).

Reference	Journal	Year	Complete response (%)
TRIALS ADOPTING EUS FOR STAGING OF GASTRIC MALT LYMPHOMA			
Bayerdorffer et al.[95]	Lancet	1995	70
Roggero et al.[94]	Ann Intern Med	1995	60
Pavlick et al.[103]	J Clin Oncol	1997	0
Levy et al.[105]	Gastrointest Endosc	1997	–
Sackmann et al.[99]	Gastroenterology	1997	54
Nobre-Leitao et al.[102]	Am J Gastroenterol	1998	100
Steinbach et al.[104]	Ann Intern Med	1999	41
Ohashi et al.[98]	Cancer	2000	82
Fischbach et al.[33]	Gastroenterology	2000	89
Ruskoné-Fourmestraux et al.[100]	Gut	2001	43
Nakamura et al.[101]	Gut	2001	71
Levy et al.[106]	Am J Gastroenterol	2002	69
Caletti et al.[118]	Aliment Pharmacol Ther	2002	55
Puspok et al.[115]	Gut	2002	82
Yeh et al.[116]	J Gastroenterol Hepatol	2003	82
Fischbach et al.[107]	Gut	2004	62

Table 13.9 Trials adopting EUS for staging of gastric MALT lymphoma

For low-grade lymphomas, which account for approximately 35% of primary gastric lymphomas, the accuracy of EUS staging and follow-up is crucial for optimal treatment. In fact, EUS can predict the outcome of treatment of MALT lymphoma by simple eradication of *H. pylori*. Although encouraging results by antibiotic treatment have been reported, many authors failed either to include EUS in their staging methods or to correlate EUS staging results, when available, with remission rates.[34,90–98]

In fact, remission rates reported by different trials in which patients with MALT lymphoma were not differentiated according to EUS stage have shown striking disparities. If these papers are examined in detail, it can be seen that remission rates should not be considered cumulatively for the whole group of patients just because they suffer from low-grade (as opposed to high-grade) MALT lymphoma, but for each subgroup identifiable by EUS TNM staging. By doing so, it becomes evident that papers that reported a complete response rate of up to 100% included patients with disease limited to the mucosa and/or submucosa at EUS.[99–102] However, very few patients with deeper infiltration showed a complete response.[103,104]

Sackmann et al.[99] studied whether staging by EUS predicted the outcome of treatment of MALT lymphoma by eradication of *H. pylori*. The infection was eradicated in all 22 patients with a

2-week course of oral omeprazole and amoxicillin. Twelve of 14 patients with lymphoma limited to the second or third layer (mucosa or submucosa) at EUS, but none of 10 patients with deeper infiltration, showed a complete response ($P<0.01$). As remission may occur even 14 months after antimicrobial therapy, EUS appeared to be a reliable method for selecting in advance patients who may benefit from antibiotics, and for referring the others to chemotherapy or surgery. Levy et al.[105] showed that patients with a thick gastric wall at EUS follow-up were highly likely to have persistent tumor infiltration, even when endoscopic biopsies were negative.

Another important trial that aimed to explain the discrepancies in remission rates mentioned above, and to determine the factors predictive of gastric lymphoma regression after anti-*H. pylori* treatment, was published by Ruskoné-Fourmestraux et al.[100] These authors enrolled 44 consecutive patients with localized gastric MALT lymphoma (Ann Arbor stages IE and IIE), all of whom underwent EUS. Overall, histologic regression of the lymphoma was obtained in only 43% of the patients; median follow-up for these 19 responders was as long as 35 months. However, there was a significant difference between the response of the lymphoma restricted to the mucosa and other more deep-seated lesions ($P<0.006$). Moreover, the complete response rate of the lymphoma increased from 56% to 79% when there was no nodal involvement at EUS. As a result, in patients carefully evaluated by EUS, without any lymph node involvement, a complete response was obtained in 79%.

Nakamura et al.[101] found that 26 (93%) of 28 MALT lymphomas restricted to the mucosa, but only 3 (23%) of 13 lymphomas that invaded the deep portion of the submucosa or beyond, regressed completely after therapy. As opposed to EUS staging, neither the presence of a high-grade component, perigastric lymphadenopathy, nor clinical staging prior to eradication correlated with the probability of lymphoma regression.

Levy et al.[106] obtained a 69% overall complete response rate in 48 treated patients. Interestingly, they found that the response did not correlate with endoscopic features or histologic grade. In contrast, it was related to EUS features: remission was achieved in 76% of patients in whom no perigastric lymph node was detected, compared with only 33% when EUS showed presence of lymph nodes ($P=0.025$). Another important point from this study is that remission could be achieved with chlorambucil monochemotherapy in 58% of patients who did not respond to anti-*H. pylori* treatment. The most recent trial came from Fischbach et al.,[107] who aimed to determine the long-term outcome of patients undergoing exclusive *H. pylori* eradication therapy. Ninety patients with a low-grade gastric MALT lymphoma were enrolled in this multicenter study and followed for at least 12 months. Long-term outcome was characterized by a complete response in 56 patients (62%), minimal residual disease in 17 (19%), partial remission in 11 (12%), no change in four (4%), and progressive disease in two patients (2%). Once again, the authors found that EUS was

fundamental for establishing the prognosis, as the regression rate was higher in stage I1 disease compared with stage I2, as assessed by EUS.

Finally, Lugering et al.[108] confirmed previous findings on the use of mini-probes for the staging and follow-up of gastric lymphoma, providing accurate staging compared with dedicated echoendoscopes. They recommended the use of mini-probes in clinical practice because the examination can be performed as a single-step procedure during diagnostic endoscopy.

In conclusion, the ability of EUS to stage lesions accurately is of paramount importance as it allows for determination of the best mode of therapy for individual patients. Although many therapies are available for gastric MALT lymphoma, they cannot be assigned randomly to an individual patient. Although early-stage lesions, T1m and T1sm, may regress following anti-*H. pylori* therapy alone, more advanced lesions (T2–T4) may require more aggressive treatment protocols. Thus, for more advanced lesions, rather than losing precious time with antibiotic treatment or single-drug chemotherapy, one may proceed directly to combination chemotherapy, radiation therapy, and/or surgery.[109–111]

In patients with more advanced disease, the optimal treatment regimen is less clear and may consist of various modalities, including antibiotics, combination chemotherapy, radiotherapy, or surgical resection.[112,113] A stepwise approach starting with antibiotics and advancing to chemotherapy with chlorambucil was investigated in a European trial.[114] Combination therapy with antibiotics and anti-CD20 monoclonal antibody therapy may be an alternative mode of therapy that needs further investigation.

It is important to note that the assessment of response to therapy requires long-term follow-up with interval upper endoscopy with biopsies as well as EUS. When biopsies remain positive for lymphoma but EUS does not reveal further changes in the wall structure, it may be appropriate to 'wait and see', as anti-*H. pylori* therapy may take up to 18 months to achieve remission.

ROLE OF EUS IN FOLLOW-UP

The importance of EUS lies not only in its ability to stage MALT lymphoma before treatment, but also in systematic follow-up, as interval EUS may determine response to therapy and detect relapse early (Fig. 13.27). At times, EUS may show restoration of normal gastric wall layers prior to histologic remission, and at other times recurrent wall thickening or disruption may be seen in individuals who were previously in remission. For patients who persist in having a thickened gastric wall on EUS despite antibiotic therapy, other treatment modalities should be considered, even if endoscopic biopsies are negative. These patients most likely have persistent lymphoma.

Many of the authors of trials adopting EUS for the pretreatment staging of gastric MALT lymphoma agree on the importance of EUS for follow-up too. However, given the relative lack of long-term follow-up case series, this issue is still

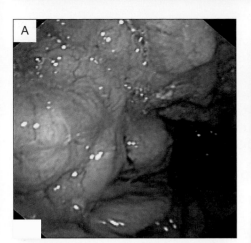

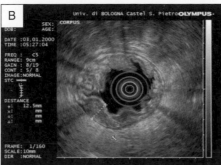

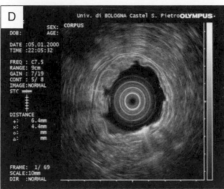

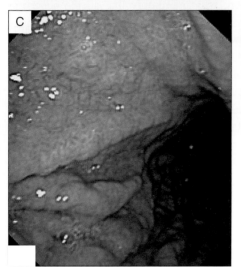

Fig. 13.27 A, Hypertrophic irregular folds on the anterior face of the gastric corpus. Histology showed low-grade MALT lymphoma. **B,** Radial scanning at the same level, showing involvement of the second and third layers. Although very close to it, there is still no lymphomatous infiltration of the fourth layer (stage T1sm N0). **C,** Improvement of the endoscopic picture 6 months after *H. pylori*-eradicating therapy. However, biopsies showed persistence of a low-grade MALT lymphoma. **D,** EUS showed improvement as well, with a significant reduction of overall wall thickness and restoration of the distinction between the second and third layers. This peculiar EUS finding suggests that the patient is responding well to antibiotics, despite histologic persistence of lymphoma, and that further follow-up without more aggressive treatments is warranted.

under debate for some conditions. For instance, Puspok et al.[115] maintain that EUS is less accurate than endoscopy with biopsies for routine follow-up. They enrolled 33 patients with primary gastric lymphoma, performing pretreatment and follow-up EUS every 3–6 months after non-surgical treatment. A total of 158 EUS examinations was performed. Within a median follow-up of 15 months, 82% of patients achieved histologic remission, whereas EUS remission was found in only 64%. Eighteen patients achieved both histologic and EUS remission, with EUS remission occurring later than histological remission (35 versus 18 weeks). Moreover, histologic relapse was demonstrated by EUS in only 1 of 5 cases. However, this trial does have some weaknesses. In particular, the authors did not use the TNM classification for EUS assessment of disease in the gastric wall; in view of the reasons cited above, this may have led to underpowering of EUS parameters in predicting remission.

Another trial, which specifically addressed the issue of the role of EUS in follow-up, came to different conclusions. Yeh et al.[116] studied 20 patients with low-grade gastric MALT lymphoma before and after eradication therapy. Of 17 patients who were *H. pylori* positive, 14 (82%) obtained histologic remission. These authors found that, although pretreatment EUS, performed with a 12-MHz miniature probe, showed significantly greater wall thickness in patients with MALT lymphoma than in controls (6.1 versus 2.8 mm), follow-up mini-probe EUS showed a comparative and statistically significant reduction in wall thickness. Interestingly, for patients with a significant reduction in wall thickness just after *H. pylori* eradication, the probability of a complete response of the MALT lymphoma was 40% at 12 months and 84% at 24 months. Thus, according to the authors, EUS plays a valuable role not only in the initial staging of gastric MALT lymphoma but also in long-term follow-up. Nevertheless, the present authors believe that EUS should not be regarded as an alternative to endoscopy with histology; on the contrary, these two techniques should always be adopted together to maximize the diagnostic yield for staging and follow-up of patients affected by gastric MALT lymphoma.

THE ITALIAN MALT LYMPHOMA STUDY GROUP EXPERIENCE

The highest incidence of gastric MALT lymphoma has been reported in north-eastern Italy, where the prevalence of *H. pylori* infection is particularly high.[117] A multicenter study[118] was carried out to determine the EUS findings that may predict regression of low-grade gastric MALT lymphoma after anti-*H. pylori* therapy.

Inclusion criteria were low-grade primary gastric MALT lymphoma stages IE (IE1–IE2) or IIE1, and *H. pylori*-positive status. The diagnosis of MALT was supported by histologic and immunohistochemical findings. EUS staging was performed according to the TNM classification. All patients were treated with a 7-day course of anti-*H. pylori* therapy consisting of omeprazole 40 mg four times daily, clarithromycin 250 mg twice daily, and tinidazole 500 mg twice a day. Repeat upper endoscopy with gastric mucosal biopsies and EUS were performed 3 months after antibiotic therapy, then at 3–4-month intervals until resolution of MALT lymphoma had been documented, then at 6-month intervals. Patients who failed to respond to anti-*H. pylori* therapy at 2-year follow-up, and those who had progressive disease, were referred for evaluation for surgery and/or chemotherapy.

Fifty-one patients (31 men, 20 women, median age 63 [range 21–88] years) met the inclusion criteria and formed the study sample. After antibiotic therapy, eradication of *H. pylori* was seen in 45 (88%) of the 51 patients. Six (12%) of the patients had persistent infection despite two courses of anti-*H. pylori* therapy. Interestingly, three of them had a complete response anyway.

Two years after therapy, regression of lymphoma was seen in 28 (55%) of the 51 patients: 25 patients were *H. pylori* negative and 3 remained *H. pylori* positive despite therapy. Twenty-three patients (45%) had either no lymphoma regression following anti-*H. pylori* therapy or lymphoma relapse after initial regression. The median time to lymphoma regression was 6 (range 1–14) months.

As for EUS staging, 12 (75%) of 16 patients with stage T1m N0 disease and 11 (58%) of 19 with stage T1sm N0 disease achieved a complete response, compared with only 4 (50%) of 8 with stages T1m N1 and T1sm N1, and 1 (25%) of 4 patients with stage T2 N0. None of the patients in stage T2 N1 achieved a complete response (Table 13.10).

H. pylori eradication was seen in 88% of cases. Among the total population, 55% of patients had histologic regression of MALT lymphoma 1–14 (median 6) months after anti-*H. pylori* therapy. Although in the majority of reported cases *H. pylori* eradication precedes MALT lymphoma regression, rare case reports of MALT lymphoma regression despite the persistence of *H. pylori* following antibiotic therapy have been published.[27,28] In fact, in the Italian MALT Lymphoma Study Group experience, 3 of the 28 patients with persistent lymphoma regression remained *H. pylori* positive despite anti-*H. pylori* therapy. We agree with other authors who postulate that, in addition to eradicating *H. pylori*, antibiotics may have a directly cytotoxic effect, leading to regression of MALT lymphoma. Moreover, it is possible that an as yet unidentified organism, closely related to *H. pylori*, may be implicated in these rare cases of MALT lymphoma.

INTEROBSERVER AGREEMENT IN THE STAGING OF GASTRIC LYMPHOMA BY EUS

There is a strict correlation between EUS staging and prognosis. For this reason, it is mandatory that all the observers agree on the same parameters of staging. This is of particular importance in EUS, which is an operator-dependent technique. Good interobserver agreement is essential to compare clinical trials conducted at different units, to stratify patients within studies, and to establish the best treatment for every patient, even when not included in clinical trials.

To ensure optimal EUS staging, the Italian MALT Lymphoma Study Group conducted a study to determine interobserver agreement among different endosonographers in judging gastric wall infiltration.[119] A multicenter evaluation of interobserver agreement was undertaken in patients with MALT lymphoma of the stomach. Our evaluation was conducted on the same patients both before and after treatment in order to assess the interobserver agreement for EUS both in initial staging and in follow-up after therapy. In the baseline group, 54 patients were studied. In the follow-up group, 42 patients were re-evaluated 6 months after medical therapy. EUS examinations were carried on at 10 italian GI units. Interobserver agreement was estimated using kappa statistics.

Overall interobserver agreement for T stage was fair, both before and after treatment ($\kappa = 0.38$ and $\kappa = 0.37$ respectively). Overall interobserver agreement for N stage was substantial before treatment, but only fair after treatment ($\kappa = 0.63$ and $\kappa = 0.34$ respectively).

When interobserver agreement relative to a single T category in the baseline group was considered, the lowest value (fair interobserver agreement) was detected for stage T2 before therapy ($\kappa = 0.33$) and for stage T1sm after therapy ($\kappa = 0.20$). However, agreement was substantial for stages N0 and N1 before treatment, but only fair after treatment.

RESPONSE ACCORDING TO EUS STAGING						
	T1m N0	T1sm N0	T2 N0	T1m N1	T1sm N1	T2 N1
Complete response	12 (75%)	11 (58%)	1 (25%)	2 (50%)	2 (50%)	0
Persistent or relapse	4 (25%)	8 (42%)	3 (75%)	2 (50%)	2 (50%)	4 (100%)

Table 13.10 Response according to EUS staging

It should be emphasized that gastric EUS is not such an easy and straightforward technique as might commonly be thought, as many factors can influence its outcome. First, the stomach must be explored in its entirety, from pylorus to cardia, with a 360° view; however, the antrum and part of the fundus can be difficult to image because of inadequate water-filling. Second, mucus and blood can interfere with ultrasound, creating artifacts or simply making the wall more difficult to explore. Third, adequate distension of the viscus is not always complete despite the administration of antispasmodics, thus making it difficult to assess the degree of infiltration of the greater curvature of the body, particularly when LGFs are present. Many of these factors are not encountered in esophageal and rectal cancer staging. Thus, all these variables should be considered to optimize interobserver agreement (Fig. 13.28).

As a secondary endpoint, we also compared the performance of each observer with that of the nine other examiners, using the Kendall system. This showed that physicians with either ≤6 years of EUS experience or ≤450 gastric EUS procedures had the lowest rates of interobserver agreement among our group of experts.

This analysis suggests that 100 gastric EUS examinations may be enough to 'initiate' a physician in this field, but not to consider him or her an expert. Surely many more than 100 procedures are required to acquire all the technical skills and subtleties needed. Moreover, accurate guidelines must be observed in patient preparation, administration of antispasmodics during the procedure, water filling of the stomach, and tilting of the endoscopic bed adequately to fill with water first the antrum and then the fundus.

CONCLUSIONS

Before EUS became available, a combination of upper endoscopy, abdominal ultrasonography, and CT was used to stage gastric lymphomas. The advent of EUS has led to a marked improvement in accuracy in the diagnosis and staging of GI lymphomas and LGFs. Currently, EUS is regarded as the most accurate imaging modality for evaluating and staging infiltrative gastric lesions. EUS allows a close and sharp visualization of each of the five layers of the gastric wall, and an accurate assessment of perigastric structures and lymph nodes.

The ability of EUS accurately to stage gastric lymphoma according to the TNM system is of paramount importance, as it allows the best mode of therapy for the individual patient to be determined. Although many therapies are now available for gastric MALT lymphoma, they cannot be randomly assigned to patients. EUS makes a difference by helping the clinician to make the right choice. Although early lesions, staged by EUS as T1m and T1sm, may regress after anti-*H. pylori* therapy alone, more advanced lesions, staged from T2 to T4 by EUS, usually require more aggressive treatment protocols.

The importance of EUS lies not only in its ability to stage MALT lymphoma before treatment, but also in follow-up, as EUS aids in determining response to therapy and in detecting relapse early. At times, EUS may show restoration of normal gastric wall layers prior to evident histologic remission, and at other times recurrent wall thickening or disruption may be seen in individuals who were previously in remission. For patients with a persistently thickened gastric wall on EUS despite antibiotic therapy, other treatment modalities should be considered, even if endoscopic biopsies are negative. In fact, these patients are likely to have persistent lymphoma.

EXAMINATION CHECKLIST

Layer of origin of wall thickening (second, third, or fourth layers, or a combination of multiple layers)

Mucosal appearance, mucosal defects

Depth of penetration of focal mass

Presence of local lymph nodes

Celiac axis

Liver

Hilum of the spleen

Gastrohepatic ligament (between stomach and liver)

Perform large-bite endoscopic biopsies

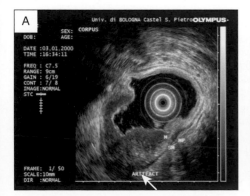 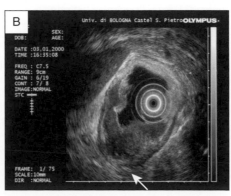

Fig. 13.28 A, Lymphomatous infiltration of the mucosa (M), submucosa (SM), and muscularis propria (MP). This image appears also to show penetration of the serosa. However, this is only an artifact due to oblique scanning of the gastric wall (arrow). **B,** After proper repositioning of the echoendoscope, it is evident that there are no interruptions in the fifth layer (arrow). As a result, T2 is the correct staging. Faultless technique is fundamental to good interobserver agreement in EUS staging of gastric lymphoma.

REFERENCES

1 Ries LAG, Eisner MP, Kosary CL, et al. SEER cancer statistics review, 1973–1999. Bethesda, MD: National Cancer Institute; 2002.

2 Solidoro A, Salazar F, De La Flor J, et al. Endoscopic tissue diagnosis of gastric involvement in the staging of non-Hodgkin's lymphoma. Cancer 1981; 48:1053–1057.

3 Valentini M, Bortolozzi F, Cannizzaro R, et al. Gastrointestinal involvement in staging nodal non-Hodgkin's lymphomas: a clinical and endoscopic prospective study of 235 patients. Am J Gastroenterol 1995; 90:1959–1961.

4 Kolve M, Fischbach W, Greiner A, et al. for the German Gastrointestinal Lymphoma Study Group. Differences in endoscopic and clinicopathological features of primary and secondary gastric non-Hodgkin's lymphoma. Gastrointest Endosc 1999; 49:307–315.

5 Isaacson P, Spencer J. Malignant lymphoma of the mucosa-associated lymphoid tissue. Histopathology 1987; 11:445–462.

6 Thieblemont C, Bastion Y, Berger F, et al. Mucosa-associated lymphoid tissue gastrointestinal and nongastrointestinal lymphoma behavior: analysis of 108 patients. J Clin Oncol 1997; 15:1624–1630.

7 Zinzani PL, Magagnoli M, Galieni P, et al. Nongastrointestinal low-grade mucosa-associated lymphoid tissue lymphoma: analysis of 75 patients. J Clin Oncol 1999; 17:1254–1258.

8 Spencer J, Finn T, Pulford KAF, et al. The human gut contains a novel population of B-lymphocytes which resemble marginal zone cells. Clin Exp Immunol 1985; 62:607–610.

9 Levine EG, Arthur DC, Machnicki J, et al. Four new recurring translocations in non-Hodgkin lymphoma. Blood 1989; 74:1796–1800.

10 Isaacson P, Wright DH. Extranodal malignant lymphoma arising from the mucosa-associated lymphoid tissue. Cancer 1984; 53:2515–2524.

11 Harris LN, Jaffe ES, Stein H, et al. A revised European American classification of lymphoid neoplasms: a proposal from the International Lymphoma Study Group. Blood 1994; 84:1361.

12 Schroy, P. Polyps, adenocarcinomas and other intestinal tumors. In: Wolfe M, Cohen S, Davis G, et al., eds. Therapy of digestive disorders. Philadelphia: W B Saunders; 2000:662–665.

13 Isaacson PG. Mucosa-associated lymphoid tissue lymphoma. Semin Hematol 1999; 36:139–147.

14 Dayal Y, De Lellis R. The gastrointestinal tract. In: Cotran R, Kumar V, Robbins S, eds. Robbin's pathologic basis of disease, 4th edn. Philadelphia: WB Saunders; 1989:858–859.

15 Wotherspoon AC, Ortiz-Hidalgo C, Falzon MR, et al. *Helicobacter pylori*-associated gastritis and primary B-cell gastric lymphoma. Lancet 1991; 338:1175–1176.

16 Feldman M, Scharschmidt B, Sleisenger M. Gastrointestinal and liver disease, 6th edn. Philadelphia: WB Saunders; 1998:1845–1846.

17 Crump M, Gospodarowicz M, Shepherd FA. Lymphoma of the gastrointestinal tract. Semin Oncol 1999; 26:324–337.

18 Hussel T, Isaacson PG, Crabtree JE, et al. *Helicobacter pylori*-specific tumour-infiltrating T cells provide contact dependent help for the growth of malignant B-cells in low grade gastric lymphoma of mucosa-associated lymphoid tissue. J Pathol 1996; 178:122–127.

19 Bertoni F, Gisi M, Roggero E, et al. Molecular detection of circulating neoplastic cells in patients with clinically localized gastric and non-gastric mucosa-associated lymphoid tissue lymphoma. Digest Liver Dis 2000; 32:188–191.

20 Wotherspoon AC, Doglioni C, Isaacson PG. Low-grade B-cell lymphoma of mucosa-associated lymphoid tissue (MALT): a multifocal disease. Histopathology 1992; 20:29.

21 Bayerdorffer E, Morgner A. Gastric marginal zone B-cell lymphoma of the mucosa-associated lymphoid tissue type: management of the disease. Digest Liver Dis 2000; 32:192–194.

22 Caletti G, Togliani T, Fusaroli P, et al. Consecutive regression of concurrent laryngeal and gastric MALT lymphoma after anti-*Helicobacter pylori* therapy. Gastroenterology 2003; 124:537–543.

23 Nagashima R, Takeda H, Maeda K, et al. Regression of duodenal mucosa-associated lymphoid tissue lymphoma after eradication of *Helicobacter pylori*. Gastroenterology 1996; 111:1674–1678.

24 Fischbach W, Tacke W, Greiner A, et al. Regression of immunoproliferative small intestine disease after eradication of *Helicobacter pylori*. Lancet 1997; 349:31–32.

25 Raderer M, Pfeffel F, Pohl G, et al. Regression of colonic low grade B cell lymphoma of the mucosa associated lymphoid tissue type after eradication of *Helicobacter pylori*. Gut 2000; 46:133–135.

26 Gupte S, Nair R, Naresh KN, et al. MALT lymphoma of nasal mucosa treated with antibiotics. Leuk Lymphoma 1999; 36:195–197.

27 Yoshikane H, Yokoi T, Hidano H, et al. Regression of superficial gastric MALT lymphoma with unsuccessful eradication therapy for *Helicobacter pylori* infection. J Gastroenterol 1997; 32:812–816.

28 Nebiki H, Harihara S, Tsukuda H, et al. Regression of gastric MALT lymphoma after unsuccessful anti-*H. pylori* therapy. Am J Gastroenterol 2000; 95:3684–3686.

29 Radaszkiewicz T, Dragosics B, Bauer P. Gastrointestinal malignant lymphomas of the mucosa-associated lymphoid tissue: factors relevant to prognosis. Gastroenterology 1992; 102:1628–1638.

30 Al-Akwaa AM, Siddiqui N, Al-Mofleh IA. Primary gastric lymphoma. World J Gastroenterol 2004; 10:5–11.

31 Fung CY, Grossbard ML, Linggood RM, et al. Mucosa-associated lymphoid tissue lymphoma of the stomach: long-term outcome after local treatment. Cancer 1999; 85:9–17.

32 Salvagno L, Soraru M, Busetto M, et al. Gastric non-Hodgkin's lymphoma: analysis of 252 patients from a multicenter study. Tumori 1999; 85:113–121.

33 Fischbach W, Dragosics B, Kolve-Goebeler ME, et al. Primary gastric B-cell lymphoma: results of a prospective multicenter study. Gastroenterology 2000; 119:1191–1202.

34 Salles G, Herbrecht R, Tilly H, et al. Aggressive primary gastrointestinal lymphomas: review of 91 patients treated with LNH-84 regimen. Am J Med 1991; 90:77–84.

35 Popescu RA, Wotherspoon AC, Cunningham D, et al. Surgery plus chemotherapy or chemotherapy alone for primary, intermediate, and high grade gastric non-Hodgkin's lymphoma: the Royal Marsden Hospital experience. Eur J Cancer 1999; 35:928–934.

36 Koch P, Del Valle F, Berdel WE, et al. Primary gastrointestinal non-Hodgkin's lymphoma: II. Combined surgical and conservative or conservative management only in localized gastric lymphoma – results of the prospective German multicenter study. The German multicenter study group on GIT-NHL. J Clin Oncol 2001; 19:3874–3883.

37 Maor MH, Velasquez WS, Fuller LM, et al. Stomach conservation in stage IE and IIE gastric non-Hodgkin's lymphoma. J Clin Oncol 1990; 8:266–271.

38 Raderer M, Valencak J, Osterreicher C, et al. Chemotherapy for the treatment of patients with primary high grade gastric B-cell lymphoma of modified Ann Arbor stages IE and IIE. Cancer 2000; 88:1979–1985.

39 Ferreri AJ, Cardio S, Ponzoni M, et al. Non-surgical treatment with primary chemotherapy, with and without radiation therapy of stage I–II high grade lymphoma. Leuk Lymphoma 1999; 33:531–541.

40 Ruskoné-Fourmestraux A, Aegerter P, Delmer A, et al. Primary digestive tract lymphoma: a prospective multicenter study of 91 patients. Gastroenterology 1993; 105:1662–1671.

41 Schechter NR, Portlock CS, Yahalom J. Treatment of mucosa-associated lymphoid tissue lymphoma of the stomach with radiation alone. J Clin Oncol 1998; 16:1916–1921.

42 Winawer SJ, Posner G, Lightdale CJ, et al. Endoscopic diagnosis of advanced gastric cancer. Gastroenterology 1975; 69:1183–1187.

43 Andriulli A, Recchia A, De Angelis C, et al. Endoscopic ultrasonographic evaluation of patients with biopsy negative gastric linitis plastica. Gastrointest Endosc 1990; 36:611–615.

44 Fork FTh, Haglund U, Hogstrom H, et al. Primary gastric lymphoma v. gastric cancer. An endoscopic and radiographic study of differential diagnostic possibilities. Endoscopy 1985; 17:5–7.

45 Caletti G, Fusaroli P, Bocus P. Endoscopic ultrasonography in large gastric folds. Endoscopy 1998; 30(Suppl 1):S72–S75.

46 Komorowski RA, Caya JG, Geenen JE. The morphologic spectrum of large gastric folds: utility of the snare biopsy. Gastrointest Endosc 1986; 32:190–192.

47 Martin TR, Onstad GR, Silvis SE, et al. Lift and cut biopsy technique for submucosal sampling. Gastrointest Endosc 1976; 23:29.

48 Tio TL. Large gastric folds evaluated by endoscopic ultrasonography. Gastrointest Endosc Clin N Am 1995; 5:683–691.

49 Vander Noot MR III, Eloubeidi MA, Chen VK, et al. Diagnosis of gastrointestinal tract lesions by endoscopic ultrasound-guided fine-needle aspiration biopsy. Cancer 2004; 102:157–163.

50 Caletti GC, Brocchi E, Ferrari A, et al. Guillotine needle biopsy as a supplement to endosonography in the diagnosis of gastric submucosal tumors. Endoscopy 1991; 23:251–254.

51 Caletti GC, Ferrari A, Bocus P, et al. Endoscopic ultrasonography in gastric lymphoma. Schweiz Med Wochenschr 1996; 126:819–825.

52 Bolondi L, Casanova P, Caletti GC, et al. Primary gastric lymphoma versus gastric carcinoma: endoscopic US evaluation. Radiology 1987; 165:821–826.

53 Caletti GC, Zani L, Bolondi L, et al. Impact of endoscopic ultrasonography on diagnosis and treatment of primary gastric lymphoma. Surgery 1988, 103:315–320.

54 Fusaroli P, Vallar R, Togliani T, et al. Scientific publications in endoscopic ultrasonography: a 20-year global survey of the literature. Endoscopy 2002; 34:451–456.

55 Suekane H, Iida M, Yao T, et al. Endoscopic ultrasonography in primary gastric lymphoma: correlation with endoscopic and histologic findings. Gastrointest Endosc 1993; 39:139–145.

56 Palazzo L, Roseau G, Ruskoné-Fourmestraux A, et al. Endoscopic ultrasonography in the local staging of primary gastric lymphoma. Endoscopy 1993; 25:502–508.

57 Van Dam J. The role of endoscopic ultrasonography in monitoring treatment: response to chemotherapy in lymphoma. Endoscopy 1994; 26:772–773.

58 Hordijk ML. Restaging after radiotherapy and chemotherapy: value of endoscopic ultrasonography. Gastrointest Endosc Clin N Am 1995; 5:601–608.

59 Caletti G, Fusaroli P, Togliani T, et al. Endosonography in gastric lymphoma and large gastric folds. Eur J Ultrasound 2000; 11:32–40.

60 Caletti G, Ferrari A, Brocchi E, et al. Accuracy of endoscopic ultrasonography in the diagnosis and staging of gastric cancer and lymphoma. Surgery 1993; 113:14–27.

61 Fischbach W, Goebeler-Kolve ME, Greiner A. Diagnostic accuracy of EUS in the local staging of primary gastric lymphoma: results of a prospective, multicenter study comparing EUS with histopathologic stage. Gastrointest Endosc 2002; 56:696–700.

62 Shimodaira M, Tsukamoto Y, Niwa Y, et al. A proposed staging system for primary gastric lymphoma. Cancer 1994; 73:2709–2715.

63 American Joint Committee on Cancer. AJCC cancer staging manual, 6th edn. New York: Springer; 2002.

64 Musshoff K, Schmidt-Vollmer H. Prognosis of non Hodgkin's lymphomas with special emphasis on staging classification. Z Krebsforshung 1975; 83:323–328.

65 Rohatiner A, D'Amore F, Coiffier B, et al. Report on a workshop convened to discuss the pathological and staging classifications of gastrointestinal tract lymphoma. Ann Oncol 1994; 5:397–400.

66 Rohatiner A, D'Amore F, Coiffier B, et al. Report on a workshop convened to discuss the pathological and staging classifications of gastrointestinal tract lymphoma. Ann Oncol 1994; 5:397–400.

67 Ruskoné-Fourmestraux A, Dragosics B, Morgner A, et al. Paris staging system for primary gastrointestinal lymphomas. Gut 2003; 52:912–913.

68 Catalano MF, Sivak MV, Rice T, et al. Endosonographic features predictive of lymph node metastasis. Gastrointest Endosc 1994; 40:442–446.

69 Bjork JT, Geenen JE, Soergel KH, et al. Endoscopic evaluation of large gastric folds. A comparison of biopsy techniques. Gastrointest Endosc 1977; 24:22–23.

70 Vilardell F. Gastritis. In: Berk JE, ed. Gastroenterology, 4th edn. Philadelphia: WB Saunders; 1985:941–974.

71 Ménétrièr P. Des polyadenomes gastriques et leurs rapports avec le cancer de stomach. Arch Physiol Norm Path 1888; 1:32–35, 236–262.

72 Kimmey MB, Martin RW, Hagitt RC, et al. Histologic correlates of gastrointestinal ultrasound images. Gastroenterology 1989; 96:433–441.

73 Gordon SJ, Rifkin MD, Goldberg BB. Endosonographic evaluation of mural abnormalities of the upper gastrointestinal tract. Gastrointest Endosc 1986; 32:193–198.

74 Botet JF, Lightdale CJ. Endoscopic sonography of the gastrointestinal tract. AJR Am J Roentgenol 1991; 156:63–68.

75 Reeder MM, Olmstead WW, Cooper PH. Large gastric folds, local or widespread. JAMA 1974; 230:273–274.

76 Fisher JR, Sanowski RA. Disseminated histoplasmosis producing hypertrophic gastric folds. Am J Dig Dis 1978; 23:282–285.

77 Morin ME, Tan A. Diffuse enlargement of gastric folds as a manifestation of secondary syphilis. Am J Gastroenterol 1980; 74:170–172.

78 Kusuhura T, Watanabe K, Fukuda M. Radiographic studies of acute gastric anisakiasis. Gastrointest Radiol 1984; 9:305–309.

79 Avunduk C, Navab F, Hampf F, et al. Prevalence of *Helicobacter pylori* infection in patients with large gastric folds: evaluation and follow-up with endoscopic ultrasound before and after antimicrobial therapy. Am J Gastroenterol 1995; 90:1969–1973.

80 Sakanari JA, McKerrow JH. Anisakiasis. Clin Microbiol Rev 1989; 2:278–284.

81 Caletti GC, Brocchi E, Ferrari A, et al. Value of endoscopic ultrasonography in the management of portal hypertension. Endoscopy 1992; 24(Suppl 1):342–346.

82 Gandolfi L, Colecchia A, Leo P, et al. Endoscopic ultrasonography in the diagnosis of gastrointestinal amyloid deposits: clinical case report. Endoscopy 1995; 27:132–134.

83 Levine MS, Kong V, Rubeswin SE, et al. Scirrhous carcinoma of the stomach: radiologic and endoscopic diagnosis. Radiology 1990; 175:151–154.

84 Nelson RS, Lanza FL. The endoscopic diagnosis of gastric lymphoma. Gross characteristics and histology. Gastrointest Endosc 1974; 21:66–68.

85 Hizawa K, Kawasaki M, Yao T, et al. Endoscopic ultrasound features of protein-losing gastropathy with hypertrophic gastric folds. Endoscopy 2000; 32:394–397.

86 Mendis RE, Gerdes H, Lightdale CJ, et al. Large gastric folds: a diagnostic approach using endoscopic ultrasonography. Gastrointest Endosc 1994; 40:437–441.

87 Songur Y, Takashi O, Watanabe H, et al. Endosonographic evaluation of giant gastric folds. Gastrointest Endosc 1995; 41:468–474.

88 Maunoury V, Klein O, Houcke ML, et al. Endoscopic ultrasonography in the diagnosis of hypertrophic gastropathy. Gastroenterology 1994; 106:820.

89 Okada M, Lizuka Y, Oh K, et al. Gastritis cystica profunda presenting as giant gastric mucosal folds: the role of endoscopic ultrasonography and mucosectomy in the diagnostic work-up. Gastrointest Endosc 1994; 40:640–644.

90 Thiede C, Morgner A, Alpen B, et al. What role does *Helicobacter pylori* eradication play in gastric MALT and gastric MALT lymphoma? Gastroenterology 1997; 113:S61–S64.

91 Parsonnet J, Hansen S, Rodriguez L, et al. *Helicobacter pylori* infection and gastric lymphoma. N Engl J Med 1994; 330:1267–1271.

92 Hussell T, Isaacson PG, Crabtree LE, et al. The response of cells from low-grade B-cell gastric lymphomas of mucosa-associated lymphoid tissue to *Helicobacter pylori*. Lancet 1993; 342:571–574.

93 Wotherspoon AC, Doglioni C, Diss TC, et al. Regression of primary low-grade B-cell gastric lymphoma of mucosa-associated lymphoid tissue type after eradication of *Helicobacter pylori*. Lancet 1993; 342:575–577.

94 Roggero E, Zucca E, Pinotti G, et al. Eradication of *Helicobacter pylori* infection in primary low-grade gastric lymphoma of mucosa-associated lymphoid tissue. Ann Intern Med 1995; 122:767–769.

95 Bayerdorffer E, Neubauer A, Rudolph B, et al. Regression of primary gastric lymphoma of mucosa-associated lymphoid tissue type after cure of *Helicobacter pylori* infection. Lancet 1995; 345:1591–1594.

96 Neubauer A, Thiede C, Morgner A, et al. Cure of *Helicobacter pylori* infection and duration of remission of low-grade gastric mucosa-associated lymphoid tissue lymphoma. J Natl Cancer Inst 1997; 89:1350–1355.

97 Weber DM, Dimopoulos MA, Anandu DP, et al. Regression of gastric lymphoma of mucosa-associated lymphoid tissue with antibiotic therapy for *Helicobacter pylori*. Gastroenterology 1994; 107:1835–1838.

98 Ohashi S, Segawa K, Okamura S, et al. A clinicopathologic study of gastric mucosa-associated lymphoid tissue lymphoma. Cancer 2000; 88:2210–2219.

99 Sackmann M, Morgner A, Rudolph B, et al. and MALT Lymphoma Study Group. Regression of gastric MALT lymphoma after eradication of *Helicobacter pylori* is predicted by endosonographic staging. Gastroenterology 1997; 113:1087–1090.

100 Ruskoné-Fourmestraux A, Lavergne A, Aegerter PH, et al. Predictive factors for regression of gastric MALT lymphoma after anti-*Helicobacter pylori* treatment. Gut 2001; 48:297–303.

101 Nakamura S, Matsumoto T, Suekane H, et al. Predictive value of endoscopic ultrasonography for regression of gastric low grade and high grade MALT lymphomas after eradication of *Helicobacter pylori*. Gut 2001; 48:454–460.

102 Nobre-Leitao C, Lage P, Cravo M, et al. Treatment of gastric MALT lymphoma by *Helicobacter pylori* eradication: a study controlled by endoscopic ultrasonography. Am J Gastroenterol 1998; 93:732–736.

103 Pavlick AC, Gerdes H, Portlock CS. Endoscopic ultrasound in the evaluation of gastric small lymphocytic mucosa-associated lymphoid tumors. J Clin Oncol 1997; 15:1761–1766.

104 Steinbach G, Ford R, Glober G, et al. Antibiotic treatment of gastric lymphoma of mucosa-associated lymphoid tissue. An uncontrolled trial. Ann Intern Med 1999; 131:88–95.

105 Levy M, Hammel P, Lamarque D, et al. Endoscopic ultrasonography for the initial staging and follow-up in patients with low-grade gastric lymphoma of mucosa-associated lymphoid tissue treated medically. Gastrointest Endosc 1997; 46:328–333.

106 Levy M, Copie-Bergman C, Traulle C, et al. Conservative treatment of primary gastric low-grade B-cell lymphoma of mucosa-associated lymphoid tissue: predictive factors of response and outcome. Am J Gastroenterol 2002; 97:292–297.

107 Fischbach W, Goebeler-Kolve M-E, Dragosics B, et al. Long term outcome of patients with gastric marginal zone B cell lymphoma of mucosa associated lymphoid tissue (MALT) following exclusive *Helicobacter pylori* eradication therapy: experience from a large prospective series. Gut 2004; 53:34–37.

108 Lugering N, Menzel J, Kucharzik T, et al. Impact of miniprobes compared to conventional endosonography in the staging of low-grade gastric malt lymphoma. Endoscopy 2001; 33:832–837.

109 Hammel P, Haioun C, Chaumette MT, et al. Efficacy of single-agent chemotherapy in low-grade B-cell mucosa-associated lymphoid tissue lymphoma with prominent gastric expression. J Clin Oncol 1995; 13:2524–2529.

110 Fung CY, Grossbard ML, Linggood RM, et al. Mucosa-associated lymphoid tissue lymphoma of the stomach: long-term outcome after local treatment. Cancer 1999; 85:9–17.

111 Schechter NR, Portlock CS, Yahalom J. Treatment of mucosa-associated lymphoid tissue lymphoma of the stomach with radiation alone. J Clin Oncol 1998; 16:1916–1921.

112 Zinzani PL, Frezza G, Bendandi M, et al. Primary gastric lymphoma: a clinical and therapeutic evaluation of 82 patients. Leuk Lymphoma 1995; 19:461–466.

113 Cogliatti SB, Schmid U, Schumacher U, et al. Primary B-cell gastric lymphoma: a clinicopathological study of 145 patients. Gastroenterology 1991; 101:1159–1170.

114 Zucca E, Roggero E, Traulle C, et al. Early interim report of the LY03 randomised cooperative trial of observation vs chlorambucil after anti-*Helicobacter* therapy in low-grade gastric lymphoma. Ann Oncol 1999; 10:25.

115 Puspok A, Raderer M, Chott A, et al. Endoscopic ultrasound in the follow up and response assessment of patients with primary gastric lymphoma. Gut 2002; 51:691–694.

116 Yeh H-Z, Chen G-H, Chang W-D, et al. Long-term follow up of gastric low-grade mucosa-associated lymphoid tissue lymphoma by endosonography emphasizing the application of a miniature ultrasound probe. J Gastroenterol Hepatol 2003; 18:162–167.

117 Doglioni C, Wotherspoon AC, Moschini A, et al. High incidence of primary gastric lymphoma in northeastern Italy. Lancet 1992; 339:834–835.

118 Caletti G, Zinzani PL, Fusaroli P, et al. The Italian Gastric Lymphoma Study Group. The importance of endoscopic ultrasonography in the management of low-grade gastric mucosa-associated lymphoid tissue lymphoma. Aliment Pharmacol Ther 2002; 16:1715–1722.

119 Fusaroli P, Buscarini E, Peyre S, et al. Interobserver agreement in staging gastric MALT lymphoma by EUS. Gastrointest Endosc 2002; 55:662–668.

PANCREAS AND BILIARY TREE

Chapter

14

How to Perform EUS in the Pancreas, Bile Duct, and Liver

Robert H. Hawes and Paul Fockens

PANCREAS

Successful pancreatic imaging requires the ability to image the entire gland. In general, the body and tail of the pancreas are imaged through the posterior wall of the stomach and, in most cases, the transgastric approach will provide images of the genu (or neck) of the pancreas as well. Imaging of the pancreatic head, however, requires positioning of the transducer potentially in three different positions within the duodenum: the apex of the duodenal bulb, directly opposite the papilla, and distal to the papilla for the uncinate process. These 'stations' are applicable to both radial and linear array imaging.

For the body and tail, the examination begins at the gastro-esophageal (GE) junction. Either the endoscopic properties of the echoendoscope can be used visually to locate the squamocolumnar junction, or the esophagogastric junction can be located by imaging the crurae of the diaphragm endosonographically. With a radial scanning instrument, the aorta is immediately visible as a round structure directly adjacent to the GE junction. Using the rotation mode on the ultrasound console, after the endosonographer has assumed a comfortable position with the echoendoscope, the image should be rotated such that the aorta is displayed at the 6 o'clock position of the viewing field. Once this position is achieved, the echoendoscope is gently advanced, keeping the aorta in its round configuration. If the aorta becomes elongated on advancement, this is an indication that the tip of the echoendoscope is being pushed laterally or embedded in the gastric wall. This occurs usually when the tip is caught within a hiatal hernia pouch. If this occurs, the tip must be realigned, as it is important to keep the aorta in its round configuration. As the echoendoscope is advanced, eventually (usually 2–5 cm beyond the GE junction) a branch is seen to come off the aorta; this represents the celiac artery (Fig. 14.1A,B). With further advancement, the celiac artery is seen to branch into the splenic and hepatic arteries. Just beyond the bifurcation of the celiac artery, the pancreas comes into view and usually, at the same time, the portal vein confluence is seen deep to the pancreas. Once the pancreas has been identified, it needs only to be traced. In general, counterclockwise torque and further advancement of the scope will demonstrate the genu area, whereas clockwise rotation of the scope and withdrawal will demonstrate the body and tail. During these maneuvers, some left and right tip deflection may be required to obtain an elongated view of the pancreas.

Once the elongated view of the pancreas is achieved, very slow and purposeful advancement and withdrawal of the scope will demonstrate the entire width of the pancreas including the pancreatic duct. The scope should be torqued clockwise and withdrawn (along with some upward tip deflection) until the splenic artery and splenic vein are seen to course directly by the transducer. This generally indicates the area of the hilum of the spleen and, when this is identified, examination of the pancreatic tail is complete. This maneuver – of beginning at the GE junction and tracing the celiac artery until the pancreas is found – should be repeated as many times as necessary until the endosonographer is confident that the pancreatic body and tail have been examined completely.

The basic maneuvers to look at the body and tail of the pancreas are essentially the same when utilizing the linear array echoendoscope. When beginning at the GE junction with the linear echoendoscope, the aorta is seen in its longitudinal confirmation. The echoendoscope is advanced, while at the same time slowly torquing counterclockwise and clockwise looking for the take-off of the celiac artery. It is necessary to torque the scope as it is slowly advanced; otherwise, if the celiac artery comes off the side of the aorta, it can be missed. Once the celiac artery has been identified, it is traced until it bifurcates and, with another centimeter of advancement, the pancreas will come into view (perhaps with some slight clockwise torque) (Fig. 14.1B,C). From this point, the pancreas is simply traced, but with a linear echoendoscope a constant clockwise and counterclockwise torquing is required, and perhaps some adjustments of the left and right tip deflection. When the scope is withdrawn until the celiac artery and vein course directly underneath the transducer, this signals complete examination of the tail of the pancreas.

To examine the entire head of the pancreas confidently, all three positions – the apex, the papilla, and distal to the papilla – should be achieved (Fig. 14.2). The most efficient position is the apex of the duodenal bulb. This position allows imaging of the entire head of the pancreas (sometimes with the exception of the uncinate process) and also includes efficient imaging of the distal common bile duct. With the radial echoendoscope, the instrument should be slowly advanced through the stomach and allowed to 'bow' along the greater curve. Once the pylorus has been visualized, the tip is advanced through the pylorus, at

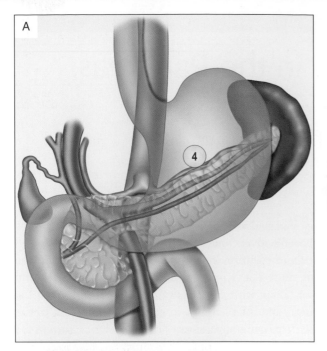

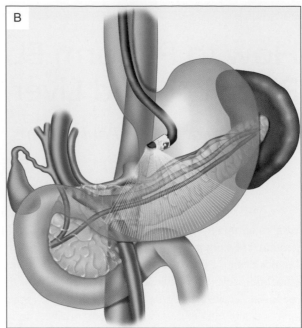

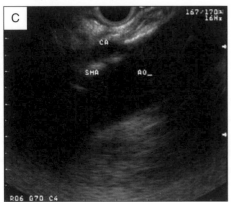

Fig. 14.1   These figures (**A,B**) and EUS image (**C**) illustrate station 4. This represents the starting point for imaging the pancreatic body and tail. The transducer is advanced while tracing the aorta, starting at the gastroesophageal junction. The first branch from the aorta represents the celiac axis; by tracing along the celiac axis, the pancreatic body can be found.

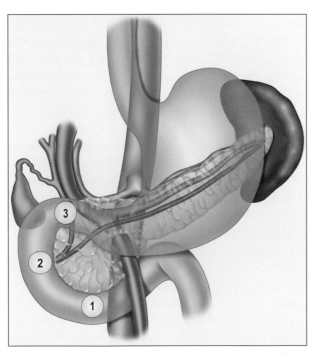

Fig. 14.2   This illustration depicts the three stations of the transducer that enable full viewing of the pancreatic head.

which point air is instilled into the duodenal bulb and some gentle downward deflection is applied to the tip of the echo-endoscope. This allows direct endoscopic visualization of the apex of the duodenal bulb. Once visualized, the tip of the echoendoscope should be advanced until it is at the level of the apex, and the balloon is inflated until it gently occludes the lumen of the duodenum. When imaging is begun, one should first look for the liver. Once the liver has been identified, the image should be rotated such that the liver is positioned in the upper left-hand corner of the screen. This will allow the endosonographers to have a uniform orientation of the image from the apical viewpoint, and will enhance learning and recognition of normalcy and pathology. Once this position is achieved, ultrasound imaging begins. From this position, there are four landmarks that one should look for. The most important is what we term the 'duodenal fall-off'. This essentially represents visualization of the muscularis propria of the duodenal wall and is seen to course downward and away from the transducer. The second landmark is the common bile duct, a tubular anechoic structure that extends from the duodenal wall towards the liver and courses closest to the transducer. This typically has a three-

.ayer echo appearance. The third landmark is the pancreatic duct. This may or may not be seen in the same plane of imaging as the bile duct. Often, gentle advancement of the scope beyond the bile duct is required in order to see the pancreatic duct. During these maneuvers to identify both the bile duct and the pancreas, the endosonographers should be prepared to use some gentle downward tip deflection. The fourth landmark is the portal vein, which is seen to course in the far left of the imaging field and is the biggest tubular structure to be seen. Once the apical position is achieved, multiple small movements that can include clockwise and counterclockwise torquing, forward advancement withdrawal of the scope, upward and downward tip deflection, as well as left and right positioning of the tip are all required completely to define the anatomy from this position. In general, however, once the bile duct has been identified, withdrawal of the scope will allow imaging of the bile duct toward the hilum (bifurcation), whereas inward advancement of the scope will allow tracing of the bile duct down to the ampulla.

The second position for pancreatic head imaging is from the level of the papilla. This position is best achieved by, first, using endoscopic visualization to localize the ampulla of Vater. Once seen, the balloon is inflated until it 'kisses' the papilla. It is best to try to orient the transducer so it is perpendicular to the papilla, and to position it in a way that upward tip deflection will result in the balloon pressing against the papilla. Once this position has been achieved, ultrasound imaging should begin. We generally recommend rotating the ultrasound image so that the papilla is located at the 6 o'clock position. From this point, the head of the pancreas is a crescent-shaped structure. As the transducer is moved gently in and out, one looks to see the bile duct and pancreatic duct coursing to the duodenal wall. The pancreatic duct will be deep to the bile duct relative to the position of the transducer. This is also the position required for imaging the ampulla of Vater specifically. This would be indicated for evaluation of an ampullary adenoma or carcinoma, and to look for an impacted stone, perhaps in a patient with gallstone pancreatitis. To image the papilla itself, the duodenum should be paralyzed with buscopan or glucagon. Once the duodenum is paralyzed, water should be infused into the duodenum so as to achieve good coupling without needing to press the balloon against the papilla. Exquisite views of the ampulla of Vater can be obtained if one can achieve perpendicular positioning of the transducer relative to the papilla, obtain good water coupling, and have the duodenum motionless. The critical anatomic landmark when staging ampullary neoplasms is the muscularis propria of the duodenal wall. If the process disrupts this layer, invasion can be predicted.

The uncinate process can be imaged with positioning of the transducer distal to the ampulla of Vater. The critical anatomic structure in this circumstance is the aorta. With a radial scanning echoendoscope, the aorta may be seen initially in its longitudinal confirmation, but after slow withdrawal the aorta becomes cross-sectional in orientation. Once this position is achieved, the pancreas will be seen just to the right of the aorta. Once again, we recommend assuming a standard image display that, in this circumstance, would have the aorta at the 7 o'clock position, with the pancreas emerging (to the right of the aorta) in the 6 o'clock position. From this point, the echoendoscope is slowly withdrawn. One problem that can be encountered with withdrawal from this position is that the echoendoscope can suddenly flip back into the duodenal bulb. This can be avoided by manipulating the echoendoscope as one would with a colonoscope. That is, instead of slow, steady withdrawal, the echoendo-

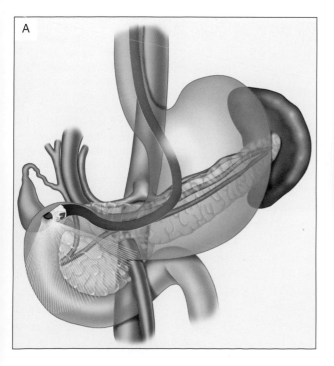

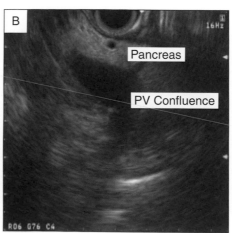

Fig. 14.3 This figure (**A**) and EUS image (**B**) illustrate station 3. This is perhaps the most important station for viewing and performing fine-needle aspiration of the pancreatic head. The transducer is placed at the level of the apex of the duodenal bulb and, after some manipulation of the scope tip, the neck of the pancreas can be viewed with the portal vein confluence deep to the pancreas.

scope is withdrawn a slight amount and then advanced a slight amount. If one can maintain one-to-one reaction of the echoendoscope to the manipulation of the shaft, then rapid uncontrolled withdrawal can be avoided.

The imaging stations are the same whether a radial or linear echoendoscope is used. Obviously, however, the anatomy that is displayed is different. With the linear echoendoscope, the apical position is the same. The scope should be advanced along the greater curve and through the pylorus, where air is instilled and gentle downward tip deflection is applied. Once the apex has been identified, the tip of the linear scope is nestled into the apex of the bulb (Fig. 14.3). At this point, however, torquing is required – generally in a counterclockwise direction. From this position, the entire head of the pancreas (perhaps minus the uncinate process) can be achieved simply by torquing the echoendoscope. The ampullary position is exactly the same with the linear as with the radial echoendoscope. The papilla is visualized endoscopically and then the transducer should be positioned perpendicular to the ampulla (Fig. 14.4). The orientation should be such that upward tip deflection should press the transducer against the papilla. If detailed images of the papilla are required, the duodenum should be paralyzed and water infused into the duodenal lumen, just as with the radial instrument. In some circumstances, however, using either the radial or the linear echoendoscope, if the curvature of the duodenum is too acute it may be impossible to obtain sufficient upward tip deflection to achieve pressing of the transducer against the papilla. This creates a situation where, inevitably, the imaging of the ampulla itself is somewhat tangential; this degrades the overall image quality and precision of interpretation. The imaging of the uncinate process remains the same with the linear echoendoscope. The transducer should be

passed just distal to the ampulla and the instrument shaft should be rotated clockwise or counterclockwise, as necessary, to locate the aorta (Fig. 14.5). Once the aorta has been visualized, the echoendoscope should be torqued (usually clockwise) and slowly withdrawn. With this maneuver, the uncinate process will come into the image adjacent to the transducer.

It is not possible to 'read a book' and translate the reading to successful imaging of the pancreas. There are innumerable nuances to successful imaging, and each patient's anatomy is a little bit different. Each case presents it own unique challenges and no endosonographer, no matter how experienced, achieves successful and complete imaging in all patients. One is always limited by the patient's individual anatomy, and these limitations must be accepted by the endosonographer.

BILE DUCT

Endoscopic ultrasound imaging of the bile duct is relatively straightforward, but overall is easier and more efficiently performed with a radial scanning echoendoscope. There are basically two positions that must be achieved to evaluate fully the extra-hepatic portion of the bile duct. The first position has been mentioned above, and is called the 'apical' position. The second position, which is important to achieve full visualization of the bile duct, is where the transducer 'kisses' the papilla. With a radial scanning echoendoscope, the apical position will usually enable a very broad section of the bile duct to be visualized at one time.

Achieving the apical position begins with the tip of the instrument in the stomach. The echoendoscope is advanced along the greater curve of the stomach with a little downward tip deflection to enable visualization of the pylorus. Slight upward

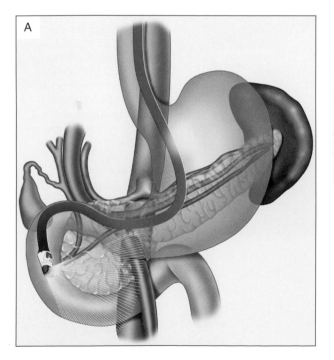

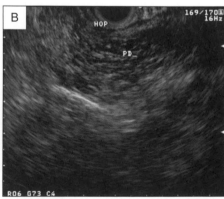

Fig. 14.4   This figure (**A**) and EUS image (**B**) illustrate station 2. The transducer is placed at a perpendicular angle to the papilla of Vater. From this position, the pancreas has a crescent shape and, with gentle movement in or out with the scope and possibly some torque, the bile duct and pancreatic duct can be seen to emerge from the papilla.

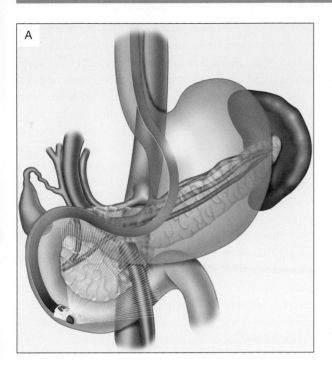

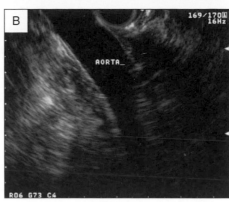

Fig. 14.5   This figure shows the position (**A**) and standard image (**B**) associated with station 1. The transducer is placed distal to the papilla and the tip of the echoendoscope is moved 'up'. From this position, the aorta can be sought; the pancreas will be viewed adjacent to it.

tip deflection is applied just before entering the pylorus and, once within the duodenal bulb, air is instilled along with slight downward tip deflection in order to visualize the apex of the duodenal bulb. The tip of the scope is then positioned in the area of the apex, the balloon is inflated until it occludes the lumen, and slight clockwise torque is then applied to the instrument shaft. Ultrasound imaging then begins. The first structure to look for is the liver. The image should be rotated such that the liver is positioned in the upper left-hand portion of the screen. From this position, at least a portion of the bile duct can usually be visualized, although slight advancement or withdrawal of the echoendoscope may be required. The bile duct will be seen as an anechoic tubular structure coursing right, adjacent to the transducer. The most important landmark of the apical position is what is called the 'duodenal fall-off'. This represents the muscularis propria of the duodenum and will be seen to course just adjacent to the transducer and then fall away directly from it in the 6 o'clock position of the screen. Once the bile duct is visualized, one should recognize that it typically has three layers. Withdrawal and counterclockwise torque of the echoendoscope will allow visualization of the bile duct toward the hilum, and clockwise torque and insertion of the endoscope shaft will allow visualization of the distal bile duct as it enters the papilla. The most common mistake made with apical imaging is that the endosonographer allows the transducer to slip back into the bulb. Some gentle pressure should be kept against the shaft of the instrument to prevent this from occurring. It is also possible that, if too much pressure is applied, the tip will slip around the apex into the second portion of the duodenum. If there is a tendency for this to occur, the balloon should be further inflated on the bulb side of the apex. Once one begins imaging from the apical position, if the bile duct is not recognized within 30 seconds, endoscopic control should be used to reposition the

transducer in the apex and ultrasound imaging restabilized. Three to four repositionings within the apex may sometimes be required to achieve proper imaging of the bile duct.

There are some cases in which a stone is impacted in the distal bile duct. In this circumstance, the only way to detect the stone may be to position the transducer directly perpendicular to the papilla. This is achieved by advancing the echoendoscope into the second portion of the duodenum and then pulling back, as one would do with an endoscopic retrograde cholangiopancreatography (ERCP) scope to achieve the 'straight scope position'. The papilla should be visualized endoscopically, the duodenum paralyzed, and water instilled within the duodenal lumen. The balloon is then slightly inflated, but not enough to press firmly against the papilla. One then scans back and forth across the papilla looking for the bile duct to emerge from the papilla. One must look carefully because, if a small stone is impacted in the ampulla, only shadowing may be seen, without the intensely echogenic rim typically observed with stones in the bile duct or gallbladder. As always, complete imaging of the bile duct may require multiple attempts at each position before success is achieved.

The technique for imaging the bile duct with the linear echoendoscope is the same as that described for the radial instrument. The two positions remain the same: apical and opposite the papilla. Because the plane of imaging for the linear scope is more restricted than that of the radial, it may be difficult to obtain long views of the bile duct. The linear instrument should be positioned in the apex of the duodenal bulb, but usually counterclockwise torque is required to image the bile duct and some left/right tip deflection may be required. The principle remains the same, however, that withdrawal of the instrument from this position generally gives views towards the hilum, whereas advancing the echoendoscope obtains views towards the papilla. Use of the linear scope for biliary imaging requires much more careful tracing as one single position provides only a small section of the bile duct. Sometimes it is easier to obtain perpendicular views of the papilla with the linear scope than with the radial. Of course, color Doppler can be used to help differentiate the bile duct from surrounding vascular structures.

LIVER

There are basically three positions to enable imaging of the liver. No matter how diligent the endosonographer, the extent to which the liver can be imaged is dependent largely on the patient's anatomy. In general, one should utilize the lowest frequency available with the instrument used to maximize penetration, and the various liver imaging positions should be repeated several times before declaring that the examination is complete. Electronic scanning echoendoscopes, whether radial or linear, generally have deeper penetration in liver tissue than mechanical rotating echoendopes.

The first 'liver' position is in the duodenal bulb. If using the radial scope, the balloon should be overinflated so that one is 'locked' in the bulb. From this position, the tip should be deflected so that is presses as firmly as possible against the right lobe of the liver. The echoendoscope is then advanced and withdrawn to its fullest extent, while at the same time utilizing a clockwise and counterclockwise torquing. The instrument should be advanced until the liver disappears and withdrawn until firm pressure is felt against the pylorus. The duodenal bulb is also the best position for imaging the gallbladder, and again the technique of balloon overinflation should be utilized to obtain full views of the gallbladder. Once imaging from this position has been exhausted, the balloon should be deflated and the transducer repositioned in the antrum. With the tip of the scope

in the antrum and the balloon inflated, the echoendoscope tip again should be pressed as firmly as possible against the wall of the stomach that lies next to the liver. Once again, the scope should be advanced and withdrawn to its fullest extent while continuously imaging the liver. The third position is from the fundus of the stomach. Beginning at the GE junction, the transducer is pressed against the gut wall in the direction of the left lobe of the liver. From this position, the scope is slowly advanced while at the same time applying clockwise and counterclockwise torque to sweep across the extent of the liver. The scope should be advanced until no further imaging of the liver can be achieved.

The technique and positions are the same whether a radial or linear instrument is used. With the latter, it takes more effort via torquing of the scope shaft to accomplish as complete an examination as possible.

The anatomy of the liver is relatively simple. Branching structures with echogenic walls represent the portal venous system, whereas anechoic structures running alongside the portal venous system and without the echogenicity (and without color Doppler signal) represent branches of the biliary tree. Hepatic cysts are common and anechoic, and have a characteristic echo enhancement along the border of the cyst further from the transducer. Hepatic metastases are generally echo-poor, without a distinct border. They can be quite subtle, and thus the endosonographer should scan slowly and carefully. Hepatic veins also lack wall echogenicity and run towards the cranial part of the liver, where they can usually be seen entering the caval vein.

Liver imaging can be a frustrating aspect of endosonography because one can never be sure that the liver has been imaged completely. As a result, the various positions mentioned above should be repeated until the endosonographer is satisfied that the extent of the examination has been as full as possible.

Chapter
15

EUS in Inflammatory Disease of the Pancreas

Joseph Romagnuolo

KEY POINTS

- Endoscopic ultrasound (EUS) is highly accurate in the diagnosis of chronic pancreatitis when five or more of nine criteria are present. The finding of 0–2 criteria has high negative predictive value. The finding of three or four criteria is often associated with abnormal histology and/or abnormal endoscopic retrograde cholangiopancreatography (ERCP); it may also indicate subtle pancreatic disease not immediately visible with conventional tests such as ERCP.

- Fine-needle aspiration (FNA) does not appear to add incremental benefit, with added risks of post-FNA pancreatitis.

- Consistency in terminology will be the key to further research in the area of chronic pancreatitis, as current agreement on terms and criteria is moderate, and interobserver agreement is barely satisfactory.

- Performance of magnetic resonance cholangiopancreatography (MRCP) in chronic pancreatitis is at an early stage, and results are variable.

- EUS in the diagnosis or staging of acute pancreatitis has not been studied.

- EUS appears to be accurate in the diagnosis of pancreas divisum, gallbladder sludge, tumors, and other causes of apparently 'idiopathic' acute pancreatitis; inability to obtain a stack sign raises suspicion of divisum, but following the duct from the major papilla to the dorsal gland is more reliable at ruling out divisum.

- EUS can help predict the value of more invasive tests, such as ERCP, in chronic pancreatitis and in divisum, but direct study of this is limited.

- Although not perfect, EUS is very useful in distinguishing inflammatory pseudotumors from neoplastic masses, even without FNA; positron emission tomography (PET) is also promising.

KEY POINTS

- Therapeutic EUS, through celiac plexus blocks and cyst drainage, plays a role in the treatment of chronic pancreatitis-related symptoms and EUS may have a role in predicting response to ERCP-guided therapy.

INTRODUCTION

Endoscopic ultrasound (EUS) is well suited to examine the pancreas because of the proximity of the probe to the pancreatic parenchyma, and was originally developed for this purpose in the early 1980s.[1–3] EUS boasts dynamic imaging, together with the fine resolution of parenchyma that real-time ultrasound is capable of, resulting in a huge advantage over static cross-sectional imaging. At the same time, EUS avoids the intervening air and fat that degrade the quality of transabdominal ultrasonography, and generally can use higher frequencies. Because higher frequency means lower depth of penetration, transabdominal ultrasound is restricted to a lower frequency (with associated lower resolution), to overcome the distance between the skin and the retroperitoneum. Because of its non-invasive nature, it avoids the risk of pancreatitis associated with endoscopic retrograde cholangiopancreatography (ERCP). The literature regarding chronic pancreatitis, which is detailed below, suggests that EUS is probably at least as sensitive as the conventional gold standard of ERCP, and may identify patients with earlier stages of disease that evade standard testing.

Grading of acute pancreatitis with EUS has not yet been studied. However, EUS appears to have a role in otherwise idiopathic recurrent pancreatitis, identifying unrecognized chronic pancreatitis, biliary sludge, small tumors, or pancreas divisum. Acute inflammatory masses can be distinguished from neoplasia to a greater extent than other imaging options because of the fine parenchymal detail seen in inflammatory masses but not in cancer. The addition of fine-needle aspiration (FNA) to EUS, in order to sample equivocal masses and lymph nodes, provides an invaluable dimension to the assessment of the pancreas that other imaging cannot currently match.

In addition, in established inflammatory diseases of the pancreas, interventional EUS can offer unique therapeutic options. These include EUS-guided transgastric celiac plexus blocks and EUS-guided pancreatic pseudocyst drainage. EUS-guided decompression of intraductal hypertension in the setting of an obstructed main pancreatic duct is being investigated in experimental models and in small patient series.

This systematic review was derived from review of the existing literature. A PubMed search (1966 to December 2004) using the MESH terms 'endosonography' and 'pancreatitis', revealed 148 abstracts; these were reviewed individually for relevance. Multiple topic reviews were also examined,[4–13] including their bibliographies, to identify missing articles.

THE NON-INFLAMED PANCREAS ON EUS

The technique for examining the pancreas by EUS is outlined in Chapter 14. Once good position and good images have been obtained, one needs to be able to recognize what is normal. Briefly, the normal non-inflamed pancreas appears to be a homogeneous structure with a single anechoic (Doppler negative) smooth ductular structure running within it in the genu, body, and tail, representing the main pancreatic duct. The pancreas has a fine diffusely speckled pattern (so-called 'salt and pepper') that is, on average, more echogenic (brighter) than the liver owing to its higher fat content; thus, a small amount of fine diffuse heterogeneity is normal. Caution should be exercised when making note of small echogenic foci or short echogenic strands when a high degree of magnification is used, as may be needed for imaging of an atrophic gland or a gland with a very small duct. The gland contour is generally smooth. The duct wall is barely perceptible, with similar echotexture to surrounding pancreatic tissue. Side-branches, other than in the head, are generally not visible. However, Catalano et al.[14] noted side-branches in 17 of 25 controls, and the mean size of side-branches was no different from that of normal controls in a study by Wiersema et al.[15] The mean sizes in the latter study were 0.7, 0.5, and 0.4 mm in the head, body, and tail, respectively. The course of the main duct can be mildly tortuous, but should remain smooth, and the duct should taper from the head to the tail with upper limits of normal of 3, 2, and 1 mm in the head, body, and tail, respectively. Above the age of 60 years, an extra 1 mm for the main duct in each section is generally allowed, due to atrophy. However, control groups have had ductal diameters up to 1 mm higher than these normal values in each category, and it may be more appropriate to say that these limits should be defined as up to 1 mm above these 'normal sizes'.[15] The anterior–posterior thickness of the pancreas is approximately 10–15 mm.[14,15] The dorsal pancreas is generally more echogenic (brighter) than the ventral pancreas, and the ventral anlage along with the transition zone can be seen on EUS in 45–75% of people.[14–16] In contrast, computed tomography (CT) and transabdominal ultrasonography note the anlage in only 25% of patients.[17,18] Finally, the normal head is generally more heterogeneous than the body and tail.

DIAGNOSIS AND STAGING OF CHRONIC PANCREATITIS

The diagnosis of chronic pancreatitis is difficult. CT and magnetic resonance imaging (MRI) must rely on main pancreatic duct dilatation, moderate-sized cysts, and calcifications for the diagnosis, all of which generally occur in more advanced disease. Magnetic resonance cholangiopancreatography (MRCP) can make some further inferences regarding main duct irregularity and the presence of dilated side-branches, but the resolution is likely still too poor at present to be accurate in this assessment, unless the duct is very irregular and the branches are very dilated. ERCP carries the risk of causing further pancreatic damage, and must rely on ductal and intraductal abnormalities alone.

In contrast, EUS uses parenchymal criteria in addition to ductal criteria to make a diagnosis of chronic pancreatitis. Smaller cysts and more subtly dilated or clubbed side-branches can also be identified more reliably. Even calcifications a few millimeters in size can be readily identified as bright/hyperechoic reflections, both because of the high resolution and the even more obvious acoustic shadowing (dark/hypoechoic wedge behind the stone) that is present when ultrasound waves are reflected by an abrupt change in acoustic impedance (e.g., a stone next to tissue or fluid).

Defining the criteria and identifying them reliably

The great difficulty with the EUS literature regarding chronic pancreatitis is that the diagnosis relies on tallying the number of criteria present, generally giving equal weighting to those criteria, and each study uses a different denominator and selection criteria, albeit with great overlap (Table 15.1). There are generally considered to be nine accepted criteria,[19] including four parenchymal criteria (hyperechoic foci, hyperechoic strands, hypoechoic lobules [also known as reduced echogenicity foci, pseudolobularity], and cysts) and five ductal criteria (dilatation, dilated side-branches, main duct irregularity, hyperechoic duct margins, and stones).

Figure 15.1 shows a few examples of these criteria. The actual histologic correlation of these criteria is unknown, but theoretical correlations have been proposed (Table 15.1). Two studies using intraductal ultrasound in comparison to surgical or autopsy specimens suggested that hyperechoic strands might represent bands around cystic structures, that lobullary might correspond to interlobular fibrosis, and that hyperechoic duct margins might correspond to periductal fibrosis.[20,21] The earliest comparative study, by Wiersema et al.,[15] initially examined 11 criteria, of which five were found to be significant independent predictors of abnormal ERCP in logistic regression analysis: (1) areas of reduced echogenicity, (2) irregular duct contour, (3) main duct dilatation, (4) dilated side-branches, and (5) echogenic foci greater than 3 mm. Three other criteria (echogenic duct wall, 'accentuated lobular pattern', and cysts) were significant individually but not in multivariate analysis.

CRITERIA AND THRESHOLDS USED BY STUDIES IN DIAGNOSING CHRONIC PANCREATITIS

Reference	Threshold no. of criteria	PARENCHYMAL CRITERIA						DUCT CRITERIA				
		Hyperechoic foci	Hyperechoic strands	Hypoechoic lobules, foci, or areas	Accentuation of lobular pattern	Irregular gland margin or increased size	Cyst	Irregular duct contour	Visible side-branches	Hyperechoic duct margin	Dilated main duct	Stone
Chong 2005 (DDW 2005)	Calcification; 3 or more, if no calcification (by ROC)	✓	✓	✓			✓	✓	✓	✓	✓	✓
Kahl et al.[29] (2002)	1 or more	✓ >3 mm	✓[e]	✓	[e]	✓ Increased gland size	✓	✓	✓	✓	✓	✓
Hollerbach et al.[34] (2001)	2 or more	✓ Hyperechoic lobules	✓ Septa				✓	✓	✓	✓		✓
Hastier et al.[55] (1999)	1 or more?	✓	✓	✓			✓	✓	✓	✓	✓	✓
Catalano et al.[14] (1998)	No criteria rules out disease; >5 criteria rules in disease; 3–5 criteria abnormal ERCP in 92%	✓[d]	✓ Septa	[c]	[c]	✓ Irregular margin	✓	✓	'Ectatic'[c]	✓	✓	✓
Sahai et al.[19] (1998)	<3 criteria rules out disease; >4 criteria rules in disease	✓ 1–2 mm	✓	✓ 2–5 mm			✓ >2 mm	✓	✓	✓	✓[f]	✓
Buscail et al.[46] (1995)	Not reported	[b]	[b]	✓			✓	✓	✓	✓[b]	✓	✓
Wiersema et al.[15] (1993)	3 or more (by ROC)	✓[a] >3 mm		✓[a]	✓		✓	✓[a]	✓[a]	✓	✓[a]	✓

Table 15.1 Criteria and thresholds used by studies in diagnosing chronic pancreatitis

✓Indicates that this criterion was sought where applicable alternate terminology and size specifications used in the publications are provided.

ERCP, endoscopic retrograde cholangiopancreatography; ROC, receiver–operator characteristic curve analysis.

[a]Significant in multivariate analysis.

[b]Diffusely heterogeneous, diffusely hyperechoic, and hypertrophic were other parenchymal criteria used in this study, and heterogeneous appears to refer to hyperechoic strands and foci; an echogenic duct wall was considered normal but a hyperechogenic duct wall was recorded as abnormal.

[c]Heterogeneous parenchyma was an additional criterion, separate from strands and foci.

[d]Foci were called 'calcifications' parenthetically in this paper, but it is not clear whether or not acoustic shadowing was required.

[e]Focal reduced echogenicity and hypoechoic areas surrounded by septae were considered two different criteria.

[f]>3 mm in the head, >2 mm in the body, >1 mm in the tail.

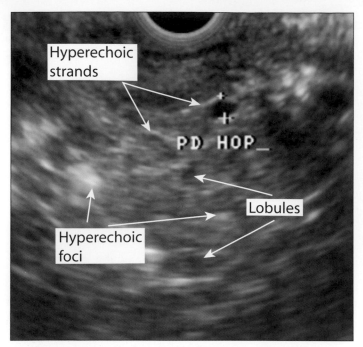

Fig. 15.1 Linear EUS of the head of pancreas (7.5 MHz) in a 52-year-old man presenting with a 2-month history of weight loss, raised lipase levels, and increased epigastric pain for 5 days. There was a remote history of heavy alcohol use. The patient had had an enhanced helical computed tomography (CT) suggestive of a mass (up to 5 cm in size) in the pancreatic head and an associated large cyst. EUS showed chronic pancreatitis, with no focal mass. Note the parenchymal reticular pattern throughout the head of the pancreas (HOP), with hypoechoic lobules and hyperechoic foci, and the preserved main pancreatic duct (PD). The pancreatic duct measured 3.1 mm in the head. Stones were seen in other parts of the gland, as were cysts. Fine-needle aspiration was not considered to be indicated, and follow-up CT a month later showed resolution of the presumed acute-on-chronic inflammatory mass. His weight stabilized.

There was only one patient with calcifications and, although this person did have chronic pancreatitis, calcification was too rare in this cohort to be considered in the model. In this latter study, patients with pancreatic-type abdominal pain and paid volunteers were assessed (echogenic foci with and without shadowing were one criteria, and focal areas of hypo-echogenicity and 'accentuation of the gland's lobular pattern' were two separate criteria). The presence of echogenic strands was not a criterion on its own, and was not separated from echogenic foci; however, echogenic strands, beginning to form lobules, may have been what was meant by the 'accentuation of lobular pattern' referred to in this study. Foci also had to be greater than 3 mm to be considered abnormal. Narrowing was also a duct criteria, in addition to irregularity of contour.

Other EUS criteria have been used in chronic pancreatitis. Some endosonographers also comment on gland contour (lobular versus smooth) and separate 'enhanced' or 'reduced' echogenic foci.[14] Loss of a distinct ventral anlage occurs in inflammatory disorders of the pancreas, and only 29% of patients with abnormal pancreatic head parenchyma (mass or chronic pancreatitis) had a visible anlage (compared with 75%

of those undergoing EUS for non-pancreatic indications).[16] However, this not been tested formally as a 'criterion' for chronic pancreatitis.

It can already be seen that there is a problem with consistency. Minimal standard terminology (MST) has been developed for these criteria and other EUS findings in the pancreas and other organs (Table 15.2).[22] The different criteria and thresholds used are summarized in Table 15.1.

The first assessment of a diagnostic test, after pilot studies defining what is normal and what is abnormal, involves measurement of reproducibility and interobserver reliability of the assessment and criteria, as determined by the κ statistic (a measure of agreement beyond what is expected by chance alone).[23] In the study by Wiersema et al.,[15] concordance for the five criteria that achieved significance in multivariate analysis was seen in 83–94% for the three reviewers. Wallace et al.[24] measured the interobserver reliability of 11 experienced endosonographers at κ=0.45, with even poorer reliability for individual criteria.[24] In this study, it was found that neither having completed a third tier fellowship, nor having performed more than 1000 pancreatic procedures, improved agreement.[24] Only two of the nine criteria had κ>0.40 (good agreement or better): main duct dilatation (0.61) and lobularity (0.51).[24] There was poor agreement on the relative importance of criteria, except that everyone considered stones to be the most important. Unfortunately, this most important criterion had a κ statistic of only 0.38 for its identification.[24]

It is difficult to understand why simple, relatively objective, criteria such as duct dilatation with preset upper limits of normal (2 mm in body, 1 mm in tail)[24] were not associated with complete agreement. However, it is possible that individual endosonographers used a different threshold for older patients,

PROPOSED THEORETICAL HISTOLOGIC CORRELATES OF EUS CRITERIA FOR CHRONIC PANCREATITIS	
EUS finding	**Proposed histologic correlate**
Hyperechoic/thickened duct margin	Periductal fibrosis
Dilated duct and/or side-branches	Dilated duct and/or side-branches
Irregular duct contour	Irregularity due to periductal fibrosis
Stones	Stones
Cysts	Cysts and/or cystic side-branches
Hyperechoic foci and strands	Focal or linear areas of fibrosis; round foci may also represent strands cut in cross-section, small calcifications, or protein plugs that are not dense enough to cause an acoustic shadow
Hypoechoic lobules	Focal edema, often surrounded by linear fibrosis

Table 15.2 Proposed theoretical histologic correlates of EUS criteria for chronic pancreatitis

and feel uncomfortable (perhaps rightly so) calling a duct abnormal if it is only a few tenths of a millimeter above the upper limit of normal, in one section of the pancreas. Although these values for reliability appear poor at first glance, the authors[24] point out that identification of bleeding ulcer stigmata (0.34–0.66),[25] stroke localization by radiologists using brain CT (0.56–0.62),[26] and heart sounds interpretation (0.05–0.18)[27] have comparable or poorer interobserver reliability as measured with the κ statistic. MRCP may have slightly better agreement.[28]

Although the reliability of the overall diagnosis of chronic pancreatitis is more clinically relevant than agreement on the individual criteria, the 'overall' κ is more difficult to interpret because: (1) one's threshold for calling chronic pancreatitis (e.g., number of criteria) and weighting criteria (e.g., calcification, cysts, ductal dilatation) may be different from that used in the study, and (2) because this κ is prone to bias. This bias occurs because, in almost all studies, endosonographers are not blinded to clinical information (e.g., alcohol history, type of pain, history of recurrent pancreatitis, etc.), and this tends artificially to improve agreement on the 'overall impression' of chronic pancreatitis.

Despite an attempt at MST,[22] there is still controversy on the definition of criteria. Should an irregular outside gland margin (what some call a 'lobular gland', different from 'lobularity') be a criterion? Does any pancreas with hypoechoic lobules, because of the echogenic strands that define the lobules and the echogenic foci that often separate them from other lobules, automatically have three criteria? Should hyperechoic foci have a size criterion, and, if so, is it >3 mm[15,29] or 1–2 mm[19]? Does a duct that has, for example, less than 10% of its course marked by an echogenic wall meet the criteria for 'echogenic and/or thickened duct wall'? How much irregularity of the pancreatic duct is 'irregular', and how does gross tortuosity differ from fine and course irregularity; do they mean the same thing? Does a side-branch have to be a certain size, be ectatic,[14] or be clubbed to be considered abnormal; or does it have to be simply 'visible'[22,30] – if the latter, at what imaging frequency and magnification should this assessment be made? Is a duct that is 2.8 mm in the head, 2.1 mm in the body, and 0.8 mm in the tail 'dilated' just because in the body it was >2 mm (2 mm in body, 1 mm in tail were the upper limits of normal in the interobserver reliability studies of Wallace et al.[24] and Sahai et al.[30])? It is not clear that this is really abnormal; the control group (n=20) in the study by Wiersema et al.[15] had ducts in the three regions measuring up to 3.6, 3, and 2 mm, respectively, despite a mean age of only 34 (range 21–52) years. Perhaps ducts need to be 0.5 to 1 mm larger than these 'upper limits of normal' to be considered truly abnormal. Lastly, it is generally recommended that the diagnosis of chronic pancreatitis be concentrated on the body and tail, and that, apart from calcifications, most other features for chronic pancreatitis when limited to the head alone are felt to be non-specific. However, what does it mean when multiple, reasonably convincing, criteria for chronic pancreatitis are met in the head alone – is this normal

or is this focal chronic inflammation (Figs 15.2 and 15.3)? These are questions that are difficult to answer but remain a significant barrier to training and research, as well as to comparing and pooling studies for meta-analysis. The MST[22] offers an excellent step towards uniformity (Table 15.3), but work still needs to be done to answer these common questions.

How many criteria are there? How many are abnormal?

The literature with respect to this issue is variable, and a summary of the different criteria sought and the thresholds used or suggested is presented in Table 15.1. One can see that the thresholds vary from one or more to six or more, and that the denominator of criteria sought also varies from five to ten or more. The most consistent criteria are the ductal ones. Of

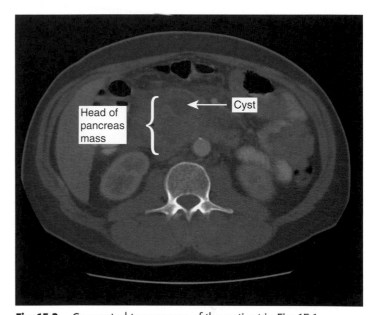

Fig. 15.2   Computed tomogram of the patient in Fig. 15.1.

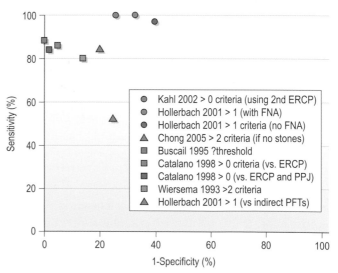

Fig. 15.3   Test performance (receiver–operator characteristics) of various studies of EUS in chronic pancreatitis, plotted as sensitivity (true positive rate) against 1-specificity (false-positive rate).

MINIMUM STANDARD TERMINOLOGY (MST) RELEVANT TO INFLAMMATORY PANCREATIC EUS CRITERIA[22]		
Term	Definition	Comments
Cyst	Abnormal anechoic (i.e., without echoes), round or oval structure	Specify size, septations, wall thickening or mural nodules, debris, connection with main duct or side-branch, and associated solid mass Inflammatory cysts are generally thin-walled, have single or no septations, often contain debris, and are often in communication with the main pancreatic duct
Calcification	Hyperechoic lesion with acoustic shadowing (reduction in echo due to strongly attenuating or reflecting structure) within a parenchymal organ or mass	Generally not recommended for describing the pancreas, unless describing components of a cyst or mass Stone is a preferred term
Stone	Hyperechoic lesion with acoustic shadowing (reduction in echo due to strongly attenuating or reflecting structure) within a duct or gallbladder	All calcifications in the pancreas (excluding masses and cysts) are by definition intraductal, although the side-branch duct in which they reside may be too small to appreciate Generally stones and pancreatic 'calcifications' are both considered 'ductal' features Size measurement may be inaccurate because, typically, only the proximal interface with the lesion is seen (as echogenic) Specify number, approximate size, location in gland (head/body/tail), and whether present within main duct
Hyperechoic foci	Small distinct reflectors	Some studies separate <3 mm and ≥3 mm sizes, but relative significance is not known Generally do not have acoustic shadowing Specify extent, location
Hyperechoic strands	Small, string-like, hyperechoic (echoes brighter than normal and/or brighter than surrounding tissues) structures	Specify extent, location
Hypoechoic lobules	Rounded homogeneous areas separated by strands of a different echogenicity	Almost by definition, lobules and strands coexist (foci also frequently coexist) The term 'lobulated' can be used to describe a gland with lobules, but is sometimes confused with a 'lobular gland margin' and so is probably best avoided There is no recommended size criterion, but care must be taken to ensure that lobules >1 cm are not in fact small masses Specify extent, location
Irregular duct contour	Coarse, uneven outline of the duct	Specify extent, location
Tortuous duct	Duct with numerous twists and bends	To be distinguished from 'irregular'. Not necessarily abnormal
Hyperechoic duct wall	Region of duct where wall echoes are brighter than normal and/or brighter than surrounding tissues	A normal pancreatic duct wall is barely perceptible (very faint interface) on ultrasonography, and is essentially isoechoic to surrounding parenchyma
Dilated duct	Abnormal increase in caliber	Duct size should be measured from the *closest* echo of the wall closest to the probe to the *closest* echo of the wall furthest from the probe Size and location, beading (alternating small and large calibers), and localized narrowings (strictures) or abrupt changes in caliber should be noted

Table 15.3 Minimum Standard Terminology (MST) relevant to inflammatory pancreatic EUS criteria[22]
The terms hypoechoic foci and accentuation of lobular pattern are not listed in the MST paper.

the parenchymal criteria, the most consistently used are hyperechoic foci (although the size criterion is not consistent), cysts, and hypoechoic lobules.

Wiersema et al.[15] used receiver–operator characteristic (ROC) curve analysis to determine the number of criteria that mathematically balance sensitivity and specificity, and the result was three or more criteria (100% sensitivity, 79% specificity). Sahai et al.[19] looked informally at different thresholds for identifying different Cambridge classes of chronic pancreatitis at the Medical University of South Carolina (MUSC). This study showed that finding fewer than three criteria effectively excludes moderate and severe chronic pancreatitis on ERCP, and that five or more criteria strongly suggests at least mild chronic pancreatitis on ERCP. Finding three to four criteria was considered equivocal but in the presence of alcohol abuse[19] or symptoms suggestive of pancreatic disease[29] may indicate a significant finding.

Another MUSC study[30] of 156 dyspeptic patients and 27 controls showed that even asymptomatic controls had a mean of 1.9 ± 1.8 criteria out of the nine listed above; no controls had more than six criteria. Only 67% of control patients had fewer than four criteria. Controls with a history of alcohol use had approximately double the number of criteria, on average, than those without an alcohol history. This study suggests that, although a few criteria are likely normal in most patients, asymptomatic chronic pancreatitis may exist in patients with a significant alcohol history; this has implications for choosing 'controls' for EUS studies on chronic pancreatitis criteria.

Rajan et al.[31] from Mayo Rochester recently showed data that suggested that the frequency of EUS findings of chronic pancreatitis increased slightly, with age. However, in contrast to the title and abstract, their multivariate analysis clearly states that the only significant predictor was male gender, not age. Although it is true that an age-related association was seen in univariate analysis, age did not end up being an independent predictor in their multivariate analysis. This apparent association, therefore is likely due to confounding by male gender (males in the study were significantly older than females).[33] The authors do not provide a table showing number of criteria for different age groups, stratified by gender. The reason why males would have a higher number of criteria is not clear; it could be due to under-reported alcohol use in males, but other possibilities exist.

Recently, our group at MUSC compared EUS findings with surgical pathology in a group of 71 patients undergoing pancreatic surgery for abdominal pain and suspected chronic pancreatitis.[33] In patients without calcifications ($n=41$), ROC curve analysis revealed that three or more EUS criteria provided the best balance of sensitivity (83%) and specificity (80%) with an area under the curve of 0.8; its ability to separate severe from non-severe disease was poorer (sensitivity 83%, specificity 53%), with the best cutoff for this severe fibrosis outcome being four or more criteria.

Accuracy and test performance

After one is confident with the reliability of a test, the next step is to assess its accuracy against a gold standard.[23] Unfortunately, for chronic pancreatitis, the gold standard is also a problem. Although histology is the gold standard, the number of histologic criteria required is also arbitrary. In addition, one rarely has the opportunity to compare test results to tissue in chronic pancreatitis, as a minority of patients undergoes resection. FNA appears unreliable and does not increase accuracy significantly.[34] We are then left with ERCP and secretin-stimulated pancreatic juice analysis, both of which likely miss early disease. Not all chronic pancreatitis results in ductal disease sufficient to be seen at ERCP, and the pancreas has tremendous functional reserve which results in false-negative secretin tests until late in the disease process. Although

advanced Bayesian statistical techniques exist to try to account for imperfect reference standards,[35] they have not been used in this literature to date.

The reference standards

ERCP relies on ductal (main and side-branch) irregularity and dilatation, intraductal filling defects or stones, and inflammatory cysts that communicate with the main pancreatic duct. These features are currently graded using the widely accepted Cambridge classification (Table 15.4).[36] These criteria were arrived at mainly by expert consensus, rather than comparison with histology, and the interobserver reliability of this gold standard has not been well studied. Fibrotic or inflammatory parenchymal changes are not able to be assessed with ERCP until they cause ductal irregularity and/or obstruction. Furthermore in some studies, equivocal or mild chronic pancreatitis on ERCP was called abnormal;[29] in others, only moderate to severe disease on ERCP was considered abnormal.[19]

There are multiple types of function testing, including measurement of stool enzymes,[37] assessing the cleavage of promarkers by proteases by measuring the markers in urine,[37] and breath tests.[38] However, the test most commonly compared with EUS and ERCP is secretin-stimulated bicarbonate; intraductal or intraduodenal collections may be used. A 1-U/kg dose (maximum 70 U) of secretin is given intravenously, and a 10–15-min collection is tested for bicarbonate; the thresholds for the intraductal (pure pancreatic juice; PPJ) and intraduodenal tests are different. Although pancreatic function testing is viewed by some as the most sensitive and reliable test for chronic pancreatitis and pancreatic insufficiency with an accuracy of 80–90%,[37] this perception may or may not be true. Because of pancreatic functional reserve, loss of exocrine function is likely

CAMBRIDGE CLASSIFICATION OF CHRONIC PANCREATITIS BY ERCP[33]	
Class	Definition
0 – Normal	Visualization of entire duct system with uniform filling of side-branches without acinar opacification, with a normal main duct and normal side-branches
1 – Equivocal	Normal main duct 1–3 abnormal side-branches
2 – Mild	Normal main duct >3 abnormal side-branches
3 – Moderate	Dilated main duct with irregularity >3 abnormal side-branches Small cysts (<10 mm)
4 – Marked or severe	Large cysts (>10 mm) Gross irregularity of main pancreatic duct Intraductal calculus or calculi Stricture(s) Obstruction with severe dilatation

Table 15.4 Cambridge classification of chronic pancreatitis by ERCP[33]

not an early phenomenon, and the apparent performance depends to some extent on the disease stage and/or case-mix of the study cohort. Sensitivity frequently drops to less than 40% in studies of early disease.[6] One recent moderate-sized study from Japan comparing the secretin test to histology in 108 patients (abnormal histology in 39) showed a sensitivity of less than 70%.[39] This study used consensus-derived histology scoring system (grades 0–4) from the Japanese Society of Gastroenterology.[40] Other older comparisons with histology have found similarly moderate sensitivity.[41,42]

Histology is an obvious reference standard, but the grading and diagnosis are unfortunately also not standardized and the literature is limited to small series.[34,43] The correlation of surgical specimens with core biopsies and FNA specimens is not clear and is likely prone to sampling error, as has been well documented in liver cirrhosis.[45] Most people with chronic pancreatitis do not need resection and so access to a surgical specimen is limited, except in advanced disease. Local data from MUSC suggest that, even in patients clinically suspected of having disease sufficiently severe to be referred for surgery, only 65 (92%) of 71 pancreas resection specimens had significant fibrosis (2 or more of 12 histologic fibrosis criteria from Ammann et al) for the diagnosis of chronic pancreatitis.[33] Therefore, histology may not even be a perfect reference standard.

Test performance

Studies without follow-up

EUS has been compared to both ERCP and secretin-stimulated pancreatic function testing as the best available reference standards for chronic pancreatitis, notwithstanding the above limitations. Studies without clinical follow-up are summarized in Table 15.5 and Fig. 15.3.

In 1993, Wiersema et al.[15] examined a sample of 20 normal, paid, healthy volunteers qualitatively. Subsequently, 69 patients with pancreaticobiliary pain were used to examine the usefulness of EUS in diagnosing chronic pancreatitis. Subjects also underwent ERCP and 16 had secretin testing. Thirty had chronic pancreatitis by ERCP (n=19), ERCP and PPJ (n=3), PPJ alone (n=6), and clinical (n=2) criteria. The sensitivity and specificity of EUS in chronic pancreatitis (three or more criteria) compared with ERCP were 100% and 79%, respectively (80% and 86%, respectively when ERCP, secretin testing, and/or 'clinical criteria' were used together). A total of five criteria (of 11 proposed initially) were found to be significant independent predictors, plus three others in univariate analysis alone. ROC curve analysis was used to select the number of criteria representing the best cut-off balancing sensitivity and specificity, using a composite gold standard. In the subgroup of patients (n=16) with secretin testing, nine were abnormal. EUS had a sensitivity and specificity of only 67% and 29%, respectively, using secretin technologies as a gold standard; however, for ERCP, these values were 33% and 86%. The apparent lack of specificity of EUS here may be due to false negative secretin tests. Although this design is acceptable for pilot data, it is

prone to bias when the cut-off for the diagnostic test is only internally validated, that is, the sensitivity and specificity reported, with respect to the composite gold standard, were based on the ideal cut-off on ROC analysis and then tested on the same group of patients on which it was derived.[23]

Other studies include one by Buscail et al.,[46] which comprised 81 consecutive patients referred for suspected pancreatic disease and compared the results of 44 who had ERCP with 18 controls. They defined a normal duct as having 'echogenic walls', (in contrast to other studies that list this as a criterion favoring a diagnosis of chronic pancreatitis). The other parenchymal criteria were also non-standard and not well defined (e.g. diffusely heterogeneous, diffusely hyperechoic, hypoechoic areas, and hypertrophic). The threshold (which criteria, how many criteria) for making a diagnosis of chronic pancreatitis was vague, but the authors reported the sensitivity and specificity as 88% and 100%, respectively. Although this design is again acceptable for pilot data, it is prone to spectrum bias, because of the inclusion of frankly normal patients (healthy controls are generally easier to separate from abnormal patients than those with clinical suspicion of disease seen in real life).[23,47,48]

Catalano et al.[14] compared 80 consecutive patients with recurrent pancreatitis in a prospective comparative trial. Patients waited at least 6 weeks after their last acute pancreatitis attack before undergoing EUS, with ERCP and secretin testing. ERCP was performed after EUS, and, although endosonographers were thereby effectively blinded from the gold standard results, ERCP endoscopists were not necessarily blinded to the EUS result. Of ten criteria, including one termed 'heterogeneity', mild chronic pancreatitis by EUS was defined (controversially) as the presence of one or two features, moderate as three to five criteria, and severe as more than five criteria. A normal pancreas by EUS was defined as having no criteria in this study. EUS had an 86% sensitivity and 95% specificity with ERCP, and an 84% sensitivity and 98% specificity when compared with ERCP plus secretin. A normal EUS (no criteria) and severe chronic pancreatitis (more than five criteria) on EUS had 100% agreement with normality or abnormality on ERCP and secretin testing, respectively; the grades also often agreed (κ=0.82). This means that a normal EUS had a negative predictive value of 100%, and an EUS showing 'severe pancreatitis' had a positive predictive value of 100%. Moderate pancreatitis (three to five criteria) by EUS was associated with 92% agreement with ERCP and 50% agreement with secretin testing. Curiously, what the authors termed 'mild pancreatitis' (one or two criteria) had a 17% rate of positivity with ERCP and 13% with secretin, despite most endosonographers considering one to two criteria as being within normal limits. This study suggested that a small percentage of patients with fewer than three criteria may actually have chronic pancreatitis.

The largest and only double-blind prospective study is from MUSC, by Sahai et al.[19] in 1998. In this study, 126 patients with unexplained abdominal pain or suspected pancreatitis referred

REVIEW OF THE LITERATURE ON THE PERFORMANCE OF EUS IN THE DIAGNOSIS OF CHRONIC PANCREATITIS, WITHOUT CLINICAL FOLLOW-UP				
Reference	*n*	Design	Results	Comments
Wiersema et al.[15] (1993)	69	69 patients with pancreatic or biliary pain studied; all had ERCP, 16 had PPJ testing 20 controls examined	30 had chronic pancreatitis by ERCP (19), ERCP and PPJ (3), PPJ alone (6), and clinical (2) SN 80%, SP 86% for ≥3 criteria (of 11) as per ROC curve analysis SN 100%, SP 79% (versus ERCP) SN 67%, SP 29% (versus PPJ (for EUS)) SN 33%, SP 86% (versus PPJ (for ERCP))	11 total criteria, 5 significant in logistic regression Called foci >3 mm 20 controls not used in accuracy calculation
Buscail et al.[46] (1995)	44	81 consecutive patients; 44 had ERCP 18 controls	SN 88%, SP 100%	Non-consecutive enrolment and 'hand-picked' normals Echogenic duct wall considered normal Non-standard terms and criteria No threshold reported
Catalano et al.[14] (1998)	80	Consecutive patients with recurrent pancreatitis	SN 86%, SP 95% (versus ERCP) SN 84%, SP 98% (versus ERCP and PPJ testing) 0 criteria: 100% NPV ≥6 criteria: 100% PPV 3–5 criteria: 92% positive ERCP, 50% positive secretin 1–2 criteria: 17% positive ERCP, 13% positive secretin	Even 1 criterion was considered abnormal Waited for 6 weeks from last acute pancreatitis attack Blinded EUS (not ERCP)
Sahai et al.[19] (1998)	126	Double-blind prospective study Patients with unexplained pain or suspected pancreatitis referred for ERCP	<3 criteria: NPV >85% ≥6 criteria: PPV >85% SN and SP not specified	9 total criteria Head ignored Sizes specified for most criteria (e.g. foci <3 mm)
Hollerbach et al.[34] (2001)	37	Suspicion of chronic pancreatitis, with FNA in 27 patients	SN 97%, SP 60% (versus ERCP, without FNA) SN 100%, SP 67% (versus ERCP, with FNA (n=27)) SN 52%, SP 75% (versus indirect pancreatic function tests)	5 total criteria Weighted criteria 7% post-FNA pancreatitis
Chong (2005, abstract)	71	Retrospective review of patients who had pancreatic surgery and preoperative EUS 92% chronic pancreatitis histologically	SN 83%, SP 80% if calcifications excluded (n=40) ≥3 criteria ideal on ROC SN 83%, SP 57% for ≥4 criteria 93% PPV for calcifications (53% missed on prior imaging)	9 total EUS criteria 12 total histologic criteria (≥2 abnormal; ≥7 severe)

Table 15.5 Review of the literature on the performance of EUS in the diagnosis of chronic pancreatitis, without clinical follow-up
ERCP, endoscopic retrograde cholangiopancreatography; SN, sensitivity; SP, specificity; PPJ, secretin-stimulated bicarbonate testing on pure pancreatic juice; ROC, receiver–operator characteristic; PPV, positive predictive value; NPV; negative predictive value; FNA, fine-needle aspiration.

for ERCP underwent EUS first, and then ERCP blinded to EUS results. Five parenchymal criteria and four ductal criteria were used. Criteria in the head were ignored. This study specified size criteria for echogenic foci (1–2 mm), hypoechoic lobules (2–5 mm), ductal size (>3 mm in head, >2 mm in body, >1 mm in tail), and cysts (>2 mm). Abnormal ERCP was defined as Cambridge 3 (25%) or higher (21%); classes 0–1 (24%) and 2 (29%) were considered normal for the purposes of their analysis (see Table 15.1). For the primary analysis, fewer than three criteria had a negative predictive value 'greater than 85%', and more than six criteria had a positive predictive value 'above 85%'. Multivariate logistic regression analysis found that, although all EUS criteria significantly predicted the presence of Cambridge 3–4 chronic pancreatitis, except hyperechoic duct margin, and

cysts, none of the criteria, nor the number of criteria, was apparently significant in multivariate analysis. In a secondary analysis, attempting to predict Cambridge 2 or more at ERCP, the number of parenchymal criteria (excluding ductal criteria, stones, cysts) were the only independent EUS predictors for chronic pancreatitis on ERCP; alcohol abuse predicted chronic pancreatitis in multivariate analysis independently of the EUS findings. In summary, this study illustrated that one to two criteria are uncommon in moderate or severe chronic pancreatitis (by ERCP), and that seven or more criteria are frequently associated with moderate or severe chronic pancreatitis on ERCP. Eliminating Cambridge class 4 (wherein, the authors argued, endosonographers may see features on EUS, such as dilated ducts and stones, that make them feel certain of chronic pancreatitis, and as a result, stop looking for other criteria), five or more criteria predicted a greater than 85% probability of finding mild or moderate chronic pancreatitis on ERCP. Disappointingly, although thresholds that are associated with predictive values '>85%' are discussed, neither sensitivity, specificity nor exact predictive values were actually reported.

In 2001, the usefulness of EUS and FNA in chronic pancreatitis was studied by Hollerbach et al.[34] This group studied 37 German patients suspected clinically of having chronic pancreatitis. Patients underwent EUS with or without FNA, ERCP, and indirect pancreatic function testing (fecal chymotrypsine and elastase-1, and urinary pancreolauryl testing). Thirty-one (84%) of 37 had abnormal ERCP. Only five criteria were used in this study – hyperechoic lobules, hyperechoic strands ('septae'), ductal irregularity, calcifications, and cysts. EUS was graded into three categories, and criteria were somewhat weighted. Grade 1 had lobularity and strands, grade 2 had findings of grade 1 plus ductal irregularities, and grade 3 had findings of grades 1–2 plus stones or cysts. For comparison with the more widely accepted list of 9 criteria, grade 1 roughly corresponds to two or three criteria, and grade 2 to three or four criteria. EUS (2 or more criteria) had a sensitivity of 97% and specificity of 60% compared with ERCP, and 52% and 75%, respectively, compared with indirect pancreatic function testing. When FNA was added (27 patients), the sensitivity and specificity increased to only 100% and 67%, respectively, using ERCP as a gold standard. Three patients who had EUS-FNA had a normal ERCP, one of these three had cytologic findings of chronic pancreatitis. Two (7%) of 27 cases were complicated by post-FNA pancreatitis requiring fluids and analgesia for 1 day.

At MUSC, we recently reviewed retrospectively 71 eligible patients who had pancreatic surgery for pain from clinically suspected chronic pancreatitis and had a preoperative EUS within 12 months. Chronic pancreatitis was diagnosed histologically (2 or more of 12 histologic criteria) in 65 (92%) of the 71 patients. In those with calcifications (n=30), 53% had their calcififations missed on previous imaging, and calcifications on EUS had a 93% positive predictive value for significant fibrosis and an 80% positive predictive value for severe fibrosis (7 or more histologic criteria). In patients without calcifications (n=41), ROC curve analysis revealed that three or more EUS criteria provided the best balance of sensitivity (83%) and specificity (80%). Correlation between the number of EUS criteria of chronic pancreatitis and the histologic fibrosis score was low, but statistically significant (r=0.4, P=0.01). On average, each additional EUS criterion correlated with a 0.8 increase in the fibrosis score. The best cutoff value for the ability to diagnose *severe* chronic pancreatitis (fibrosis score of 7 or more) was 4 or more EUS criteria, but for this outcome, EUS was less accurate, mainly due to problems with specificity (sensitivity 83%, specificity 57%).

Although studies[49,50] have shown that the pancreatic duct is seen reasonably well with MRCP, especially with secretin, comparative studies are rare and involve small numbers of patients. Calvo et al.[51] showed an 86% sensitivity compared

with ERCP for ductal abnormalities in 78 patients. Only four of these patients had chronic pancreatitis and all were correctly diagnosed; there was a 94% specificity for a normal pancreatic duct. In contrast, Alcaraz et al.[52] studied 81 patients undergoing both MRCP and ERCP, but showed only a 50% sensitivity for chronic pancreatitis (99% specificity). A novel approach by Czako et al.[53] involved comparing changes in T2 gland signal intensity and duodenal filling at secretin-stimulated MRCP with the Lundh test for exocrine pancreatic function in 20 patients and 10 volunteers. The increase in T2 intensity was lower in those with chronic pancreatitis than in normal volunteers. Duodenal filling on MR after secretin was reduced in patients with abnormal function testing, but the degree of insufficiency did not correlate with duodenal dilatation.[53] Overall, the volume of comparative literature regarding MRCP in chronic pancreatitis is far less than that of EUS.

Studies with follow-up

Because our gold standards are somewhat 'tarnished', there have been a few studies aimed at following up patients with so-called 'false-positive EUS' to see whether there is progression of early chronic pancreatitis that may have been missed on the traditional gold standards. The results are conflicting (Table 15.6 and Fig. 15.3).

An abstract from MUSC[54] in 2002 suggested that of 51 patients with normal ERCP but abnormal EUS, six underwent repeat ERCP more than 12 months later, and five of the ERCPs were subsequently abnormal. Of 248 patients with both normal EUS and normal ERCP, 13 underwent ERCP more than 12 months later, and only 8% of these (one patient) had an abnormal ERCP on follow-up.

Hastier et al.[55] studied 72 French patients with alcoholic cirrhosis (without symptoms of pancreatitis) and 32 age- and sex-matched controls with abdominal pain and a normal ERCP, with no history of pancreatitis or alcohol abuse. Five ductal criteria and three parenchymal (cysts, lobules, foci) criteria were used. Eighteen patients with one or more parenchymal criteria alone, and either a failed (n=1) or normal (n=18) ERCP, underwent repeat EUS (n=18) with or without ERCP (n=10) in follow-up 12–38 months later. In all patients, EUS findings were unchanged; in the ten who underwent repeat ERCP, it remained normal.

A second German study by Kahl et al.[29] studied 92 symptomatic patients with known or suspected chronic pancreatitis. Thirty-eight had a normal ERCP, and of these 32 (84%) had an abnormal finding on EUS. Of the 38 patients, 57% drank alcohol during the follow-up period of 6–25 months. Five parenchymal EUS criteria (including 'gland size', focal hypoechoic areas, hyperechoic areas >3 mm, cysts, and hypoechoic areas surrounded by echogenic septae) and five ductal criteria were used. All patients had lobules and septations, and 15% had duct wall hyperechogenicity. Sixteen of 38 did not have a follow-up ERCP. Twenty-two (69%) of the 32 with abnormal EUS had an ERCP on follow-up. All 22 ERCPs were abnormal, approximately half of which had Cambridge 1 only and half had Cambridge 2 grades. If the abnormal second ERCP is used as a gold standard, the

Reference	n	Design	Results	Comments
REVIEW OF THE LITERATURE ON THE PERFORMANCE OF EUS IN THE DIAGNOSIS OF CHRONIC PANCREATITIS, WITH CLINICAL FOLLOW-UP				
Hastier et al.[55] (1999)	18	72 patients with alcoholic cirrhosis without pancreatic symptoms 32 controls with abdominal pain and normal ERCP, without history of pancreatitis or alcohol 18 had EUS parenchymal criteria only, and either follow-up EUS or ERCP	No patient with only parenchymal criteria on EUS had either progression on follow-up EUS or new abnormalities on ERCP (n=10)	8 criteria sought Kasugai ERCP grading No blinding Denominator was 104 patients Selection bias likely, due to confounding by the clinical factors leading to repeat EUS or ERCP
Chen et al.[54] (2002) (abstract)	19	Retrospective study of patients with normal EUS and ERCP repeated >12 months later	5 of 6 patients with normal ERCP, but abnormal EUS, had abnormal ERCP on follow-up 1 of 13 with normal EUS and normal ERCP had abnormal ERCP on follow-up	Denominator was 299 patients Selection bias likely, due to confounding by the clinical factors leading to repeat ERCP
Kahl et al.[29] (2002)	92	Symptomatic with known or suspected chronic pancreatitis 32 had abnormal EUS 22 of the 22 who had follow-up ERCP had abnormal findings on second ERCP	Half of abnormal second ERCPs were Cambridge 1, half Cambridge 2 Using second ERCP as a gold standard in those with abnormal EUS, ERCP had an 81% SN EUS had 100% SN; 16% SP (74% SP using second ERCP as gold standard)	10 criteria sought Cambridge ERCP grading No blinding Most ERCP 'progression' was subtle (Cambridge 1) with similar selection biases to studies above regarding selective repeat ERCP
Singh et al.[56] (2004) (abstract)	39	Retrospective study of EUS patients with ≤3 criteria	18% developed diabetes over a mean of 5 years' follow-up, (much higher than the age–sex–matched expected rate)	No data on whether ERCP was normal at baseline Suggests 1–3 criteria may mean structural damage

Table 15.6 Review of the literature on the performance of EUS in the diagnosis of chronic pancreatitis, with clinical follow-up
ERCP, endoscopic retrograde cholangiopancreatography; SN, sensitivity; SP, specificity

first ERCP had an 81% sensitivity. EUS had 100% sensitivity and 16% specificity if one did not take into account that some of the ERCPs may have been 'false negatives'; specificity was 74% if this is taken into account. This study's results conflict with those of Hastier et al.,[55] possibly due to different diagnostic criteria for chronic pancreatitis by EUS, by ERCP (Kasugai[55] vs. Cambridge[29]), and asymptomatic[55] versus symptomatic[29] patient cohort. Another explanation may be that many of the abnormalities on follow-up ERCP were subtle (Cambridge 1; see Table 15.1). A critical source of bias that threatens the internal validity of both studies is the apparent lack of blinding of the physician interpreting the follow-up imaging. This leaves both studies prone to bias, especially with respect to subtle and/or subjective findings.[23,47]

Comparison and follow-up with respect to endocrine pancreatic function has generally not been reported, mainly because endocrine insufficiency (impaired glucose tolerance or diabetes) is a late finding due to the extensive endocrine reserve of the gland. At the Digestive Disease Week in 2004, an abstract described the follow-up of a number of patients with a low probability of chronic pancreatitis by EUS (three or fewer criteria) for the development of diabetes.[56] The incidence of diabetes in this cohort (n=39) over follow-up (mean 5 years) was calculated, and compared with age- and sex-matched standardized incidence. The conclusion was that low to moderate probability of chronic pancreatitis was associated with an increased risk of diabetes in the years to follow (seven patients, 18%). This is another piece of evidence that suggests that a 'low probability' by EUS may in fact correlate with pancreatic structural and functional damage in some patients.

Chronic pancreatitis criteria in kindreds at high risk for pancreatic cancer

The interpretation of 'chronic pancreatitis criteria' in kindreds with familial pancreatic cancer and Peutz–Jeghers should be cautious. These same endosonographic findings may have very different histologic correlates. Canto et al.[57] from Johns Hopkins have raised a concern that, in this group of patients, criteria for chronic pancreatitis may be associated with dysplasia rather than with inflammation and fibrosis. Of their cohort of 38 patients, 45% had three or more criteria; 35% of the subgroup that did not drink any alcohol had this finding. Brentnall et al.,[58] from Seattle, found evidence of pancreatic intraepithelial neoplasia in patients with ERCP and/or EUS findings of 'chronic pancreatitis' in high-risk individuals.

DIAGNOSIS OF PANCREAS DIVISUM

A MUSC study by Bhutani et al.[59] showed that the inability to obtain a 'stack sign' duodenal apical view resulting in a long-axis view of the portal vein, pancreatic duct, and common bile duct simultaneously) suggested pancreas divisum. It was hypothesized that, because the ventral pancreatic duct is rudimentary in divisum, a good stack sign would not be able to be obtained in these patients. A stack sign was seen in 83% of 30 patients without divisum and in only two (33%) of six patients with divisum; in these two patients, a dilated ventral duct and an unusually long ventral duct were thought to account for the ability to see the stack sign ('false negative' EUS for divisum).

In 2002, Chen et al.[60] showed that a stack sign could be obtained in only 51% of patients with divisum (compared with 6% in patients without divisum). A prominent dorsal duct was more common (16% versus 0%), as was a 'cross-duct' sign (8% versus 0%). The latter sign represents the visualization of the Santorini cutting across horizontally from the minor papilla to the dorsal pancreas, perpendicular to the common bile duct.

A more recent study of 162 patients from Minneapolis, with a 14% divisum prevalence, has shown high accuracy for linear EUS in excluding divisum.[61] The technique involves following the main pancreatic duct from the major papilla to the body of the pancreas and/or noting the pancreatic duct crossing from ventral to dorsal pancreas. Thirty-five patients (22%) had incomplete visualization. Classifying these 35 as 'negative exams', the sensitivity, specificity, and positive and negative predictive values were 82%, 98%, 86%, and 97%, respectively. Excluding patients in whom the assessment could not be done, the sensitivity rose to 95%. False-positive EUS examinations included a pancreatic duct stricture between the head and body, and two patients with ansa pancreatica. In comparison, 41 patients had MRCP, 12% of whom had divisum on ERCP; the sensitivity and specificity were 60% and 89%, respectively, for MRCP. One pseudo-divisum (correctly diagnosed as an adenocarcinoma by EUS-FNA), was a false positive on MRCP for divisum.

DIAGNOSIS AND STAGING OF ACUTE PANCREATITIS

Idiopathic acute pancreatitis

Acute pancreatitis is most commonly due to either alcohol abuse or stones obstructing the common bile duct; together, these account for the etiology in 80% of cases. The role of EUS in choledocholithiasis is discussed in Chapter 18. The other 20% are generally considered idiopathic, but up to half of these cases can be explained by a variety of causes, including medication, microlithiasis, tumors (especially in those aged over 60 years), sphincter dysfunction (biliary and/or pancreatic), pancreas divisum, occult chronic pancreatitis (intermittently obstructing protein plugs or stones, with or without strictures), viruses, metabolic causes (hypercalcemia, hypertriglyceridemia),

autoimmune disease, genetic causes, and others. Because 80% of 'idiopathic' cases do not recur, after ruling out obvious causes (medications, metabolic causes, and, in older patients, tumors), a more extensive work-up is generally not arranged until the problem recurs.[62] Because some of these causes are structural, EUS could theoretically be helpful in the work-up of recurrent idiopathic cases. Pancreas divisum has been discussed above. Fig. 15.4 shows an example of gallbladder sludge on EUS, missed by CT and EUS.

Yusoff et al.[63] recently published results of 370 patients with idiopathic pancreatitis undergoing EUS in Montreal; 169 of the cases were recurrent. Of the 370 patients, 124 (34%) had previously undergone cholecystectomy. Thirty-two per cent of patients with a gallbladder, and 24% of those without a gallbladder, had a possible explanation shown by EUS; when chronic pancreatitis was included as a potential 'etiology', these proportions rose to 63% and 51%. Chronic pancreatitis was seen significantly more commonly (approximately twice as often) in the recurrent than in the single-episode subgroups. The prevalence of stones in the gallbladder or common bile duct varied from 0% in the recurrent subgroup of those who had had a previous cholecystectomy, to 9% in those with a single episode and who still had their gallbladder. Eleven per cent of patients with a gallbladder had sludge within it. Divisum was seen in 5.3% when the gallbladder was present, compared with 11.3% when absent. Neoplasms were seen in 2.8% versus 4.8%, respectively. Limitations of the study include that EUS was done as close as 4 weeks to the previous attack, and may account to some extent for the apparent doubling of the prevalence of inflammatory criteria in the recurrent group; it is more difficult to wait a significant time after an attack in patients who may be having frequent attacks. This group may therefore be more

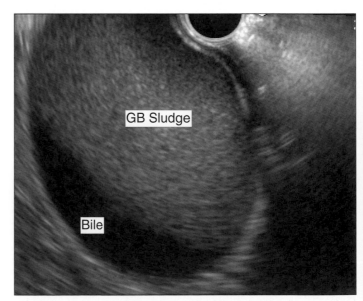

Fig. 15.4   Extensive sludge in the gallbladder (GB) in a patient with acute idiopathic pancreatitis. A normal gallbladder was noted on computed tomography and abdominal ultrasonography within 1 week prior to this linear EUS (7.5 MHz).

likely to have residual acute inflammatory changes mimicking chronic ones. The mean, median, and range of time since the last attack was not given for the single-episode and recurrent subgroups. The other main limitation was the very liberal definition of idiopathic; a patient had to have had a binge of more than 12 alcoholic drinks (>120 g/day) within 14 days for alcohol to be considered a possible cause. This may also explain the high prevalence of chronic changes. It is possible that EUS would pick up abnormalities with a different frequency in a more homogeneously idiopathic group.

Tandon and Topazian[64] reviewed their experience of EUS in idiopathic acute pancreatitis (not necessarily recurrent) and showed that in 21 of 31 subjects a potential cause for pancreatitis was identified. Most (90%) had their gallbladder in situ. The causes included microlithiasis (16%), chronic pancreatitis (45%), divisum (6%), and cancer (3%). ERCP was performed in 29% for persistent or recurrent pancreatitis over a mean of 16 months. One limitation to this study is that it is not clear whether the group is homogeneous. Some 50% of patients had had only one attack. Many would argue this group does not need extensive investigation, except to rule out tumors in the older subset,[62] as the majority do not recur or need treatment. In addition, it is also not clear that this group was truly idiopathic. Sixteen (52%) had moderate to heavy alcohol use and, not surprisingly, two-thirds of these had chronic pancreatitis on EUS. Almost 10% had never had even a single abdominal ultrasound to investigate for cholelithiasis or sludge, bile duct dilatation, and choledocholithiasis. Lastly, the 2–3-week minimum delay from the acute attack until EUS is likely too short to have allowed acute pancreatitis changes to resolve, and may (along with the alcohol history) have accounted for the high prevalence of chronic pancreatitis in this study.

Norton and Alderson[65] reported their results for 44 consecutive patients with idiopathic pancreatitis. Previous cholecystectomy had been performed in 18%. Findings included gallbladder stones (50%), choledocholithiasis (9%), divisum (2%), mass (2%), and chronic pancreatitis (9%). Again, only 23% of these patients had recurrent disease (at least one previous attack). All had had at least one abdominal ultrasound, which was often repeated after resolution of the attack if no stones were seen or if views were inadequate.

Coyle et al.[66] from the MUSC group published results of a series of 90 patients with idiopathic pancreatitis, 66 of which were recurrent. A much higher proportion had had a cholecystectomy in this cohort (50% versus 10–18%[64,65] and 34%[63]). Patients underwent EUS (62%) with duodenal bile sampling (after intravenous cholecystokinin; CCK) and ERCP (99%) with bile sampling and an attempt at dual sphincter manometry (70%). In 18 patients, chronic pancreatitis was diagnosed on both ERCP and EUS, and in nine others EUS alone showed chronic pancreatitis (30% overall) when a minimum of three criteria were used for this diagnosis; 12% further had chronic changes only on ERCP. Causes were found in 80% of patients by ERCP, including 31% with sphincter of Oddi dysfunction

(SOD). Four patients had isolated pancreatic sphincter hypertension. There was a high rate of post-ERCP complications, with pancreatitis occurring in 14%. Eighteen patients had a biliary cause, of which only three were seen by EUS. It is not clear what the concordance between CCK-stimulated duodenal sampling and direct biliary sampling was for the assessment of biliary crystals. The details of preprocedural imaging were not given, although it appears that most had abdominal ultrasonography and CT.

Liu et al.[67] prospectively evaluated the prevalence of occult cholelithiasis in idiopathic pancreatitis. Of 89 patients, 18 were found to be idiopathic after ultrasonography was performed in all patients, including a repeat ultrasound in 50%. Thirty-three percent had CT, and even had an ERCP. Stones ranging in size from 1 to 9 mm stones were seen in the gallbladder in 14 (78%) of the 18 patients; three (17%) also had choledocholithiasis. All of these diagnoses were confirmed by ERCP and cholecystectomy.

Duodenal sampling at EUS, with or without CCK, is easy to do but has not been well studied. Lee et al.[68] and Ros et al.[69] showed that crystals or sludge were seen duodenal aspirates of 73–74% of patients with so-called idiopathic pancreatitis. It appears that EUS itself may be more sensitive than duodenal fluid crystal analysis (96% versus 67%).[70] More study is needed to determine whether this is a useful adjunct to the EUS for idiopathic pancreatitis, when sludge and stones are not seen.

Staging of acute pancreatitis

Identification of fluid collections and the proportion of gland with necrosis, traditionally by contrast-enhanced CT, are important predictors of outcome in acute pancreatitis.[71] There are essentially no published data on the ability of EUS to detect or stage acute pancreatitis. Except for calcifications, all of the criteria used to detect and grade chronic pancreatitis can also be seen in acute pancreatitis, including cysts and mild ductal and side-branch dilatation. Although the standard for detecting necrosis is contrast-enhanced pancreatic-protocol CT, echo-enhanced EUS has not been studied to assess for focal hypoperfusion of the pancreas; this could in theory be possible. In comparison, MRI with and without enhancement and secretin stimulation has been studied for this purpose and appears comparable to enhanced CT.[72,73] Both MRI and EUS would potentially have a useful role in staging acute pancreatitis, especially in those with renal failure and/or diabetes in whom intravenous CT contrast may be harmful.

Differentiating inflammatory pseudotumors from neoplastic masses

Acute pancreatitis and acute inflammatory exacerbations of chronic pancreatitis can result in focal edema. This focal edema can be indistinguishable from a neoplastic mass on CT if no local invasion is seen, and a 16–23% error rate has been reported in this setting.[74,75] Although the presence of signs of chronic pancreatitis raises the suspicion of an inflammatory condition, 2–4% of patients with chronic pancreatitis develop pancreatic cancer after 10–20 years.[76] Both false negatives (missed opportunities to remove a resectable cancer) and false positives (unnecessary Whipple pancreaticoduodenectomy) have serious consequences.

Lymph nodes, including celiac nodes, can occur in both benign and neoplastic pancreatic diseases. Biliary and/or pancreatic duct dilatation is also common in both benign and malignant disease. Pancreatic duct irregularity is common in this scenario, and even if a pancreatic duct stricture is seen on ERCP this may not be a helpful finding.[77] Acute and chronic benign pancreatic duct strictures can be tight and irregular, and the yield of duct cytology is low in neoplasia. The accuracy of EUS, with or without FNA, for pancreatic cancer has been well studied,[78] and is detailed in Chapter 16, but most studies do not have a good mix of neoplastic and non-neoplastic cases. As an example, the study by Mallery et al.[79] had a 92% prevalence of malignancy.

Other imaging methods have been studied in this area. Intraductal ultrasonography may be a helpful adjunct in some cases because of its high imaging resolution. Fluorodeoxyglucose positron emission tomography (FDG-PET) also appears promising, with a sensitivity of up to 88%, and uses metabolic activity to distinguish inflammatory and neoplastic lesions.[80–83] In one review of over 200 pancreatic masses, eight false negatives were seen.[83] Up to 20% of cancer cases had decreased delayed uptake,[83] which is one of the PET features seen in benign lesions.[84] Yamaguchi et al.[85] achieved a high sensitivity when K-ras and p53 suppressor gene mutations were used together (92%) to test pancreatic juice of pancreatic cancer patients, however, there was a low sensitivity for the latter alone (42%) and no control group was provided to gauge specificity.

Painless versus painful presentations, frank jaundice, persistent cholestasis, recent worsening of or onset of diabetes, weight loss, or obvious invasion on cross-sectional imaging can all be helpful in distinguishing benign and malignant causes of the mass. The presentation in benign cases can uncommonly be accompanied by weight loss. In smoldering long-lasting acute pancreatitis or in chronic pancreatitis, because of decreased intake, there may be nausea, pain, and/or pancreatic insufficiency. Diabetes can also worsen abruptly in someone with acute-on-chronic inflammation if endocrine function is borderline at baseline. Because of this overlap, management decisions can be very difficult.

EUS is uniquely able to view parenchymal detail in pancreatic tissue, and does not rely solely on size, asymmetry of the gland, or upstream ductal dilatation to make an assessment of pseudotumors. The usual fine speckling and reticular pattern of the pancreas and other inflammatory features (stranding, lobules, etc.), and ducts and side-branches, are generally lost in neoplastic masses, which are generally more homogeneous and are distinctly hypoechoic from surrounding tissue. In addition, the assessment for invasion is very accurate (this is discussed in Chapter 16), and vascular invasion is highly suggestive of malignancy. In come cases, inflammation-related compression of vascular structures and thrombosis unfortunately can increase the error in assessment. One significant limitation to EUS is that acoustic shadowing from calcifications in advanced chronic pancreatitis can obscure variable proportions of the gland from assessment. An example of a difficult case with a falsely positive EUS (true negative FNA) is shown in Fig. 15.5.

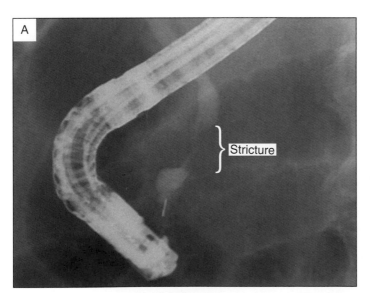

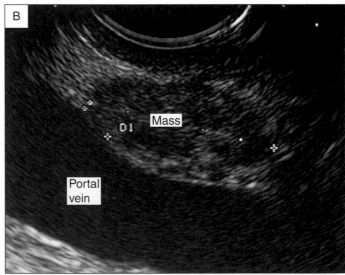

Fig. 15.5   ERCP and linear EUS of a 70-year-old man with painless jaundice, mild weight loss, and no past history of alcohol or pancreatitis. **A,** ERCP showed a tight, shouldered biliary stricture, but cytology from biliary brushings were negative. CT of the pancreas was normal. **B,** A 5 × 25-mm hypoechoic mass, distinct from adjacent non-inflamed parenchyma, can be seen in the head, abutting the portal vein with a preserved fat plane except for a very short break in the interface. The rest of the pancreas appeared normal (no chronic pancreatitis criteria). Fine-needle aspiration showed benign cells. Despite the negative cytology findings, the patient underwent a Whipple resection because of the suspicious cholangiogram and presentation. Surgical pathology was consistent with focal chronic pancreatitis of the head.

Barthet et al.[86] studied five French patients (aged 62–66 years) with suspected pancreatic cancer complicating chronic pancreatitis of a total of 85 patients in whom EUS showed chronic pancreatitis. All five patients had weight loss, calcifications seen on plain radiography, and jaundice. Masses of 2–3.5 cm were seen as irregular hypoechoic areas. Two patients were FNA-negative and did not show progression 2 years later; the other three had histologic confirmation of adenocarcinoma. One patient with a benign inflammatory mass had an increased level of CA19-9 (282 U/l), but the two other patients with confirmed malignancy and CA19-9 measured, had levels above 4000 U/l. One of the inflammatory tumors had central calcification. Four patients underwent ERCP, and all had 'double duct signs', including the two inflammatory masses. Although a 'sensitivity' for EUS was quoted in this paper, it is not really appropriate as no data were provided on the follow-up of other patients with chronic pancreatitis whom the authors did not consider to have a mass (so-called verification bias).[47,87]

Kaufman and Sivak[88] studied 25 patients, ten of whom were ultimately found to have cancer. There was one false negative (90% sensitivity) and two false positives (87% specificity). Nattermann et al.[89] studied 130 consecutive patients, 61 (47%) of whom had pancreatic cancer. These investigators found several non-significant predictors of cancer versus focal inflammation: 7% versus 23% hyperechoic foci, 30% versus 7% loss of demarcation with the luminal wall, 28% versus 9% loss of separation between vascular structures, and 11% frank invasion of a vessel versus 0%. Becker et al.[77] published results using an echo-enhanced EUS approach; this is described further in the corresponding section below.

Glasbrenner et al.[90] studied 95 consecutive patients, 50 (53%) of whom had cancer. The endosonographer was blinded to previous imaging results, but may not have been blinded to clinical data. EUS without FNA had 78% sensitivity and 93% specificity.

Finally, there appear to be genes that are overexpressed in pancreatic cancer,[91–100] and some genes that are overexpressed and/or differentially expressed in chronic pancreatitis.[101–105] MUSC has shown that real-time reverse transcription–polymerase chain reaction (RT-PCR) can detect genetic abnormalities with EUS-derived FNA samples in lung cancer.[106] Therefore, there is potential for RT-PCR to complement cytologic findings in these diagnostic dilemmas as well.

EUS-GUIDED THERAPY OF THE INFLAMED PANCREAS AND PREDICTORS OF RESPONSE TO ENDOSCOPIC THERAPY

Predicting response to endoscopic therapy

Catalano et al.[103] studied 40 subjects with symptomatic chronic pancreatitis with (n=15) and without (n=25) duct obstruction. Of those obstructed, 15 had strictures, three had stones, and two had papillary stenosis. Sensitivity and specificity were 80% and 96%, respectively, using the criterion of a secretin-induced pancreatic duct dilatation of 1 mm or more that persisted for at least 15 min. The interobserver reliability was excellent (κ=0.78). This, in theory, would help predict those who would potentially benefit from ERCP and endoscopic therapy. However, the ability to detect sphincter dysfunction was less impressive (57% and 92%, respectively), as was the interobserver reliability in this regard (κ=0.53). Of the 20 control subjects, 80% had no change in pancreatic duct diameter, but 20% had ductal dilatation that began in 3–4 min and lasted for less than 10 min.

Catalano et al.[107] also studied 22 patients with divisum, attempting to predict who would respond to pancreatic duct stenting using retin-stimulated EUS. Although they showed an 81% sensitivity and 83% specificity, interobserver reliability was only fair (κ=0.58) and their definition of clinical response was not clear.

EUS-guided celiac plexus block for chronic pancreatitis pain

This area is covered in more detail in Chapter 24, but a brief overview of celiac blocks in benign pancreatic disease is appropriate here. Chronic narcotic-dependent or medically refractory pain is a debilitating problem in chronic pancreatitis, resulting in very poor quality of life. Endoscopic and surgical ductal decompression is performed when feasible, but a large group of patients does not qualify; furthermore, a proportion of those who do qualify do not respond, or respond initially and then recur. For these patients, celiac plexus nerve blockage is a reasonable option to consider. Posterior, anterior, and transaortic CT-guided techniques have been used and are generally safe; however, rare reports of vascular damage and even paraplegia exist with alcohol neurolysis.[108] This should in theory be avoided with the EUS-guided transgastric approach with color Doppler. The latter approach involves traversing only a few centimeters of tissue, with no significant intervening vessels or organs. Generally, for benign disease, bupivacaine and steroid are used rather than alcohol, but those who have responded to repeated bupivacaine blocks are sometimes candidates for a more permanent treatment (e.g., alcohol neurolysis) to avoid the risks, costs, and inconvenience of repeated therapies but the resultant significant scarring might complicate plans for any pancreatic surgery in the future.

The procedure, performed with a linear echoendoscope, can take less than 10 min to perform; propofol is often needed for sedation because of the chronic pain, previous substance abuse issues, and narcotic dependence that are frequent in these patients. After color Doppler confirmation, a non-vascular route is planned, and the needle is placed through the gastric wall, usually torquing slightly off the celiac artery. A 22-G needle is commonly used, but injection is easier, with less resistance, with a 19-G needle and is probably just as safe; however, no comparative safety data exist. A spraying needle with side-holes is also now available. There is no compelling evidence to suggest that injecting on both sides of the celiac artery is any better than injecting the entire solution anteriorly, and in many patients the celiac artery comes off so abruptly to the right, towards the liver, that injecting on both sides is not feasible. A recent non-randomized series presented in abstract form has suggested that a bilateral approach might be superior, but this observation remains to be confirmed.[109] There are few data on whether the steroid component is necessary, but the author's institution and others[110] use bupivacaine (25%, 20 ml) mixed with triamcinolone (80 mg, 2 ml). Transient increases in pain (up to 33%), diarrhea (0–15%), and hypotension (1%) can occur;[110,111] because of the latter, and because blood pressure often falls by 10–15% during the procedure,[111] generous intravenous saline is given during and after the procedure, with boluses as needed for any drop in blood pressure. Patients are kept for observation for 2 h in the author's institution. More detail on technique (and use in malignant indications) is available in Chapter 24.

In a large prospective series of 64 patients undergoing EUS-guided celiac block or neurolysis, seven of whom had chronic pancreatitis, the median duration of pain control was only 2-weeks in the chronic pancreatitis group; this duration was significantly shorter than that of the group with malignancy (20 weeks).[111] A small randomized trial has compared EUS-guided and CT-guided approaches for pain in chronic pancreatitis.[110] The solution used was 0.75% bupivacaine (10 ml) and 30 mg triamcinolone (3 ml), injected on either side of the celiac artery with a 22-G needle via EUS. The CT-guided approach was a posterior one with a 15-cm long 22-G spinal needle but used the same solution as the EUS-guided approach. A drop of 3 or more points on a 0–10 visual analog scale was considered a 'positive response', and relapse was considered to have occurred when pain returned to the baseline level. Despite the rather subjective primary outcome the coordinator assessing the outcome in follow-up was unfortunately not blinded, cointerventions, such as changes in narcotic prescriptions, were also not standardized. The minimum time for which patients needed to maintain a 'positive result' to be considered significant was also not stated. In the EUS arm, 50% had a positive result, with persistent benefit in 40% at 8 weeks, and 30% at 24 weeks. For CT, a positive result was achieved in only 25%. At 4 weeks, the median pain scores dropped from 8 to 1 in the EUS group, and from 10 to 9 in the CT group (P=0.02). Costs were slightly lower with EUS ($1100 versus $1400). Based on assessing patient preference in the 9 patients randomized to EUS who had previous experience with the CT-guided approach, and 12 patients who crossed over from EUS to CT or vice versa, the EUS approach was preferred in two-thirds of cases.

EUS-guided cystenterostomy and pancreaticogastrostomy

Mature symptomatic pseudocysts

Endoscopic drainage of pancreatic pseudocysts has become one of the preferred strategies for mature and symptomatic pseudocysts, without large amounts of debris, and with less than 1 cm between the lumen and the cyst cavity.[112,113] As such, EUS-guided therapy plays an important role in benign inflammatory pancreatic disease. Differentiating these collections from cystic neoplasms is of great importance, and is discussed in Chapter 17. To target the transgastric or transduodenal puncture, a visible bulge is required. In addition, even when liver disease is absent because of splenic vein thrombosis that may accompany acute or chronic pancreatitis or splenic vein compression by a large pseudocyst, gastric varices may develop. These varices and the associated perigastric venous collateralization increase the risk of bleeding with a blind puncture. Because cysts are easily targeted with EUS, and because linear EUS with color Doppler accurately allows the detection of intervening vessels, EUS is theoretically helpful in this setting. 'Marking' a spot with EUS is theoretically attractive, but in practice is difficult and does not necessarily guarantee that the needle will follow the same avascular route as was planned with real-time EUS.

Two studies from Amsterdam and the Mayo Clinic describe the role of predrainage EUS for assessing the feasability and safety of endoscopic cyst drainage.[114,115] Findings significant enough to change management were seen in 18–38% of patients. Of these findings, the most common were intervening collaterals, large interluminal distances atypical features suspicious of a cystic neoplasm, or interval resolution of the cyst. EUS can also rule out large amounts of debris or septations that might complicate successful long-term cyst resolution, after endoscopic therapy.[107,108]

Therapeutic linear EUS scopes made by both Pentax and Olympus allow passage of 10-Fr stents and have an elevator to assist with stent and dilator insertion. Unfortunately, because of the oblique view of the echoendoscope, rather than the side view of the duodenoscope, endoscopic therapy using a therapeutic linear echoendoscope remains more awkward than the same therapy via a duodenoscope. It is possible to exchange the echoendoscope for a duodenoscope over a wire after cyst puncture, but this is time consuming and risks loss of wire access. Because of this, the EUS-guided approach is generally reserved for non-bulging cysts, failed blind punctures, or known gastric varices or perigastric collaterals.

Since a case report in 1992,[116] there has been a moderate experience published with EUS guided cystenterostomy.[117–124] A technique involving loading a 7-Fr stent on a 1-mm outer diameter beveled needle, connected with a thread to a stent pusher, has been described in six patients.[117] A similar technique with a one-step puncture and stenting protocol was described in three patients by Inui et al.,[125] and in one patient by Vilmann et al.[118] These techniques potentially allow a one-step stent insertion after EUS-guided puncture, without dilatation, cautery, or even fluoroscopy, but do not allow larger and/or multiple stents to be placed. It is not known whether this approach is adequate compared to conventional drainage with multiple and/or larger stents, with respect to either infection or recurrence due to occlusion of the single small (7–8.5 Fr) stent by debris.

In a non-blinded study, it appeared that complications (especially bleeding) occurred less frequently with a Seldinger technique (passing a guidewire through a larger (18–19 G) needle) without cautery than an approach with cautery;[126] the former approach is feasible through an echoendoscope, and use of a linear scope with a larger 'therapeutic' channel permits 10-Fr stents to be inserted over a guidewire after tract dilatation. The success rate has been reported as 94%.[119] Complications occurred in 8% in one series.[119] Stents are generally pulled after radiologic confirmation of cyst resolution 1–3 months later.

Acute fluid collections, abscesses, and necrosis

It can be difficult to differentiate secondary inflammatory cysts in acute pancreatitis from cystic neoplasms that are the cause of the acute pancreatitis (see Ch. 17). It is usually wise to hold off on imaging, allowing inflammatory cysts to mature or regress, before trying to make this differentiation. However, some acute fluid collections are so symptomatic that it may not be feasible to wait the recommended 4–6 weeks.

In 2000, Fuchs et al.[127] reported three German cases with success in EUS-guided drainage of infected pancreatic pseudocysts. Giovannini et al.[124] then reported the results in 35 French patients with pancreatic cysts who had EUS-guided drainage, 20 of whom had infected collections. EUS-guided puncture was performed, and a 7-Fr nasocystic tube was attempted to be placed over a guidewire in all abscesses. No bleeding complications occurred, and 18 of the 20 cysts were able to be drained. The two remaining patients, and two others who relapsed, had surgery (overall success rate 80%).

The safety of draining collections that contain significant particulate matter, such as pseudocysts with large amounts of debris or partially liquefied necrosis, is not clear.[112] It appears reasonable to restrict endoscopic treatment to symptomatic collections and, perhaps selectively, to infected collections. Those seen on imaging to have significant debris should likely have a flushing nasocystic tube, at least temporarily, ideally placed alongside one or two large pigtail stents. Before stent placement, the fistula should be dilated to a reasonable size to allow debris to exit alongside and within the stents when the nasocystic catheter is flushed. There are insufficient data at the present time concerning infected necrosis with respect to the choice between surgical and endoscopic intervention. There is no evidence that endoscopic intervention of sterile necrosis is of benefit, and it certainly has tremendous theoretical risks of infection.

Pancreaticogastrostomy in chronic pancreatitis

François et al.[128] have published experience of four patients with chronic pancreatitis, pain, and a dilated pancreatic duct with EUS-guided pancreaticogastrostomy. Ductal diameter was not given for all four patients, but was up to 15 mm (these were very

large ducts). Stent insertion was performed under fluoroscopy, using a cut portion of a 6-Fr nasobiliary catheter after puncture with a 19-G needle and dye injection. A 6.5-Fr prototype diathermy sheath was exchanged over a guidewire for the needle, and the stent was then inserted. None of the cases was associated with acute pancreatitis, bleeding, or infection. One patient had stent migration, a second had a stricture and required a second procedure and trans-fistula stricture dilatation, and a third did not achieve pain relief. Stents were not removed systematically, and a recommendation of how long stents should remain was not given; long-term follow-up was not available. This is certainly an interesting and exciting approach, but longer systematic follow-up of these patients and further study, perhaps in an animal model, and comparison with surgical drainage are needed.

'ENHANCED' EUS AND INTRADUCTAL ULTRASONOGRAPHY IN PANCREATITIS

Echo-enhanced EUS

Assessing the perfusion of lesions with intravascular micro-bubbles and accentuating functional or mechanical obstruction of the pancreatic duct with secretin are both possible with EUS. The latter was studied in the setting of predicting response to endoscopic therapy by Catalano et al.[107] The former has been studied in the evaluation of lymph nodes, but the setting most relevant here is the differentiation of benign and malignant masses of the pancreas.

Becker et al.[77] studied German patients with the addition of an acoustic contrast agent to distinguish inflammatory and neoplastic masses in the pancreas – so-called 'echo-enhanced' or 'contrast-enhanced' EUS. In this study, an albumin-based product (Optison; Mallinckrodt Incorporated, St Louis, Missouri) with stabilized 2–8 μm-sized micro-bubbles was used to increase backscatter in small blood vessels perfusing the pancreas. The resulting bubbles are the size of a red blood cell and can flow through lung capillaries; this product has been approved for echocardiography in the USA. When injected intravenously, it takes 15–25 s to reach the pancreatic circulation and then persists for approximately 3 min. A 1:10, 10-ml solution was first injected. A second injection and evaluation was performed 5 min after the first. The rationale for this approach was to make use of the relative hypoperfusion and hyperperfusion status of malignant and benign tissue, respectively, that assists the differentiation of benign and malignant processes on contrast-enhanced CT.

Twenty-three consecutive patients with non-cystic pancreatic masses were studied.[77] Surgical pathology or lack of progression for 6 months was considered the outcome. Five patients had a history of acute pancreatitis, 80% of whom had inflammatory masses as the final diagnosis. All 15 hypoperfused masses were malignant, and seven of eight hyperperfused masses were inflammatory (100% positive predictive value, 88% negative predictive value). FNA was positive in the one hyperperfused mass that was malignant; of note, CT had also shown a hyperperfused lesion. ERCP incorrectly classified two of the 16 patients with carcinoma as having had chronic pancreatitis (false negatives), and four of the 7 patients with inflammation were thought to have had cancer by ERCP (false positive).

Intraductal ultrasonography

Intraductal ultrasonography is performed with a high-frequency radial mini-probe that fits down the accessory channel of the side-viewing duodenoscope, at ERCP. It therefore assumes the associated risks of diagnostic ERCP (e.g., post-ERCP pancreatitis). The added risk associated with intraductal ultrasound imaging itself is felt to be low but is truly unknown. Once cannulation is achieved, a guidewire is inserted (size dependent on the duct being examined) under fluoroscopic control after dye has been injected, and the mini-probe is passed over the guidewire into the duct. Minimal application of the elevator is used, and the probe should be frozen (i.e., not rotating) while outside the duct, to minimize trauma to the moving parts of the probe. A sphincterotomy is not usually needed. Generally, when performed in the pancreas, the probe is pulled back slowly from the tail, keeping the guidewire in place, with a view of the anechoic splenic vein in cross-section (Fig. 15.6). On pull-back, the splenic vein enlarges at the genu as it joins the portal vein, and just below this point the intrapancreatic portion of the bile duct becomes visible, again in cross-section.

Furukawa et al.[129] have studied 26 Japanese patients with pancreatic strictures, 12 of whom had chronic pancreatitis. A 30-MHz ultrasound mini-probe was used; patients were examined prior to resection and the pancreatic ducts of the ex vivo specimens were re-imaged within a few hours of resection.

The images were categorized into two groups: (1) hyperechoic ring surrounded by a band of hypoechoic tissue (without a reticular pattern), and (2) hypoechoic ring surrounded by relatively hyperechoic tissue with a reticular pattern. Fourteen (93%) of 15 type 1 cases represented pancreatic cancer, and all 11 type 2 cases were inflammatory. Correlation was made with histology. A prospective study is needed to test this interesting observation.

SUMMARY

EUS is highly accurate in the diagnosis of chronic pancreatitis. There or more (of nine) criteria appears to be the best cut-off (balancing sensitivity and specificity). When multiple criteria (generally five or more) are present correlation is very high with both ERCP and pancreatic exocrine function testing. However, a normal EUS (two criteria or fewer) effectively rules out chronic pancreatitis. Intermediate probability by EUS (three or four criteria) still appears to increase the risk of functional abnormalities (exocrine and endocrine), even when standard tests (including ERCP) are normal. This is especially true when there is a history of alcohol or other clinical suspicion of chronic pancreatitis. FNA is not recommended to confirm or rule out chronic pancreatitis. Unfortunately, because the treatment for chronic pancreatitis without ductal dilatation is relatively ineffective, the clinical relevance of finding these abnormalities in someone with unexplained, pancreatic-sounding pain is unclear. Apart from sphincter dysfunction, EUS is reasonably good at predicting the presence of pancreatic duct abnormalities (e.g. stones or strictures) that may respond to endoscopic therapy. Because of this, it is likely the diagnostic test of choice for pancreatic-sounding pain to

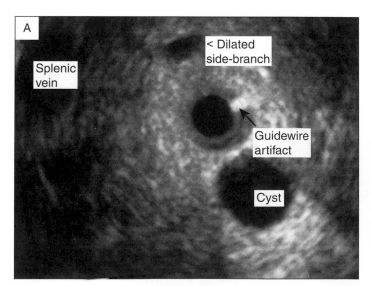
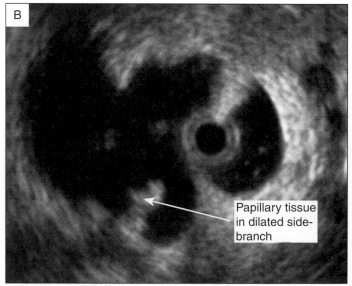

Fig. 15.6   A, Pancreatic intraductal ultrasonography (IDUS) showing a 5-mm anechoic cyst (with distal acoustic enhancement) in the tail of the pancreas with a dilated side-branch but normal-sized main pancreatic duct. **B,** A more obvious side-branch intraductal papillary mucinous neoplasm (IPMN) can be seen in the head of the pancreas (20 MHz). On resection, the small cyst was also found to be a small IPMN (i.e., multifocal). The parenchyma was otherwise normal on IDUS.

diagnose chronic pancreatitis and assess for candidacy for endoscopic or surgical decompression. The addition of secretin stimulation may eventually prove to make this assessment even better. The main limitation to the use of EUS is consistency in the definition of, and therefore the threshold number of, the criteria being assessed.

Although the literature is in its early phase, the diagnosis of divisum by EUS appears accurate, comparable to our experience with the performance of MRCP with secretin, and superior to MRCP without secretin.[130] An inability to achieve a 'stack sign' raises suspicion of divisum, but following the pancreatic duct from the major ampulla is more reliable. In addition, EUS for the identification of possible etiologies for idiopathic pancreatitis (tumors, gallbladder, or bile duct crystals and sludge, idiopathic chronic pancreatitis, divisum) appears to have a reasonable yield. This is especially true in older patients at risk for neoplasia and for patients who have not had a cholecystectomy and have normal right upper quadrant extracorporeal ultrasound findings.

Therapy for inflammatory pancreatic disease is increasingly possible via EUS. For non-bulging pseudocysts, pseudocysts associated with gastric varices, or pseudocysts that have failed blind endoscopic puncture, EUS-guided drainage is a reasonable next step. Although an entirely EUS-guided (no fluoroscopy) one-step drainage approach appears feasible, it is not clear whether this is as effective as dilatation and insertion of multiple stents and/or nasocystic drainage. EUS-guided celiac plexus blocks with bupivicaine are also effective for chronic pain in chronic pancreatitis, and appeared in a small randomized trial[110] to be more effective than the CT-guided approach. Recurrence of pain is the rule, with more than two-thirds of patients returning to their baseline pain by 6 months; repeat procedures are therefore expected. If surgery is a possible future consideration, alcohol injection should likely be avoided.

Although not perfect, EUS is one of the best tests available to distinguish inflammatory (pseudotumors) from neoplastic masses in the pancreas. Often FNA is not required, as the EUS appearance is that of bulkiness and inflammatory changes alone or without any perceptible discrete mass. In indeterminate masses, FNA is definitely helpful. Most cases in this category require some type of follow-up imaging in approximately a month's time to pick up the rare EUS false negatives, and to confirm resolution or stability of benign masses.

EUS is an emerging gold standard for both diagnosis and therapy in inflammatory diseases of the pancreas. Future directions will include making histologic correlation with individual chronic pancreatitis criteria and clusters of criteria, in addition to collecting more follow-up data in those patients with so-called 'false positive' EUSs for chronic pancreatitis. Gaining more consistency in our criteria and terminology for chronic pancreatitis is also key. For celiac plexus blocks, more research is needed to determine the best technique and the simplest effective injection solution. EUS-guided transgastric pancreatic therapy for pseudocysts and obstructed pancreatic ducts is evolving rapidly, and is an exciting addition to our endoscopic repertoire in inflammatory pancreatic disease.

EXAMINATION CHECKLIST

Examine body and tail of pancreas beginning with visualization of celiac trunk (station 4)

Examine the head of the pancreas from the apex of the duodenal bulb (station 3), opposite the papilla (station 2), and uncinate process (station 1)

REFERENCES

1 Hisanaga K, Hisanaga A, Nagata K, et al. High sped rotating scanner for transgastric sonography. Am J Radiol 1980; 135:627–639.

2 DiMagno EP, Buxton JL, Regan PT, et al. Ultrasonic endoscope. Lancet 1980; ii:629–631.

3 DiMagno EP, Regan PT, Clain JE, et al. Human endoscopic ultrasonography. Gastroenterology 1982; 83:824–829.

4 Snady H. Endoscopic ultrasonography in benign pancreatic disease. Surg Clin North Am 2001; 81:329–344.

5 Inui K, Nakazawa S, Yoshino J, et al. Endoluminal ultrasonography for pancreatic diseases. Gastroenterol Clin North Am 1999; 28:771–781.

6 Clain JE, Pearson RK. Diagnosis of chronic pancreatitis. Is a gold standard necessary? Surg Clin North Am 1999; 79:829–845.

7 Raimondo M, Wallace MB. Diagnosis of early chronic pancreatitis by endoscopic ultrasound. Are we there yet? JOP 2004; 5:1–7.

8 Etemab B, Whitcomb DC. Chronic pancreatitis: diagnosis, classification, and new genetic developments. Gastroenterology 2001; 120:682–707.

9 Bhutani MS. Endoscopic ultrasound in pancreatic diseases: Indications, limitations and the future. Gastroenterol Clin 1999; 28:747–770.

10 Wallace MB, Hawes RH. Endoscopic ultrasound in the evaluation and treatment of chronic pancreatitis. Pancreas 2001; 23:26–35.

11 Dancygier H. Endoscopic ultrasonography in chronic pancreatitis. Gastrointest Endosc Clin North Am 1995; 5:795–804.

12 Wiersema MJ, Wiersema LM. Endosonography of the pancreas: normal variation versus changes of early chronic pancreatitis. Gastrointest Endosc Clin North Am 1995; 5:487–496.

13 Kahl S, Glasbrenner B, Zimmerman S, et al. Endoscopic ultrasound in pancreatic diseases. Dig Dis 2002; 20:120–126.

14 Catalano MF, Lahoti S, Geenen JE, et al. Prospective evaluation of endoscopic ultrasonography, endoscopic retrograde pancreatography, and secretin test in the diagnosis of chronic pancreatitis. Gastrointest Endosc 1998; 48:11–17.

15 Wiersema MJ, Hawes RH, Lehman G, et al. Prospective evaluation of endoscopic ultrasonography and endoscopic retrograde cholangiopancreatography in patients with chronic abdominal pain of suspected pancreatic origin. Endoscopy 1993; 25:555–564.

16 Savides TJ, Gress FG, Zaidi SA, et al. Detection of embryologic ventral pancreatic parenchyma with endoscopic ultrasound. Gastrointest Endosc 1996; 43:14–19.

17 Donald JJ, Shorvon PJ, Lees WR. A hypoechoic area within the head of the pancreas – a normal variant. Clin Radiol 1990; 41:337–338.

18 Atri M, Nazarnia S, Mehio A, et al. Hypoechogenic embryologic ventral aspect of the head and uncinate process of the pancreas: in vitro correlation of US with histopathologic findings. Radiology 1994; 190:441–444.

19 Sahai AV, Zimmerman M, Aabakken L, et al. Prospective assessment of the ability of endoscopic ultrasound to diagnose, exclude, or establish the severity of chronic pancreatitis found by endoscopic retrograde cholangiopancreatography. Gastrointest Endosc 1998; 48:18–25.

20 Menzel J, Foerster EC, Ubrig B, et al. Ex vivo examination of the pancreas by intraductal ultrasonography (IDUS). Endosonography 1993; 25:571–576.

21 Furukawa T, Tsukamoto Y, Naitoh Y, et al. Differential diagnosis of pancreatic diseases with an intraductal ultrasound system. Gastrointest Endosc 1994; 40:213–219.

22 International Working Group for Minimum Standard Terminology for Gastrointestinal Endoscopy. Reproduction of minimum standard terminology in gastrointestinal endosonography. Dig Endosc 1998; 10:158–184.

23 Romagnuolo J, Joseph L, Barkun AN. Interpretation of diagnostic tests. In: Rosenberg L, Joseph L, Barkun AN, eds. Surgical arithmetic: epidemiological, statistical, and outcome-based approach to surgical practice. Georgetown, Texas: Landes Bioscience; 2000:64–83.

24 Wallace MB, Hawes RH, Durkalski V, et al. The reliability of EUS for the diagnosis of chronic pancreatitis: interobserver agreement among experienced endosonographers. Gastrointest Endosc 2001; 53:294–299.

25 Lau JY, Sung JJ, Chan AC, et al. Stigmata of hemorrhage in bleeding peptic ulcers: an interobserver agreement study among international experts. Gastrointest Endosc 1997; 46:33–36.

26 von Kummer R, Holle R, Gizyska U, et al. Interobserver agreement in assessing early CT signs of middle cerebral artery infarction. Am J Neuroradiol 1996; 17:1743–1748.

27 Lok CE, Moragan CD, Ranganathan N. The accuracy and interobserver agreement in detecting the 'gallop sounds' by cardiac auscultation. Chest 1998; 114:1283–1288.

28 Takehara Y, Ichijo K, Tooyama N, et al. Breath-hold MR cholangiopancreatography with a long-echo-train fast spin-echo sequence and a surface coil in chronic pancreatitis. Radiology 1994; 192:73–78.

29 Kahl S, Glasbrenner B, Leodolter A, et al. EUS in the diagnosis of early chronic pancreatitis: a prospective follow-up study. Gastrointest Endosc 2002; 55:507–511.

30 Sahai AV, Mishra G, Penman ID, et al. EUS to detect evidence of pancreatic disease in patients with persistent or nonspecific dyspepsia. Gastrointest Endosc 2000; 52:153–159.

31 Rajan E, Clain JE, Levy MJ, et al. Age-related changes in the pancreas identified by EUS: a prospective evaluation. Gastrointest Endosc 2005; 61:401–406.

32 Chong AK, Romagnuolo J, Lewin D, et al. Diagnosis of chronic pancreatitis with endoscopic ultrasound: a comparison with histopathology. Gastrointest Endosc 2005; 61:AB77.

33 Chong A, Romagnuolo J. Gender-related changes in the pancreas by EUS. Gastrointest Endosc 2005; 62:475(letter).

34 Hollerbach S, Klamann A, Topalidis T, et al. Endoscopic ultrasonography (EUS) and fine-needle aspiration (FNA) cytology for diagnosis of chronic pancreatitis. Endoscopy 2001; 33:824–831.

35 Joseph L, Gyorkos TW, Coupal L. Bayesian estimation of disease prevalence and the parameters of diagnostic tests in the absence of a gold standard. Am J Epidemiol 1995; 141:263–272.

36 Axon AT, Classen M, Cotton PB, et al. Pancreatography in chronic pancreatitis: international definitions. Gut 1984; 25:1107–1112.

37 Forsmark CE. Chronic pancreatitis. In: Feldman M, Tschumy WOJ, Friedman LS, Sleisenger MH, eds. Sleisenger & Fordtran's Gastrointestinal and Liver Disease, 7th edn. Philadelphia: Elsevier; 2002:943–969.

38 Romagnuolo J, Schiller D, Bailey RJ. Using breath tests wisely in a gastroenterology practice: an evidence-based review of indications and pitfalls in interpretation. Am J Gastroenterol 2002; 97:1113–1126.

39 Hayakawa T, Kondo T, Shibata T, et al. Relationship between pancreatic exocrine function and histological changes in chronic pancreatitis. Am J Gastroenterol 1992; 87:1170–1174.

40 Research Committee for Chronic Pancreatitis in Japanese Society of Gastroenterology. In: Yamagata S, ed. Clinical diagnostic criteria for chronic pancreatitis. Tokyo: Igakutosho; 1984.

41 Heij HA, Obertop H, van Blankenstein M, et al. Relationship between functional and histological changes in chronic pancreatitis. Dig Dis Sci 1986; 31:1009–1013.

42 Heij HA, Obertop H, van Blankenstein M, et al. Comparison of endoscopic retrograde pancreatography with functional and histologic changes in chronic pancreatitis. Acta Radiol 1987; 28:289–293.

43 Fekete PS, Nunez C, Pitlik DA. Fine-needle aspiration biopsy of the pancreas: a study of 61 cases. Diagn Cytopathol 1986; 2:301–306.

44 Ammann RW, Heitz PU, Kloppel G. Course of alcoholic chronic pancreatitis: a prospective clinicomorphological long-term study. Gastroenterology 1996; 111(1):224–231.

45 Regev A, Berho M, Jeffers LJ, et al. Sampling error and intraobserver variation in liver biopsy in patients with chronic HCV infection. Am J Gastroenterol 2002; 97:2614–2618.

46 Buscail L, Escourrou J, Moreau J, et al. Endoscopic ultrasonography in chronic pancreatitis: a comparative prospective study with conventional ultrasonography, computed tomography, and ERCP. Pancreas 1995; 10:251–257.

47 Begg CB. Biases in the assessment of diagnostic tests. Stat Med 1987; 6:411–423.

48 Lachs MS, Nachamkin I, Edelstein PH, et al. Spectrum bias in the evaluation of diagnostic tests: lessons from the rapid dipstick test for urinary tract infection. Ann Intern Med 1992; 117:135–140.

49 Lomas DJ, Bearcroft PW, Gimson AE. MR cholangiopancreatography: prospective comparison of a breath-hold 2D projection technique with diagnostic ERCP. Eur Radiol 1999; 9:1411–1417.

50 Manfredi R, Costamagna G, Brizi MG, et al. Severe chronic pancreatitis versus suspected pancreatic disease: dynamic MR cholangiopancreatography after secretin stimulation. Radiology 2000; 214:849–855.

51 Calvo MM, Bujanda L, Calderon A, et al. Comparison between magnetic resonance cholangiopancreatography and ERCP for evaluation of the pancreatic duct. Am J Gastroenterol 2002; 97:347–353.

52 Alcaraz MJ, de la Morena EJ, Polo A, et al. A comparative study of magnetic resonance cholangiography and direct cholangiography. Rev Esp Enferm Digest 2000; 92:427–438.

53 Czako L, Endes J, Takacs T, et al. Evaluation of pancreatic exocrine function by secretin-enhanced magnetic resonance cholangiopancreatography. Pancreas 2001; 23:323–328.

54 Chen RYM, Hino S, Aithal GP, et al. Endoscopic ultrasound (EUS) features of chronic pancreatitis predate subsequent development of abnormal endoscopic retrograde pancreatogram (ERP). Gastrointest Endosc 2002; 55:AB242 (abstract).

55 Hastier P, Buckley MJ, Francois E, et al. A prospective study of pancreatic diseases in patients with alcoholic cirrhosis: comparative diagnostic value of ERCP and EUS and long-term significance of isolated parenchymal abnormalities. Gastrointest Endosc 1999; 49:705–709.

56 Singh P, Vela S, Agrawal D, et al. Long term outcome in patients with endosonographic findings suggestive of mild chronic pancreatitis. Gastrointest Endosc 2004; 59:AB231 (abstract).

57 Canto MI, Goggins M, Yeo CJ, et al. Screening for pancreatic neoplasia in high-risk individuals: an EUS-based approach. Clin Gastroenterol Hepatol 2004; 2:606–621.

58 Brentnall TA, Bronner MP, Byrd DR, et al. Early diagnosis and treatment of pancreatic dysplasia in patients with a family history of pancreatic cancer. Ann Intern Med 1999; 131:247–255.

59 Bhutani MS, Hoffman B, Hawes RH. Diagnosis of pancreas divisum by endoscopic ultrasonography. Endoscopy 1999; 31:167–169.

60 Chen RYM, Hawes RH, Wallace MB, et al. Diagnosing pancreas divisum in patients with abdominal pain and pancreatitis: is endoscopic ultrasound (EUS) accurate enough? Gastrointest Endosc 2002; 55:AB96 (abstract).

61 Lai R, Freeman ML, Cass OW, et al. Accurate diagnosis of pancreas divisum by linear-array endosonography. Endoscopy 2004; 36:705–709.

62 Ballinger AB, Barnes E, Alstead EM, et al. Is intervention necessary after a first episode of acute idiopathic pancreatitis? Gut 1996; 38:293–295.

63 Yusoff IF, Raymond G, Sahai AV. A prospective comparison of the yield of EUS in primary vs. recurrent idiopathic acute pancreatitis. Gastrointest Endosc 2004; 60:673–678.

64 Tandon M, Topazian M. Endoscopic ultrasound in idiopathic acute pancreatitis. Am J Gastroenterol 2001; 96:705–709.

65 Norton SA, Alderson D. Endoscopic ultrasonography in the evaluation of idiopathic acute pancreatitis. Br J Surg 2000; 87:1650–1655.

66 Coyle WJ, Pineau BC, Tarnasky PR, et al. Evaluation of unexplained acute and acute recurrent pancreatitis using endoscopic retrograde cholangiopancreatography, sphincter of Oddi manometry and endoscopic ultrasound. Endoscopy 2002; 34:617–623.

67 Liu CL, Lo CM, Chan JK, et al. EUS for detection of occult cholelithiasis in patients with idiopathic pancreatitis. Gastrointest Endosc 2000; 51:28–32.

68 Lee SP, Nicholls JF, Park HZ. Biliary sludge as a cause of acute pancreatitis. N Engl J Med 1992; 326:589–593.

69 Ros E, Navarro S, Bru C, et al. Occult microlithiasis in 'idiopathic' acute pancreatitis: prevention of relapses by cholecystectomy or ursodeoxycholic acid therapy. Gastroenterology 1991; 101:1701–1709.

70 Dahan P, Andant C, Levy P, et al. Prospective evaluation of endoscopic ultrasonography and microscopic examination of duodenal bile in the diagnosis of cholecystolithiasis in 45 patients with normal conventional ultrasonography. Gut 1996; 38:277–281.

71 DiMagno EP, Chari S. Acute pancreatitis. In: Feldman M, Tschumy WOJ, Friedman LS, Sleisenger MH, eds. Sleisenger & Fordtran's gastrointestinal and liver disease, 7th edn. Philadelphia: Elsevier Science; 2002:913–942.

72 Lecesne R, Taourel P, Bret PM, et al. Acute pancreatitis: interobserver agreement and correlation of CT and MR cholangiopancreatography with outcome. Radiology 1999; 211:727–735.

73 Arvanitakis M, Delhaye M, De Maertelaere V, et al. Computed tomography and magnetic resonance imaging in the assessment of acute pancreatitis. Gastroenterology 2004; 126:715–723.

74 Delhaze M, Jonard P, Gigot JF, et al. Chronic pancreatitis and pancreatic cancer. an often difficult differential diagnosis. Acta Gastroenterol Belg 1989; 52:458–466.

75 DelMaschio A, Vanzulli A, Sironi S, et al. Pancreatic cancer versus chronic pancreatitis: diagnosis with CA 19-9 assessment, US, CT, and CT-guided fine-needle biopsy. Radiology 1991; 178:95–99.

76 Lowenfels AB, Maisonneuve P, Cavallini G, et al. Pancreatitis and the risk of cancer. N Engl J Med 1993; 328:1433–1437.

77 Becker D, Strobel D, Bernatik T, et al. Echo-enhanced color- and power-Doppler EUS for the discrimination between focal pancreatitis and pancreatic carcinoma. Gastrointest Endosc 2001; 53:784–789.

78 Kochman ML. EUS in pancreatic cancer. Gastrointest Endosc 2002; 56:S6–S12.

79 Mallery JS, Centeno BA, Hahn PF, et a l. Pancreatic tissue sampling guided by EUS, CT/US, and surgery: a comparison of sensitivity and specificity. Gastrointest Endosc 2002; 56:218–224.

80 Keogan MT, Tyler D, Clark L, et al. Diagnosis of pancreatic carcinoma: role of FDG PET. AJR Am J Roentgenol 1998; 171:1565–1570.

81 Rajput A, Stellato TA, Faulhaber PF, et al. The role of fluorodeoxyglucose and positron emission tomography in the evaluation of pancreatic disease. Surgery 1998; 124:793–797.

82 Bares R, Klever P, Hauptmann S, et al. F-18 fluorodeoxyglucose PET in vivo evaluation of pancreatic glucose metabolism for detection of pancreatic cancer. Radiology 1994; 192:79–86.

83 Higashi T, Saga T, Nakamoto Y, et al. Diagnosis of pancreatic cancer using fluorine-18 fluorodeoxyglucose positron emission tomography (FDG PET) – usefulness and limitations in 'clinical reality'. Ann Nucl Med 2003; 17:261–279.

84 Nakamoto Y, Higashi T, Sakahara H, et al. Delayed (18)F-fluoro-2-deoxy-D-glucose positron emission tomography scan for differentiation between malignant and benign lesions in the pancreas. Cancer 2000; 89:2547–2554.

85 Yamaguchi K, Chijiiwa K, Noshiro H, et al. Ki-*ras* codon 12 point mutation and *p53* mutation in pancreatic diseases. Hepatogastroenterology 1999; 46:2575–2581.

86 Barthet M, Portal I, Boujaoude J, et al. Endoscopic ultrasonographic diagnosis of pancreatic cancer complicating chronic pancreatitis. Endoscopy 1996; 28:487–491.

87 Sackett DL, Haynes RB, Guyatt GH, et al. Clinical epidemiology: a basic science for clinical medicine, 2nd edn. Boston, MA: Little Brown; 1991.

88 Kaufman AR, Sivak MV Jr. Endoscopic ultrasonography in the differential diagnosis of pancreatic disease. Gastrointest Endosc 1989; 35:214–219.

89 Nattermann C, Goldschmidt AJ, Dancygier H. Endosonography in the assessment of pancreatic tumors. A comparison of the endosonographic findings of carcinomas and segmental inflammatory changes. Dtsch Med Wochenschr 1995; 120:1571–1576.

90 Glasbrenner B, Schwartz M, Pauls S, et al. Prospective comparison of endoscopic ultrasound and endoscopic retrograde cholangiopancreatography in the preoperative assessment of masses in the pancreatic head. Dig Surg 2000; 17:468–474.

91 Yu XJ, Long J, Fu DL, et al. Analysis of gene expression profiles in pancreatic carcinoma by using cDNA microarray. Hepatobiliary Pancreat Dis Int 2003; 2:467–470.

92 Chhieng DC, Benson E, Eltoum I, et al. *MUC1* and *MUC2* expression in pancreatic ductal carcinoma obtained by fine-needle aspiration. Cancer 2003; 99:365–371.

93 Crnogorac-Jurcevic T, Missiaglia E, Blaveri E, et al. Molecular alterations in pancreatic carcinoma: expression profiling shows that dysregulated expression of S100 genes is highly prevalent. J Pathol 2003; 201:63–74.

94 Iacobuzio-Donahue CA, Ashfaq R, Maitra A, et al. Highly expressed genes in pancreatic ductal adenocarcinomas: a comprehensive characterization and comparison of the transcription profiles obtained from three major technologies. Cancer Res 2003; 63:8614–8622.

95 Jonckheere N, Perrais M, Mariette C, et al. A role for human *MUC4* mucin gene, the ErbB2 ligand, as a target of TGF-beta in pancreatic carcinogenesis. Oncogene 2004; 23:5729–5738.

96 Juuti A, Nordling S, Louhimo J, et al. Loss of *p27* expression is associated with poor prognosis in stage I–II pancreatic cancer. Oncology 2003; 65:371–377.

97 Missiaglia E, Blaveri E, Terris B, et al. Analysis of gene expression in cancer cell lines identifies candidate markers for pancreatic tumorigenesis and metastasis. Int J Cancer 2004; 112:100–112.

98 Su SB, Motoo Y, Iovanna JL, et al. Expression of *p8* in human pancreatic cancer. Clin Cancer Res 2001; 7:309–313.

99 Maacke H, Jost K, Opitz S, et al. DNA repair and recombination factor Rad51 is over-expressed in human pancreatic adenocarcinoma. Oncogene 2000; 19:2791–2795.

100 Biankin AV, Morey AL, Lee CS, et al. *DPC4/Smad4* expression and outcome in pancreatic ductal adenocarcinoma. J Clin Oncol 2002; 20:4531–4542.

101 Boltze C, Schneider-Stock R, Aust G, et al. CD97, CD95 and Fas-L clearly discriminate between chronic pancreatitis and pancreatic ductal adenocarcinoma in perioperative evaluation of cryocut sections. Pathol Int 2002; 52:83–88.

102 Casey G, Yamanaka Y, Friess H, et al. *p53* mutations are common in pancreatic cancer and are absent in chronic pancreatitis. Cancer Lett 1993; 69:151–160.

103 Di Sebastiano P, di Mola FF, Di Febbo C, et al. Expression of interleukin 8 (IL-8) and substance P in human chronic pancreatitis. Gut 2000; 47:423–428.

104 Liao Q, Kleeff J, Xiao Y, et al. Preferential expression of cystein-rich secretory protein-3 (CRISP-3) in chronic pancreatitis. Histol Histopathol 2003; 18:425–433.

105 Logsdon CD, Simeone DM, Binkley C, et al. Molecular profiling of pancreatic adenocarcinoma and chronic pancreatitis identifies multiple genes differentially regulated in pancreatic cancer. Cancer Res 2003; 63:2649–2657.

106 Mitas M, Cole DJ, Hoover L, et al. Real-time reverse transcription-PCR detects KS1/4 mRNA in mediastinal lymph nodes from patients with non-small cell lung cancer. Clin Chem 2003; 49:312–315.

107 Catalano MF, Lahoti S, Alcocer E, et al. Dynamic imaging of the pancreas using real-time endoscopic ultrasonography with secretin stimulation. Gastrointest Endosc 1998; 48:580–587.

108 Davies DD. Incidence of major complications of neurolytic coeliac plexus block. J R Soc Med 1993; 86:264–266.

109 Lemelin V, Lam E, Sahai A. A prospective trial of central versus bilateral celiac plexus block neurolysis in 160 patients: bilateral injection is safe and is more effective. Gastroenterol Endosc 2005; 61:AB77.

110 Gress F, Schmitt C, Sherman S, et al. A prospective randomized comparison of endoscopic ultrasound- and computed tomography-guided celiac plexus block for managing chronic pancreatitis pain. Am J Gastroenterol 1999; 94:900–905.

111 Wiersema MJ, Harada N, Wiersema LM. Endosonography-guided celiac plexus neurolysis: efficacy in chronic pancreatitis and malignant disease. Acta Endosc 1998; 28:67–79.

112 Baron TH. Endoscopic drainage of pancreatic fluid collections and pancreatic necrosis. Gastrointest Endosc 2003; 13:743–764.

113 Fockens P. EUS in drainage of pancreatic pseudocysts. Gastrointest Endosc 2002; 56:S93–S97.

114 Fockens P, Johnson TG, van Dullemen HM, et al. Endosonographic imaging of pancreatic pseudocysts before endoscopic transmural drainage. Gastrointest Endosc 1997; 46:412–416.

115 Norton ID, Clain JE, Wiersema MJ, et al. Utility of endoscopic ultrasonography in endoscopic drainage of pancreatic pseudocysts in selected patients. Mayo Clin Proc 2001; 76:794–798.

116 Grimm H, Binmoeller KF, Soehendra N. Endosonography-guided drainage of a pancreatic pseudocyst. Gastrointest Endosc 1992; 38:170–171.

117 Seifert H, Dietrich C, Schmitt T, et al. Endoscopic ultrasound-guided one-step transmural drainage of cystic abdominal lesions with a large-channel echo endoscope. Endoscopy 2000; 32:255–259.

118 Vilmann P, Hancke S, Pless T, et al. One-step endosonography-guided drainage of a pancreatic pseudocyst: a new technique of stent delivery through the echo endoscope. Endoscopy 1998; 30:730–733.

119 Cortes ES, Maalak A, Le Moine O, et al. Endoscopic cystenterostomy of nonbulging pancreatic fluid collections. Gastrointest Endosc 2002; 56:380–386.

120 Wiersema MJ, Baron TH, Chari ST. Endosonography-guided pseudocyst drainage with a new large-channel linear scanning echoendoscope. Gastrointest Endosc 2001; 53:811–813.

121 Giovannini M, Bernardini D, Seitz JF. Cystogastrotomy entirely performed under endosonography guidance for pancreatic pseudocyst: results in six patients. Gastrointest Endosc 1998; 48:200–203.

122 Dohmoto M, Akiyama K, Lioka Y. Endoscopic and endosonographic management of pancreatic pseudocyst: a long-term follow-up. Rev Gastroenterol Peru 2003; 23:269–275.

123 Vosoghi M, Sial S, Garrett B, et al. EUS-guided pancreatic pseudocyst drainage: review and experience at Harbor-UCLA Medical Center. MedGenMed 2002; 4:2.

124 Giovannini M, Pesenti C, Rolland AL, et al. Endoscopic ultrasound-guided drainage of pancreatic pseudocysts or pancreatic abscesses using a therapeutic echo endoscope. Endoscopy 2001; 33:473–477.

125 Inui K, Yoshino J, Okushima K, et al. EUS-guided one-step drainage of pancreatic pseudocysts: experience in 3 patients. Gastrointest Endosc 2001; 54:87–89.

126 Monkemuller KE, Baron TH, Morgan DE. Transmural drainage of pancreatic fluid collections without electrocautery using the Seldinger technique. Gastrointest Endosc 1998; 48:195–200.

127 Fuchs M, Reimann FM, Gaebel C, et al. Treatment of infected pancreatic pseudocysts by endoscopic ultrasonography-guided cystogastrostomy. Endoscopy 2000; 32:654–657.

128 François E, Kahaleh M, Giovannini M, et al. EUS-guided pancreaticogastrostomy. Gastrointest Endosc 2002; 56:128–133.

129 Furukawa T, Tsukamoto Y, Naitoh Y, et al. Differential diagnosis between benign and malignant localized stenosis of the main pancreatic duct by intraductal ultrasound of the pancreas. Am J Gastroenterol 1994; 89:2038–2041.

130 Borak G, Bohler JD, Cotton PB, et al. MRCP frequently misses divisum in routine practice. Gastrointest Endosc 2005; 61:AB187.

Chapter

16

EUS in Pancreatic Neoplasms

John DeWitt

KEY POINTS

- Endoscopic ultrasound (EUS) is the most sensitive imaging modality for the detection of pancreatic masses. It is particularly useful for identification of tumors undetected by other methods, such as computed tomography (CT).

- A normal-appearing pancreas without a mass essentially rules out the possibility of pancreatic cancer. If cancer is expected but EUS demonstrates chronic pancreatitis with or without a focal mass, follow-up EUS, CT, or referral for possible surgery should be considered.

- Recent studies have failed to confirm early studies that suggested EUS was superior to CT for staging pancreatic neoplasms. The differences may be due to improved CT technology, changing criteria for surgical exploration, or different staging classifications used in the various studies.

- Due to anatomic and equipment limitations, CT and magnetic resonance imaging (MRI) are superior to EUS for detection of metastatic cancer. EUS-guided fine-needle aspiration (EUS-FNA) of liver metastases, ascites, or celiac adenopathy may prevent the need for surgical exploration.

- EUS is superior to CT and angiography for detection of tumor invasion of the portal vein or confluence. CT appears to be superior to EUS for invasion of the superior mesenteric vessels and major arteries of the upper abdomen.

- Among proposed criteria for vascular invasion, the identification of an irregular vessel wall, visible tumor within the vessel lumen, or the presence of venous collaterals may maximize the specificity for detection of true involvement by pancreatic cancer.

- EUS-FNA of pancreatic tumors has a sensitivity of 85% and a specificity approaching 100%. Diagnostic yield appears to be maximized by the presence of on-site cytopathology interpretation. The role of EUS-guided Tru-Cut biopsy for pancreatic tumors is currently best reserved for transgastric biopsy following negative or non-diagnostic EUS-FNA.

KEY POINTS

- Most studies comparing EUS, CT, and MRI have demonstrated no significant differences between these modalities for determination of resectability of pancreatic cancer. However, EUS is usually used before surgery in combination with CT or MRI to evaluate vascular invasion or previously undetected metastases. Optimal preoperative evaluation of these patients is dependent on referral patterns and availability of EUS, but should be individualized on a case-by-case basis.

- EUS is the most accurate modality for detection of pancreatic neuroendocrine tumors (PNETs), particularly tumors smaller than 2.0 cm in diameter. Optimal workup of patients with suspected PNETs should incorporate EUS, EUS-FNA, and somatostatin receptor scintigraphy.

- EUS-FNA may rarely identify pancreatic metastases in patients with a simultaneous or remote history of malignancy. These tumors are more likely to have well defined margins compared to primary pancreatic cancer.

- Endoscopy and EUS are the most accurate imaging modalities for ampullary tumor detection. EUS is more accurate than CT or MRI for staging ampullary cancers, but accuracy may be diminished by the presence of a biliary stent.

INTRODUCTION

Endosonographers are frequently asked for further evaluation of known or suspected pancreatic masses detected by other cross-sectional imaging studies. Examination of the pancreas and other upper abdominal retroperitoneal structures by endoscopic ultrasound (EUS) is generally considered the most technically demanding region to visualize and master reproducibly. This difficulty arises for several reasons. First, it is necessary to learn the normal appearance and anatomic relationships of multiple organs, vessels, and other structures in the upper abdomen. Second, precise placement of the echoendoscope in the stomach and duodenum is required for complete examination of the pancreas and its surrounding structures. Third, an excellent working knowledge of retroperitoneal imaging by linear array endosonography is required to utilize other techniques such as EUS-guided fine-needle aspiration (EUS-FNA) or EUS-guided celiac plexus neurolysis or injection. However, once these skills are learned, EUS permits the most detailed non-operative view of the pancreas that is available. This chapter summarizes the role of EUS in the evaluation of solid pancreatic neoplasms.

DETECTION OF PANCREATIC TUMORS

EUS is the most sensitive non-operative imaging method for the detection of benign or malignant pancreatic lesions (Fig. 16.1). When summarizing the results of 22 studies containing 1003 patients over a 17-year period, the sensitivity of EUS for detection of a pancreatic mass was 96% (range 85–100%) (Table 16.1).[1–22] Some of these studies, however, included benign pancreatic disease and ampullary tumors,[1–4,11,12,17–19] and this may bias the analysis of tumor detection in favor of EUS. Therefore, caution must be exercised when extrapolating these data to pancreatic malignancy. In 16 studies that compared EUS and CT over the same time period,[3,4,6,7–13,16–19,21,22] the sensitivity of EUS for mass detection was superior to that of CT (98% versus 77%, respectively; $P < 0.0001$) (Table 16.2). EUS is clearly superior to conventional CT[3,4,6,16] and transabdominal ultrasonography[2–4,6,12] for pancreatic tumor detection. Compared to single-detector helical CT, however, EUS has been reported to be either equivalent[13] or superior[11,17–19] for tumor detection. Current state-of-the-art CT utilizes a 32 or 64-row detector that enables the acquisition of multiple images with very thin collimation.[23] Furthermore, volumetric data may be obtained by this method to construct multiplanar reformations of pancreatic anatomy.

The first two comparative studies between EUS and multidetector-row CT (MDCT) for pancreatic tumors have

SENSITIVITY OF EUS FOR DETECTION OF PANCREATIC TUMORS

Reference	No. of patients	Sensitivity (%)
Yasuda et al.[1] (1988)[a]	50	100
Lin et al.[2] (1989)[b]	33	94
Rosch et al.[3] (1991)[c]	102	99
Rosch et al.[4] (1992)[d]	60	98
Snady et al.[5] (1992)	60	85
Palazzo et al.[6] (1993)	49	91
Muller et al.[7] (1994)	33	94
Marty et al.[8] (1995)	37	92
Melzer et al.[9] (1996)	12	100
Dufour et al.[10] (1997)	24	92
Howard et al.[11] (1997)[e]	21	100
Sugiyama et al.[12] (1997)[f]	73	96
Legmann et al.[13] (1998)	30	100
Akahoshi et al.[14] (1998)	37	89
Harrison et al.[15] (1999)	19	89
Gress et al.[16] (1999)	81	100
Midwinter et al.[17] (1999)[g]	34	97
Mertz et al.[18] (2000)	31	93
Rivadeneira et al.[19] (2003)[h]	44	100
Ainsworth et al.[20] (2003)	22	87
Agarwal et al.[21] (2004)	71	100
DeWitt et al.[22] (2004)	80	98
Total	1003	96

Table 16.1 Sensitivity of EUS for detection of pancreatic tumors
[a] Includes 8 patients with chronic pancreatitis.
[b] Includes 15 patients with benign disease.
[c] Includes 26 patients with benign disease.
[d] Includes 14 patients with ampullary cancer.
[e] Includes 6 patients with ampullary cancer.
[f] Includes 19 patients with bile duct cancer.
[g] Includes 6 patients with ampullary cancer and 4 with benign disease.
[h] Includes 4 patients with ampullary cancer.

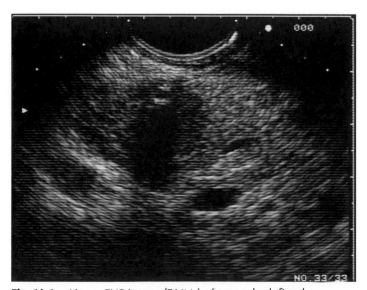

Fig. 16.1   Linear EUS image (5 MHz) of a poorly defined, hypoechoic, 22 × 21-mm ductal adenocarcinoma in the head of the pancreas adjacent to, but not involving, the superior mesenteric artery and vein. A plastic biliary stent is present. Multidetector CT with dual-phase imaging did not visualize any tumor.

recently been published. Each study compared EUS with four-row CT scanners. Agarwal et al.[21] retrospectively reviewed 81 consecutive patients who underwent EUS, EUS-FNA, and multidetector spiral CT for clinical suspicion of a pancreatic cancer. The sensitivity of EUS for the diagnosis of cancer was 100%. For MDCT, however, even when 'probable' masses were considered as positive, the sensitivity was 86%. Similarly, for a prospective cohort of 80 patients with pancreatic cancer, DeWitt et al.[22] reported that the sensitivity of EUS (98%) was statistically superior to that of MDCT (86%) for identification of pancreatic tumors. It appears, therefore, that EUS is still superior to MDCT for tumor detection. There are relatively few comparative data between EUS and MRI for tumor detection. EUS has been reported to be either superior[7] or inferior[20] to MRI for the

SENSITIVITY OF EUS COMPARED WITH OTHER IMAGING MODALITIES FOR DETECTION OF PANCREATIC MASSES							
		SENSITIVITY (%)					
Reference	No. of patients	EUS	CT	MRI	US	PET	ERCP
Lin et al.[2] (1989)	33	94			91		
Rosch et al.[3] (1991)	102	99	77		67		90
Rosch et al.[4] (1992)	60	98	85		78		
Palazzo et al.[6] (1993)	49	91	66		64		
Muller et al.[7] (1994)	33	94	69	83			
Marty et al.[8] (1995)	37	92	63				
Melzer et al.[9] (1996)	12	100	83				
Dufour et al.[10] (1997)	24	92	88				
Howard et al.[11] (1997)	21	100	67				
Sugiyama et al.[12] (1997)	73	96	86		81		
Legmann et al.[13] (1998)	30	100	92				
Gress et al.[16] (1999)	81	100	74				
Midwinter et al.[17] (1999)	34	97	76				
Mertz et al.[18] (2000)	31	93	53			87	
Rivadeneira et al.[19] (2003)	44	100	68				
Ainsworth et al.[20] (2003)	22	87		96			
Agarwal et al.[21] (2004)	71	100	86				
Dewitt et al.[22] (2004)	80	98	86				
Total no. of subjects	837	837	782	55	317	31	102
Overall sensitivity	–	98	77	88	76	87	90

Table 16.2 Sensitivity of EUS compared with other imaging modalities for detection of pancreatic masses

diagnosis of pancreatic tumors. Future studies comparing EUS to MRI (3.0 Tesla or higher) are needed to define the roles of each modality in the diagnosis of pancreatic masses.

EUS is particularly useful for identification of tumors smaller than 30 mm in size that have been undetected by other imaging modalities.[1,3,7,13,17,21,22] For tumors of 15–35 mm, Legmann et al.[13] reported that EUS and helical CT both detected 14 of 14 tumors (100%). For tumors smaller than 15 mm, however, EUS detected 6 of 6 (100%), whereas CT detected 4 of 6 (67%). Muller et al.[7] found that the sensitivity of EUS, CT, and MRI for identification of tumors smaller than 3 cm was 93%, 53%, and 67%, respectively. Similarly, for tumors less than 2 cm, the sensitivity of each was 90%, 40%, and 33%. With thinner slice imaging and precisely timed contrast administration, coupled with multiplanar reconstruction,[24] CT may now be able to identify small pancreatic masses that previously may have been undetected by conventional or even single-detector dual-phase imaging. Indeed, DeWitt et al.[22] recently reported a non-significant trend toward improved detection by EUS compared with MDCT for 19 tumors smaller than 25 mm (89% versus 53%, respectively; P=0.08). More comparative studies using state-of-the-art imaging are needed to evaluate the role of preoperative imaging of small pancreatic tumors. Nevertheless, EUS should be performed in all patients with obstructive jaundice in whom CT or MRI does not definitively identify a pancreatic lesion, both to detect any tumor and to exclude non-neoplastic diseases.

Although EUS is the most accurate imaging study for pancreatic mass detection, clearly some lesions are undetected. Bhutani et al.[25] retrospectively examined 20 cases of pancreatic neoplasms missed by nine experienced endosonographers to identify possible associated factors that may have contributed to failed detection. The most common etiology (60%) for a false-negative EUS was associated features of chronic pancreatitis. Other less common associated factors were a diffusely infiltrating carcinoma, a prominent ventral/dorsal anlage split, and a recent episode (<4 weeks) of acute pancreatitis. Five patients with a negative initial EUS underwent a follow-up EUS after 2–3 months, with a pancreatic mass being found in all cases. In another study, Catanzaro et al.[26] retrospectively identified 80 patients with clinical suspicion of pancreatic cancer and a normal EUS. After a mean follow-up of 24 months, one patient with EUS evidence of chronic pancreatitis was found to have pancreatic cancer at surgery. No patient with a normal pancreatic EUS developed cancer during the follow-up period. From these two studies by experienced endosonographers in patients with suspected cancer, two important conclusions may be drawn.

First, follow-up EUS or other imaging study is indicated when EUS evidence of chronic pancreatitis is present without other evidence of a mass or malignancy. Second, a normal-appearing pancreas by EUS essentially rules out the presence of pancreatic cancer. Caution should also be exercised during EUS examination of a patient with obstructive jaundice and an indwelling biliary or pancreatic stent, as acoustic shadowing caused by the stent may impede visualization of a small pancreatic mass.

Owing to the ability of EUS to provide high-resolution images, there has been interest in using this technique to screen asymptomatic high-risk cohorts for early cancer detection. Brentnall et al.[27] first reported the use of endoscopic retrograde cholangiopancreatography (ERCP), EUS, spiral CT, serum carcinoembryonic antigen, and CA19-9 analysis in 14 patients from three kindreds with a history of familial pancreatic cancer. Seven of the 14 patients were believed to have dysplasia on the basis of clinical history and abnormalities on EUS and ERCP. EUS findings noted in these seven included changes suggestive of chronic pancreatitis. At surgery, all seven patients had histologic evidence of dysplasia. Using a decision-analysis model, the same group[28] concluded that endoscopic screening of pancreatic cancer in high-risk individuals was cost-effective, with an incremental cost-effectiveness ratio of $16 885 per life-year saved. Screening remained cost-effective if the prevalence of dysplasia was greater than 16% or if the sensitivity of EUS was greater than 84%. Canto et al.[29] recently evaluated an EUS-based screening approach in a prospective cohort of 38 asymptomatic individuals with Peutz–Jeghers syndrome ($n=1$) or from kindreds with three or more ($n=31$) or two affected relatives ($n=6$) with pancreatic cancer. Six pancreatic masses were found by EUS: one invasive ductal adenocarcinoma, one benign intraductal papillary mucinous neoplasm, two serous cystadenomas, and two non-neoplastic masses. The diagnostic yield for detecting clinically significant pancreatic neoplasms was 5.3% (2 of 38). False-positive changes consistent with chronic pancreatitis were found in some individuals with or without alcohol consumption. These studies illustrate that EUS-based screening of asymptomatic high-risk individuals for pancreatic cancer is feasible and may be cost-effective. At this time, however, there are insufficient data to recommend endoscopic screening for these patients. Multicenter studies using this same screening approach are currently under way to evaluate further use of this testing.

STAGING OF PANCREATIC TUMORS

Preoperative staging of pancreatic neoplasms is believed to be one of the most difficult tasks an endosonographer performs. Staging of pancreatic malignancy is done using the American Joint Committee for Cancer (AJCC) tumor node metastasis (TNM) classification, which describes the tumor extension (T), lymph node (N), and distant metastases (M) of tumors. Reported accuracies of T staging by EUS range from 62% to 94% (Table 16.3).[6,7,13,14,16,22,30,31,33,36–40] Initial studies published prior to 1997[6,7,30,31,33,36] indicated EUS T-staging accuracies of 82–94% for pancreatic tumors. Although some reports after 1997 demonstrated similar results,[13,16] most others[14,22,37–40] could not replicate the encouraging results from earlier studies. Therefore, previous enthusiasm over the excellent staging accuracy of EUS staging may need to be tempered.

Several reasons may explain the apparent tumor staging discrepancies between initial publications and more recent reports. First, earlier studies[6,31,32] enrolled relatively small numbers of patients, most of whom went to surgery, presumably to correlate EUS data with intraoperative findings. Recent studies,[14,16,22,37,39] however, have usually restricted surgical exploration to patients with suspected operable disease. Consequently, surgical exploration in these later reports[14,16,22,37,39] is limited to 36–67% of enrolled patients. The non-operative management of patients with suspected irresectable malignancy limits statistical analysis to those most likely not to have vascular invasion (except the splenic vessels, which are readily removed surgically). Overall accuracy of T staging by EUS may therefore be underestimated. The second possible reason for the apparent discrepancies is the improved preoperative cross-sectional imaging available in recent years. Earlier studies used conventional CT with wider slice thickness, which may have missed distant metastases or incorrectly assessed vascular invasion. Currently available state-of-the-art CT, which utilizes a dual-phase, contrast-enhanced, multidetector-row CT protocol with available multiplanar reconstruction, has improved staging and detection of pancreatic tumors and distant metastases.[21–23,40–42] Therefore, tumors that previously may have had surgical correlation in older studies are now managed without surgery. Third, the earliest 1987 TNM classification[43] utilized for most studies incorporated a T1–T3 tumor staging system. A modification in the 1993 system added stages T1a and T1b for tumors smaller than or greater than 2 cm in dimension confined to the pancreas, respectively. The 1997 AJCC staging system,[44] which has been utilized by most recent studies, added stage T4 for suspected inoperable malignancy. Four recent series[22,38–40] with surgical exploration in 226 patients with pancreatic cancer that utilized the 1997 TNM classification found EUS T-staging accuracies of between 63% and 69%. Ahmad et al.[38] reported staging accuracies of 61% and 78% for T4 and T3 malignancy, respectively. Furthermore, these authors found that EUS T staging was unable reliably to predict tumor resectability. DeWitt et al.[22] reported accuracies of 88% and 74% for T4 and T3 disease, respectively, but only 11% for nine patients with T1–T2 malignancy. One of the criticisms of the 1997 staging system was the poor correlation between the tumor stage and its resectability at surgery and after histopathologic evaluation. For example, splenic vessels may be easily removed intraoperatively. In addition, some tertiary referral centers routinely attempt reconstruction of the portal vein or superior mesenteric vein in patients without thrombosis or occlusion to achieve completely negative surgical margins.[45] To distinguish better potentially resectable (T3) from irresectable (T4) tumors, the current AJCC 2003 staging criteria[46] classify

ACCURACY OF EUS FOR TUMOR (T) AND NODAL (N) STAGING OF PANCREATIC CANCER				
			ACCURACY (%)	
Reference	No. of enrolled patients	No. of patients to surgery with pancreatic cancer	T stage	N stage
Tio et al.[30] (1990)	43	36	92	74
Grimm et al.[31] (1990)	NA	26	85	72
Mukai et al.[32] (1991)	26	26	NR	65
Rosch et al.[4] (1992)	60	40	NR	72
Rosch et al.[33] (1992)	46	35	94	80
Palazzo et al.[6] (1993)	64	49	82	64
Yasuda et al.[34] (1993)	NA	29	NR	66
Muller et al.[7] (1994)	49	16	82	50
Giovannini & Seitz[35] (1994)	90	26	NR	80
Tio et al.[36] (1996)	70	52	84	69
Akahoshi et al.[14] (1998)	96	37	64	50
Legmann et al.[13] (1998)	30	22	90	86
Buscail et al.[37] (1999)	73	26	73	69
Midwinter et al.[17] (1999)	48	23	NR	74
Gress et al.[16] (1999)	151	75	85	72
Ahmad et al.[38] (2000)	NA	89	69	54
Rivadeneira et al.[19] (2003)	NA	44	NR	84
Soriano et al.[39] (2004)	127	62	62	65
Ramsay et al.[40] (2004)	27	22	63	69
DeWitt et al.[22] (2004)	104	53	67	41

Table 16.3 Accuracy of EUS for tumor (T) and nodal (N) staging of pancreatic cancer
NA, not applicable; NR, not reported.

only vascular invasion of the celiac or superior mesenteric arteries as T4 cancer (Table 16.4). These needed changes should improve overall staging accuracies of pancreatic cancer in future studies. To date, however, no studies have been published that incorporate this new classification.

Despite the variations in T-staging criteria described for pancreatic cancer, nodal (N) metastases have uniformly been classified as absent (N0) or present (N1) across all AJCC editions, including the latest edition.[46] The accuracy of EUS for N staging of pancreatic tumors ranges from 41% to 86% (Table 16.5).[4,6,7,13,14,16,17,19,22,30–40] Various criteria have been proposed for endosonographic detection of metastatic lymph nodes, including: size greater than 1cm, hypoechoic echogenicity, distinct margins, and round shape. When all four features are present within a lymph node, there is an 80–100% chance of malignant invasion.[47,48] The sensitivity of EUS alone for the diagnosis of metastatic adenopathy in pancreatic cancer is 28–92%;[6,7,14,17,19,36,39,40] however, most report sensitivities of less than 65%. This low sensitivity presumably occurs for two reasons. First, most metastatic lymph nodes do not have all four endosonographic features described above,[47] and may therefore be incorrectly assumed to be benign. Second, peritumoral inflammation and large tumor size may contribute to poor

detection of adenopathy.[49] The specificity of EUS alone for the diagnosis of metastatic adenopathy in pancreatic cancer is 26–100;[6,7,14,17,19,36,39,40] however, most report specificities above 70%. As false-positive assessments of metastatic adenopathy do occur, it may be presumed that the addition of EUS-FNA for suspicious lymph nodes may increase the specificity of detection. Unfortunately, there are few data that describe the impact of EUS-FNA in addition to EUS alone for the diagnosis of metastatic lymphadenopathy in pancreatic cancer. Cahn et al.[50] reported that EUS-FNA diagnosed lymph node metastasis in seven of the 13 patients (54%) with pancreatic cancer in whom sampling was performed. For tumors involving the head of the pancreas, malignant lymph nodes are removed en bloc with the surgical specimen. Therefore, accurate detection of these lymph nodes is not essential[22] and routine EUS-FNA of peritumoral lymph nodes with pancreatic head cancers may not be necessary. As preoperative identification and EUS-FNA of celiac nodes may preclude surgery, meticulous survey of this region is critical during staging of all pancreatic tumors. In one series, mediastinal lymph node metastases were reported to occur in 7% of patients undergoing EUS evaluation of pancreatic masses.[51] Therefore, a brief survey of this region may be helpful during staging of pancreatic lesions.

AMERICAN JOINT COMMITTEE ON CANCER 2003 TNM STAGING CLASSIFICATION FOR PANCREATIC CANCER[46]	
Stage	Description
Primary tumor (T)	
TX	Primary tumor cannot be assessed
T0	No evidence of primary tumor
Tis	Carcinoma in situ
T1	Tumor limited to the pancreas, 2 cm or less in greatest dimension
T2	Tumor limited to the pancreas, more than 2 cm in greatest dimension
T3	Tumor extends beyond the pancreas but without involvement of the celiac axis or the superior mesenteric artery
T4	Tumor involves the celiac axis or the superior mesenteric artery (unresectable primary tumor)
Regional lymph nodes (N)	
NX	Regional lymph nodes cannot be assessed
N0	No regional lymph node metastasis
N1	Regional lymph node metastasis
Distant metastasis (M)	
MX	Distant metastasis cannot be assessed
M0	No distant metastasis
M1	Distant metastasis
AJCC stage groupings	
Stage 0	Tis, N0, M0
Stage IA	T1, N0, M0
Stage IB	T2, N0, M0
Stage IIA	T3, N0, M0
Stage IIB	T1, N1, M0 or T2, N1, M0 or T3, N1, M0
Stage III	T4, any N, M0
Stage IV	Any T, any N, M1

Table 16.4 American Joint Committee on Cancer 2003 TNM staging classification for pancreatic cancer[46]
Bach CM, et al. Melanoma of the skin. In: Greene FL, Page DL, Fleming ID, et al., editors. AJCC Cancer Staging Manual, Sixth Edition. New York: Springer-Verlag, 2002:209-220. Used with permission of the American Joint Committee on Cancer (AJCC), Chicago, Illinois. The original source for this material is the AJCC Cancer Staging Manual. Sixth Edition (2002) published by Springer-Verlag New York, www.springeronline.com.

Early studies found that EUS was superior to conventional CT for tumor[6,7] and nodal[4,6,7,32] staging of pancreatic cancer (Table 16.6). Although one recent study has reported that EUS is superior to CT for T staging,[22] most have confirmed that the two are equivalent for both tumor[17,39,40] and nodal[13,17,19,22,39,40] staging of these tumors. Soriano et al.,[39] however, found that helical CT was superior to EUS in the assessment of locoregional extension among 62 patients with pancreatic cancer. Similar to CT, early studies showed that EUS was superior to MRI for staging of pancreatic tumors.[6,7] However, two recent studies[39,40] found no difference between EUS and MRI for both T and N staging. Clearly, the initial advantage demonstrated by EUS over other imaging modalities for the staging of pancreatic tumors has narrowed considerably. Future studies that compare EUS to MDCT and higher-tesla MRI are needed to confirm these findings and further define the role of EUS for the locoregional staging of pancreatic tumors.

For detection of non-nodal metastatic cancer, CT and MRI are superior to EUS, due to both anatomic limitations of normal upper gastrointestinal anatomy and the limited range of EUS imaging even at lower frequencies such as 5 or 6 MHz. Although the entire left lobe of the liver may be seen by transgastric imaging in most patients, most of the right lobe may not be visualized by either transgastric or transduodenal imaging. Therefore, EUS clearly cannot replace, but may supplement, other modalities for staging of hepatic metastases. The principal advantages of EUS for the evaluation of liver metastases are the detection of small lesions missed by other imaging modalities[52-55] and the ability to sample visualized accessible masses by EUS-FNA.[52-56] The sensitivity of EUS-FNA for benign and malignant liver masses reportedly ranges from 82% to 94%,[53,56] and the diagnosis of liver metastases from pancreatic cancer precludes surgical resection.[53] Similar to EUS-FNA of pancreatic masses, however, a negative or non-diagnostic biopsy does not rule out the presence of metastatic disease.[53,56] Therefore,

TEST CHARACTERISTICS OF EUS FOR DETECTION OF MALIGNANT LYMPHADENOPATHY IN PANCREATIC CANCER

Reference	No. of patients	Sensitivity (%)	Specificity (%)	PPV (%)	NPV (%)	Accuracy (%)
Tio et al.[30] (1990)	43					74
Grimm et al.[31] (1990)	NA					72
Mukai et al.[32] (1991)	26					65
Rosch et al.[4] (1992)	40			82	61	72
Rosch et al.[33] (1992)	35					80
Palazzo et al.[6] (1993)	49	62				74
Yasuda et al.[34] (1993)	29					66
Muller et al.[7] (1994)	16	33	71	60	45	50
Giovannini & Seitz[35] (1994)	26					80
Tio et al.[36] (1996)	52	92	26			69
Akahoshi et al.[14] (1998)	32	28	79	56	46	50
Legmann et al.[13] (1998)	30					86
Buscail et al.[37] (1999)	26					69
Midwinter et al.[17] (1999)	23	44	93	80	72	74
Gress et al.[16] (1999)	75					72
Ahmad et al.[38] (2000)	89					54
Rivadeneira et al.[19] (2003)	44	61	100			84
Soriano et al.[39] (2004)	62	36	87	67	65	65
Ramsay et al.[40] (2004)	22	43	89			69
DeWitt et al.[22] (2004)	53					41

Table 16.5 Test characteristics of EUS for detection of malignant lymphadenopathy in pancreatic cancer
PPV, positive predictive value; NPV, negative predictive values; NA, not applicable.

COMPARISON OF THE ACCURACY OF EUS WITH CT, MRI AND US FOR TUMOR AND NODAL STAGING OF PANCREATIC CANCER

Reference	No. of patients	Accuracy of EUS (%)		Accuracy of CT (%)		Accuracy of MRI (%)		Accuracy of US (%)	
		T	N	T	N	T	N	T	N
Mukai et al.[32] (1991)	26		65		38				58
Rosch et al.[4] (1992)	40		72		38				53
Palazzo et al.[6] (1993)	64	82	64	45	50	50	56		37
Muller et al.[7] (1994)	16	82	50	56	38	57	50		
Legmann et al.[13] (1998)	22	90	86	86	77				
Midwinter et al.[17] (1999)	23		74		65				
Rivadeneira et al.[19] (2003)	44		84		68				
Soriano et al.[39] (2004)	62	63	67	73	56	62	60		
Ramsay et al.[40] (2004)	27	63	69	76	63	83	56		
DeWitt et al.[22] (2004)	53	67	44	41	47				

Table 16.6 Comparison of the accuracy of EUS with CT, MRI and US for tumor and nodal staging of pancreatic cancer

repeat EUS or percutaneous FNA or surgery is recommended if clinically necessary to confirm metastatic disease. EUS may also identify and aspirate ascites either previously detected or undetected by other imaging studies.[57,58] Small amounts of peritoneal fluid usually appear as a triangle-shaped anechoic region outside an otherwise normal gastrointestinal wall. EUS-guided paracentesis may confirm the diagnosis of suspected malignant ascites and prevent the need for surgical exploration. These data demonstrate that meticulous examination for liver masses, ascites as well as celiac adenopathy should always be performed during EUS evaluation of suspected pancreatic tumors. When detected, EUS-FNA should be performed to rule out the presence of metastatic malignancy.

VASCULAR INVASION BY PANCREATIC TUMORS

Accurate preoperative assessment of any vascular invasion by a pancreatic tumor is a critical component to determine both the T stage and potential resectability. The placement of an echoendoscope into the duodenum and stomach provides a unique opportunity to evaluate peritumoral arterial and venous structures (Figs 16.2–16.5). Interpretation of data regarding the accuracy of EUS for vascular invasion, however, is difficult for several reasons. First, there is little histologic correlation with intraoperative findings regarding vascular invasion in most studies. True vascular invasion may be overestimated or underestimated by intraoperative findings,[59,60] and therefore give false information regarding the accuracy of EUS staging. Second, there is no established consensus among endosonographers on the optimal criteria to be utilized for EUS assessment of vascular invasion by pancreatic or other tumors. Consequently, multiple criteria have been proposed by various authors for this indication. Nevertheless, evaluation of these studies may yield some important conclusions regarding assessment of malignant invasion by pancreatic tumors.

For overall vascular invasion, the accuracy of EUS ranges from 40% to 100% (Table 16.7).[9,10,16,18,19,32,37,39,40] Sensitivity

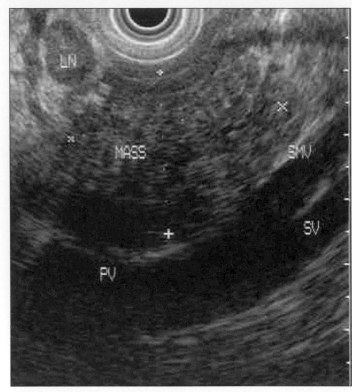

Fig. 16.3 Radial image (7.5 MHz) of a large pancreatic head mass with invasion into the superior mesenteric vein (SMV) at the portal vein confluence. A malignant appearing lymph node is seen adjacent to the mass. Invasion into the SMV was confirmed at surgery.

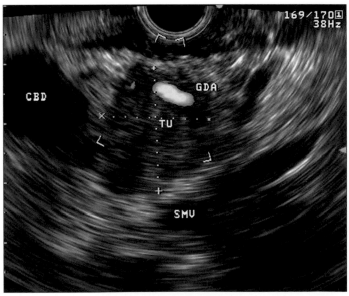

Fig. 16.2 Linear EUS image (6 MHz) of a 2.5-cm mass in the head of the pancreas encasing the gastroduodenal artery (GDA). Doppler imaging demonstrates preserved blood flow within the vessel. The mass does not invade the duodenal wall or the superior mesenteric vein (SMV) on this image. The common bile duct (CBD) is obstructed and dilated above the mass.

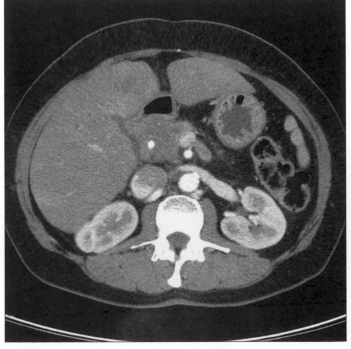

Fig. 16.4 Axial CT image of the same patient as in Fig. 16.3, demonstrating invasion into the portal confluence by the pancreatic head mass.

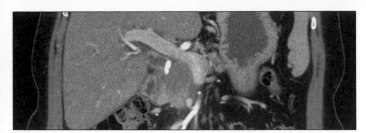

Fig. 16.5 Multiplanar reconstruction of the axial CT image in the same patient as in Fig. 16.3 along the portal vein and superior mesenteric vein (SMV). Invasion of the confluence portal vein can be seen.

and specificity of EUS for malignant vascular invasion range from 42–91% and 89–100% respectively.[16,37,39,40,61] Although some studies demonstrate that EUS is more accurate[9,16,18,19,32] than CT for vascular invasion, other authors have reported that the accuracy of CT is superior[10,39,40] to that of EUS. Overall accuracy of MRI is reportedly equivalent[39] or superior[40] to

EUS. For overall venous invasion, EUS is reportedly superior[6] or equivalent[8] to CT. Overall sensitivity and accuracy of EUS for arterial invasion are 56%[8] and 50%[6] respectively. Angiography is consistently inferior to EUS and CT for assessment of vascular infiltration by tumor, and therefore has no current role in the staging of pancreatic tumors.[4,32,39]

The sensitivity of EUS for tumor invasion of the portal vein (PV) or PV confluence is 60–100% (Table 16.8),[1,4,12,17,33,62] with most studies demonstrating sensitivities of more than 80%. The sensitivity of EUS for PV invasion is also consistently superior to that of CT[4,12,17,33] and angiography.[4,12,33,62] For the superior mesenteric vein (SMV), superior mesenteric artery (SMA), and celiac artery, the sensitivity of EUS is only 17–83%,[37] 17%,[18] and about 50%,[4,33] respectively. The sensitivity of CT for staging of the SMA[17,18] and celiac artery[4,33] appear to be better than with EUS. EUS staging of the superior mesenteric vessels may be difficult, due to either the inability to visualize the entire course of the vessel or the obscuring of these vessels by a large tumor in the uncinate or inferior portion of the pan-

COMPARISON OF THE OVERALL ACCURACY OF EUS WITH CT, US, ANGIOGRAPHY AND MRI FOR VASCULAR INVASION BY PANCREATIC CANCER							
References	No. of patients	Modality	Sensitivity (%)	Specificity (%)	PPV (%)	NPV (%)	Accuracy (%)
Mukai et al.[32] (1991)[a]	26	EUS					77
		CT					38
		US					50
		Angiography					56
Melzer et al.[9] (1996)	13	EUS					92
		CT					61
Dufor et al.[10] (1997)	24	EUS					40
		CT					90
Buscail et al.[37] (1999) [b]	32	EUS	67	100	100	83	88
Gress et al.[16] (1999)	75	EUS	91	96	94	93	93
		CT	15	100	100	60	62
Mertz et al.[18] (2000)	6	EUS					100
		CT					50
Tierney et al.[61] (2001)	45	EUS	87				
		CT	33				
Rivadeneira et al.[19] (2003)	9	EUS					100
		CT					45
Ramsay et al.[40] (2004)	19	EUS	56	89			68
		CT	80	78			89
		MRI	56	100			78
Soriano et al.[39] (2004)	62	EUS	42	97	89	74	76
		CT	67	94	89	80	83
		MRI	59	84	72	74	74
		Angiography	21	100	100	64	67

Table 16.7 Comparison of the overall accuracy of EUS with CT, US, angiography and MRI for vascular invasion by pancreatic cancer
[a] Retroperitoneal vasculature.
[b] Includes some patients with ampullary cancer.

TEST CHARACTERISTICS OF EUS FOR VASCULAR INVASION OF INDIVIDUAL BLOOD VESSELS BY PANCREATIC CANCER

Reference	No. of patients	Vessel	Modality	Sensitivity (%)	Specificity (%)	PPV (%)	NPV (%)	Accuracy (%)
Yasuda et al.[1] (1988)		PV	EUS	91				
		SV	EUS	64				
Rosch et al.[33] (1992)	35	PV	EUS	93				
			CT	36				
			Angiography	36				
			US	14				
		SV	EUS	92				
			CT	69				
			US	39				
		Celiac	EUS	57				
			CT	71				
			Angiography	86				
			US	29				
Rosch et al.[4] (1992)[a]	40	PV/SMV	EUS	91	97	91	97	
			CT	36	85	50	78	
			US	9	72	11	68	
			Angiography	45	100	100	83	
Brugge et al.[62] (1996)[b]	28	PV	EUS	60–78	31–100			
			Angiography	20–33	52–100			
		SMV	EUS	17–83	33–100			
			Angiography	20–83	75–94			
		SV	EUS	67–100	33–100			
			Angiography	60	80–100			
Sugiyama et al.[12] (1997)[c]	73	PV	EUS	95				93
			US	55				57
			CT	65				74
			Angiography	75				79
Midwinter et al.[17] (1999)	34	PV/SMV	EUS	81	86	87	80	83
			CT	56	100	100	67	77
		SMA	EUS	17	67	17	67	55
			CT	50	100	100	83	86

Table 16.8 Test characteristics of EUS for vascular invasion of individual blood vessels by pancreatic cancer
PV, portal vein; SMA, superior mesenteric artery; SMV, superior mesenteric vein; SV, splenic vein.
[a] Includes 12 patients with ampullary cancer.
[b] Test characteristics vary for criteria used for vascular invasion.
[c] Includes 54 patients with pancreatic and 19 with biliary cancer.

creatic head.[63] This is in contrast to the splenic artery and vein, which are generally easily seen and staged well by EUS.[1,33,62,63] For assessment of the celiac artery, previous studies[4,33] have utilized a radial array echoendoscope, which may provide a suboptimal assessment of this vessel compared with a linear array instrument. Clearly, more data are needed regarding the role of EUS for staging the superior mesenteric vessels, celiac artery, and hepatic artery. Until then, assessment of tumor resectability for these vessels by EUS is best done in combination with CT or MRI, rather than by EUS alone.

The reportedly good accuracy of EUS for assessment of vascular invasion of pancreatic tumors has been questioned recently by Rosch et al.[63] In a blinded fashion, one author reviewed previously recorded videotapes of 75 patients with pancreatic head cancer made over a 5-year period. The authors sought to determine the value of EUS criteria and any potential bias introduced by the availability of previous clinical information. Interestingly, this study found that the overall sensitivity and specificity of EUS for the diagnosis of venous invasion were 43% and 91%, respectively. These values were lower than those reported previously by the same authors,[4] and raise concerns about whether previously reported data may have been biased. Although complete withholding of information from an endosonographer for study purposes alone is impractical, future work is needed to elucidate the accuracy of EUS for vascular invasion.

Several authors have attempted to describe the accuracy of various endosonographic findings to assess vascular invasion by malignant pancreatic tumors (Table 16.9). Using the criteria 'rough-edged vessel with compression', Yasuda et al.[1] found a sensitivity, specificity, and accuracy of 79%, 87%, and 81%, respectively, for malignant invasion of the portal venous system. Rosch et al.[4] found a sensitivity, specificity, and accuracy of 91%, 96%, and 94%, respectively, for invasion of the portal vein using the criteria 'abnormal contour, loss of hyperechoic interface, and close contact'. In a further blinded videotape review,[63] these same authors found that no single criterion was able to predict venous invasion with a sensitivity and specificity exceeding 80%. However, they found that both complete vascular obstruction and the presence of collaterals demonstrated a specificity of 94% for vascular invasion. Depending on the EUS criteria chosen, Brugge et al.[62] found a sensitivity and

specificity of 40–80% and 23–100%, respectively, for malignant invasion of the portal vein. From these data, it is clear that there is a trade-off between sensitivity and specificity for vascular invasion. However, criteria with the highest specificity are needed in order to optimize the selection of patients most likely to benefit from surgical exploration. Therefore, the findings of an irregular vascular wall, venous collaterals, and visible tumor within the vessel should be the preferred EUS criteria utilized for assessment of vascular invasion. More data with EUS alone and comparative studies with state-of-the-art imaging are needed to assess the role of EUS in assessment of vascular invasion by pancreatic tumors.

RESECTABILITY OF PANCREATIC TUMORS

Complete surgical removal of pancreatic cancer and locoregional disease with negative histopathologic margins (R0 resection) is the only potential curative treatment. Furthermore, complete tumor removal is an independent predictor of postoperative survival.[65,66] Therefore, the principal role of preoperative evaluation is accurately to identify patients with resectable disease who may benefit from surgery while avoiding surgery in patients with suspected irresectable disease. Unlike tumor staging classifications, which change periodically, the definition of complete resectability has generally remained constant over time. However, some disagreement among experts exists about the resectability

EVALUATION OF INDIVIDUAL EUS CRITERIA FOR VASCULAR INVASION BY PANCREATIC CANCER							
Reference	No. of patients	EUS criteria for vascular invasion	Sensitivity (%)	Specificity (%)	PPV (%)	NPV (%)	Accuracy (%)
Yasuda et al.[1] (1988)	37	Rough-edged vessel with compression	79	87			81
Rosch et al.[4] (1992)	40	Close contact, abnormal contour, loss of hyperechoic interface	91	96			94
Snady et al.[64] (1994)	33	Venous collaterals	19	100			55
		Tumor in lumen	38	100			66
		Loss of hyperechoic interface	33	100			63
Brugge et al.[62] (1996)	28	Irregular vein wall	40	100			85
		Loss of hyperechoic interface	50	85			77
		Proximity of mass	87	55			73
		Size of mass	80	23			33
Rosch et al.[63] (2000)	12	Irregular interface between tumor and vessel	12	79	42	41	41
	11	Tumor in vessel lumen	10	79	36	41	40
	10	Complete vascular obstruction	19	94	80	48	52
	17	Visualization of collaterals	36	94	88	53	61
	24	Tumor/vessel contact but preservation of echo-rich vessel wall	52	83	71	67	69
	18	Separation between tumor and vessel	49	95	89	70	75

Table 16.9 Evaluation of individual criteria for vascular invasion by pancreatic cancer

of neoplasms that involve the portal vein and its confluence with the SMV. Despite this, the general consensus concerning the definition of an R0 resection makes assessment of EUS accuracy and comparisons with other imaging modalities more uniform and easier to interpret than tumor staging. Furthermore, although staging of tumor extension and nodal metastasis of pancreatic tumors is important, in reality determination of resectability is the more clinically relevant preoperative assessment. Currently, however, there is no consensus on the optimal diagnostic preoperative testing necessary for a patient with suspected pancreatic cancer.

In a pooled analysis of nine studies involving 377 patients (Table 16.10), the sensitivity and specificity of EUS for resectability of pancreatic cancer was 69% and 82%, respectively.[11,13,16,22,37,39,40,67,68] Ranges of reported sensitivities and specificities were 23–95% and 63–100%, respectively. Overall EUS accuracy for tumor resectability was 77%. Eight of the nine studies also compared the accuracy of EUS to one or more imaging modalities (Table 16.11). Howard et al.[11] concluded that, compared with EUS and angiography, for 21 patients with pancreatic (n=15) and ampullary (n=6) cancer, CT was the 'best single test of those evaluated to determine resectability of periampullary carcinoma', despite a low sensitivity for tumor detection. This study, however, did not use statistical comparison to evaluate each modality; therefore it is difficult to evaluate the assertion reached by these authors. Soriano et al.[39] found that in 62 patients with pancreatic cancer CT had a higher sensitivity, negative predictive value (NPV), and accuracy for tumor resectability compared with EUS, CT, and angiography. In a large retrospective study, Gress et al.[16] reported that the sensitivities of EUS (95%) and CT (97%) for resectability of pancreatic cancer were similar. However, these authors found

that the overall accuracy of EUS (93%) was superior to that of CT (60%) (P<0.001), principally due to the poor specificity of CT (19%) compared with EUS (92%). Compared with helical CT[13,68] and multidetector CT,[22] other studies reported that the accuracies of EUS and helical CT were equivalent for resectability. Ramsay et al.[40] found that the sensitivity, NPV, and accuracy of MRI for resectability appeared superior to both EUS and CT, but these results were not statistically significant. Two other studies have also shown that EUS and MRI appear to be equivalent for determination of resectability of pancreatic tumors.[39,67]

As most studies have reported that EUS is similar to both CT and MRI for assessment of resectability, some authors have proposed that optimal preoperative imaging of pancreatic cancer requires the use of multiple modalities. Using a decision analysis, Soriano et al.[39] found that accuracy for tumor resectability was maximized and costs were minimized when CT or EUS was performed initially, followed by the other test in those with potentially resectable neoplasms. Ahmad et al.[67] proposed that, although individually EUS and MRI are not sensitive for tumor resectability, the use of both modalities may increase positive predictive value of resectability compared with either test alone. Tierney et al.[68] suggested that CT should be performed initially, but that EUS should also be utilized in most patients because of its improved detection of vascular invasion. When surgery was performed only when the findings on MDCT and EUS agreed with respect to tumor resectability, DeWitt et al.[22] reported that there was a non-significant trend toward improved accuracy of resectability compared with either modality alone. Other studies have suggested that EUS should be incorporated into preoperative imaging to prevent unnecessary surgery[37] and to aid detection and staging of tumors missed by CT.[13,22]

TEST CHARACTERISTICS OF EUS FOR RESECTABILITY OF PANCREATIC CANCER						
Reference	No. of patients	Sensitivity (%)	Specificity (%)	PPV (%)	NPV (%)	Accuracy (%)
Howard et al.[11] (1997)[a]	21	75	77	67	83	76
Legmann et al.[13] (1998)	27	90	83	95	75	92
Buscail et al.[37] (1999)	26	47	100	100	50	65
Gress et al.[16] (1999)	75	95	92	93	94	93
Ahmad et al.[67] (2000)	63	61	63	69	55	62
Tierney et al.[68] (2001)	24	93	67	82	83	83
Soriano et al.[39] (2004)	62	23	100	100	64	67
Ramsay et al.[40] (2004)	26	56	83	91	38	63
DeWitt et al.[22] (2004)	53	88	68	71	86	77
Total	377	69	82	86	72	77

Table 16.10 Test characteristics of EUS for resectability of pancreatic cancer
[a] Includes 6 patients with ampullary cancer.

COMPARISON OF EUS WITH CT, MRI, AND ANGIOGRAPHY FOR RESECTABILITY OF PANCREATIC CANCER							
Reference	No. of patients	Modality	Sensitivity (%)	Specificity (%)	PPV (%)	NPV (%)	Accuracy (%)
Howard et al.[11] (1997)[a]	22	EUS	75	77	67	83	76
		CT	63	100	100	80	86
		Angiography	38	92	75	71	71
Legmann et al.[13] (1998)	27	EUS	90	83	95	75	92
		CT	90	100	100	77	93
Gress et al.[16] (1999)	75	EUS	95	92	93	94	93
	58	CT	97	19	58	83	60
Ahmad et al.[67] (2000)	63	EUS	61	63	69	55	62
		MRI	73	72	77	68	73
Tierney et al.[68] (2001)	24	EUS	93	67	82	83	83
		CT	100	33	71	100	75
Ramsay et al.[40] (2004)	26	EUS	56	83	91	38	63
		CT	79	67	88	50	76
		MRI	81	83	93	67	83
Soriano et al.[39] (2004)	62	EUS	23	100	100	64	67
		CT	67	97	95	77	83
		MRI	57	90	81	73	75
		Angiography	37	100	65	71	
DeWitt et al.[22] (2004)	53	EUS	88	68	71	86	77
		CT	92	64	70	90	77

Table 16.11 Comparison of EUS with CT, MRI, and angiography for resectability of pancreatic cancer
[a] Includes 6 patients with ampullary cancer.

Clearly, there is no consensus on the best test or tests necessary for preoperative staging of suspected pancreatic tumors. The role of EUS, therefore, is likely to be dependent on its availability, referral patterns, and local expertise. Further cost and decision analysis, and comparative studies of EUS with state-of-the-art CT and MRI, are required to optimize surgical exploration in appropriate patients.

EUS-FNA OF PANCREATIC CANCER

Prior to the advent of EUS, FNA or core biopsy of pancreatic masses was performed either during surgery[69,70] or percutaneously under CT or ultrasound (US)[71–74] guidance. Intraoperative FNA of pancreatic tumors is an accurate technique with a low complication rate. This technique, however, may increase operating time considerably, especially with on-site interpretation of specimens. US- and CT-guided percutaneous FNA are also highly accurate techniques, with reported sensitivities of about 80%.[74] Previous enthusiasm for the use of percutaneous FNA, however, has decreased, because of reports of needle-track seeding[75–77] and the development of EUS-FNA.

The first reported use of EUS-FNA of a pancreatic mass was made by Villman et al.[78] in 1992. Chang et al.[79] subsequently reported successful EUS-FNA of a 1.6-cm adenocarcinoma in the head of the pancreas. Since these initial reports, multiple authors have documented their experience of EUS-FNA of pancreatic tumors[21,50,80–96] in nearly 1700 patients (Table 16.12, Figs 16.6–16.13). The overall sensitivity and specificity of EUS-FNA for the diagnosis of pancreatic tumors are 85% and 98%, respectively. Some authors have even reported a sensitivity of EUS-FNA for pancreatic cancer exceeding 90% in patients following negative or non-diagnostic sampling from previous ERCP or percutaneous approach.[92,93] Despite excellent sensitivity, the NPV of EUS-FNA for pancreatic tumors is 55%.[21,81,82,84,89,91,93,94,96] Therefore, a negative or non-diagnostic biopsy does not completely exclude the possibility of malignancy. Fritscher-Ravens et al.[97] found in a series of 207 consecutive patients with focal pancreatic lesions that the sensitivity of EUS-FNA for the diagnosis of malignancy in patients with normal parenchyma (89%) was superior to that in patients with parenchymal evidence of chronic pancreatitis (54%). The authors concluded that surgery is often still required to confirm malignancy in patients with chronic pancreatitis and a focal mass. The presence of chronic pancreatitis may also hinder cytologic interpretation of pancreatic biopsy, thus decreasing specificity of EUS-FNA of pancreatic masses.[98]

SUMMARY OF ARTICLES SUMMARIZING THE TEST CHARACTERISTICS OF EUS-GUIDED FINE-NEEDLE ASPIRATION OF PANCREATIC CANCER						
Reference	No. of patients	Sensitivity (%)	Specificity (%)	PPV (%)	NPV (%)	Accuracy (%)
Giovannini et al.[80] (1995)	43	75				
Wegener et al.[81] (1995)	11	44	100	100	29	55
Cahn et al.[50] (1996)	50	85	100			
Faigel et al.[82] (1997)	45	94	100		82	
Chang et al.[83] (1997)	47	83	80			88
Bhutani et al.[84] (1997)	47	64	100	100	16	
Wiersema et al.[85] (1997)	124	86	100			88
Gress et al.[86] (1997)	121	80	100			85
Binmoeller et al.[87] (1998)	45	76	100			
Hunerbein et al.[88] (1998)	26	88	100			
Fritscher-Ravens et al.[89] (1999)	45	80	100	100	80	
Williams et al.[90] (1999)	144	82	100			85
Voss et al.[91] (2000)	90	75	88	98	26	
Gress et al.[92] (2001)	102	93	100			
Harewood & Wiersema[93] (2002)	185	94		96	63	92
Ylagan et al.[94] (2002)	80	78	100	100	78	
Raut et al.[95] (2003)	233	91	100			92
Eloubeidi et al.[96] (2003)	158	84	97	99	64	84
Agarwal et al.[21] (2004)	81	89	100	100	56	90
Total	1677	85	98	98	55	88

Table 16.12 Summary of articles summarizing the test characteristics of EUS-guided fine-needle aspiration of pancreatic cancer

As most studies document an overall sensitivity above 80% for EUS-FNA of pancreatic tumors, most endosonographers should expect eventually to achieve this level of competency. There are few data, however, that document the experience required to achieve this goal. Mertz and Gautam[99] recently reported that at least 40 procedures were required for a novice endosonographer to achieve at least 80% sensitivity for the diagnosis of pancreatic cancer. Short mentored training of EUS-FNA appears to permit significant improvements in EUS-FNA accuracy, principally by decreasing the number of inadequate specimens.[100] The current American Society of Gastrointestinal Endoscopy guidelines recommend that at least 25 supervised EUS-FNA procedures be performed during monitored training in order to maximize proficiency. These studies suggest that these recommendations appear reasonable. Although not always available, training for EUS-FNA is best accomplished by expert formal instruction in a high-volume referral practice.

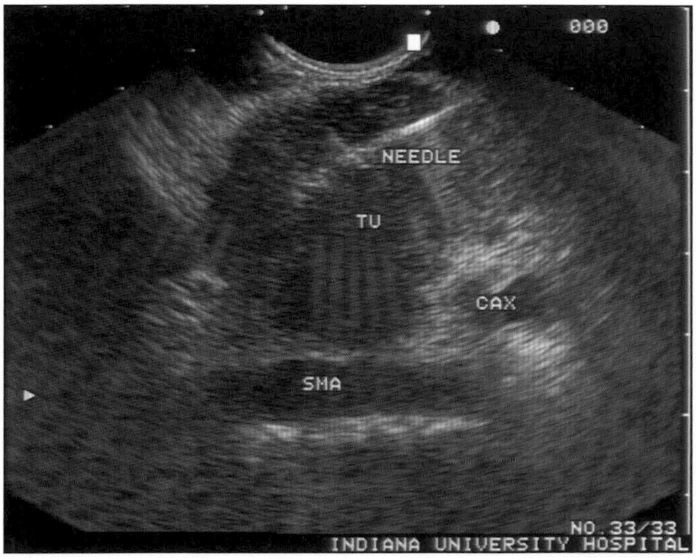

At most tertiary referral centers, on-site cytopathology assistance is provided to offer immediate feedback to the endosonographer about the quality of EUS-FNA specimens obtained. Furthermore, there are now data to suggest that this practice is beneficial. Klapman et al.[101] reported that on-site specimen interpretation following EUS-FNA could both improve diagnostic certainty and minimize diagnostic uncertainty. However, some endosonographers do not have the benefit of on-site cytopathology assessment during these procedures. Two studies[102,103] reported that at least five to seven EUS-FNA passes should be performed for pancreatic masses in order to

Fig. 16.6   EUS-FNA (5 MHz) of a 4-cm pancreatic body mass.

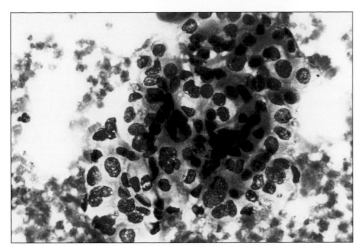

Fig. 16.7   Cytology from EUS-FNA in the same patient (hematoxylin and eosin stain; 20×). Pleomorphic, overlapping cells with increased nuclear to cytoplasmic ratio are present, consistent with adenocarcinoma.

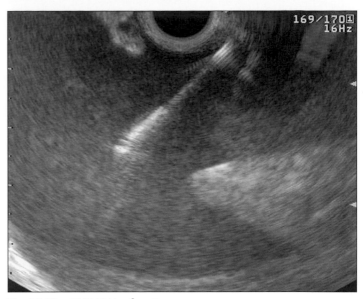

Fig. 16.10   EUS-FNA of ascites.

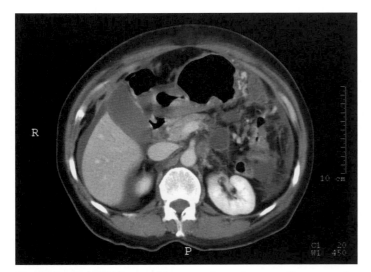

Fig. 16.8   Axial CT image demonstrating a 3-cm cystic pancreatic body mass and perihepatic ascites.

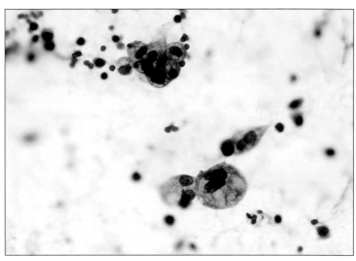

Fig. 16.11   Cytology specimen from ascites fluid, demonstrating metastatic adenocarcinoma (Diff-Quik stain; 100×).

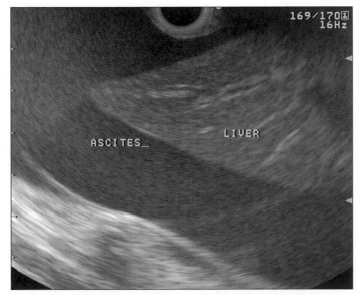

Fig. 16.9   Linear EUS image (6.0 MHz) of perihepatic ascites.

maximize diagnostic yield during EUS-FNA of suspected pancreatic cancer. This information may prove helpful to endosonographers performing EUS-FNA when rapid pathology interpretation is not available. It must be emphasized, however, that on-site assessment of specimen adequacy increases the diagnostic yield of EUS-FNA, thereby decreasing overall procedure time. Therefore, hospital and personnel resources should be utilized to provide this service when feasible.

Major complications following EUS-FNA of solid pancreatic masses occur in 0.5–2.5% of patients.[85,86,96,104,105] A multicenter experience of EUS-FNA of 124 pancreatic mass lesions demonstrated an overall complication rate of 1.1%, which was higher for cystic (14%) than for solid (0.5%) pancreatic lesions.[85] Therefore, antibiotics are always recommended following pancreatic cyst aspiration, but are not usually required following EUS-FNA of solid lesions. Gress et al.[86] reported a 1.7% (2 of

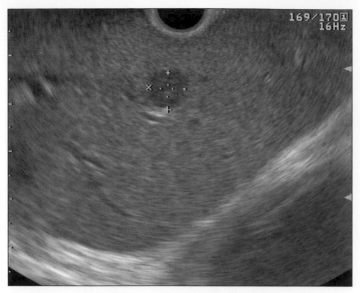

Fig. 16.12   Linear EUS image (6 MHz) of a 6-mm hypoechoic mass in the left lobe of the liver in a patient with a 2.5-cm mass in the head of the pancreas. The liver lesion was not seen on CT.

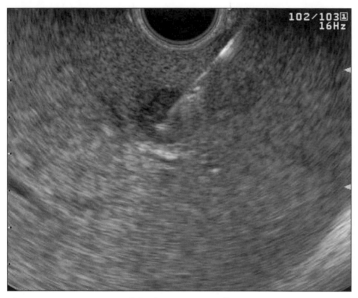

Fig. 16.13   EUS-FNA of the liver mass in the same patient. Cytology confirmed metastatic adenocarcinoma, thus making the tumor irresectable.

121) risk of pancreatitis and a 0.8% (1 of 121) risk of severe bleeding following EUS-FNA of solid pancreatic masses. In this series, the overall complication rate following EUS-FNA of all lesions (including non-pancreatic masses) was higher for radial (4.0%; 3 of 75) than for linear array (0.8%; 1 of 133) echoendoscopes. This apparent discrepancy in complication rates is due to the inability to image the entire length of the biopsy needle during real-time EUS-FNA using a radial array echoendoscope. Therefore, EUS-FNA using radial EUS endoscopes is not recommended. A prospective trial reported 2 (2%) of 100 patients developed acute pancreatitis following EUS-

FNA of a pancreatic mass; both of the patients had a history of recent pancreatitis.[104] Therefore, caution should be exercised when performing EUS-FNA in these patients. Following EUS-FNA of the pancreas, Eloubeidi et al.[96] reported self-limiting immediate postprocedure complications in 10 (6.3%) of 158 patients, including: hypoxia requiring the use of reversal medication ($n=1$), abdominal pain ($n=6$), excessive bleeding at biopsy site but not clinically manifested ($n=2$), and sore throat ($n=1$). In 78 (86.6%) of 90 patients contacted up to 3 days after EUS-FNA, 20 patients reported at least one minor symptom, one patient had mild acute pancreatitis, and two had visited the emergency room, one of whom was admitted with dehydration. No additional complications were reported at 30 days after EUS-FNA. When classified according to the severity of the complication, four (2.5%) complications were classified as major including: oversedation ($n=1$), self-limiting acute pancreatitis ($n=1$), and emergency room visits ($n=2$), one of which led to admission. In a series of 248 patients who underwent EUS-FNA of solid ($n=134$) and cystic ($n=114$) lesions, O'Toole et al.[105] reported a rate of complications of 0% (0 of 134) and 3.5% (4 of 114), respectively. Complications following EUS-FNA of cystic lesions included acute pancreatitis ($n=3$) and aspiration pneumonia ($n=1$), and all cases of pancreatitis resulted from FNA of lesions in the head/uncinate process. The risk of peritoneal seeding of tumor cells following EUS-FNA (2.2%) appears to be less than for CT-guided FNA (16.3%).[106]

To date, there have been no large prospective trials comparing the accuracy of EUS-FNA with that of percutaneous FNA of pancreatic masses. Qian and Hecht[107] reported that CT-FNA was superior to EUS-FNA of pancreatic masses. However, these results are difficult to generalize owing to selection bias, in that tumors sampled by EUS-FNA in this study were generally smaller than those assessed by CT. Mallery et al.[108] found no significant difference between the accuracy of surgically directed, CT-FNA, and EUS-FNA of pancreatic masses. Similar to the findings of Qian and Hecht,[107] however, the lesions sampled by EUS-FNA by Mallery et al.[108] were more difficult to sample than for the other methods studied. It appears that percutaneous FNA is an acceptable option for sampling of pancreatic tumors that are visible, accessible, and clearly inoperable based on imaging findings. For all other lesions, EUS-FNA is preferable to percutaneous FNA. Furthermore, the initial use of EUS and EUS-FNA appears to be a more cost-effective initial strategy for the initial work-up of patients with suspected pancreatic malignancy.[109,110]

Despite excellent accuracy and a low incidence of major complications, EUS-FNA of pancreatic masses has several limitations. First, an on-site cytopathologist during EUS-FNA is recommended for assessment of specimen adequacy. Second, primary pancreatic lymphomas and well differentiated ductal adenocarcinomas are often difficult to diagnose by use of cytology alone. Finally, the low negative predictive value of EUS-FNA does not permit exclusion of malignancy in negative specimens. To overcome these limitations, a spring-loaded 19-G Tru-Cut core biopsy needle (Quick-Core; Wilson-Cook, Winston-Salem, North Carolina, USA) has been developed to obtain histologic tissue samples using a standard linear array echoendoscope.[111] Larghi et al.[112] evaluated the role of EUS-guided Tru-Cut biopsy (EUS-TCB) in 23 consecutive patients with solid pancreatic masses detected on previous CT. Pancreatic tissue was obtained in 17 (74%) of 23 patients. EUS-TCB was successful in 13 of 13 and in 4 (40%) of 10 when a transgastric and transduodenal biopsy was performed, respectively. The authors reported that transduodenal biopsy was difficult when required upward deflection of the echoendoscope to bring the target lesion into appropriate position precluded extension of the needle from the accessory channel. The overall accuracy of EUS-TCB was 61% (14 of 23). Another study that compared EUS-TCB with EUS-FNA for multiple sites found no difference in diagnostic accuracy between the two devices.[113] In this study, two patients with pancreatic head cancer had the diagnosis made by EUS-FNA following non-diagnostic EUS-TCB. These data collectively demonstrate that EUS-TCB of pancreatic masses is best reserved for patients requiring transgastric biopsy after a negative EUS-FNA. Its utility for pancreatic head masses requires further study (perhaps with improved device design) before general recommendations can be made for this indication.

Some investigators have evaluated whether analysis of abnormal genes or expression of certain proteins on epithelial cells may increase the diagnostic yield of EUS-FNA of pancreatic masses. Tada et al.[114] quantitatively analyzed mutant K-ras gene expression from EUS-FNA specimens in 34 patients with adenocarcinoma ($n=26$) and chronic pancreatitis ($n=8$). Mutant gene was detected at high amounts (more than 2% of total ras genes) in 20 (77%) of 26 specimens. In contrast, mutant gene was absent or low level despite suspicious cytology in patients with benign pancreatic lesion. The authors concluded that the quantitative analysis of K-ras gene expression augments the yield of EUS-FNA of pancreatic masses, and that levels of the mutant gene may help predict the malignant potential of these lesions. Chhieng et al.[115] evaluated the expression of glycoproteins MUC1 and MUC2 from cell blocks previously obtained from EUS-FNA specimens in patients with malignant ($n=28$) or benign ($n=11$) pancreatic masses. Twenty-three (96%) of 24 pancreatic ductal carcinomas demonstrated positive staining with MUC1. The sensitivity and specificity of MUC1 as a marker for pancreatic ductal carcinomas were 96% and 94%, respectively. In contrast, only 1 of 11 benign lesions demonstrated weak MUC1 staining. Three pancreatic ductal carcinomas and one chronic pancreatitis specimen demonstrated cytoplasmic staining with MUC2. These studies suggest that molecular analysis of cytology specimens from EUS-FNA may increase the overall diagnostic yield. Larger studies examining other candidate markers and the cost of these additional tests are needed before these techniques may be recommended for general use.

PANCREATIC NEUROENDOCRINE TUMORS

Pancreatic neuroendocrine tumors (PNETs) represent less than 10% of pancreatic tumors. They are rare neoplasms with an overall prevalence of 10 per million.[116] Between 70% and 85% of these tumors are classified as functional PNETs (fPNETs), in which excessive tumor hormone production produces a distinct clinical syndrome. The two most clinically important fPNETs are gastrinomas and insulinomas. When a distinct series of symptoms is present (i.e., refractory hypoglycemia for insulinoma; or abdominal pain, diarrhea and peptic ulcer disease for gastrinoma) and imaging reveals a pancreatic mass, the clinical suspicion of PNET is relatively straightforward. Excessive secretory products are then easily measured to confirm the suspected diagnosis. When PNETs do not produce a clinical syndrome (15–30% overall), they are classified as non-functional (nfPNETs).[117] Due to a lack of characteristic symptoms related to hormone excess, nfPNETs are usually recognized later with larger tumors and produce non-specific symptoms such as jaundice, weight loss, abdominal pain, or pancreatitis.[118,119] Differentiation between benign and malignant PNETs is difficult with surgical pathology alone.[120] Therefore, malignancy is usually confirmed by the presence of distant metastases, and benign disease is confirmed by clinical follow-up.[121] Similar to primary ductal adenocarcinoma, surgical resection is the only cure for these tumors.[122,123] Therefore, a high index of suspicion coupled with a stepwise preoperative evaluation for localization may optimize patient selection for potentially curative surgery.

In a series of studies that compared EUS to other imaging modalities, the sensitivity of EUS for detection of PNETs was 77–94% (Table 16.13).[124–131] EUS appears especially useful for detection of small PNETs (<2.5 cm) missed by other imaging studies (Fig. 16.14). The sensitivity of transabdominal ultrasound detection of PNETs is between 7% and 29%.[125,126,128] Similarly, early studies with CT demonstrated poor detection, with reported sensitivities of 14–30%.[125,126,128] Recently, Gouya et al.[131] demonstrated that CT localization of PNETs is highly dependent on the optimal CT technique utilized. In a series of 30 patients with 32 insulinomas imaged over 13 years by three different techniques, overall diagnostic sensitivity for non-helical CT ($n=7$) and dual-phase MDCT without thin sections ($n=8$) were 29% and 57%, respectively. For the remaining 15 patients imaged with thin-slice, dual-phase MDCT, sensitivity increased to 94%. For the same group of 30 patients, the sensitivity of EUS was 94%. Early studies that compared EUS with MRI[126,128] demonstrated a sensitivity of MRI for PNET detection of 25–29%. Recent studies, however, have demonstrated a sensitivity of 85–100%[132,133] and a positive predictive value (PPV) of 96%[134] for PNET detection. As PNETs are hypervascular tumors, angiography sometimes demonstrates a 'blushing' pattern in the pancreas in suspected PNET. The sensitivity of diagnostic angiography for tumor detection is less than 30%.[124,128] Utilizing selective arterial calcium stimulation and hepatic venous sampling (ASVS), some authors have reported

COMPARISON OF EUS WITH CT, US, MRI, SRS AND ANGIOGRAPHY FOR DETECTION OF PANCREATIC NEUROENDOCRINE TUMORS

Reference	No. of patients	Tumor type[a]	Modality	Sensitivity (%)	Specificity (%)	PPV (%)	NPV (%)	Accuracy (%)
Rosch et al.[124] (1992)	37	Insulinomas (31)	EUS	82	95			
		Gastrinomas (7)	CT	0				
		Glucagonoma (1)	US	0				
			Angiography	27				
Palazzo et al.[125] (1993)	30	Insulinoma (13)	EUS	79				
		Gastrinoma (17)	CT	14				
			US	7				
			EUS	79				
Zimmer et al.[126] (1996)	20	Gastrinoma (10)	EUS	79				
		Insulinoma (10)	CT	29				
			MRI	29				
			US	29				
			SRS	86				
			EUS	93				
			CT	21				
			MRI	7				
			US	7				
			SRS	14				
Proye et al.[127] (1998)[b]	41	All PNETs	EUS					
		Insulinoma (20)	SRS			94		
		Gastrinoma (21)	SRS	77		100		
		Insulinoma (9)	EUS + SRS	60		100		
		Gastrinoma (14)		25				
				89				
				93				
De Angelis et al.[128] (1999)	23	Insulinoma (12)	EUS	87				
			CT	30				
			MRI	25				
			US	17				
			SRS	15				
			Angiography	27				
Ardengh et al.[129] (2000)	12	Insulinoma (12)	EUS	83				
			CT	17				
Anderson et al.[130] (2000)	75	Gastrinoma (36)	EUS	100	94	95	100	97
	14	Insulinoma (36)	EUS	88	100	100	43	89
			Angiography	44				
Gouya et al. [131](2003)[c]	38	Insulinoma (38)	EUS	94				
			CT	29–94				

Table 16.13 Comparison of EUS with CT, US, MRI, SRS and angiography for evaluation of pancreatic neuroendocrine tumors

SRS, somatostatin receptor scintigraphy; PNET, pancreatic neuroendocrine tumor.

[a] Vaues in parentheses are numbers of each tumor type.

[b] Overall sensitivity of combined EUS and SRS was 89% for insulinoma (n=9) and 93% for gastrinoma (n=14).

[c] Sensitivity of CT for non-helical CT, thick-section multidetector row computed tomography (MDCT) and thin-section MDCT was 79%, 57%, and 94%, respectively.

a sensitivity of 89–96% for detection of hyperinsulinemic hypoglycemia,[135,136] even superior to conventional CT and MRI. Its role, however, requires further study, including comparison to EUS. The clinical utility of somatostatin receptor scintigraphy (SRS) for identification of insulinomas is limited, with sensitivities ranging from 14% to 60%.[126–128] For other PNETs, SRS has a reported sensitivity of up to 58–86% for tumor detection.[126,137,138] Proye et al.[127] found that, for a series of patients

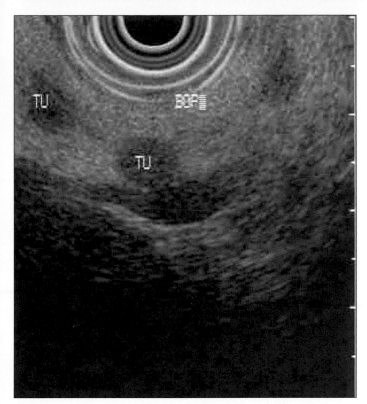

Fig. 16.14 Two subcentimeter hypoechoic pancreatic body masses in a patient with multiple endocrine neoplasia (MEN) type 1. CT demonstrated no masses in the pancreas.

demonstrate that EUS may not only identify but accurately sample PNETs. Preoperative EUS-guided injection of India ink has been demonstrated to aid in localization of an insulinoma.[142] This information may confirm clinically suspected tumors and aid in appropriate planning of medical or surgical management.

PANCREATIC METASTASES

Isolated pancreatic masses are usually due to either focal chronic pancreatitis or benign or malignant primary pancreatic tumors.

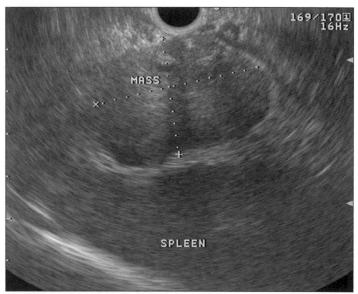

Fig. 16.15 Linear EUS image (6.0 MHz) of a 4.5-cm, well defined, hypoechoic mass in the tail of the pancreas. The patient's only symptoms were left-sided abdominal pain.

with histologically proven insulinoma ($n=20$) or gastrinoma ($n=21$), the sensitivity and PPV of EUS were, respectively, 77% and 94% for pancreatic tumors. For the same patients, the sensitivity and PPV of SRS for insulinoma and gastrinoma were 60% and 100%, and 25% and 100%, respectively. When both tests were combined for patients with insulinoma ($n=9$) and gastrinoma ($n=14$), the overall sensitivity of combined EUS and SRS was 89% and 93%, respectively. It appears that the combination of EUS and SRS may optimize preoperative identification of PNETs and limit the need for more invasive tests such as angiography. Similar to pancreatic adenocarcinoma,[109,110] the early incorporation of EUS into the preoperative localization of PNETs appears to be cost effective, principally by decreasing the need for more invasive tests and morbidity.[139]

The use of EUS-FNA permits tissue confirmation of a suspected PNET (Figs 16.15–16.18). In a retrospective study of 30 patients with fPNET ($n=16$), nfPNET ($n=7$), peripancreatic lymph nodes ($n=5$), or other ($n=2$), Ardengh et al.[140] reported a sensitivity, specificity, PPV, NPV, and accuracy of EUS-guided FNA of 83%, 86%, 95%, 60%, and 83%, respectively, for tumor diagnosis. There was one false-positive diagnosis by EUS-guided FNA, and four false-negative diagnoses. In two of the latter cases, EUS-guided FNA was unsuccessful. Ginès et al.[141] demonstrated a sensitivity of 90% for EUS-FNA in ten patients with fPNETs with a mean tumor size of 12 (range 4–25) mm. These studies

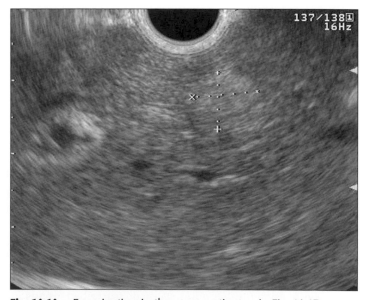

Fig. 16.16 Examination in the same patient as in Fig. 16.15 demonstrated multiple hyperechoic masses in the left lobe of the liver, suggestive of metastases.

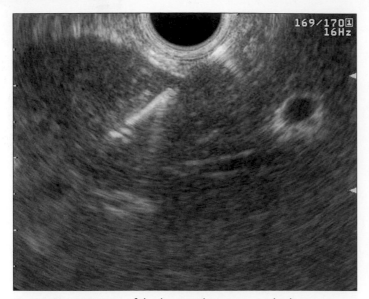

Fig. 16.17 EUS-FNA of the hyperechoic mass in the liver.

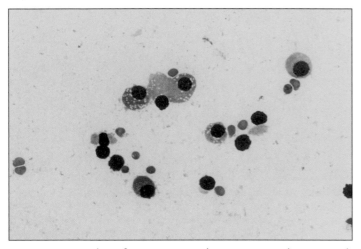

Fig. 16.18 Cytology from EUS-FNA demonstrating plasmacytoid cells with eccentric nuclei, consistent with a metastatic neuroendocrine tumor. As the patient had no symptoms, this was classified as a non-functional pancreatic neuroendocrine tumor with liver metastases.

Rarely, secondary involvement of the pancreas by systemic malignancy may occur, and has been reported in 2–3% of pancreatic resections.[142–144] Accurate identification of isolated pancreatic metastases is clinically important because aggressive surgical resection in selected patients may permit long-term survival.[145–147] In other patients, however, proper diagnosis may avoid unnecessary surgery and permit triage to more appropriate non-operative therapy.

EUS features of pancreatic metastases appear to be different from those observed in cases of primary pancreatic cancer. In seven patients with metastatic pancreatic lesions, Palazzo et al.[148] described homogeneous, round, well circumscribed lesions in 15 of 16 masses observed. Compared to patients with primary cancer (n=80), DeWitt et al.[149] found that pancreatic metastases

(n=24) were more likely to have well defined than irregular margins. In a recent report of 11 patients with metastatic renal cell carcinoma (RCC) to the pancreas, Béchade et al.[150] found that 10 had well defined borders. Therefore, it appears that EUS visualization of a well defined pancreatic mass in a patient with a history of malignancy should raise suspicion for a metastatic lesion.

EUS-FNA permits an accurate cytologic diagnosis of metastatic lesions to the pancreas (Figs 16.19–16.21).[149–153] In a series of 12 patients, Fritscher-Ravens et al.[151] reported metastatic lesions from primary RCC (n=3), breast cancer (n=2), esophageal cancer (n=2), colonic cancer (n=2), non-small cell lung cancer (n=1), non-Hodgkin lymphoma (n=1), and ovarian cancer (n=1). DeWitt et al.[149] reported the use of EUS-FNA for the diagnosis of metastasis from primary kidney (n=10), skin (n=6), lung (n=4), colon (n=2), liver (n=1), and stomach (n=1) cancer in 24 patients. Metastasis to the pancreas may occur many years (especially for RCC) after diagnosis of the primary tumor. Obtaining a detailed medical history for previous malignancy may raise suspicion for this diagnosis. In patients with a remote history of malignancy, obtaining additional cytologic material for cell block and the use of immunocytochemistry may be helpful to confirm the diagnosis of pancreatic metastases and recurrent malignancy.[149]

AMPULLARY TUMORS

Cancer of the ampulla or major papilla often produces the same clinical symptoms as tumors of the pancreatic head, including jaundice, weight loss, and duodenal obstruction. Survival with ampullary cancer is better than pancreatic cancer,[154–156] as locoregional invasion usually occurs later with ampullary

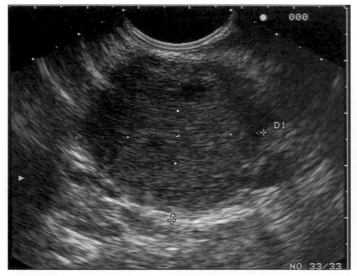

Fig. 16.19 Linear EUS view (5.0 MHz) demonstrating a well defined, hypoechoic, 4-cm mass in the head of the pancreas in a patient with a remote history of renal cell carcinoma removed 12 years previously.

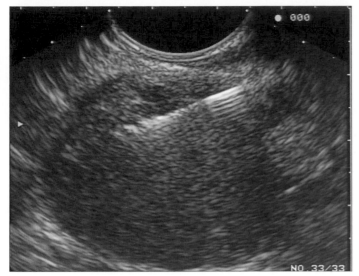

Fig. 16.20   EUS-FNA of the pancreatic head mass of the patient in Fig. 16.19.

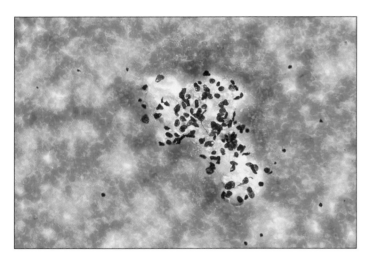

Fig. 16.21   Cytology from EUS-FNA demonstrating clear cells, consistent with metastatic, recurrent renal cell carcinoma. These findings were confirmed by surgical resection.

cancer. Treatment of benign tumors and superficial ampullary cancers may include endoscopic resection[157] or transduodenal excision,[158] but more invasive malignancies are usually managed with more aggressive surgical excision such as pancreaticoduodenectomy.[155,156] Therefore, accurate staging and detection of ampullary neoplasms may permit triage to appropriate endoscopic or surgical management (Figs 16.22 & 16.23).

In an analysis of 11 studies in 286 patients (Table 16.14), the accuracy of EUS for assessment of tumor extension and nodal metastasis of ampullary cancer was 78%[7,36,37,160–166] and 62%,[36,37,159–161,163–166] respectively. This is significantly superior to CT, which has reported T- and N-staging accuracies of 24% and 48%, respectively.[7,162–166] In the only two studies[7,163] to date in 17 patients that compared EUS and MRI, the T- and N-

staging accuracies of MRI were 35% and 77%, respectively. EUS is also the most sensitive imaging tests for the detection of ampullary neoplasms (Table 16.15). For a series of 121 patients, the sensitivity of EUS for ampullary cancer was 89%, which is

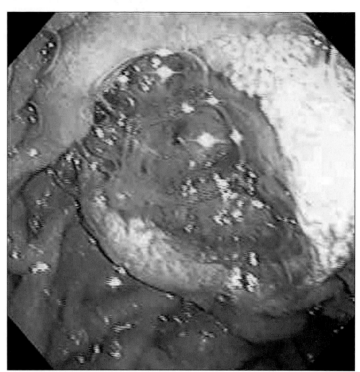

Fig. 16.22   Endoscopic image of an ampullary mass.

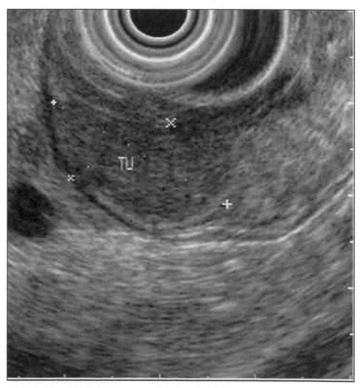

Fig. 16.23   Radial EUS view (7.5 MHz) of the same mass as in Fig. 16.22, demonstrating a 2.0 × 1.5-cm hypoechoic mass invading the submucosa of the duodenal wall. The muscularis propria was not invaded by the mass. Surgical resection confirmed a T1sm ampullary cancer.

ACCURACY OF EUS FOR TUMOR (T) AND NODAL (N) STAGING OF AMPULLARY CANCER				
Reference	No. of patients	Modality	T-stage accuracy (%)	N-stage accuracy (%)
Mitake et al.[159] (1990)	28	EUS	89	69
Muller et al.[7] (1994)	6	EUS	100	
	6	CT	17	
	4	MRI	25	
Zhang et al.[160] (1996)	22	EUS	82	59
Tio et al.[36] (1996)	32	EUS	84	53
Sauvanet et al.[161] (1997)	26	EUS	75	69
Buscail et al.[37] (1999)	6	EUS	83	100
Menzel et al.[162] (1999)	15	IDUS	87	
	5	EUS	40	
	5	CT	60	
Cannon et al.[163] (1999)[a]	50	EUS	78	68
	37	CT	24	59
	13	MRI	46	77
Kubo et al.[164] (1999)	35	EUS	74	69
Chen et al.[165] (2001)	56	EUS	72	47
	56	CT	22	33
	56	US	11	7
Skordilis et al.[166] (2002)	20	EUS	82	71
	20	CT	24	65
	20	US	12	47
Total	286	EUS	78	62
	124	CT	24	48
	17	MRI	35	77
	76	US	12	17
	15	IDUS	87	n/a

Table 16.14 Accuracy of EUS for tumor (T) and nodal (N) staging of ampullary cancer
IDUS, intraductal ultrasonograph; n/a, not applicable.
[a] Includes 9 adenomas with high-grade dysplasia, 1 carcinoid, 1 somatostatinoma.

higher than that for both CT (32%) and transabdominal ultrasonography (18%).[4,19,162,165,166]

Menzel et al.[162] reported that the addition of intraductal ultrasonography (IDUS) improves both tumor detection and staging of ampullary neoplasms. In 27 consecutive patients with benign (n=12) and malignant (n=15) ampullary tumors, these authors found that IDUS (100%) was significantly superior to standard transduodenal EUS (59%) and CT (30%) for tumor detection. Furthermore, the accuracy of IDUS was superior to EUS for differentiating benign adenomas from carcinomas (89% versus 56% respectively). The accuracy of IDUS in assessing T stage was 87% (13 of 15). The authors hypothesized that the increased accuracy of detection and staging by IDUS was due to the ability of the IDUS probe to image perpendicular the bile duct instead of perpendicular to the duodenal wall as is required with EUS. Furthermore, accurate imaging by EUS may be compromised by air artifact and extrinsic compression onto the ampullary mass. Although IDUS is not used at all referral centers, it appears to be a useful adjunct to EUS and CT for locoregional staging of these tumors.

As patients with ampullary tumors usually present initially with jaundice, ERCP and stent placement is often performed prior to EUS evaluation. Two studies have demonstrated that stent placement and consequential acoustic shadowing may decrease accuracy of EUS staging of ampullary neoplasms. Cannon et al.[163] found that the presence of a biliary stent caused a non-significant decrease in accuracy in tumor and nodal staging of ampullary cancers. In this study, stent insertion decreased T staging from 84% to 72%, and N staging from 76% to 64%. The decrease in tumor staging was primarily due to under-staging T2 and T3 cancers as T1 tumors. Chen et al.[165] also reported that the presence of a biliary stent decreased the

COMPARISON OF SENSITIVITY OF EUS WITH OTHER MODALITIES FOR DETECTION OF AMPULLARY NEOPLASMS

Reference	No. of patients	Modality	Sensitivity (%)
Rosch et al.[4] (1992)	12	EUS	92
		CT	25
		US	0
Menzel et al.[162] (1999)[a]	27	EUS	59
		IDUS	100
		CT	30
Chen et al.[165] (2001)	56	EUS	97
		CT	39
		US	24
Skordilis et al.[166] (2002)	20	EUS	100
		CT	20
		US	15
Rivadeneira et al.[19] (2003)	6	EUS	100
Total	121	EUS	89
	115	CT	32
	88	US	18
	27	IDUS	100

Table 16.15 Comparison of sensitivity of EUS with other modalities for detection of ampullary neoplasms
IDUS, intraductal ultrasonography.
[a] Includes 12 benign and 15 malignant ampullary tumors.

accuracy of T staging from 81% to 65%, and N staging from 80% to 70%. Therefore, caution must be exercised when staging ampullary cancers with an indwelling biliary stent. It also remains unclear whether an initial attempt at transduodenal excision following EUS staging of an ampullary cancer with an indwelling stent should be attempted. When available, simultaneous ERCP with IDUS staging followed by stenting (if needed) may optimize staging and preoperative management of these tumors.

EXAMINATION CHECKLIST

Primary tumor and peripancreatic region
Liver
Presence or absence of ascites
Celiac axis
Portal vein, superior mesenteric vein, splenic vein, and confluence
Superior mesenteric artery

REFERENCES

1 Yasuda K, Mukai H, Fujimoto S, et al. The diagnosis of pancreatic cancer by endoscopic ultrasonography. Gastrointest Endosc 1988; 34:1–8.
2 Lin JT, Wang JT, Wang TH. The diagnostic value of endoscopic ultrasonography in pancreatic disorders. Taiwan Yi Xue Hui Za Zhi 1989; 88:483–487.
3 Rosch T, Lorenz R, Braig C, et al. Endoscopic ultrasound in pancreatic tumor diagnosis. Gastrointest Endosc 1991; 37:347–352.
4 Rosch T, Braig C, Gain T, et al. Staging of pancreatic and ampullary carcinoma by endoscopic ultrasonography. Comparison with conventional sonography, computed tomography, and angiography. Gastroenterology 1992; 102:188–199.
5 Snady H, Cooperman A, Siegel J. Endoscopic ultrasonography compared with computed tomography with ERCP in patients with obstructive jaundice or small peri-pancreatic mass. Gastrointest Endosc 1992; 38:27–34.
6 Palazzo L, Roseau G, Gayet B, et al. Endoscopic ultrasonography in the diagnosis and staging of pancreatic adenocarcinoma. Results of a prospective study with comparison to ultrasonography and CT scan. Endoscopy 1993; 25:143–150.
7 Muller MF, Meyenberger C, Bertschinger P, et al. Pancreatic tumors: evaluation with endoscopic US, CT, and MR imaging. Radiology 1994; 190:745–751.
8 Marty O, Aubertin JM, Bouillot JL, et al. Prospective comparison of ultrasound endoscopy and computed tomography in the assessment of locoregional invasiveness of malignant ampullary and pancreatic tumors verified surgically. Gastroenterol Clin Biol 1995; 19:197–203.
9 Melzer E, Avidan B, Heyman Z, et al. Preoperative assessment of blood vessel involvement in patients with pancreatic cancer. Isr J Med Sci 1996; 32:1086–1088.
10 Dufour B, Zins M, Vilgrain V, et al. Comparison between spiral X-ray computed tomography and endosonography in the diagnosis and staging of adenocarcinoma of the pancreas. Clinical preliminary study. Gastroenterol Clin Biol 1997; 21:124–130.
11 Howard TJ, Chin AC, Streib EW, et al. Value of helical computed tomography, angiography, and endoscopic ultrasound in determining resectability of periampullary carcinoma. Am J Surg 1997; 174:237–241.
12 Sugiyama M, Hagi H, Atomi Y, et al. Diagnosis of portal venous invasion by pancreatobiliary carcinoma: value of endoscopic ultrasonography. Abdom Imaging 1997; 22:434–438.
13 Legmann P, Vignaux O, Dousset B, et al. Pancreatic tumors: comparison of dual-phase helical CT and endoscopic sonography. AJR Am J Roentgenol 1998; 170:1315–1322.
14 Akahoshi K, Chijiiwa Y, Nakano I, et al. Diagnosis and staging of pancreatic cancer by endoscopic ultrasound. Br J Radiol 1998; 71:492–496.
15 Harrison JL, Millikan KW, Prinz RA, et al. Endoscopic ultrasound for diagnosis and staging of pancreatic tumors. Am Surg 1999; 65:659–664, discussion 664–665.

16 Gress FG, Hawes RH, Savides TJ, et al. Role of EUS in the preoperative staging of pancreatic cancer: a large single-center experience. Gastrointest Endosc 1999; 50:786–791.

17 Midwinter MJ, Beveridge CJ, Wilsdon JB, et al. Correlation between spiral computed tomography, endoscopic ultrasonography and findings at operation in pancreatic and ampullary tumours. Br J Surg 1999; 86:189–193.

18 Mertz HR, Sechopoulos P, Delbeke D, et al. EUS, PET, and CT scanning for evaluation of pancreatic adenocarcinoma. Gastrointest Endosc 2000; 52:367–371.

19 Rivadeneira DE, Pochapin M, Grobmyer SR, et al. Comparison of linear array endoscopic ultrasound and helical computed tomography for the staging of periampullary malignancies. Ann Surg Oncol 2003; 10:890–897.

20 Ainsworth AP, Rafaelsen SR, Wamberg PA, et al. Is there a difference in diagnostic accuracy and clinical impact between endoscopic ultrasonography and magnetic resonance cholangiopancreatography? Endoscopy 2003; 35:1029–1032.

21 Agarwal B, Abu-Hamda E, Molke KL, et al. Endoscopic ultrasound-guided fine needle aspiration and multidetector spiral CT in the diagnosis of pancreatic cancer. Am J Gastroenterol 2004; 99:844–850.

22 DeWitt J, Devereaux B, Chriswell M, et al. Comparison of endoscopic ultrasound and multidetector computed tomography for the detection and staging of pancreatic cancer. Ann Intern Med 2004; 141:753–763.

23 Prokesch RW, Schima W, Chow LC, et al. Multidetector CT of pancreatic adenocarcinoma: diagnostic advances and therapeutic relevance. Eur Radiol 2003; 13:2147–2154.

24 Bronstein YL, Loyer EM, Kaur H, et al. Detection of small pancreatic tumors with multiphasic helical CT. AJR Am J Roentgenol 2004; 182:619–623.

25 Bhutani MS, Gress FG, Giovannini M, et al. The No Endosonographic Detection of Tumor (NEST) Study: a case series of pancreatic cancers missed on endoscopic ultrasonography. Endoscopy 2004; 36:385–389.

26 Catanzaro A, Richardson S, Veloso H, et al. Long-term follow-up of patients with clinically indeterminate suspicion of pancreatic cancer and normal EUS. Gastrointest Endosc 2003; 58:836–840.

27 Brentnall TA, Bronner MP, Byrd DR, et al. Early diagnosis and treatment of pancreatic dysplasia in patients with a family history of pancreatic cancer. Ann Intern Med 1999; 131:247–255.

28 Rulyak SJ, Kimmey MB, Veenstra DL, et al. Cost-effectiveness of pancreatic cancer screening in familial pancreatic cancer kindreds. Gastrointest Endosc 2003; 57:23–29.

29 Canto MI, Goggins M, Yeo CJ, et al. Screening for pancreatic neoplasia in high-risk individuals: an EUS-based approach. Clin Gastroenterol Hepatol 2004; 2:606–621.

30 Tio TL, Tytgat GN, Cikot RJ, et al. Ampullopancreatic carcinoma: preoperative TNM classification with endosonography. Radiology 1990; 175:455–461.

31 Grimm H, Maydeo A, Soehendra N. Endoluminal ultrasound for the diagnosis and staging of pancreatic cancer. Baillieres Clin Gastroenterol 1990; 4:869–888.

32 Mukai H, Nakajima M, Yasuda K, et al. Preoperative diagnosis and staging of pancreatic cancer by endoscopic ultrasonography (EUS) – a comparative study with other diagnostic tools. Nippon Shokakibyo Gakkai Zasshi 1991; 88:2132–2142.

33 Rosch T, Dittler HJ, Lorenz R, et al. The endosonographic staging of pancreatic carcinoma. Dtsch Med Wochenschr 1992; 117:563–569.

34 Yasuda K, Mukai H, Nakajima M, et al. Staging of pancreatic carcinoma by endoscopic ultrasonography. Endoscopy 1993; 25:151–155.

35 Giovannini M, Seitz JF. Endoscopic ultrasonography with a linear-type echoendoscope in the evaluation of 94 patients with pancreatobiliary disease. Endoscopy 1994; 26:579–585.

36 Tio TL, Sie LH, Kallimanis G, et al. Staging of ampullary and pancreatic carcinoma: comparison between endosonography and surgery. Gastrointest Endosc 1996; 44:706–713.

37 Buscail L, Pages P, Berthelemy P, et al. Role of EUS in the management of pancreatic and ampullary carcinoma: a prospective study assessing resectability and prognosis. Gastrointest Endosc 1999; 50:34–40.

38 Ahmad NA, Lewis JD, Ginsberg GG, et al. EUS in preoperative staging of pancreatic cancer. Gastrointest Endosc 2000; 52:463–468.

39 Soriano A, Castells A, Ayuso C, et al. Preoperative staging and tumor resectability assessment of pancreatic cancer: prospective study comparing endoscopic ultrasonography, helical computed tomography, magnetic resonance imaging, and angiography. Am J Gastroenterol 2004; 99:492–501.

40 Ramsay D, Marshall M, Song S, et al. Identification and staging of pancreatic tumours using computed tomography, endoscopic ultrasound and mangafodipir trisodium-enhanced magnetic resonance imaging. Australas Radiol 2004; 48:154–161.

41 Tamm EP, Silverman PM, Charnsangavej C, et al. Diagnosis, staging, and surveillance of pancreatic cancer. AJR Am J Roentgenol 2003; 180:1311–1323.

42 Vargas R, Nino-Murcia M, Trueblood W, et al. MDCT in pancreatic adenocarcinoma: prediction of vascular invasion and resectability using a multiphasic technique with curved planar reformations. AJR Am J Roentgenol 2004; 182: 419–425.

43 Sobin LH, Hermanek P, Hutter RP. TNM classification or malignant tumors. Cancer 1988; 61:2310–2314.

44 American Joint Committee on Cancer. Exocrine pancreas. In: Greene FL, Page DL, Fleming ID, et al., eds. AJCC cancer staging manual, 5th edn. Philadelphia: Lippincott-Raven; 1997:121–126.

45 Howard TJ, Villanustre N, Moore SA, et al. Efficacy of venous reconstruction in patients with adenocarcinoma of the pancreatic head. J Gastrointest Surg 2003; 27:1089–1095.

46 Greene FL, Page DL, Fleming ID, et al. AJCC Cancer Staging Manual, Sixth Edition. New York: Springer-Verlag, 2002:209-220.

47 Bhutani MS, Hawes RH, Hoffman BJ. A comparison of the accuracy of echo features during endoscopic ultrasound (EUS) and EUS-guided fine-needle aspiration for diagnosis of malignant lymph node invasion. Gastrointest Endosc 1997; 45:474–479.

48 Catalano MF, Sivak MV Jr, Rice T, et al. Endosonographic features predictive of lymph node metastases. Gastrointest Endosc 1994; 40:442–446.

49 Nakaizumi A, Uehara H, Iishi H, et al. Endoscopic ultrasonography in diagnosis and staging of pancreatic cancer. Dig Dis Sci 1995; 40:696–700.

50 Cahn M, Chang K, Nguyen P, et al. Impact of endoscopic ultrasound with fine-needle aspiration on the surgical management of pancreatic cancer. Am J Surg 1996; 172:470–472.

51 Hahn M, Faigel DO. Frequency of mediastinal lymph node metastases in patients undergoing EUS evaluation of pancreaticobiliary masses. Gastrointest Endosc 2001; 54:331–335.

52 Nguyen P, Feng JC, Chang KJ. Endoscopic ultrasound (EUS) and EUS-guided fine-needle aspiration (FNA) of liver lesions. Gastrointest Endosc 1999; 50:357–361.

53 DeWitt J, LeBlanc J, McHenry L, et al. Endoscopic ultrasound-guided fine needle aspiration cytology of solid liver lesions: a large single-center experience. Am J Gastroenterol 2003; 98:1976–1981.

54 Prasad P, Schmulewitz N, Patel A, et al. Detection of occult liver metastases during EUS for staging of malignancies. Gastrointest Endosc 2004; 59:49–53.

55 tenBerge J, Hoffman BJ, Hawes RH, et al. EUS-guided fine needle aspiration of the liver: indications, yield, and safety based on an international survey of 167 cases. Gastrointest Endosc 2002; 55:859–862.

56 Hollerbach S, Willert J, Topalidis T, et al. Endoscopic ultrasound-guided fine-needle aspiration biopsy of liver lesions: histological and cytological assessment. Endoscopy 2003; 35:743–749.

57 Chang KJ, Albers CG, Nguyen P. Endoscopic ultrasound-guided fine needle aspiration of pleural and ascitic fluid. Am J Gastroenterol 1995; 90:148–150.

58 Nguyen PT, Chang KJ. EUS in the detection of ascites and EUS-guided paracentesis. Gastrointest Endosc 2001; 54:336–339.

59 Furukawa H, Kosuge T, Mukai K, et al. Helical computed tomography in the diagnosis of portal vein invasion by pancreatic head carcinoma: usefulness for selecting surgical procedures and predicting the outcome. Arch Surg 1998; 133:61–65.

60 Ishikawa O, Ohigashi H, Sasaki Y, et al. Intraoperative cytodiagnosis for detecting a minute invasion of the portal vein during pancreatoduodenectomy for adenocarcinoma of the pancreatic head. Am J Surg 1998; 175:477–481.

61 Tierney WM, Francis IR, Eckhauser F, et al. The accuracy of EUS and helical CT in the assessment of vascular invasion by peripapillary malignancy. Gastrointest Endosc 2001; 53:182–188.

62 Brugge WR, Lee MJ, Kelsey PB, et al. The use of EUS to diagnose malignant portal venous system invasion by pancreatic cancer. Gastrointest Endosc 1996; 43:561–567.

63 Rosch T, Dittler HJ, Strobel K, et al. Endoscopic ultrasound criteria for vascular invasion in the staging of cancer of the head of the pancreas: a blind revaluation of videotapes. Gastrointest Endosc 2000; 52:469–477.

64 Snady H, Bruckner H, Siegel J, et al. Endoscopic ultrasonographic criteria of vascular invasion by potentially resectable pancreatic tumors. Gastrointest Endosc 1994; 40:326–333.

65 Richter A, Niedergethmann M, Sturm JW, et al. Long-term results of partial pancreaticoduodenectomy for ductal adenocarcinoma of the pancreatic head: 25-year experience. World J Surg 2003; 27:324–329.

66 Benassai G, Mastrorilli M, Quarto G, et al. Factors influencing survival after resection for ductal adenocarcinoma of the head of the pancreas. J Surg Oncol 2000; 73:212–218.

67 Ahmad NA, Lewis JD, Siegelman ES, et al. Role of endoscopic ultrasound and magnetic resonance imaging in the preoperative staging of pancreatic adenocarcinoma. Am J Gastroenterol 2000; 95:1926–1931.

68 Tierney WM, Francis IR, Eckhauser F, et al. The accuracy of EUS and helical CT in the assessment of vascular invasion by peripapillary malignancy. Gastrointest Endosc 2001; 53:182–188.

69 Saez A, Catala I, Brossa R, et al. Intraoperative fine needle aspiration cytology of pancreatic lesions. A study of 90 cases. Acta Cytol 1995; 39:485–488.

70 Schadt ME, Kline TS, Neal HS, et al. Intraoperative pancreatic fine needle aspiration biopsy. Results in 166 patients. Am Surg 1991; 57:73–75.

71 Sperti C, Pasquali C, Di Prima F, et al. Percutaneous CT-guided fine needle aspiration cytology in the differential diagnosis of pancreatic lesions. Ital J Gastroenterol 1994; 26:126–131.

72 Brandt KR, Charboneau JW, Stephens DH, et al. CT- and US-guided biopsy of the pancreas. Radiology 1993; 187:99–104.

73 Di Stasi M, Lencioni R, Solmi L, et al. Ultrasound-guided fine needle biopsy of pancreatic masses: results of a multicenter study. Am J Gastroenterol 1998; 93:1329–1333.

74 Bret PM, Nicolet V, Labadie M. Percutaneous fine-needle aspiration biopsy of the pancreas. Diagn Cytopathol 1986; 2:221–227.

75 Ferrucci JT, Wittenberg J, Margolies MN, et al. Malignant seeding of the tract after thin-needle aspiration biopsy. Radiology 1979; 130:345–346.

76 Smith FP, Macdonald JS, Schein PS, et al. Cutaneous seeding of pancreatic cancer by skinny-needle aspiration biopsy. Arch Intern Med 1980; 140:855.

77 Caturelli E, Rapaccini GL, Anti M, et al. Malignant seeding after fine-needle aspiration biopsy of the pancreas. Diagn Imaging Clin Med 1985; 54:88–91.

78 Vilmann P, Jacobsen GK, Henriksen FW, et al. Endoscopic ultrasonography with guided fine needle aspiration biopsy in pancreatic disease. Gastrointest Endosc 1992; 38:172–173.

79 Chang KJ, Albers CG, Erickson RA, et al. Endoscopic ultrasound-guided fine needle aspiration of pancreatic carcinoma. Am J Gastroenterol 1994; 89:263–266.

80 Giovannini M, Seitz JF, Monges G, et al. Fine-needle aspiration cytology guided by endoscopic ultrasonography: results in 141 patients. Endoscopy 1995; 27:171–177.

81 Wegener M, Pfaffenbach B, Adamek RJ. Endosonographically guided transduodenal and transgastral fine-needle aspiration puncture of focal pancreatic lesions. Bildgebung 1995; 62:110–115.

82 Faigel DO, Ginsberg GG, Bentz JS, et al. Endoscopic ultrasound-guided real-time fine-needle aspiration biopsy of the pancreas in cancer patients with pancreatic lesions. J Clin Oncol 1997; 15:1439–1443.

83 Chang KJ, Nguyen P, Erickson RA, et al. The clinical utility of endoscopic ultrasound-guided fine-needle aspiration in the diagnosis and staging of pancreatic carcinoma. Gastrointest Endosc 1997; 45:387–393.

84 Bhutani MS, Hawes RH, Baron PL, et al. Endoscopic ultrasound guided fine needle aspiration of malignant pancreatic lesions. Endoscopy 1997; 29:854–858.

85 Wiersema MJ, Vilmann P, Giovannini M, et al. Endosonography-guided fine-needle aspiration biopsy: diagnostic accuracy and complication assessment. Gastroenterology 1997; 112:1087–1095.

86 Gress FG, Hawes RH, Savides TJ, et al. Endoscopic ultrasound-guided fine-needle aspiration biopsy using linear array and radial scanning endosonography. Gastrointest Endosc 1997; 45:243–250.

87 Binmoeller KF, Thul R, Rathod V, et al. Endoscopic ultrasound-guided, 18-gauge, fine needle aspiration biopsy of the pancreas using a 2.8 mm channel convex array echoendoscope. Gastrointest Endosc 1998; 47:121–127.

88 Hunerbein M, Dohmoto M, Haensch W, et al. Endosonography-guided biopsy of mediastinal and pancreatic tumors. Endoscopy 1998; 30:32–36.

89 Fritscher-Ravens A, Schirrow L, Atay Z, et al. Endosonographically controlled fine needle aspiration cytology – indications and results in routine diagnosis. Z Gastroenterol 1999; 37:343–351.

90 Williams DB, Sahai AV, Aabakken L, et al. Endoscopic ultrasound guided fine needle aspiration biopsy: a large single centre experience. Gut 1999; 44:720–726.

91 Voss M, Hammel P, Molas G, et al. Value of endoscopic ultrasound guided fine needle aspiration biopsy in the diagnosis of solid pancreatic masses. Gut 2000; 46:244–249.

92 Gress F, Gottlieb K, Sherman S, et al. Endoscopic ultrasonography-guided fine-needle aspiration biopsy of suspected pancreatic cancer. Ann Intern Med 2001; 134:459–464.

93 Harewood GC, Wiersema MJ. Endosonography-guided fine needle aspiration biopsy in the evaluation of pancreatic masses. Am J Gastroenterol 2002; 97:1386–1391.

94 Ylagan LR, Edmundowicz S, Kasal K, et al. Endoscopic ultrasound guided fine-needle aspiration cytology of pancreatic carcinoma: a 3-year experience and review of the literature. Cancer 2002; 96:362–369.

95 Raut CP, Grau AM, Staerkel GA, et al. Diagnostic accuracy of endoscopic ultrasound-guided fine-needle aspiration in patients with presumed pancreatic cancer. J Gastrointest Surg 2003; 7:118–126, discussion 127–128.

96 Eloubeidi MA, Chen VK, Eltoum IA, et al. Endoscopic ultrasound-guided fine needle aspiration biopsy of patients with suspected pancreatic cancer: diagnostic accuracy and acute and 30-day complications. Am J Gastroenterol 2003; 98:2663–2668.

97 Fritscher-Ravens A, Brand L, Knofel WT, et al. Comparison of endoscopic ultrasound-guided fine needle aspiration for focal pancreatic lesions in patients with normal parenchyma and chronic pancreatitis. Am J Gastroenterol 2002; 97:2768–2775.

98 Schwartz DA, Unni KK, Levy MJ, et al. The rate of false-positive results with EUS-guided fine-needle aspiration. Gastrointest Endosc 2002; 56:868–872.

99 Mertz H, Gautam S. The learning curve for EUS-guided FNA of pancreatic cancer. Gastrointest Endosc 2004; 59:33–37.

100 Harewood GC, Wiersema LM, Halling AC, et al. Influence of EUS training and pathology interpretation on accuracy of EUS-guided fine needle aspiration of pancreatic masses. Gastrointest Endosc 2002; 55:669–673.

101 Klapman JB, Logrono R, Dye CE, et al. Clinical impact of on-site cytopathology interpretation on endoscopic ultrasound-guided fine needle aspiration. Am J Gastroenterol 2003; 98:1289–1294.

102 Erickson RA, Sayage-Rabie L, Beissner RS. Factors predicting the number of EUS-guided fine-needle passes for diagnosis of pancreatic malignancies. Gastrointest Endosc 2000; 51:184–190.

103 LeBlanc JK, Ciaccia D, Al-Assi MT, et al. Optimal number of EUS-guided fine needle passes needed to obtain a correct diagnosis. Gastrointest Endosc 2004; 59:475–481.

104 Gress F, Michael H, Gelrud D, et al. EUS-guided fine-needle aspiration of the pancreas: evaluation of pancreatitis as a complication. Gastrointest Endosc 2002; 56: 864–867.

105 O'Toole D, Palazzo L, Arotcarena R, et al. Assessment of complications of EUS-guided fine-needle aspiration. Gastrointest Endosc 2001; 53:470–474.

106 Micames C, Jowell PS, White R, et al. Lower frequency of peritoneal carcinomatosis in patients with pancreatic cancer diagnosed by EUS-guided FNA vs. percutaneous FNA. Gastrointest Endosc 2003; 58:690–695.

107 Qian X, Hecht JL. Pancreatic fine needle aspiration. A comparison of computed tomographic and endoscopic ultrasonographic guidance. Acta Cytol. 2003; 47:723–726.

108 Mallery JS, Centeno BA, Hahn PF, et al. Pancreatic tissue sampling guided by EUS, CT/US, and surgery: a comparison of sensitivity and specificity. Gastrointest Endosc 2002; 56:218–224.

109 Harewood GC, Wiersema MJ. A cost analysis of endoscopic ultrasound in the evaluation of pancreatic head adenocarcinoma. Am J Gastroenterol 2001; 96:2651–2656.

110 Chen VK, Arguedas MR, Kilgore ML, et al. A cost-minimization analysis of alternative strategies in diagnosing pancreatic cancer. Am J Gastroenterol 2004; 99:2223–2234.

111 Levy MJ, Jondal ML, Clain J, et al. Preliminary experience with an EUS-guided Trucut biopsy needle compared with EUS-guided FNA. Gastrointest Endosc 2003; 57:101–106.

112 Larghi A, Verna EC, Stavropoulos SN, et al. EUS-guided Trucut needle biopsies in patients with solid pancreatic masses: a prospective study. Gastrointest Endosc 2004; 59:185–190.

113 Varadarajulu S, Fraig M, Schmulewitz N, et al. Comparison of EUS-guided 19-gauge Trucut needle biopsy with EUS-guided fine-needle aspiration. Endoscopy 2004; 36:397–401.

114 Tada M, Komatsu Y, Kawabe T, et al. Quantitative analysis of K-ras gene mutation in pancreatic tissue obtained by endoscopic ultrasonography-guided fine needle aspiration: clinical utility for diagnosis of pancreatic tumor. Am J Gastroenterol 2002; 97:2263–2270.

115 Chhieng DC, Benson E, Eltoum I, et al. MUC1 and MUC2 expression in pancreatic ductal carcinoma obtained by fine-needle aspiration. Cancer 2003; 99:365–371.

116 Jensen RT, Norton JA. Pancreatic endocrine tumors. In: Feldman M, Scharschmidt BF, Sleisenger MH, eds. Sleisenger and Fordtran's gastrointestinal and liver disease, 7th edn. Philadelphia: WB Saunders; 2002:988–1016.

117 Modlin IM, Tang LH. Approaches to the diagnosis of gut neuroendocrine tumors: the last word (today). Gastroenterology 1997; 112:583–590.

118 Madura JA, Cummings OW, Wiebke EA, et al. Nonfunctioning islet cell tumors of the pancreas: a difficult diagnosis but one worth the effort. Am Surg 1997; 63:573–578.

119 Lam KY, Lo CY. Pancreatic endocrine tumor: a 22-year clinicopathological experience with morphological, immunohistochemical observation and a review of the literature. Eur J Surg Oncol 1997; 23:36–42.

120 Kloppel G, Heitz PU. Pancreatic endocrine tumors. Pathol Res Pract 1988; 183:155–168.

121 Schindl M, Kaczirek K, Kaserer K, et al. Is the new classification of neuroendocrine pancreatic tumors of clinical help? World J Surg 2000; 24:1312–1318.

122 Akerstrom G, Hellman P, Hessman O, et al. Surgical treatment of endocrine pancreatic tumours. Neuroendocrinology. 2004; 80(Suppl 1):62–66.

123 Azimuddin K, Chamberlain RS. The surgical management of pancreatic neuroendocrine tumors. Surg Clin North Am 2001; 81:511–525.

124 Rosch T, Lightdale CJ, Botet JF, et al. Localization of pancreatic endocrine tumors by endoscopic ultrasonography. N Engl J Med 1992; 326:1721–1726.

125 Palazzo L, Roseau G, Chaussade S, et al. Pancreatic endocrine tumors: contribution of ultrasound endoscopy in the diagnosis of localization. Ann Chir 1993; 47:419–424.

126 Zimmer T, Stolzel U, Bader M, et al. Endoscopic ultrasonography and somatostatin receptor scintigraphy in the preoperative localisation of insulinomas and gastrinomas. Gut 1996; 39:562–568.

127 Proye C, Malvaux P, Pattou F, et al. Noninvasive imaging of insulinomas and gastrinomas with endoscopic ultrasonography and somatostatin receptor scintigraphy. Surgery 1998; 124:1134–1143, discussion 1143–1144.

128 De Angelis C, Carucci P, Repici A, et al. Endosonography in decision making and management of gastrointestinal endocrine tumors. Eur J Ultrasound 1999; 10:139–150.

129 Ardengh JC, Rosenbaum P, Ganc AJ, et al. Role of EUS in the preoperative localization of insulinomas compared with spiral CT. Gastrointest Endosc 2000; 51:552–555.

130 Anderson MA, Carpenter S, Thompson NW, et al. Endoscopic ultrasound is highly accurate and directs management in patients with neuroendocrine tumors of the pancreas. Am J Gastroenterol 2000; 95:2271–2277.

131 Gouya H, Vignaux O, Augui J, et al. CT, endoscopic sonography, and a combined protocol for preoperative evaluation of pancreatic insulinomas. AJR Am J Roentgenol 2003; 181:987–992.

132 Semelka RC, Custodio CM, Cem Balci N, et al. Neuroendocrine tumors of the pancreas: spectrum of appearances on MRI. Magn Reson Imaging 2000; 11:141–148.

133 Van Nieuwenhove Y, Vandaele S, Op de Beeck B, et al. Neuroendocrine tumors of the pancreas. Surg Endosc 2003; 17:1658–1662.

134 Thoeni RF, Mueller-Lisse UG, Chan R, et al. Detection of small, functional islet cell tumors in the pancreas: selection of MR imaging sequences for optimal sensitivity. Radiology 2000; 214:483–490.

135 Baba Y, Miyazono N, Nakajo M, et al. Localization of insulinomas. Comparison of conventional arterial stimulation with venous sampling (ASVS) and superselective ASVS. Acta Radiol 2000; 41:172–177.

136 Wiesli P, Brandle M, Schmid C, et al. Selective arterial calcium stimulation and hepatic venous sampling in the evaluation of hyperinsulinemic hypoglycemia: potential and limitations. J Vasc Interv Radiol 2004; 15:1251–1256.

137 van Eijck CH, Lamberts SW, Lemaire LC, et al. The use of somatostatin receptor scintigraphy in the differential diagnosis of pancreatic duct cancers and islet cell tumors. Ann Surg 1996; 224:119–124.

138 Gibril F, Reynolds JC, Doppman JL, et al. Somatostatin receptor scintigraphy: its sensitivity compared with that of other imaging methods in detecting primary and metastatic gastrinomas. A prospective study. Ann Intern Med 1996; 125:26–34.

139 Bansal R, Tierney W, Carpenter S, et al. Cost effectiveness of EUS for preoperative localization of pancreatic endocrine tumors. Gastrointest Endosc 1999; 49:19–25.

140 Ardengh JC, de Paulo GA, Ferrari AP. EUS-guided FNA in the diagnosis of pancreatic neuroendocrine tumors before surgery. Gastrointest Endosc 2004; 60:378–384.

141 Ginès A, Vazquez-Sequeiros E, Soria MT, et al. Usefulness of EUS-guided fine needle aspiration (EUS-FNA) in the diagnosis of functioning neuroendocrine tumors. Gastrointest Endosc 2002; 56:291–296.

142 Roland CF, van Heerden JA. Nonpancreatic primary tumors with metastasis to the pancreas. Surg Gynecol Obstet 1989; 168:345–347.

143 Nakeeb A, Lillemoe KD, Cameron JL. The role of pancreaticoduodenectomy for locally recurrent or metastatic carcinoma to the periampullary region. J Am Coll Surg 1995; 180:180–192.

144 Sperti C, Pasquali C, Liessi G, et al. Pancreatic resection for metastatic tumors. J Surg Oncol 2003; 83:161–166.

145 Z'graggen K, Fernandez-del Castillo C, et al. Metastases to the pancreas and their surgical extirpation. Arch Surg 1998; 133:413–417, discussion 418–419.

146 Ghavamian R, Klein KA, Stephens DH, et al. Renal cell carcinoma metastatic to the pancreas: clinical and radiological features. Mayo Clin Proc 2000; 75:581–585.

147 Faure JP, Tuech JJ, Richer JP, et al. Pancreatic metastasis of renal cell carcinoma: presentation, treatment and survival. J Urol 2001; 165:20–22.

148 Palazzo L, Borotto E, Cellier C, et al. Endosonographic features of pancreatic metastases. Gastrointest Endosc 1996; 44:433–436.

149 DeWitt J, Jowell P, LeBlanc J, et al. EUS-guided FNA of pancreatic metastases: a multicenter experience. Gastrointest Endosc 2005; 61:689–696.

150 Béchade D, Palazzo L, Fabre M, et al. EUS-guided FNA of pancreatic metastasis from renal cell carcinoma. Gastrointest Endosc 2003; 58:784–788.

151 Fritscher-Ravens A, Sriram PV, Krause C, et al. Detection of pancreatic metastases by EUS-guided fine-needle aspiration. Gastrointest Endosc 2001; 53:65–70.

152 DeWitt JM, Chappo J, Sherman S. EUS-FNA of metastatic malignant melanoma to the pancreas: report of two cases and review. Endoscopy 2003; 35:219–222.

153 DeWitt J, Ghorai S, Kahi C, et al. EUS-FNA of recurrent postoperative extraluminal or metastatic malignancy. Gastrointest Endosc 2003; 58:542–548.

154 Hayes DH, Bolton JS, Wilis GW, et al. Carcinoma of the ampulla of Vater. Ann Surg 1987; 206:572–577.

155 Akwari OE, van Heerden JA, Adson MA, et al. Radical pancreatoduodenectomy for cancer of the papilla of Vater. Arch Surg 1977; 112:451–456.

156 Sperti C, Pasquali C, Piccoli A, et al. Radical resection for ampullary carcinoma: long-term results. Br J Surg 1994; 81:668–671.

157 Cheng CL, Sherman S, Fogel EL, et al. Endoscopic snare papillectomy for tumors of the duodenal papillae. Gastrointest Endosc 2004; 60:757–764.

158 Posner S, Colletti L, Knol J, et al. Safety and long-term efficacy of transduodenal excision for tumors of the ampulla of Vater. Surgery 2000; 128:694–701.

159 Mitake M, Nakazawa S, Tsukamoto Y, et al. Endoscopic ultrasonography in the diagnosis of depth invasion and lymph node metastasis of carcinoma of the papilla of Vater. J Ultrasound Med 1990; 9:645–650.

160 Zhang Q, Nian W, Zhang L, et al. Endoscopic ultrasonography assessment in preoperative staging for carcinoma of ampulla of Vater and extrahepatic bile duct. Chin Med J (Engl) 1996; 109:622–625.

161 Sauvanet A, Chapuis O, Hammel P, et al. Are endoscopic procedures able to predict the benignity of ampullary tumors? Am J Surg 1997; 174:355–358.

162 Menzel J, Hoepffner N, Sulkowski U, et al. Polypoid tumors of the major duodenal papilla: preoperative staging with intraductal US, EUS, and CT – a prospective, histopathologically controlled study. Gastrointest Endosc 1999; 50:27–33.

163 Cannon ME, Carpenter SL, Elta GH, et al. EUS compared with CT, magnetic resonance imaging, and angiography and the influence of biliary stenting on staging accuracy of ampullary neoplasms. Gastrointest Endosc 1999; 49:349–357.

164 Kubo H, Chijiiwa Y, Akahoshi K, et al. Pre-operative staging of ampullary tumours by endoscopic ultrasound. Br J Radiol 1999; 72:443–447.

165 Chen CH, Tseng LJ, Yang CC, et al. The accuracy of endoscopic ultrasound, endoscopic retrograde cholangiopancreatography, computed tomography, and transabdominal ultrasound in the detection and staging of primary ampullary tumors. Clin Ultrasound 2001; 29:313–321.

166 Skordilis P, Mouzas IA, Dimoulios PD, et al. Is endosonography an effective method for detection and local staging of the ampullary carcinoma? A prospective study. BMC Surg 2002; 2:1–8.

Chapter

17 EUS in the Evaluation of Pancreatic Cysts

Anne Marie Lennon and Ian D. Penman

KEY POINTS

- The differential diagnosis of pancreatic cystic lesions is wide: the vast majority are pseudocysts, but detection of mucinous neoplasms is most important as these may be malignant or have malignant potential.

- The diagnostic accuracy of EUS morphologic features is limited, as is the value of fluid cytology and measurement of tumor markers.

- A combination of EUS features, fluid cytology, and carcinoembryonic or amylase levels may improve accuracy in detecting (potentially) malignant lesions.

- Fine-needle aspiration of cystic lesions under antibiotic cover is safe, with low rates of bleeding, infection, and pancreatitis.

- Accurate diagnosis and management of pancreatic cystic lesions require careful evaluation of the clinical setting, other imaging modalities, and multidisciplinary collaboration.

INTRODUCTION

Pancreatic cystic lesions, once thought to be rare, are now detected more frequently as a result of the increased use of high-resolution computed tomography (CT) and magnetic resonance imaging (MRI). The vast majority (80–90%) of these lesions are pseudocysts; congenital or simple cysts and other rarities account for around 10%. Cystic neoplasms, mainly serous cystadenoma, mucinous cystadenoma, mucinous cystadenocarcinoma, and intraductal papillary mucinous neoplasia (IPMN), comprise the remaining 10%.[1]

Despite advances in CT and MRI, the ability of cross-sectional modalities to characterize these lesions correctly, and to differentiate between benign and malignant lesions, remains limited. EUS is ideally suited to imaging pancreatic lesions because of its high resolution and ability to sample cystic lesions or adjacent lymph nodes. This chapter discusses the different types of pancreatic cystic lesions, their endosonographic features, and the role of fine-needle aspiration (FNA) for cytologic and tumor marker analysis. A diagnostic approach to patients

with pancreatic cysts is also described. The EUS features of pseudocysts are described, but therapy of these is discussed further in Chapter 25 and solid pancreatic tumors are discussed in Chapter 16.

EUS AND OTHER IMAGING MODALITIES

The differential diagnosis of pancreatic cystic lesions is wide (Table 17.1). Management and outcome depend on accurate characterization of these lesions as mucinous lesions have malignant potential and should be treated by surgical excision, whereas serous cystadenomas are benign and rarely become malignant.

Most studies of the diagnostic accuracy of non-invasive imaging using ultrasonography (US), CT, and MRI have been small retrospective case series containing different lesion types, and few well designed prospective studies have been reported. Not surprisingly, therefore, reported accuracies vary widely, from 20% to 88%,[2,3] and it is difficult to draw meaningful conclusions. In a prospective study of 100 serous cystadenomas (with histologic confirmation in 68), however, the accuracies of US, CT, and MRI were 53%, 54%, and 74%, respectively,[4] highlighting the limitations of cross-sectional imaging, even in this homogeneous and well characterized study population. Published studies of the diagnostic accuracy of transabdominal US, CT, and MRI have been summarized recently by Brugge et al.[5] (Table 17.2).

Although numerous case series of the performance of EUS in evaluating these lesions have also been reported, they too suffer from the same limitations of small size, retrospective design, lack of blinding, and often lack of histologic confirmation. Furthermore, few studies directly comparing EUS and CT/MRI have been published so far. Of the two large prospective series reported to date, Brugge et al.[6] conducted a multicenter collaborative study to determine the most accurate combination of EUS features, cytologic findings, and cyst fluid tumor markers for differentiating mucinous lesions from other types. A total of 341 patients underwent EUS and FNA with measurement of carcinoembryonic antigen (CEA), CA72-4, CA125, CA19-9, and CA15-3 concentrations. Some 112 of these patients subsequently underwent surgical resection, and the accuracy of EUS morphology was only 51%, with cytology faring little better at 59%. A CEA concentration above 192 ng/ml was 79% accurate for distinguishing mucinous lesions and, perhaps surprisingly, no combination of tests performed better

CLASSIFICATION OF PANCREATIC CYSTIC LESIONS

Type of lesion	Percentage of cases
Pseudocysts	80–90
Neoplastic	5–10
Serous cystadenoma	
Mucinous cystadenoma	
Mucinous cystadenocarcinoma	
Intraductal papillary mucinous neoplasm (IPMN)	
Cystic endocrine tumor	
Solid and pseudopapillary neoplasm	
Acinar cell cystadenocarcinoma	
Congenital	5–10
'Simple' cyst	
Polycystic disease	
Cystic fibrosis	
Von Hippel–Lindau associated cysts	
Other	
Parasitic infection (e.g., amebiasis, *Ascaris*)	

Table 17.1 Classification of pancreatic cystic lesions

than cyst fluid CEA concentration alone. The role of tumor markers is discussed in more detail below.

A similar single-center French study of 67 patients found that the overall accuracy of EUS morphology for all types of cystic lesion was 73%,[7] with significant variations according to lesion type. Sensitivity for serous lesions was only 43%, whereas that for mucinous cystadenomas was 65% and for cystadenocarcinomas 88%. In contrast to the US study, the

sensitivities of cytology for mucinous, malignant mucinous, serous lesions, and pseudocysts, respectively, were 94%, 100%, 100%, and 100%. The specificity for all these lesions was, as expected, 98–100%. A broad panel of tumor markers was analyzed and, although a low CEA level (<5 ng/ml) was predictive of serous lesions and a high amylase or lipase concentration was associated with pseudocysts, tumor marker analysis contributed little to the results of cytology.

CONGENITAL OR 'SIMPLE' CYSTS

These are usually seen as a coincidental finding during CT imaging of the abdomen. They can occur as part of the spectrum of adult polycystic kidney disease and also in von Hippel–Lindau syndrome (Fig. 17.1), although serous cystadenomas also occur in the latter. The clinical importance of small, simple-looking cysts discovered incidentally (Fig. 17.2) is unknown, and no observational follow-up studies have been performed to date. At EUS, these cysts are usually small, thin walled, and uniformly anechoic, with no mural nodularity or papillary elements. The surrounding pancreas shows no features of chronic pancreatitis, and, if aspirated, the fluid is bland looking, containing only small numbers of inflammatory cells and low concentrations of CEA and amylase.

PSEUDOCYSTS

Accounting for approximately 80% of pancreatic cystic lesions, these usually occur in the setting of an episode of acute pancreatitis, or insidiously in patients with chronic pancreatitis, mostly in middle-aged men. Knowledge of the clinical presentation is therefore essential in aiding accurate differentiation of pseudocysts from cystic neoplasms. Pseudocysts lack a true

STUDIES OF DIAGNOSTIC ACCURACY OF EUS IN PANCREATIC CYSTIC LESIONS

Reference	Year	Technique	No. of patients	Histologic confirmation	Accuracy of EUS (%)	Accuracy of cytology (%)
Brugge et al.[6 a]	2004	EUS-FNA	341	112	51	59
Frossard et al.[7 a]	2003	EUS-FNA	127	67	77	97
Sedlack et al.[42]	2002	EUS-FNA	34	34	82	55
Hernandez et al.[63]	2002	EUS-FNA	43	9	Predicted malignancy in 8/9	Sensitivity for malignancy 2/9
Gress et al.[17]	2000	EUS	35	35	Not stated	–
Koito et al.[41]	1997	EUS	52	52	92–96 (for neoplastic lesions)	–
Ahmad et al.[43]	2001	EUS	98	48	No features predictive of malignancy	–
Ahmad et al.[44]	2003	EUS	31	31	40–93 Interobserver variation ++	–
Chatelain et al.[80]	2002	EUS	8	8	Not stated	–

Table 17.2 Studies of diagnostic accuracy of EUS in pancreatic cystic lesions
[a] Prospective studies.
Adapted from Brugge et al.[5] With permission from American Society for Gastrointestinal Endoscopy.

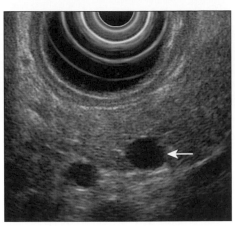

Fig. 17.1 Simple pancreatic cyst. A thin-walled and simple-looking 5-mm cyst (arrow) is seen in the pancreatic body. There is no solid mural component, no debris within the cyst, no mass lesion, and the surrounding pancreatic parenchyma is normal.

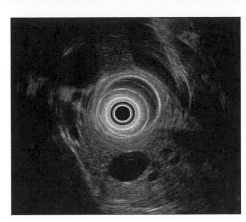

Fig. 17.2 Von Hippel–Lindau syndrome (VHL). A simple 1-cm cyst is seen in the pancreatic body in a patient with VHL. Cysts may be numerous, but are either simple or benign serous cystadenomas in the pancreas, despite the high risk of malignancy elsewhere in this condition.

epithelial lining, the wall consisting of inflammatory and fibrous tissue. This is thin in early pseudocysts but, as they mature, the wall may become thick. Pseudocysts are often extremely large, but usually unilocular and anechoic (Fig. 17.3). The fluid density, however, may increase if necrotic debris or infection is present, and occasionally this may lead to suspicion of a cystic neoplasm (Figs 17.4 & 17.5). Septations are rare but do occur (Fig. 17.6); there may be features of acute or chronic pancreatitis elsewhere in the gland; and it may be possible to demonstrate direct communication with the pancreatic duct – features that support a diagnosis of pseudocyst over neoplasm. Other features that should be noted are the distance between the intestinal wall and cyst lumen, and the presence of interposed (by Doppler examination) or collateral vessels as evidence of segmental portal hypertension secondary to portal vein or splenic vein thrombosis. Lymph nodes that appear to be inflamed may also be seen adjacent to the pseudocyst.

Because pseudocysts lack an epithelial lining, no epithelial cells should be present in FNA samples, unless there is contamination of the needle with gastric or duodenal epithelium during puncture. Aspirated fluid is of low viscosity, often dark, turbid or even bloody, and contains inflammatory cells such as macrophages and histiocytes. Raised amylase (>5000 U/ml) and lipase (>2000 U/ml) concentrations are present, but levels of other tumor markers should be low, although increased CEA levels have been reported when infection is present.

SEROUS CYSTADENOMA

Serous cystadenomas are the commonest form of cystadenoma, accounting for 10–45% of cases. They are much commoner in women and classically occur (>80%) in the body or tail of the pancreas,[8] although some authors report a greater preponderance in the head and neck.[9,10] Serous cystadenomas classically consist of well demarcated microcystic (<2 cm) lesions (Figs 17.7 & 17.8) with thin septa.[11] In a small proportion of cases, the cysts are associated with central fibrosis or calcification.[12,13] Solid and macrocystic serous cystadenomas have also been described, with the solid appearance resulting from coalescence of multiple tiny (1–2 mm) cysts.[14–16] The appearance of focal cyst wall nodularity or thickening, intracystic mucin or floating debris, echogenic ductal wall thickening, or pancreatic duct dilatation is unusual and suggests the possibility of an

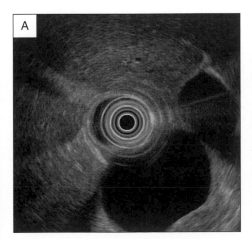

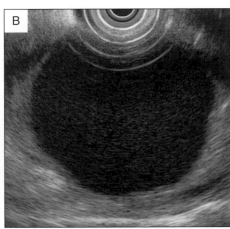

Fig. 17.3 Pseudocysts. **A,** Radial EUS in a patient with a recent episode of pancreatitis reveals a 3-cm, thin-walled, anechoic cystic lesion in close contact with the gastric wall. **B,** Similar findings in another patient with chronic abdominal pain, who presented with chronic pancreatitis and a pseudocyst.

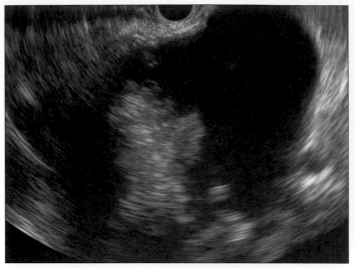

Fig. 17.4 Infected pseudocyst in a patient with severe acute pancreatitis and fever. The irregular hyperechoic material seen within the cyst raises the suspicion of a cystic neoplasm but it is not murally based. FNA cytology revealed only macrophages and debris; the amylase concentration was greater than 6000 U/ml.

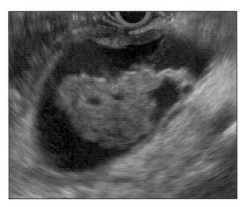

Fig. 17.5 Atypical appearance of pseudocyst. The patient presented with chronic abdominal pain and weight loss. The EUS appearances are suspicious for a mucinous neoplasm, but FNA revealed old blood-stained fluid with inflammatory cells, low CEA levels, and an amylase concentration greater than 66 000 U/ml. Because of ongoing concerns, the lesion was resected and a pseudocyst confirmed.

underlying mucinous tumor.[2,13,15,17–19] The morphologic characteristics of serous cystadenomas are often diagnostic of the lesion.[16] Nevertheless, cytology may improve the diagnostic accuracy of EUS. FNA can be difficult owing to the small size of the cysts coupled with the vascular nature of these lesions. The cytologic appearances are of a serous fluid containing small cuboidal cells that stain for glycogen but not mucin. The fluid classically contains low amylase, CA15-3, CA72-4, and CEA concentrations.[20–22] The prognosis is usually excellent, although a 3% risk of malignancy was reported in one study, with few pathologic features to differentiate benign from malignant lesions, the latter becoming apparent only when subsequent metastases appeared.[23]

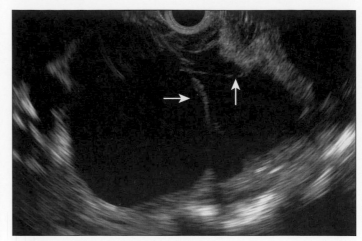

Fig. 17.6 Thin-walled internal septations (arrows) in a patient with a longstanding pseudocyst.

MUCINOUS CYSTADENOMA AND ADENOCARCINOMA

Mucinous cystic lesions are rarer than serous cystadenomas, accounting for approximately 10% of cystic neoplasms, and, unlike serous cystadenomas, are either malignant or have potential for malignant transformation. They occur most often in young or middle-aged women (90%), with solitary cysts being found in the body and tail of the pancreas. The morphologic appearances are of macrocystic (>2 cm) lesions with few septations (Fig. 17.9).[17,21] Peripheral calcification, which is found in 15% of patients, is highly suggestive but may also be seen in solid and pseudopapillary neoplasms.[13,24] The presence of other cystic lesions or a dilated pancreatic duct is

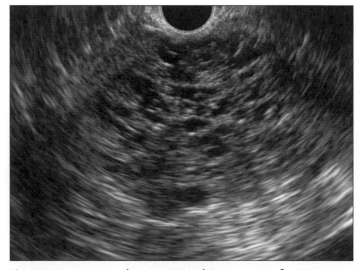

Fig. 17.7 Serous cystadenoma. Typical appearance of a 2.5-cm microcystic serous cystadenoma. There are multiple small, anechoic cystic areas and a 'honeycomb' appearance. This lesion does not show the central area of fibrosis or calcification that is sometimes present.

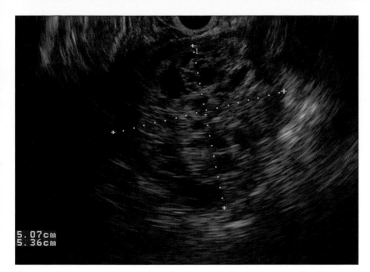

Fig. 17.8 A 5-cm serous cystadenoma in the pancreatic body. Note the numerous small cysts with thin septations.

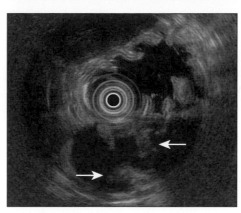

Fig. 17.10 Mucinous cystadenoma. Villiform solid tissue is seen projecting into the cyst cavity (arrows).

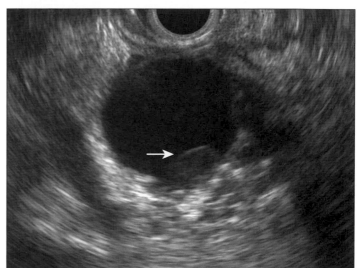

Fig. 17.11 Mucinous cystadenoma. A small mural nodule is seen (arrow) in this 15-mm lesion. Mucin stain of aspirated fluid was positive, but CEA and amylase concentrations were not raised.

unusual, and, if present, an intraductal papillary mucinous neoplasm (IPMN) should be considered. The risk of malignancy increases with larger lesions[25] and the presence of an irregular or thickened cyst wall, solid regions within the cysts, an adjacent solid mass (Figs 17.10 & 17.11), or a strictured, obstructed or displaced pancreatic duct suggests malignant transformation.[17,26,27] FNA can be useful in confirming the diagnosis. The cyst wall and septa should be sampled, in addition to aspirating the fluid. This can be difficult because of the viscous nature of the fluid, but is easier when a 19-G needle is used. Cytology demonstrates viscous fluid containing mucin and columnar epithelial cells. The presence of columnar cells is not pathognomonic as they are also found in IPMN.[28] The presence of columnar epithelial cells from the stomach or duodenum can further complicate the cytologic interpretation, and care should be taken to avoid contamination of the cyst fluid by using a stylet during initial cyst puncture.

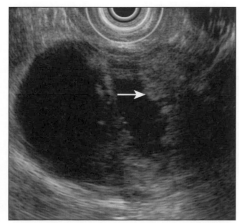

Fig. 17.9 Mucinous cystadenoma. Numerous solid, papillary projections from the cyst wall are seen (arrow). FNA revealed mucin-positive cuboidal cells, and resection confirmed a benign mucinous cystadenoma.

INTRADUCTAL PAPILLARY MUCINOUS NEOPLASIA

IPMN is relatively rare, accounting for 1–3% of pancreatic exocrine tumors.[29,30] It has a slight female preponderance, with a peak in the sixth decade, and occurs most frequently in the head of the pancreas. Endoscopic appearances include the presence of a dilated main pancreatic duct or side-branch, depending on the site of the tumor.[15,17,31] A gaping papilla extruding mucus ('mucinous ductal ectasia') is found in 25–50% of patients.[32] A communication between side and main duct branches is a feature, although this is not always present as it can be obstructed by mucin. Filling defects in the pancreatic duct at endoscopic retrograde cholangiopancreatography (ERCP) can result from tumor nodules or mucus plugs in the ducts. IPMN can sometimes present as a solid mass, although this is rare. It can be associated with parenchymal changes due to obstruction of the duct, and this can make it difficult to differentiate from chronic pancreatitis. The presence of features such as a focal hypoechoic mass, mural nodules (Fig. 17.12), or a large unilocular cystic component are suggestive of malignancy.[33] Higher-frequency intraductal ultrasound catheter probes have been used in some studies to characterize IPMN, and may be able to provide extra information about the longitudinal extent of duct involvement, the presence of mural nodules, and invasion of the pancreatic parenchyma.[34]

IPMNs are clinically and pathologically heterogeneous. The degree of cytologic atypia can vary from minimal to severe or frankly malignant, with features resembling mucinous cystic neoplasms or even ductal adenocarcinoma. Different patterns of mucin immunohistochemistry have been observed,[35] but whether or not these are prognostically important is unknown. Little is known about tumor markers in these lesions; the patterns reported are generally similar to mucinous neoplasms, although a high amylase concentration may be seen, in keeping with an origin from, or communication with, the pancreatic duct. Prognosis is generally good.

SOLID AND PSEUDOPAPILLARY NEOPLASM

Once thought to be rare, this distinctive lesion is now better recognized and increasingly reported; it accounts for 10% of cystic pancreatic tumors. It is usually discovered incidentally in young women, can occur anywhere in the pancreas, and may be very large. In some patients, symptoms related to the size of the tumor or pain from bleeding into it can be the presentation. The hallmark is central hemorrhagic cystic degeneration and a pseudocapsule that may calcify. Thus, solid, cystic, and 'pseudopapillary' areas may all be seen. The cell of origin is unknown but has eosinophilic cytoplasm and mixed immuno-

histochemical features of endocrine, epithelial, and mesenchymal differentiation. These are slow-growing tumors and, when resected, the prognosis is excellent.

Only a few case reports and small case series of either abdominal US or EUS have been reported.[36,37] Lesions are usually well demarcated, may appear solid or mixed solid–cystic, with or without septations, and peripheral calcification may limit examination of the internal echostructure. The hemorrhagic degeneration often results in a bloody, necrotic FNA sample, which can provide a clue to the diagnosis, although histology is usually characteristic.

CYSTIC ENDOCRINE TUMORS

Most neuroendocrine tumors of the pancreas are solid, but uncommonly may be cystic, either primarily or secondary to cystic degeneration. The EUS features are variable and cytology reveals a homogeneous population of small cells with little cytoplasm. Little information exists about tumor marker levels in these lesions.

OTHER CYSTIC LESIONS

Ductal adenocarcinoma of the pancreas may occasionally show cystic degeneration, which can confuse the clinical picture. Many other cystic lesions of the pancreas have been reported as rarities, including dermoid cysts, metastases to the pancreas, and parasitic infections (e.g., amebiasis, *Ascaris* infection). These possibilities should always be borne in mind, especially when the clinical and imaging features are not typical of the more common cystic lesions.

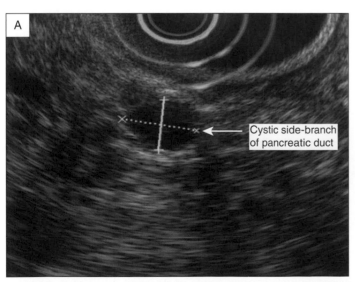

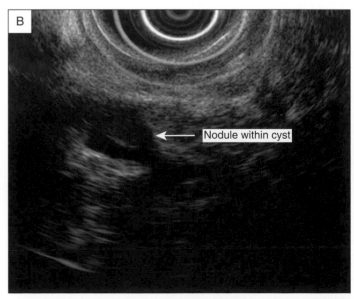

Fig. 17.12 A, This cystic dilation of a side-branch of the pancreatic duct represents the side-branch form of intraductal papillary mucinous neoplasia (IPMN). This is thought to be a more benign form of IPMN, but patients should be followed for the development of a nodule within the cyst (**B**). If this develops, it is thought to indicate a high risk of progression to cancer.

ENDOSONOGRAPHIC APPEARANCES OF CYSTIC LESIONS

A detailed description of the endosonographic approach to examining the pancreas is described in Chapter 14, and FNA techniques are described in Chapter 22. The general endosonographic approach to pancreatic cystic lesions is described below, and the appearances of specific pancreatic cystic lesions are described above.

When a cystic lesion has been identified, the size, exact location, relation to adjacent vessels and organs, and presence of locoregional or distant metastases should be noted as this information may influence management.[38–40] The cyst itself should be examined to determine the wall thickness, presence of focal irregularity, papillary projections, or an associated mass. Cyst size, thickness of any septations, the presence of echodense mucus or debris should also be assessed as these features are more often reported in malignant cystic tumors.

Several authors have tried to determine EUS features that are predictive of malignancy.[17,19,41,42] Koito et al.[41] found that a thick wall or septa, protruding tumor, or microcystic type were associated with malignancy, whereas thin septa and simple-looking cysts were benign. They found this system to have an accuracy of 96% and 92% for malignant and benign lesions, respectively. Gress et al.[17] reported that mucinous cystadenocarcinomas were more likely to be characterized by a hypoechoic cystic–solid mass or complex cyst, and were frequently associated with a dilated main pancreatic duct. Benign mucinous ductal ectasia (IPMN) was characterized by a dilated main pancreatic duct in conjunction with hyperechoic thickening of the duct wall. Intraductal papillary carcinoma had similar features, but additionally revealed a hypoechoic mass. Sedlack et al.[42] found that a wall thickness of 3 mm or more, macrosepation (cyst compartment >10 mm), a mass or intramural growth, or cystic dilation of the main pancreatic duct predicated a malignant or potentially malignant cystic lesion with an overall accuracy of 82%. Song et al.[19] examined endoscopic appearances that could differentiate cystic tumors from pseudocysts and found that parenchymal changes, septa, and mural nodules were independent predictors for cystic tumors.

Not all studies, however, have confirmed that endosonographic appearances alone can reliably differentiate benign from malignant cystic lesions.[43] Interobserver agreement in examining different endoscopic features and differentiating neoplastic from non-neoplastic pancreatic cystic lesions has been shown to be moderately good in detecting a solid component, fair for the presence of an abnormal pancreatic duct, debris, or septations, and only fair for the diagnosis of neoplastic versus non-neoplastic lesions.[44] As discussed above, a large prospective mulicenter US study[6] found that the accuracy of EUS imaging features for diagnosing mucinous lesions was only 51% and so, despite its high resolution, sonographic appearances clearly have limitations. EUS may also be technically challenging in certain situations when the anatomy is altered by previous surgery or compression by a large lesion. EUS imaging is also sometimes limited by attenuation of the ultrasound beam in lesions greater than 6 cm in diameter.

ENDOSCOPIC ULTRASOUND-GUIDED FINE-NEEDLE ASPIRATION

FNA cytology has been safely performed for many years under US, CT, or EUS guidance. The US or CT approach may be hampered when the lesion is small or, in the case of US, where there is intervening gas. Technical difficulties in acquiring specimens can also limit the usefulness of these imaging modalities. CT-guided FNA is associated with a risk of peritoneal dissemination of cancer cells[45,46] and has a false-negative rate of up to 20%.[47] EUS overcomes many of these limitations. Its high definition means that it can visualize lesions as small as 2–3 mm, as well as defining surrounding structures. Its close proximity to the lesion reduces the distance a needle has to travel and minimizes the risk of needle-tract seeding. Although one case of EUS-FNA needle-tract seeding has been reported, the risk is far less than that associated with US-or CT-guided FNA, particularly as the area through which the biopsy is taken is usually resected at any subsequent operation.

EUS-guided FNA is a safe procedure with reported complication rates of less than 1%.[48–53] The yield of fluid is usually small in serous cystadenomas because of their microcystic nature, and aspiration of fluid in mucinous lesions may be difficult because of the fluid viscosity. In this case, or where the lesion is large, aspiration to dryness is easier with a 19-G needle (Fig. 17.13). To minimize the risks of subsequent infection it is recommended that the number of cyst punctures be kept to a minimum (ideally one) and that the cyst is aspirated completely where possible. Antibiotic prophylaxis, usually with intravenous ciprofloxacin prior to the procedure, followed by 3 days of oral ciprofloxacin, is also recommended, although the evidence base to support these recommendations is not strong.

EUS-GUIDED CORE BIOPSIES

Core biopsies of pancreatic tissue and surrounding lymph nodes under US or CT guidance are safe[13,54–56] and, in recent years, needles for core biopsy under EUS guidance have been developed. These have the theoretic advantage over FNA of preserving tissue architecture and may offer diagnostic advantages for lesions such as lymphomas.[55] The reported diagnostic accuracy of EUS 'Quickcore' biopsy versus EUS-FNA for solid pancreatic lesions is variable, with some studies showing superiority over FNA whereas others have found FNA to be more sensitive.[57–59] The use of core biopsy needles may be appropriate when a mass lesion is present, but FNA is necessary to allow fluid sampling for cytology and measurement of tumor markers.

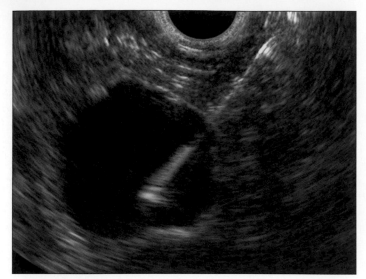

Fig. 17.13 EUS-FNA. Either a 22-G or a 19-G needle can be used. In this case a 22-G needle was sufficient to aspirate the lesion completely. Aspiration should continue until the lesion collapses or no further fluid is obtained. This may reduce the risk of infection and also facilitates FNA of the cyst walls.

COMPLICATIONS OF EUS-FNA OF CYSTIC LESIONS

These are uncommon. Intracystic hemorrhage and infection each occur in less than 1% of cases, and the reported rate of procedure-related pancreatitis is 2–3%.[7,60,61]

CYTOLOGY AND CYST FLUID ANALYSIS

The specificity of cytology in most studies is excellent and approaches 100%, but the sensitivity varies considerably in reported series, reflecting the difficulty of interpreting these lesions, especially when the cellularity of samples is low. Brandwein et al.[62] and Brugge et al.[6] reported sensitivities of 55% and 59%, respectively, for differentiating benign from malignant or potentially malignant pancreatic cystic lesions. This contrasts with studies by Hernandez et al.[63] and Frossard et al.,[7] who demonstrated sensitivities of 89% and 97%, respectively. Reasons for these widely varying results are not clear but may relate to the presence of an experienced cytopathologist in the procedure room. The sensitivity of cytologic aspiration of pancreatic duct fluid has also been examined, again with greatly varying sensitivity, ranging from 21%[64] to 75%.[65]

The sensitivity of cytology can be affected by several factors. Operator experience affects performance,[66,67] and the presence of a cytopathologist during the EUS examination can help to confirm the adequate cellularity of the sample. Sampling error may occur in both microcystic and mucinous lesions where cellular atypia is patchy, leading to false-negative results, and the presence of blood or benign epithelial cells from the gastric or duodenal mucosa can make interpretation difficult or lead to falsely positive results.

ANALYSIS OF CYST FLUID TUMOR MARKERS AND BIOCHEMISTRY

Given the limited sensitivity of cytology, the value of tumor markers in aspirated cyst fluid has been examined. Tumor markers that have been studied include CEA, CA19-9, CA72-4, CA125, and CA15-3. CEA is found in high levels in mucinous tumors, whereas levels are low in pseudocysts (unless infected) and serous cystadenomas.[10,63,68] The sensitivity and specificity of CEA vary depending on the study and the CEA threshold used. A CEA level of less than 5 ng/ml is associated with a sensitivity of 57–100% and a specificity of 77–86% for serous cystadenomas.[20,69] A cut-off of more than 400 ng/ml was associated with 100% specificity in differentiating mucinous cystic neoplasms from pseudocysts in one study,[70] but not in another, where the sensitivity (13%) and specificity (75%) were poor.[7] In the largest prospective study to date, however, Brugge et al.[6] used receiver–operator characteristic curves to determine the optimum cut-off value of CEA, and found this to be 192 ng/ml. This was associated with an accuracy of 79% for differentiating mucinous from other cyst types, significantly better than the accuracy of EUS morphology alone (51%) or cytology (59%). Interstingly, in this study no combination of morphologic features, cytology, and tumor markers was better than CEA alone.

CA19-9 is another tumor marker that has been used to identify cystic pancreatic lesions. Frossard et al.[7] found that a CA19-9 level greater than 50 000 U/ml had 15% sensitivity and 81% specificity in differentiating mucinous cysts from other cystic lesions, whereas it had 86% sensitivity and 85% specificity in distinguishing cystadenocarcinoma from other cystic lesions. The usefulness of CA19-9 may be limited, however, as it is often raised in inflammatory conditions or when biliary obstruction is present.[10,63,71]

Two other tumor markers, CA72-4 and CA15-3, have also been examined. CA72-4 was able to distinguish mucinous cystadenomas from serous cystadenomas and pseudocysts with 63% sensitivity and 98% specificity,[70] whereas others have suggested that CA72-4 is more useful than CEA or CA15-3 estimation, with a sensitivity and specificity of 87.5% and 94%.[72] CA15-3 has also been used to distinguish mucinous cystadenomas from mucinous cystadenocarcinomas. Rubin et al.[73] reported that a threshold of 30 U/ml was associated with 100% sensitivity and 100% specificity. At the present time, however, it has to be concluded that the performance of tumor markers other than CEA is inadequate for diagnostic purposes and measurement of these, outwith research studies, is not justified.

Although they are not tumor markers, amylase and lipase concentrations are often measured. Amylase is found in high concentration in pseudocysts and IPMN,[68] with levels greater than 5000 U/l having quoted sensitivities and specificities of 61–94% and 58–74% for differentiating pseudocysts from other cystic pancreatic tumors.[7,74]

FEATURES OF CYSTIC PANCREATIC LESIONS

	Serous cystadenoma	Mucinous cystadenoma/carcinoma	IPMN	Solid and pseudopapillary neoplasm	Pseudocyst	Simple cyst
Location	Body/tail > head	Body/tail > head	Arise from main duct or side-branch; head > body/tail	Anywhere	Anywhere	Anywhere
Malignant potential	Very low	High	Variable; high	Low (5–10%)	Nil	Nil
EUS features	Multiple small cysts; often microcystic 'honeycomb'; central fibrosis or calcification	Macrocystic (1–3+); can be large; septations; nodularity or papillary projections	Mural nodule or mass arising in dilated main or side-branch of PD	Mixed solid–cystic; hemorrhagic center	Unilocular, variable size and wall thickness; echogenic material; features of acute/chronic pancreatitis	Usually small, thin-walled, uniformly echopoor/anechoic
Communication with PD	Rare	Rare	Yes, often dilated ++	Rare	Sometimes	No
Vascularity	++	++	+/–	+/–	+/– (variable)	–
Cytology	Bland glycogen-positive cuboidal cells	Columnar/cuboidal, mucin-positive cells; may show atypia, dysplasia, or malignant features	Columnar/cuboidal mucin-positive cells; may show atypia, dysplasia, or malignant features	Heterogeneous; eosinophilic, papillary cells, PAS-positive deposits, vimentin positivity	Macrophages, inflammatory cells, debris	Hypocellular, mainly inflammatory cells
Cyst fluid	Small volume, low viscosity	Often large volume, high viscosity	Small volume, high viscosity	Low viscosity, bloody and necrotic	Large volume, low viscosity; may be blood-stained or turbid	Variable volume, low viscosity, pale fluid
Amylase	Low	Low	Variable, often high	Low	High	Low
CEA	Low	Variable, usually high	Variable	Unknown	Low	Low
Other markers	Low	Variable	Variable	Unknown	Variable	Low

Table 17.3 Features of cystic pancreatic lesions
CEA, carcinoembryonic antigen; IPMN, intraductal papillary mucinous neoplasia; PAS, periodic acid–Schiff stain; PD, pancreatic duct.

DIAGNOSTIC APPROACH

Most patients will have already undergone CT prior to being referred for EUS but, if not, a contrast-enhanced helical or multidetector-row CT of the pancreas, surrounding areas and liver is recommended. A standard radial or linear EUS examination of the entire pancreas and surrounding structures is performed and the cystic lesion is then carefully assessed, noting the features listed in Table 17.3 and in the examination checklist at the end of the chapter. If the lesion is clearly a pseudocyst, it is assessed for suitability for endoscopic drainage, either under EUS or endoscopically and, if not being performed at the same procedure, the optimum site for drainage is marked by diathermy, clipping, or submucosal dye injection. If a cystic neoplasm is suspected, or the diagnosis is unclear, EUS-FNA is performed, using a 19- or 22-G needle, and under antibiotic cover. The cyst is completely aspirated if at all possible and the fluid sent for cytologic examination and measurement of amylase and CEA concentrations. The wall of the cyst or any associated mass or lymph nodes also undergo FNA. The patient is observed for 2–4 h after the procedure and is allowed home if well, with written advice about complications and a 3-day supply of oral ciprofloxacin.

FUTURE DEVELOPMENTS

EUS is not without limitations in the evaluation of pancreatic cystic lesions (Table 17.4), and these need to be addressed. Enhanced-power Doppler transabdominal ultrasonography has shown promising results after injection of ultrasound contrast agents in detecting neuroendocrine tumors,[75] and initial studies using EUS are also promising.[76,77] The ability of tumor markers and amylase estimation to identify pancreatic cystic lesions is limited, and alternative markers are needed. Recent studies of molecular markers in DNA aspirated from cyst fluid[78] have described multiple allelic losses at critical sites associated with Ki-*ras* mutations, and reported that these could predict behavior. Further studies of this type are therefore awaited with interest.

At present, surgical resection is the only curative treatment for pancreatic cystic neoplasms, yet carries appreciable morbidity and even mortality, especially in patients who may be of borderline fitness. Carefully conducted long-term EUS follow-up studies of non-resected cysts would be important to understand further the natural history of cystic lesions. Recently, the possibility of endoscopic therapy under EUS has been explored. In a preliminary study, Gan et al.[79] reported the feasibility and safety of EUS-guided alcohol injection into pancreatic cystic

tumors, with short-term resolution in 62% of patients. Larger studies with longer-term follow-up are necessary, and randomized trials of surgical resection versus endoscopic alcohol ablation would also be welcome.

IMPORTANT LIMITATIONS OF EUS IN THE EVALUATION OF PANCREATIC CYSTIC LESIONS	
Procedure aspect	Limitation
Technical	Attenuation of imaging in large (>6 cm) lesions
EUS imaging	Morphologic features of lesions overlap considerably
FNA	Aspiration of viscous fluid with 22-G needles
	Small volumes obtained in microcystic lesions
	Limited accuracy of cytology: contamination with columnar gastroduodenal epithelium; sampling error – dysplasia and malignant change is patchy in mucinous lesions
Amylase concentration	May be raised in lesions that communicate with the pancreatic duct
CEA level	May be raised in infected pseudocysts
Other tumor markers (CA19-9, CA72-4, etc.)	Unproven value; investigational role

Table 17.4 Important limitations of EUS in the evaluation of pancreatic cystic lesions

EXAMINATION CHECKLIST

Localize and describe cyst
- Wall thickness
- Distance from lumen, interposed vessels
- Focal irregularity, papilliary projections, or mural nodules
- Associated mass lesion or central calcification
- Septation(s)
- Debris or echogenic material in cust
- Communication with pancreatic duct

Examine rest of pancreas (see Ch. 14)

EUS-guided FNA biopsy of all solid lesions

EUS-guided FNA of cyst fluid under antibiotic cover, preferably one pass

Empty cyst if possible

Determine CEA and amylase levels, and cytology

REFERENCES

1 Balthazar EJ, Chacko AC. Computed tomography of pancreatic masses. Am J Gastroenterol 1990; 85:343–349.

2 Torresan F, Casadei R, Solmi L, et al. The role of ultrasound in the differential diagnosis of serous and mucinous cystic tumors of the pancreas. Eur J Gastroenterol Hepatol 1997; 9:169–172.

3 Le Borgne J, de Calan L, Partensky C. Cystadenomas and cystadenocarcinomas of the pancreas: a multi-institutional retrospective study of 398 cases. French Surgical Association. Ann Surg 1999; 230:152–161.

4 Bassi C, Salvia R, Molinari E, et al. Management of 100 consecutive cases of pancreatic serous cystadenoma: wait for symptoms and see at imaging or vice versa? World J Surg 2003; 27:319–323.

5 Brugge WR. Evaluation of pancreatic cystic lesions with EUS. Gastrointest Endosc 2004; 59:698–707.

6 Brugge WR, Lewandrowski K, Lee-Lewandrowski E, et al. Diagnosis of pancreatic cystic neoplasms: a report of the cooperative pancreatic cyst study. Gastoenterology 2004; 126:1330–1336.

7 Frossard JL, Amouyal P, Amouyal G, et al. Performance of endosonography-guided fine needle aspiration and biopsy in the diagnosis of pancreatic cystic lesions. Am J Gastroenterol 2003; 98:1516–1524.

8 Pyke CM, van Heerden JA, Colby TV, et al. The spectrum of serous cystadenoma of the pancreas. Clinical, pathologic, and surgical aspects. Ann Surg 1992; 215:132–139.

9 Sarr MG, Kendrick ML, Nagorney DM, et al. Cystic neoplasms of the pancreas: benign to malignant epithelial neoplasms. Surg Clin North Am 2001; 81:497–509.

10 Siech M, Tripp K, Schmidt-Rohlfing B, et al. Cystic tumours of the pancreas: diagnostic accuracy, pathologic observations and surgical consequences. Langenbecks Arch Surg 1998; 383:56–61.

11 Procacci C, Graziani R, Bicego E, et al. Serous cystadenoma of the pancreas: report of 30 cases with emphasis on the imaging findings. J Comput Assist Tomogr 1997; 21:373–382.

12 Warshaw AL, Compton CC, Lewandrowski K, et al. Cystic tumours of the pancreas. New clinical, radiologic, and pathologic observations in 67 patients. Ann Surg 1990; 212:432–443.

13 Johnson CD, Stephens DH, Charboneau JW, et al. Cystic pancreatic tumors: CT and sonographic assessment. AJR Am J Roentgenol 1988; 151:1133–1138.

14 Lewandrowski K, Warshaw A, Compton C. Macrocystic serous cystadenoma of the pancreas: a morphologic variant differing from microcystic adenoma. Hum Pathol 1992; 23:871–875.

15 Ariyama J, Suyama M, Satoh K, et al. Endoscopic ultrasound and intraductal ultrasound in the diagnosis of small pancreatic tumours. Abdom Imaging 1998; 23:380–386.

16 Gouhiri M, Soyer P, Barbagelatta M, et al. Macrocystic serous cystadenoma of the pancreas: CT and endosonographic features. Abdom Imaging 1999; 24:72–74.

17 Gress F, Gottlieb K, Cummings O, et al. Endoscopic ultrasound characteristics of mucinous cystic neoplasms of the pancreas. Am J Gastroenterol 2000; 95:961–965.

18 Brugge WR. The role of EUS in the diagnosis of cystic lesions of the pancreas. Gastrointest Endosc 2000; 52:S18–S22.

19 Song MH, Lee SK, Kim MH, et al. EUS in the evaluation of pancreatic cystic lesions. Gastrointest Endosc 2003; 57:891–896.

20 Carlson SK, Johnson CD, Brandt KR, et al. Pancreatic cystic neoplasms: the role and sensitivity of needle aspiration and biopsy. Abdom Imaging 1998; 23:387–393.

21 Jones EC, Suen KC, Grant DR, et al. Fine needle aspiration cytology of neoplastic cysts of the pancreas. Diagn Cytopathol 1987; 3:238–243.

22 Centeno BA, Lewandrowski, KB, Warshaw AL, et al. Cyst fluid cytologic analysis in the differential diagnosis of pancreatic cystic lesions. Am J Clin Pathol 1994; 101:483–487.

23 Strobel O, Z'graggen K, Schmitz-Winnenthal FH, et al. Risk of malignancy in serous cystic neoplasms of the pancreas. Digestion 2003; 68:24–33.

24 Sarr MG, Carpenter HA, Prabhakar LP, et al. Clinical and pathologic correlation of 84 mucinous cystic neoplasms of the pancreas: can one reliably differentiate benign from malignant (or premalignant) neoplasms? Ann Surg 2000; 231:205–212.

25 Thompson LD, Becker RC, Przygodzki RM, et al. Mucinous cystic neoplasm (mucinous cystadenocarcinoma of low-grade malignant potential) of the pancreas: a clinicopathologic study of 130 cases. Am J Surg Pathol 1999; 23:1–16.

26 Zamboni G, Scarpa A, Bogina G, et al. Mucinous cystic tumors of the pancreas: clinicopathological features, prognosis, and relationship to other mucinous cystic tumors. Am J Surg Pathol 1999; 23:410–422.

27 Fernandez-del Castillo C, Warshaw AL. Cystic tumors of the pancreas. Surg Clin North Am 1995; 75:1001–1016.

28 Sperti C, Pasquali C, Guolo P, et al. Serum tumor markers and cyst fluid analysis are useful for the diagnosis of pancreatic cystic tumors. Cancer 1996; 78:237–243.

29 Kloppel G. Pancreatic, non-endocrine tumours. In: Kloppel G, Heitz PU, eds. Pancreatic pathology. Edinburgh: Churchill-Livingstone; 1984:79–113.

30 Sugiyama M, Atomi Y. Extrapancreatic neoplasms occur with unusual frequency in patients with intraductal papilary mucinous tumors of the pancreas. Am J Gastroenterol 1999; 94:470–473.

31 Inui K, Nakazawa S, Yoshino J, et al. Mucin-producing tumor of the pancreas – intraluminal ultrasonography. Hepatogastroenterology 1998; 45:1996–2000.

32 Seo DW, Kang GH. Twenty-six cases of mucinous ductal ectasia of the pancreas. Gastrointest Endosc 1999; 50:592–594.

33 Maeshiro K, Nakayama Y, Yasunami Y, et al. Diagnosis of mucin-producing tumor of the pancreas by balloon-catheter endoscopic retrograde pancreatography – compression study. Hepatogastroenterology 1998; 45:1986–1995.

34 Hara T, Yamaguchi T, Ishihara T, et al. Diagnosis and patient management of intraductal papillary–mucinous tumor of the pancreas by using peroral pancreatoscopy and intraductal ultrasonography. Gastroenterology 2002; 122:34–43.

35 Luttges J, Zamboni G, Longnecker D, et al. The immunohistochemical mucin expression pattern distinguishes different types of intraductal papillary mucinous neoplasms of the pancreas and determines their relationship to mucinous noncystic carcinoma and ductal adenocarcinoma. Am J Surg Pathol 2001; 25:942–948.

36 Lee DH, Yi BH, Lim JW, et al. Sonographic findings of solid and papillary epithelial neoplasm of the pancreas. J Ultrasound Med 2001; 20:1229–1232.

37 Nadler EP, Novikov A, Landzberg BR, et al. The use of endoscopic ultrasound in the diagnosis of solid pseudopapillary tumors of the pancreas in children. J Pediatr Surg 2002; 37:1370–1373.

38 Norton JA, Fraker DL, Alexander HR, et al. Surgery to cure the Zollinger–Ellison syndrome. N Engl J Med 1999; 341:635–644.

39 Warshaw AL, Rattner DW, Fernandez-del Castillo C, et al. Middle segment pancreatectomy: a novel technique for conserving pancreatic tissue. Arch Surg 1998; 133:327–331.

40 Wiedenmann B, Jensen RT, Mignon M, et al. Preoperative diagnosis and surgical management of neuroendocrine gastroenteropancreatic tumours: general recommendations by a consensus workshop. World J Surg 1998; 22:309–318.

41 Koito K, Namieno T, Nagakawa T, et al. Solitary cystic tumor of the pancreas: EUS–pathologic correlation. Gastrointest Endosc. 1997; 45:268–276.

42 Sedlack R, Affi A, Vazquez-Sequeiros E, et al. Utility of EUS in the evaluation of cystic pancreatic lesions. Gastrointest Endosc 2002; 56:543–547.

43 Ahmad NA, Kochman ML, Lewis JD, et al. Can EUS alone differentiate between malignant and benign cystic lesions of the pancreas? Am J Gastroenterol 2001; 96:3295–3300.

44 Ahmad NA, Kochman ML, Brensinger C, et al. Interobserver agreement among endosonographers for the diagnosis of neoplastic versus non-neoplastic pancreatic cystic lesions. Gastrointest Endosc 2003; 58:59–64.

45 Ferrucci JT, Wittenberg J, Margolies MN, et al. Malignant seeding of the tract after thin-needle aspiration biopsy. Radiology 1979; 130:345–346.

46 Caturelli E, Rapaccini GL, Anti M, et al. Malignant seeding after fine-needle aspiration biopsy of the pancreas. Diagn Imaging Clin Med 1985; 54:88–91.

47 Bret PM, Nicolet V, Labadie M. Percutaneous fine-needle aspiration biopsy of the pancreas. Diagn Cytopathol 1986; 2:221–227.

48 Giovannini M, Seitz JF, Monges G, et al. Fine needle aspiration cytology guided by endoscopic ultrasonography: results in 141 patients. Endoscopy 1995; 27:171–177.

49 Chang KJ, Katz KD, Durbin TE, et al. Endoscopic ultrasound guided fine needle aspiration. Gastrointest Endosc 1994; 40:694–699.

50 Vilmann P, Hancke S, Henriksen FW, et al. Endoscopic ultrasonography-guided fine needle aspiration biopsy of lesions in the upper gastrointestinal tract. Gastrointest Endosc 1995; 41:230–235.

51 Wiersema MJ, Kochman ML, Cramer HM, et al. Endosonography-guided real-time fine-needle aspiration biopsy. Gastrointest Endosc 1994; 40:700–707.

52 Chang KJ, Albers CG, Erickson RA, et al. Endoscopic ultrasound guided fine needle aspiration of pancreatic carcinoma. Am J Gastroenterol 1994; 89:263–266.

53 Vilmann P, Hancke S, Henriksen FW, et al. Endosonographically-guided fine needle aspiration biopsy of malignant lesions in the upper gastrointestinal tract. Endoscopy 1993; 25:523–527.

54 Ball AB, Fisher C, Pittam M, et al. Diagnosis of soft tissue tumours by Tru-Cut biopsy. Br J Surg 1990; 77:756–758.

55 Zinzani PL, Coleccchia A, Festi D, et al. Ultrasound-guided core-needle biopsy is effective in the initial diagnosis of lymphoma patients. Haematologica 1998; 83:989–992.

56 Nyman RS, Cappelen-Smith J, Brismar J, et al. Yield and complications in ultrasound-guided biopsy of abdominal lesions. Comparison of fine-needle aspiration biopsy and 1.2-mm needle core biopsy using an automated biopy gun. Acta Radiol 1995; 36:485–490.

57 Levy MJ, Jondal ML, Clain JE, et al. Preliminary experience with an EUS-guided Trucut biopsy needle compared with EUS-guided FNA. Gastrointest Endosc 2003; 57:101–106.

58 Largi A, Verna EC, Stavropoulos SN, et al. EUS-guided Trucut needle biopsies in patients with solid pancreatic masses: a prospective study. Gastrointest Endosc 2004; 59:185–190.

59 Varadarajulu S, Fraig M, Schmulewitz N, et al. Comparison of EUS-guided 19-gauge Trucut needle biopsy with EUS-guided fine-needle aspiration. Endoscopy 2004; 36:397–401.

60 O'Toole D, Palazzo L, Arotcarena R, et al. Assessment of complications of EUS-guided fine-needle aspiration. Gastrointest Endosc 2001; 53:470–474.

61 Williams DB, Sahai AV, Aabakken L, et al. Endoscopic ultrasound guided fine needle aspiration biopsy: a large single centre experience. Gut 1999; 44:720–726.

62 Brandwein SL, Farrell JJ, Centeno BA, et al. Detection and tumor staging of malignancy in cystic, intraductal, and solid tumors of the pancreas by EUS. Gastrointest Endosc 2001; 53:722–727.

63 Hernandez LV, Mishra G, Forsmark C, et al. Role of endoscopic ultrasound (EUS) and EUS-guided fine needle aspiration in the diagnosis and treatment of cystic lesions of the pancreas. Pancreas 2002; 25:222–228.

64 Maire F, Couvelard A, Hammel P, et al. Intraductal papillary mucin tumours of the pancreas: the preoperative value of cytologic and histopathologic diagnosis. Gastrointest Endosc 2003; 58:701–706.

65 Lai R, Stanley MW, Bardales R, et al. Endoscopic ultrasound-guided pancreatic duct aspiration: diagnostic yield and safety. Endoscopy 2002; 34:715–720.

66 Harewood GC, Wiersema LM, Halling AC, et al. Influence of EUS training and pathology interpretation on accuracy of EUS-guided fine needle aspiration of pancreatic masses. Gastrointest Endosc 2002; 55:669–673.

67 Mertz H, Gautam S. The learning curve for EUS-guided FNA of pancreatic cancer. Gastrointest Endosc 2004; 59:33–37.

68 Sand JA, Hyoty MK, Mattila J, et al. Clinical assessment compared with cyst fluid analysis in the differential diagnosis of cystic lesions in the pancreas. Surgery 1996; 119:275–280.

69 Hammel P, Levy P, Voitot H, et al. Preoperative cyst fluid analysis is useful for the differential diagnosis of cystic lesions of the pancreas. Gastroenterology 1995; 108:1230–1235.

70 Hammel P, Voitot H, Vilgrain V, et al. Diagnostic value of CA 72-4 and carcinoembryonic antigen determination in the fluid of pancreatic cystic lesions. Eur J Gastroenterol Hepatol 1998; 10:345–348.

71 Warshaw AL, Brugge WR, Lweandrowski KB, et al. A 75-year-old man with a cystic lesion of the pancreas. N Engl J Med 2003; 349:1954–1961.

72 Sperti C, Pasquali C, Pedrazzoli S, et al. Expression of mucin-like carcinoma-associated antigen in the cyst fluid differentiates mucinous from nonmucinous pancreatic cysts. Am J Gastroenterol 1997; 92:672–675.

73 Rubin D, Warshaw AL, Southern JF, et al. Expression of CA 15.3 protein in the cyst contents distinguishes benign from malignant pancreatic mucinous cystic neoplasms. Surgery 1994; 115:52–55.

74 American Society for Gastrointestinal Endoscopy Standards of Practice Committee. ASGE guideline: the role of endoscopy in the diagnosis and the management of cystic lesions and inflammatory fluid collections of the pancreas. Gastrointest Endosc 2005; 61:363–370.

75 Rickes S, Unkrodt K, Ocran K, et al. Differentiation of neuroendocrine tumors from other pancreatic lesions by echo-enhanced power Doppler sonography and somatosatin receptor scintigraphy. Pancreas 2003; 26:76–81.

76 Ueno N, Ozamaw Y. Pancreatic cancer evaluated by contrast-enhanced color Doppler endoscopic ultrasound. Dig Endosc 2002; 14:184.

77 Kitano M, Kudo M, Maekawa K, et al. Dynamic imaging of pancreatic diseases by contrast enhanced coded phase inversion harmonic ultrasonography. Gut 2004; 53:854–859.

78 Khalid A, Finkelstein S, Brody D, et al. Mutational allelotyping of aspirated free-floating DNA predicts the biological behavior of cystic pancreatic neoplasms. Gastrointest Endosc 2004; 59:AB95 (Abstract).

79 Gan I, Bounds B, Brugge WR. EUS-guided ethanol lavage of cystic lesions of the pancreas is feasible and safe. Gastrointest Endosc 2004; 59:AB94 (Abstract).

80 Chatelain D, Hammel P, O'Toole D, et al. Macrocystic form of serous pancreatic cystadenoma. Am J Gastroenterol 2002; 97:2566–2571.

Chapter

18

EUS in Bile Duct, Ampullary, and Gallbladder Lesions

Bertrand Napoléon, Costas Markoglou, Christine Lefort, and Gidej Durivage

KEY POINTS

- In patients with low or moderate risk of common bile duct (CBD) stones, EUS is recommended before endoscopic retrograde cholangiopancreatography (ERCP) is performed.

- In patients with acute pancreatitis of unknown origin or right hypochondrial pain with normal transabdominal ultrasonographic findings, EUS should be considered.

- In patients with a CBD stricture of unknown origin, EUS should be performed and, if inconclusive, followed by ERCP with tissue sampling with or without intraductal ultrasonography (IDUS).

- Gallbladder polyps larger than 5 mm in size may be investigated with EUS to determine the risk of malignancy and the therapeutic approach.

- Ampullary tumors can be staged with EUS and IDUS. EUS is best to differentiate between early (adenoma, T1) and advanced (T2–4) tumors. IDUS may help to stage early tumors.

BILE DUCT STONES

Endoscopic retrograde cholangiography pancreaticography (ERCP) has long been considered the best diagnostic method for common bile duct (CBD) stones. Moreover, ERCP allows stone removal during the same endoscopic session when combined with endoscopic sphincterotomy. Nevertheless it remains an invasive method, associated with substantial complications in 5% of patients, and the mortality rate is 0.1–0.2%.[1,2] Furthermore, as it can be difficult to differentiate small stones from aerobilia, a substantial proportion of ERCP procedures are completed with endoscopic sphincterotomy, in order to confirm the diagnosis of choledocholithiasis. Endoscopic sphincterotomy has a complication rate of 7–10%,[3,4] and its mortality rate ranges between 0.2% and 2.2%.[4,5] Long-term sequelae, such as stenosis and non-obstructive cholangitis, occur in 13%

of patients 6–13 years after endoscopic sphincterotomy[6] due to permanent loss of biliary sphincter function.[7] An accurate diagnostic tool associated with lower morbidity and mortality rates was awaited, to replace ERCP and to reserve endoscopic sphincterotomy for patients with CBD stones. ERCP remained the first-line examination until the appearance of transcutaneous abdominal ultrasonography (US). Nowadays, in patients presenting with clinical and/or laboratory suspicion of CBD stones, US is always used for the initial diagnostic evaluation. However, although US is very specific for the diagnosis of choledocholithiasis, it is not particularly sensitive,[8,9] even though the calcium present within CBD stones is a strong reflector of ultrasound waves. Adjacent duodenal air interferes with imaging of the distal bile duct, and the ultrasound beam is often attenuated in obese patients. Computed tomography (CT) also has an unacceptably low sensitivity.

In the past decade, helical CT, endoscopic ultrasonography (EUS), and magnetic resonance cholangiopancreatography (MRCP) have improved the diagnosis of CBD stones, avoiding the need for cholangiography (ERCP or peroperative opacification). Although helical CT remains inferior, with a sensitivity of 85–88%, specificity of 88–97%, and diagnostic accuracy of 86–94%,[10,11] EUS and MRCP are now considered as highly accurate methods for diagnosing CBD stones. Currently, what are the respective accuracies of EUS, MRCP, and ERCP? What is the respective place of each of these examinations? Examination of the abundant literature on the subject should help us to answer these questions.

EUS overcomes the limitations of US, because the examination is carried out through the wall of the second part of the duodenum and the duodenal bulb without interference from bowel gas. It provides excellent sonographic visualization of the extrahepatic biliary tree. Bile duct stones are shown as echo-rich structures (Fig. 18.1) within the ampulla or CBD, possibly moving within the bile duct, with or without acoustic shadowing or inflammatory thickening of the bile duct (Fig. 18.2). The accuracy of EUS is better than that of ERCP for the detection of small CBD stones,[12] with minimal or no invasiveness[13,14] and a lower failure rate.[15] The specificity of EUS in ruling out the presence of CBD stones was 98%[16] in some series. EUS detects bile duct sludge as well as microlithiasis (Fig. 18.3), often missed by the other imaging techniques.[17]

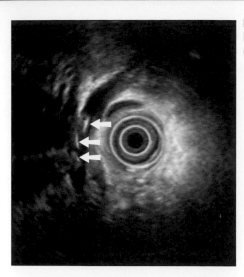

Fig. 18.1 Common bile duct stones (arrows).

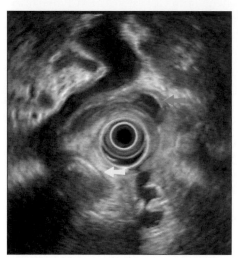

Fig. 18.2 Common bile duct stone (yellow arrow) with cystic wall thickening (green arrow).

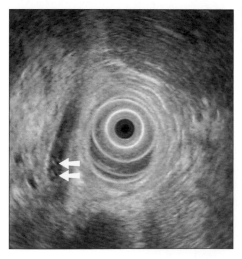

Fig. 18.3 Common bile duct microlithiasis (arrows).

MRCP is a completely non-invasive procedure regarded as more accurate than CT for the diagnosis of choledocholithiasis.[18] The two main disadvantages of this technique are the limited spatial resolution and the difficulty of diagnosing CBD stones in the peripapillary region. Moreover, MRCP is absolutely contra-

indicated in patients with a permanent pacemaker or cerebral aneurysm clips, and claustophobic patients (estimated to represent 4% of the population[19]) cannot undergo the examination. EUS offers higher resolution than MRCP (0.1 versus 1–1.5 mm), which explains the lower sensitivity of MRCP in the diagnosis of small stones.[20] Thus, it is not surprising that stones not diagnosed by MRCP were always smaller than 10 mm.[21–23] Nevertheless, improvements in imaging may in the future permit the detection of calculi smaller than 5 mm, as shown in a recent series.[24]

To compare the performance of each technique, some parameters have to be considered. The first consideration is the delay between the performance of the technique being evaluated and the 'gold standard' examination. In fact, spontaneous stone migration between the two examinations can lead to false-positive results. In a study of discrepancies between EUS and ERCP in relation to the time elapsed between the two procedures, stone migration was found to have occurred in 21% of patients within 1 month.[25] Ideally, in comparative studies the gold standard examination should be performed immediately after the evaluated technique, or at least during the subsequent 48 h. Second, the perfect 'gold standard' is a matter of debate. ERCP and peroperative cholangiography are the reference techniques most commonly chosen. Nevertheless, it is well known that opacification alone is not sufficient to exclude CBD stones, because its sensitivity is around 90% (89% in a study comparing EUS and ERCP). The best gold standard is the association of ERCP, endoscopic sphincterotomy and instrumental exploration of the CBD (with a Dormia basket or balloon). However, because of ERCP associated morbidity and mortality, it is difficult ethically to propose this approach in patients at low or moderate risk of CBD stones. Another approach in these patients would be to perform ERCP, endoscopic sphincterotomy, and bile duct exploration when a stone is evidenced, and to follow the patient when a stone has been excluded. As some patients with CBD stones missed by the investigation remain symptom-free for a long time, follow-up must be sufficiently long for adequate conclusions to be drawn. In series in which patients were followed for up to 1 year, no stone was evidenced after 6 months of follow-up.[12,26] Six months should therefore be the standard follow-up period.

Publications evaluating the respective performances of EUS and MRI can therefore be classified into three groups (Table 18.1) according to the level of proof, from the more significant to the less significant:

1 Technique compared with the gold standard (ERCP, endoscopic sphincterotomy, and CBD instrumental exploration) with a very short interval between the two examinations.[27]

2 Technique compared with ERCP and endoscopic sphincterotomy if a stone is evidenced, and with clinical and biologic follow-up of at least 6 months if not.[12,13,26,28]

3 Technique compared with cholangiography (ERCP or peroperative cholangiography).

PERFORMANCE OF EUS AND MRI IN THE DIAGNOSIS OF COMMON BILE DUCT STONES

Reference	Level of proof[a]	No. of patients	Frequency of CBD stones (%)	EUS Sensitivity (%)	EUS Specificity (%)	EUS PPV (%)	EUS NPV (%)	EUS Accuracy (%)	MRI Sensitivity (%)	MRI Specificity (%)	MRI PPV (%)	MRI NPV (%)	MRI Accuracy (%)
Prat et al.[27]	1	119	66	93	97	98	88						
Kohut et al.[32] (linear scope)	1	134	68	93	93	98	87	94					
Canto et al.[13]	2	64	30	84	98	94	93	94					
Napoléon et al.[12]	2	334	22	81	96	85	94	93					
Buscarini et al.[28]	2	463	52	98	99	99	98	97					
Shim et al.[47]	3	132	21	89.3									
Palazzo et al.[15]	3	422	36	95	98			96					
Amouyal et al.[48]	3	62	36	97	100		97	98					
Sugiyama & Atomi[38]	3	142	36	96	100			99					
Gautier et al.[49]	2	99	23				95.7	98.7	95.7	98.7			
Cervi et al.[50]	3	60	22						100	94			
Demartines et al.[51]	3	70	25						100	95.6	93	100	
Kim et al.[52]	3	121	47						95	95			95
Stiris et al.[53]	3	50	64						87.5	94.4	97	81	
Taylor et al.[54]	3	146	32						98	89	84	99	
Aubé et al.[24]	2	47	34	93.8	96.6	94	97		87.5	96.6	93	93	
Materne et al.[31]	3	50		97	88	94		94	91	94			92
De Ledinghen et al.[30]	3	32	31.2	100	95.4	91	100	96.9	100	72.7	62	100	82.2
Scheiman et al.[29]	3	30	16.6	80					40				

Table 18.1 Performance of EUS and MRI in the diagnosis of common bile duct stones

[a]Level 1: technique compared with ERCP and systematic endoscopic sphincterotomy with a very short interval between the technique and ERCP;[6] level 2: technique compared with ERCP and endoscopic sphincterotomy if positive, and clinical and biologic follow-up of at least 6 months if negative;[6,8,10,25] level 3: technique compared with ERCP or peroperative cholangiography.
PPV, positive predictive value; NPV, negative predictive value.

In the first comparative studies, EUS was found to be superior to MRCP in the detection of bile duct calculi[29,30] (Table 18.1). In another comparative study, EUS and MRCP were equally accurate in the diagnosis of extrahepatic biliary obstruction.[31] Improvements in imaging modalities may modify these findings: in the most recent series,[24] the specificity of EUS and MRCP were found to be equal (97%). Sensitivity was greater with EUS than with MRCP (94% versus 88%, respectively).[24] These good results need to be confirmed in larger series. At present, EUS can be considered to be more accurate than MRCP, especially for smaller stones.

In all of these series, radial echoendoscopes were used. Nevertheless, the accuracy seems comparable with that for linear echoendoscopes, as indicated in one series[32] that compared linear EUS with ERCP plus endoscopic sphincterotomy or choledochotomy with choledochoscopy (Table 18.1). The use of extraductal catheter probe EUS (EDUS) has also been evaluated. In a recently published prospective study, EDUS with a radial scanning catheter probe was performed before ERCP and endoscopic sphincterotomy in patients with suspected CBD stones or other bile flow obstruction of the distal CBD.[33] EDUS detected 33 of 34 bile duct stones. In eight patients the stones were missed on ERCP and seen with endoscopic sphincterotomy. Intraductal ultrasonography (IDUS) has also been proposed recently for this indication (Fig. 18.4). In a prospective study of patients with suspected CBD stones who underwent ERCP, IDUS was performed in those with equivocal cholangiograms or cholangiographic evidence of stones. IDUS revealed false-positive as well as false-negative results. No lithiasis was found in 36% of patients with a positive finding on ERCP. This, according to the authors, was partly due to the existence of aerobilia. In 35% of patients with a negative ERCP result, sludge or stones were found on IDUS and confirmed following endoscopic sphincterotomy. IDUS led to a change in management in 37% of patients.[34] However, IDUS cannot be proposed as a routine procedure because of the morbidity associated with ERCP. It might be proposed,

before endoscopic sphincterotomy, in patients in whom CBD stones have been found at EUS or MRCP, but not at ERCP.

The performance of alternative imaging procedures results in a considerable reduction in the number of inappropriate invasive investigations of the bile duct.[12,28] Given that the accuracy of EUS is greater than that of MRCP, at least in patients with microlithiasis,[23,29,30] EUS should replace diagnostic ERCP. Whenever EUS is contraindicated, as in patients with a total or Billroth II gastrectomy, or in those with digestive stenosis, MRCP might be proposed. ERCP plus endoscopic sphincterotomy should be used in patients already known to have CBD stones (shown by US, for example).

A question remains about the interest of performing an unnecessary EUS or MRI before ERCP when the probability of finding a CBD stone is high. Patients suspected of having CBD stones on clinical and laboratory criteria and/or US findings can be grouped into risk classes, ranging from low to high.[35,36] The proportion of high-risk patients that actually have CBD stones is around 70%,[27,37,38] whereas fewer than 30% of patients classified as being at moderate risk have choledocholithiasis.[13] Most authors consider that ERCP could be performed as a first-line approach in patients at high risk of bile duct stones,[12,13,15,36] although it may be impossible completely to avoid unnecessary ERCP investigations.[39] EUS as a first-line approach, even in patients at high risk for suspected CBD stones, has already found some support.[28] However, there is still no general agreement with regard to the clinical applicability of EUS, particularly when compared with ERCP.[40] The best approach is to perform EUS with or without endoscopic sphincterotomy (when a stone is evidenced) during the same endoscopic procedure. For moderate- and low-risk patients, the general consensus is to consider EUS (or MRCP) as the first-line diagnostic approach (after US). Thus, EUS could be the ideal alternative, selecting only those patients with bile duct stones for ERCP/EST. Morever, it should be mentioned that the replacement of ERCP by EUS for diagnostic purposes actually enhances the efficiency of endoscopic sphincterotomy by encouraging the use of aggressive techniques, such as pre-cut papillotomy, when appropriate. The need for ERCP could be obviated, if biliary EUS proved normal,[12] unless symptoms persisted or recurred during follow-up.

This approach was evaluated in the context of laparoscopic cholecystectomy.[26] First-line ERCP was performed in patients considered to be at high risk according to preoperative criteria, and EUS was carried out before laparoscopic cholecystectomy in intermediate-risk patients. EUS followed by EST, if needed, was performed in 35% of the patients. Choledocholithiasis was found in 19% of patients at intermediate risk and in 78% of those at high risk. This endoscopic approach for choledocholithiasis and laparoscopic approach for gallstones proved to be an efficient option, optimized by the use of EUS. After a mean follow-up of 32 months, no retained stones were found in this series of 300 patients.

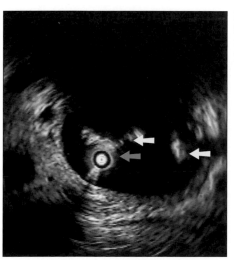

Fig. 18.4 Common bile duct stones (yellow arrows) at IDUS (green arrow).

With regard to cost-effectiveness, there is no agreement that a strategy of first-line EUS with no discrimination of patients is financially advantageous. The estimation of cost will be different in different countries and healthcare systems. In a recently published, prospective controlled study of 485 patients suspected of having CBD stones, EUS was always performed, whether the patient had been classified as at high risk or not. The positive EUS cases were confirmed by ERCP and endoscopic sphincterotomy. The mean cost for patients managed by the EUS-based strategy was significantly lower (P<0.001) than that for patients who had ERCP.[28] Others believe that EUS improves the cost-effectiveness only in patients at low, moderate, or intermediate risk.[28] The skill of the operator is crucial, not only for the accuracy of EUS, but also for the performance of ERCP. EUS and ERCP, as indicated by EUS findings, should be performed on the same day by experienced physicians in centers specialized with both procedures, in order to avoid prolonged hospital stay.

EUS and gallbladder stones

The performance of abdominal US in diagnosing gallstones is excellent, with a sensitivity and specificity of 97% and 95%, respectively, in a meta-analysis.[41] After adjustment, the sensitivity decreases to 88%. Sensitivity is lower for small stones with a diameter of less than 3 mm, for cystic stones, and in 'difficult' patients, for example those with obesity or meteorism. The use of bile crystal analysis is justified when there is discordance between negative US findings and symptoms.[42] Because of the value of EUS in diagnosing small CBD stones, this procedure has also been evaluated in the gallbladder (Fig. 18.5). The first series of Dill et al.[43] in 1995 showed that EUS was as accurate as crystal bile analysis for the diagnosis of microlithiasis (Fig. 18.6) and failed on only one occasion to demonstrate microlithiasis in a group of 58 patients with biliary-type pain and negative US findings. In another study,[44] conducted in patients with suspected gallstones and two normal US investigations, the sensitivity of EUS for the diagnosis of gallstones was 96%, with a specificity of 86%.

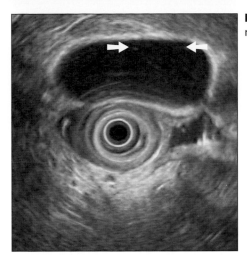

Fig. 18.6 Gallbladder microlithiasis (arrows).

In the specific and difficult case of acute pancreatitis, the superiority of EUS has been confirmed. Gallstones were found by EUS in 14 of 18 patients with negative findings on US by Liu et al.[16] in 2000. In a 1999 study performed by Chak et al.[45] that compared EUS and US, the sensitivity was 91% versus 50%, and the accuracy 97% versus 83%, respectively. In a larger series,[17] 168 patients referred with a diagnosis of idiopathic pancreatitis were evaluated. EUS identified gallbladder lithiasis (sludge or very small stones) in 40% of patients, whether or not associated with CBD stones, that had been missed by other examinations. Overall, EUS was able to find a cause for the acute pancreatitis in 80% of patients. This underlines the importance of EUS in management of unexplained acute pancreatitis[16,17,45,46] and for the diagnosis of gallbladder lithiasis.

Summary

EUS is the least invasive method for confirming the presence or absence of CBD stones. Its use in avoiding unnecessary ERCP or endoscopic sphincterotomy has been validated in patients at low or moderate risk of CBD stones. MRCP should probably be used as an alternative, with two limitations: (1) it necessitates the use of older-generation equipment; and (2) EUS is preferred in acute pancreatitis where symptomatic stones can be very small. For patients at high risk of CBD

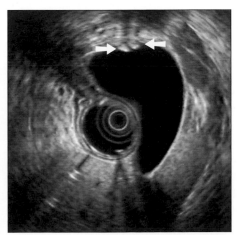

Fig. 18.5 Gallbladder stones (arrows).

DIAGNOSTIC CHECKLIST

CBD or gallbladder stone
- Hyperechoic mobile lesion with or without acoustic shadowing

Associated signs
- Dilation of extrahepatic ducts and/or cystic duct
- Thickening of the gallbladder and/or ductal walls
- Thickening of the ampulla
- Perigallbladder fluid

stones, two approaches can be considered: ERCP ± endoscopic sphincterotomy (in case of CBD stones in evidence during cholangiography) or EUS ± endoscopic sphincterotomy carried out during the same session (in case of CBD stones in evidence at EUS). The possibility of performing endoscopic sphincterotomy EST immediately after a positive EUS investigation represents the future for interventional endoscopists. EUS is now the second-line examination after US for the diagnosis of gallbladder lithiasis in patients with unexplained right hypochondrial pain, and also in those with acute pancreatitis of unknown origin.

EUS IN BILE DUCT TUMORS

Diagnosis of the nature of bile duct strictures and the staging of cholangiocarcinomas remain a challenge for the gastroenterologist. Although transcutaneous US and helical CT can reliably demonstrate dilated bile ducts, they allow assessment of the cause in only two-thirds of cases.[9,55] Apart from contiguous tumor invasion or metastasis, MRCP appears to be no better than ERCP in the diagnosis of malignancy.[56] ERCP has a high diagnostic accuracy in the confirmation of obstructive jaundice, but the diagnostic information obtained for tumor-associated obstruction is limited, as only indirect tumor signs such as stenosis or prestenotic dilation, or both, are visualized, and the tumor itself is generally not seen. Intraductal tissue samplings are commonly used at the time of ERCP. Brushing has poor results in the diagnosis of bile duct tumors, owing to their desmoplastic nature, and is frequently negative for extrinsic tumors (pancreatic cancer, gallbladder cancer, metastatic lymph nodes).[57] Forceps biopsy during ERCP has a higher sensitivity than ERCP brush cytology,[58,59] but is also limited, except in the case of malignant polypoid lesions. This has led to the development of techniques that abrade the tumor surface in order to improve cytologic yield. The combination of stricture dilation with 10-Fr endoscopic needle aspiration and biliary brush cytology has been shown significantly to improve the diagnostic yield in malignant strictures compared with brushings alone.[60] Nevertheless, these results have not been confirmed.[61] Bile duct biopsy under cholangioscopy[62,63] is the most effective method, with a sensitivity of 93–96%. However, cholangioscopy remains an invasive procedure rarely performed in Western countries, and the problem of diagnosing the nature of a biliary stricture remains, even when both invasive and non-invasive imaging procedures are available.[64,65]

How can EUS and IDUS overcome these difficulties?

EUS readily visualizes the CBD and can be used in the differential diagnosis of bile duct masses or strictures[66] (Figs 18.7 & 18.8). The main limitations are Klatskin tumors, owing to the reduced field of exploration, even though imaging has recently improved with the use of a lower frequency of 5 MHz. Otherwise, EUS has proved to be a useful tool in obstructive jaundice, as it provides direct images of the neoplasia and permits

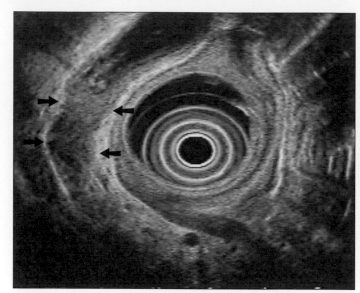

Fig. 18.7 CBD infiltrative cholangiocarcinoma (arrows).

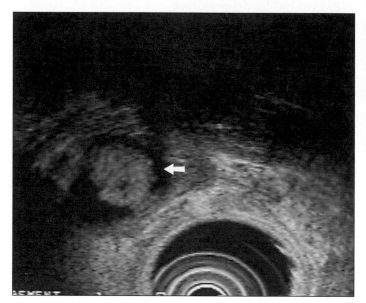

Fig. 18.8 Early CBD cholangiocarcinoma (arrow).

local tumor staging.[67–69] The decision concerning the optimal use of the various imaging modalities is still critical. In a prospective comparative study of ERCP or percutaneous transhepatic cholangiography (PTC), MRCP, CT, and EUS, 40 patients with biliary stricture underwent all four imaging tests.[70] The specificity was improved when MRCP was combined with EUS. Tissue sampling under EUS guidance should improve the diagnostic rate, depending of the origin of the stenosis. Biliary strictures due to pancreatic diseases are evaluated accurately by EUS and cytologic examination of samples obtained by EUS-guided fine-needle aspiration (EUS-FNA).[71–75] There is little information regarding the use of EUS-FNA in patients with bile duct masses or strictures. In a recent retrospective study, the diagnostic yield of EUS was improved by performing EUS-FNA, especially in patients with negative brush cytology findings.[76] However, only 3 of 23 patients had lesions localized in the hilar bile duct. Hilar lesions are often small or diffusely infiltrating, and can therefore be difficult to detect. According to a small study, EUS-FNA may aid in the diagnosis of hilar cholangiocarcinomas when standard methods of tissue diagnosis are inconclusive.[77]

With the advent of high-frequency (20 MHz) mini-probes over a guidewire, intraductal ultrasonography (IDUS) has emerged as a feasible and promising imaging technique in the diagnosis of biliary stricture. Mini-probes can now be easily inserted through the papilla without prior papillotomy. In a minority of the patients (11%) a precut is necessary to introduce the guidewire.[78] IDUS provides an accurate image of bile duct wall and surrounding tissue. Even when the penetration depth is limited (2 cm), this is sufficient to provide a precise image of an intraductal lesion and possible invasion or compression of adjacent structures. IDUS is faster and easier to learn than conventional EUS. It should be performed prior to drainage in order to avoid inflammatory artifacts, and therefore should be better performed by ERCP experts during the same procedure.[79] Complete examination of bile duct strictures is possible in the majority of patients. The literature indicates that IDUS can be used to pass through biliary strictures in 86–100% of cases,[60,78,80,81] mostly without previous dilation. Most failures were due to tight strictures of the hilum or intrahepatic ducts that the guidewire could not cross.[78,80,81] In Klatskin tumors, the examination is generally possible from the opposite side when the right or left hepatic duct stenosis cannot be crossed by the probe. The presence of the guidewire in the bile duct throughout the procedure does not often interfere with US imaging (in case of artifact, the guidewire could be removed before IDUS). The most recent generation of IDUS (3D-IDUS imaging system; Olympus Medical Systems, Tokyo, Japan) consists of an ultrasonic probe that is automatically moved for

scanning within an external tube. It carries out linear and radial scanning simultaneously in real time with one scanning operation. Three-dimensional images can be generated automatically. Comparative studies between two and three-dimensional images would be necessary to define the possible advantages of this procedure.

As with EUS, three layers are seen in the bile duct wall with IDUS. The first hyperechoic layer corresponds to the mucosa in addition to a border echo; the second hypoechoic layer is the smooth muscle fibers with fibroelastic tissue; and the third hyperechoic layer is the thin and loose connective tissue with a border echo.[82,82] The criteria for malignancy of a stricture are: disruption of the normal three-layer sonographic pattern of the bile duct wall (outer echogenic, middle hypoechoic, inner echogenic) (Fig. 18.9), a hypoechoic infiltrating lesion with irregular margins, heterogeneous echo-poor areas invading surrounding tissue, and continuation of the main hypoechoic mass into adjacent structures. Findings considered diagnostic of a benign stricture (Fig. 18.10) include preservation of the normal three-layer sonographic wall pattern, homogeneous echo patterns, smooth margins, hyperechogenic lesions, and the absence of a mass lesion. For lesions with intermediate echogenicity, asymmetric lesions are considered malignant, whereas symmetric lesions are classified as benign; however, asymmetry has not been considered by all authors as a criterion for malignancy.[62,71,80,84] The accuracy of IDUS in differentiating benign from malignant strictures ranges from 76% to 92% in series of patients with various causes of biliary stricture.[60,62,80,85] In 2002, Tamada et al.[85] proposed other IDUS criteria. Interruption of the bile duct wall is considered specific for tumoral stricture. Sessile tumors, even when they remain intraductal or extend outside the CBD wall, and tumor size greater than 10 mm are the other major positive criteria indicating malignancy. Echogenicity of the stricture, which is probably highly

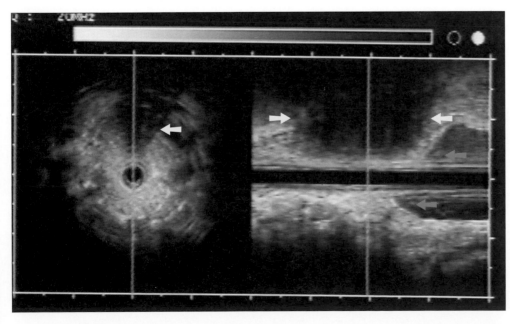

Fig. 18.9 Three-dimensional IDUS showing biliary duct stenosis (green arrows) and pancreatic adenocarcinoma (yellow arrows).

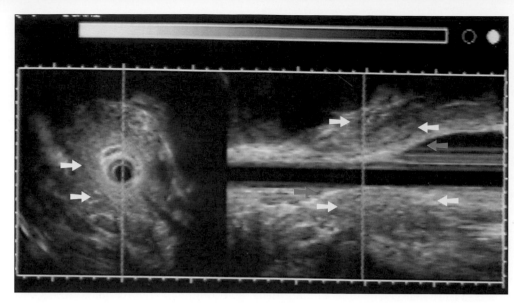

Fig. 18.10 Three-dimensional IDUS showing biliary duct stenosis (green arrows) and inflammatory extrinsic compression following acute pancreatitis (yellow arrows).

operator dependent, is no longer considered a factor predictive of malignancy.

The vast majority of patients without the above-mentioned criteria and with negative samplings do not have a malignant lesion. The presence of two of the criteria, even with negative biopsies, is highly suspicious of malignancy. The absence of IDUS criteria of malignancy and the negativity of biopsies indicates the existence of a benign lesion with 95% accuracy and 100% negative predictive value.[85] A previous history of choledocholithiasis or surgery of the biliary tract has been found to predict a benign lesion. Moreover, IDUS is very effective in confirming an extrinsic compression by a vascular structure or by a stone impacted in the cystic duct and compressing the common bile duct (Mirizzi's syndrome).[60,78,85] Biliary papillomatosis is also detected accurately by IDUS, whereas this pathology is frequently misdiagnosed with usual imaging techniques such as ERCP, EUS, or MRI. Biliary ducts with normal appearance alternating with areas covered by polypoid lesions protruding into the lumen establish the diagnosis.[86,87] In 30 patients with cholangiocarcinoma studied by IDUS, biliary papillomatosis was shown in three (10%) and

confirmed by biopsy or surgery.[86] When ERCP diagnosed a polypoid lesion inside the CBD, IDUS was the only test able to detect combined biliary papillomatosis inside the intrahepatic ducts (Fig. 18.11). The clinical impact of this diagnosis can be important, as young patients with biliary papillomatosis without advanced cholangiocarcinoma should be treated with a Whipple resection in combination with partial hepatectomy or liver transplantation.[87]

Unfortunately, IDUS and EUS are no more accurate than other imaging modalities in the diagnosis of carcinoma in patients with underlying sclerosing cholangitis. Indeed, there are no criteria that allow differentiation between an inflammatory thickening due to the cholangitis (Fig. 18.12) or to underlying early carcinoma.[88]

How to approach a bile duct stricture

If the stricture is localized at the level of the CBD, EUS should be proposed after non-invasive imaging modalities. Considering the very promising IDUS results,[60,71,85] some authors have also proposed ERCP with IDUS rather than EUS. Tissue could be biopsied at the same time. Nevertheless, the application of

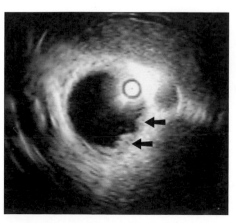

Fig. 18.11 Two-dimensional IDUS showing biliary papillomatosis with intrahepatic polypoid spread (arrows).

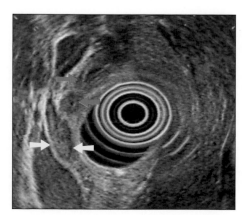

Fig. 18.12 Sclerosing cholangitis with thickened, irregular CBD (yellow arrows) and cystic wall (green arrows).

IDUS has some important drawbacks. The morbidity associated with ERCP and IDUS is higher than that with EUS. The accuracy of IDUS seems to be poor in the evaluation of metastatic lymph node staging[80] and in the full exploration of pancreatic lesions,[60] owing to limited penetration depth. Finally, performing ERCP prior to EUS is potentially disturbing, as papillotomy, drainage, or stenting may hamper the EUS interpretation. It might therefore be reasonable to propose the following algorithm for the interpretation of the bile duct strictures:[89]

- For common hepatic duct and hilar strictures: MRI plus ERCP with IDUS
- For middle and inferior bile duct strictures: EUS plus FNA followed by ERCP plus IDUS, if needed.

How to stage a cholangiocarcinoma

When a bile duct carcinoma is diagnosed, the aim of the investigation is to determine whether the patient can be treated by surgery or not. The first important criterion is the tumor (T) and node (N) staging. Histologically, early cancer presents with the deepest invasion limited to the mucosa or fibromuscular layer of the extrahepatic bile duct, regardless of lymph node metastasis. Serosa is found in part of the anterior and right posterior wall of hilar, superior, and middle bile duct. Bile duct carcinomas are staged according to the following classification, modified from the TNM staging system: T1, limited to the CBD wall; T2, invasion beyond the CBD wall; and T3, invasion of adjacent structures such as the pancreas, duodenum, and portal vein.

In a prospective study comparing EUS and IDUS in biliary strictures, the accuracy of IDUS in T staging (77.7%) was higher than that of EUS (54.1%).[71] EUS accuracy was inferior mainly in hilar or common hepatic duct strictures due to the limited field of exploration. N staging was comparable, but other authors found that the depth of penetration of the standard 20-MHz catheter probe was not adequate for the evaluation of lymph nodes associated with advanced malignant strictures.[60] EUS and IDUS were not able to differentiate T1 from T2 bile duct cancers. In fact, the main question for the staging of biliary tumors is resectability, which relies on vascular, longitudinal, and pancreatic spread. The available imaging modalities are used to try to select patients who are eligible for this very high risk and difficult surgery. Conventional investigations (MRI, helical CT) can be useful to prevent surgery in some patients, such as those with a Bismuth type IV Klatskin tumor. Nevertheless, the exact longitudinal spread of bile duct carcinoma is not easily detected. The diagnostic problem of microscopic involvement of the bile duct wall has not been overcome, resulting in understaging in terms of the resectional margins. Cholangiography and choledochoscopy with biopsy also have limitations in determining the extent of spread.[90] Although EUS is limited to staging the longitudinal extension to the hepatic side, IDUS seems promising. In an initial series, Tamada et al.[91] concluded that IDUS accuracy in

the assessment of longitudinal cancer extension to the hepatic side of the stricture was 72% with selected criteria (notching of the outer margins).[81] This accuracy was increased when asymmetric wall thickening was considered as a criterion of longitudinal tumor spread on both hepatic and duodenal sides, with an accuracy of 84% and 86%, respectively, compared with ERCP (47% and 43%).[81] The only limitation is the inflammatory thickening induced when prior drainage of the biliary tract has been performed[79] (Fig. 18.13). Consequently IDUS must be carried out at the same time as ERCP or transhepatic drainage.

IDUS is also very accurate (100%) in defining portal vein and right hepatic artery involvement (Fig. 18.14), which are the two most frequently involved vessels. Left and common hepatic arteries are more rarely involved and are not easily seen, as IDUS cannot explore the area outside the hepatoduodenal ligament.[92,93] In the two most recent preoperative studies of Tamada et al.,[92,93] the accuracy of IDUS in detecting vascular involvement was significantly higher than angiography for both the portal vein (100% versus 50%) and the right hepatic artery (100% versus 33%). Invasion of the adjacent pancreatic parenchyma by a bile duct tumor should be determined in order to propose duodenopancreatectomy in combination with bile duct resection. IDUS was also superior to EUS in identifying slight invasion of the pancreatic parenchyma (accuracy

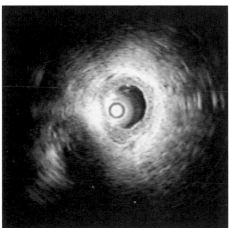

Fig. 18.13 IDUS showing inflammatory wall thickening after stenting.

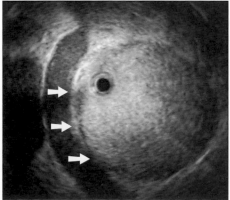

Fig. 18.14 IDUS showing vascular staging of cholangiocarcinoma with no infiltration of the right hepatic artery (arrows).

100% versus 78%),[79] but the therapeutic impact is probably small, as IDUS may understage intraductal infiltration.

Control series comparing the performance of each imaging modality (CT, MRCP, EUS, and IDUS) are lacking. A clinical approach in patients with Klatskin tumors should be to start with MRI and MR angiography. In patients with resectable tumors, ERCP plus IDUS should be the second step, carried out before surgery. For bile duct tumors, EUS remains the most effective approach. ERCP plus IDUS shoud be proposed only when the upper part of the tumor cannot be seen with EUS, or when doubt remains concerning spread to the portal vein. Finally, EUS and IDUS are useful tools in determining the nature of a biliary stenosis and for the staging of cholangiocarcinoma. As a result of their respective limitations (hilum for EUS, and need for biliary drainage with IDUS), their use depends on the clinical presentation and results of conventional imaging.

DIAGNOSTIC CHECKLIST

Cholangiocarcinoma
- Hypoechoic thickening of the wall with or without a mass
- Polypoid intraluminal tumor
- Involvement of vessels, pancreas, liver, ampulla, or duodenum
- Bile duct dilation
- Papillomatosis
- Polypoid intraluminal tumor with alternation of normal bile duct wall

Mirizzi's syndrome
- Compression of CBD by intracystic stone
- Regular thickening of bile duct wall

Other benign stenosis
- Regular thickening without wall disruption

GALLBLADDER DISEASE (EXCLUDING STONES)

Polyps

The widespread use of US has led to the identification of an increasing number of polypoid lesions of the gallbladder. Indeed, 4–7% of the healthy population has been reported to have polyps in the gallbladder.[94-96] Cholesterol, inflammatory, and fibrous polyps have no malignant potential, and surgical intervention is not required as long as the patient is asymptomatic. In contrast, adenomatous polyps must be resected as the adenoma–carcinoma sequence is well characterized in the biliary epithelium and gallbladder.[87,98] In a histologic review of a large series of 1605 sequential cholecystectomy specimens, the presence of histologic transition of adenoma into carcinoma was revealed. All in situ carcinomas were associated with adenomatous components.[97] The same association was found

in 19% of invasive carcinomas. Moreover, gallbladder carcinoma has one of the most dismal prognosis among malignancies of the digestive system, except at an early stage.

With regard to treatment, laparoscopic surgery is a minimally invasive method for removal of the gallbladder. However, the rate of procedure-related complications has been reported to be as high as 4.3%.[99,100] Moreover, postcholecystectomy syndrome develops in up to 20% of cholecystectomized patients.[101,102] It is therefore important to establish criteria to select candidates for surgery among patients with gallbladder polyps. However, it is still hard to make differential diagnoses of such lesions by US, CT, or MRI, and the incidental finding of a gallbladder polyp in an asymptomatic patient often leads to a clinical dilemma. Solitary lesions, greater than 10 mm in diameter, of sessile appearance and hypoechogenicity are findings suggestive of a neoplastic polyp,[97,103] and in these patients surgical treatment should be performed.[104,105] However, polyps smaller than 10 mm in diameter and appearing as echogenic pedunculated masses at US are generally cholesterol and inflammatory polyps, and only a follow-up should be recommended. This approach can, however, be debated. In a recent study of 70 patients with polypoid lesions smaller than 2 cm, 34.6% of non-neoplastic polyps were more than 10 mm in diameter.[106] Moreover, it has been reported that 30% of polyps measuring 11–20 mm in diameter are cholesterol polyps.[107] The indication of cholecystectomy for gallbladder polyps larger than 10 mm should therefore be re-evaluated. However, 19–29% of polyps between 5 and 10 mm of size correspond to adenomas.[103,108] A precise diagnosis of the etiology of the polyp is then necessary to determine the best therapeutic approach. Considering its higher-resolution performances, EUS should be more accurate than US for imaging gallbladder lesions.[103,108,109]

The structure of the gallbladder wall can readily be seen with EUS as a two-layered structure. The inner hypoechoic layer represents the mucosa, muscular layer, and subserosal fibrous layer. The outer hyperechoic layer represents the subserosal fat layer and serosa.[110-113] In some cases, a hyperechoic layer is demonstrated on the inner hypoechoic layer. This is considered to be mainly an interface echo. Gallbladder polyp is defined as a fixed echo structure protruding into the gallbladder lumen without acoustic shadowing on EUS. For Azuma et al.,[109] EUS was better than US in diagnosing the nature of gallbladder polyps: of 89 polyps smaller than 2 cm, 86.5% were correctly diagnosed by EUS, compared with only 51.7% by US. The sensitivity, specificity, positive predictive value, and negative predictive value of EUS in the diagnosis of carcinoma were 91.7%, 87.7%, 75.9%, and 96.6%, respectively.

Two series proposed a scoring system that relied on EUS findings in order to ascertain the risk of neoplasia.[106,108] In a retrospective analysis of EUS findings in 70 patients operated on for polypoid gallbladder lesions smaller than 20 mm, Sadamoto et al.[106] analyzed the morphologic characteristics of gallbladder polyps by multivariate stepwise logistic regression. The polypoid lesions confirmed by cholecystectomy were classified into two groups: neoplastic (adenomas and adenocarcinomas) and non-neoplastic lesions (fibrous, inflammatory, and cholesterol polyps). The EUS variables studied were the maximum diameter and height/width ratio of the largest polyps, echo level, internal echo pattern, surface patterns, number and shape of polyps, presence of hyperechoic spots, and presence of gallbladder stones. The variables of internal echo pattern and hyperechoic spots were statistically significant in addition to tumor size. All neoplastic polyps, including the smaller ones, were shown on EUS with a relatively heterogeneous internal echo pattern. In contrast, large cholesterol polyps (more than 10 mm in diameter) had a homogeneous internal echo pattern. It has been proposed that the heterogeneous internal echo pattern of neoplastic lesions corresponds to their irregular internal structure, seen in the resected specimens, due to cancerous tubular structures and mixed cellularity. The hyperechoic spotting has been reported to represent a mass of foamy histiocytes containing cholesterol.[96,107] Hyperechoic spotting is highly significant for cholesterol polyps.[106,107] However, it has been reported that, in two cases of polypoid adenocarcinomas, hyperechoic spotting representing the accumulation of foamy cells underneath cancerous epithelium was detected by EUS.[106] The overall EUS score for the risk of neoplastic polyps was calculated as follows: maximum diameter in millimeters plus internal echo pattern score plus hyperechoic spots score (heterogeneous, +4; homogeneous, 0; presence of hyperechoic spots, - 5; absence of hyperechoic spots, 0). The sensitivity, specificity, and accuracy with scores of 12 or higher were 77.8%, 82.7%, and 82.9%, respectively.[106] According to these results, polypoid lesions with a score of at least 12 have a high likelihood of being neoplastic. The sensitivity, specificity, and accuracy of a score lower than 12 for the diagnosis of non-neoplastic polyp were not evaluated.

Another scoring system based on five EUS variables has been proposed to predict the malignancy of gallbladder polyps.[108] It was based on layer structure, echo pattern, margin, stalk, and number of polyps. The EUS scoring system has been developed retrospectively using data obtained from a reference group of 79 patients, and applied to a validation group of 53 patients (26 patients with polyps of 5–15 mm in diameter). According to the results of this study, size was the most significant predictor of neoplastic polyps. All polyps with a diameter of 5 mm or less were non-neoplastic, whereas 94% of polyps larger than 15 mm were neoplastic. When the size of a gallbladder polyp exceeded 15 mm, the risk of neoplasia increased significantly compared with that of polyps measuring 5–10 or 10–15 mm in diameter. However, polyps of 5 –10 and 10–15 mm in diameter showed no significant difference in terms of risk of malignancy. For polyps measuring between 5 and 15 mm, the risk of neoplasia was significantly greater with a score of at least 6 than for those with a score of less than 6, with a sensitivity, specificity, and accuracy of 81%, 86%, and 84%, respectively. The authors concluded that use of the scoring system in patients with 5–15-mm gallbladder polyps could identify those

patients at risk of neoplasia, and that echo pattern was more important than size in the differential diagnosis of gallbladder polyps in this group of patients. Therefore, EUS should be included in the work-up of the majority of patients with gallbladder polyps.

Considering the results of these series, it would appear that gallbladder polyps may be differentiated more accurately with EUS than with US. Nevertheless, these results must be interpreted with caution as they are the result of retrospective studies including small numbers of patients. Furthermore, no interobserver agreement study has been done. Consequently, further large prospective studies are needed before EUS findings can be considered accurate enough to make the choice between surgery and follow-up. A systematic surgical approach for gallbladder polyps bigger than 1 cm remains the safest choice. Nevertheless, in patients at high surgical risk, this approach should be adapted to the complementary result of EUS. However, although it is probably unnecessary to perform EUS for polyps of 5 mm or less, it could be proposed for those between 5 and 10 mm. In cases of suspicious EUS, surgery should be performed earlier to avoid the risk of loss during follow-up. In other cases EUS would be a reference examination for polyps that exhibit growth or changes in echo patterns and shape on US follow-up.[114,115]

Gallbladder tumors

Preoperative differentiation of adenomas from adenocarcinomas is unnecessary as adenomas have malignant potential,[97] and both lesions should be treated surgically. However, with the replacement of open cholecystectomy by the laparoscopic approach, the preoperative diagnosis of gallbladder cancer is very important as recurrence of cancer in the abdominal wall[24] has occasionally been reported after laparoscopic cholecystectomy in advanced carcinomas. Recent advances in abdominal US and CT have made it possible to diagnose gallbladder carcinoma at an earlier stage. However, these modalities can stage only advanced lesions. As EUS is helpful in differentiating the benign or malignant nature of a polyp, it can help to determine the optimal surgical approach: laparoscopy for benign polyps or early cancer, and open surgery for advanced cancer.[117]

The accuracy of EUS in gallbladder cancer staging depends on the criteria chosen. The integrity of the wall layers at the base of a gallbladder polyp is the determinant criteria (Fig. 18.15). Fujita et al.[111] retrospectively divided the tumors into four groups, with good interobserver correlation. Type A was a pedunculated mass including a solid echo pattern with a fine nodular surface. Type B tumor was a broad-based mass with an irregular surface and intact outer hyperechoic layer. In type C tumors, the outer hyperechoic layer of the wall was irregular due to a mass echo, whereas in type D tumors the entire layer structure was disrupted. The definition of T staging of gallbladder carcinoma according to the International Union Against Cancer (UICC)[118] is as follows. Tis, carcinoma in situ; T1a, invasion of lamina propria; T1b, invasion of muscle layer; T2, tumor

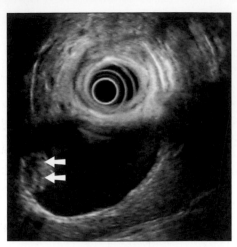

Fig. 18.15
Adenomatous gallbladder polyp 15 mm in diameter (arrows).

invades the perimuscular connective tissue without extension beyond the serosa; T3, tumor perforates the serosa or directly invades into the liver to a depth of less than 2 cm; T4, tumor penetration of more than 2 cm into the liver and/or other adjacent organs. After correlation of EUS aspect and pathology, the authors proposed that type A cancer on EUS should be classified before surgery as Tis, because cancer invasion is confined to the mucosa with no invasion of the surrounding epithelium. Type C cancer invades the adipose layer of the subserosa; therefore its preoperative T staging should be T2. Type B carcinomas can be T1 or T2, because their depth of invasion varies from mucosa to the fibrous layer of the subserosa. This is the most difficult case to classify correctly, as diagnosing the depth of invasion is difficult when the outer hyperechoic layer is preserved.

In another recent retrospective study of 41 patients with gallbladder cancer,[119] a strong correlation between EUS images and histopathologic tumor stage was found. EUS and histopathologic findings were compared, especially the depth of invasion of the lesion in the resected specimens. EUS images were classified according to the shape of the tumor and the adjacent gallbladder wall structure as follows: type A, pedunculated mass with preserved adjacent wall structure; type B, sessile and/or broad-based mass with a preserved outer hyperechoic layer of the gallbladder wall; type C, sessile and/or broad-based mass with a narrowed outer hyperechoic layer; and type D, sessile and/or broad-based mass with a disrupted outer hyperechoic layer. The four types of EUS image correlated with the histologic depth of invasion and T stage. Type A corresponded to Tis, type B to T1, type C to T2, and type D to T3–4. The corresponding accuracies of EUS classification were 100%, 75.6%, 85.3%, and 92.7% for types 1, 2, 3, and 4, respectively. The best results were found for Tis or T3–4 tumors. An extended cholecystectomy with systematic lymph node dissection and resection of the liver bed could be applied in type D tumors, and a celioscopic cholecystectomy performed for Tis tumors. The difference between T1 and T2 tumors was more difficult to establish. The differential diagnosis between T1 and T2 polypoid gallbladder tumors was easier when a hypoechoic area

within the deeper part of the tumor was found by EUS. This finding indicates subserosal invasion,[120] but is valuable only for polypoid gallbladder tumors.

The value of EUS-FNA in the diagnosis and staging of gallbladder tumors remains questionable. It appears to be a safe procedure for obtaining samples from gallbladder masses for cytologic examination.[121] It could also be used for confirming lymph node involvement, as the existence of malignant lymph nodes indicates stage III disease irrespective of T staging.[122] Nevertheless, the real impact of the FNA result remains dependent on each clinical case. Considering the limited morbidity of surgery, it is certainly not reasonable to take the risk of a false-negative FNA result in operable patients. The most valuable use would probably be in the confirmation of distant metastatic lymph nodes in patients with advanced disease, to choose a non-surgical therapy.

The place of EUS in the staging of gallbladder cancer remains questionable, as the series are scarce and retrospective. Nevertheless, EUS appears to be effective in confirmation of early tumors. In these cases, surgery should begin with a laparoscopic approach. EUS also allows the diagnosis of more advanced cases (≥T3), where open cholecystectomy with extensive resection should be considered. In other cases, open cholecystectomy with adaptation of the procedure during surgery, remains the more prudent approach.

Other etiologies of wall thickening

A large number of diseases can induce a localized or diffuse thickening of the gallbladder wall (Table 18.2). Faced with a diffuse thickening with perivesicular fluid, the main issue is to differentiate acute cholecystitis from other diagnoses. In acute cholecystitis, thickening of the wall (>3 mm) is generally combined with an intravesicular thick component, including stones, pus, or fibrin residues.[123] A comparable thickening associated or not with perivesicular fluid can be seen in ascites, portal hypertension, viral hepatitis, and hypoalbuminemia.[123,124] The internal component of the gallbladder and the clinical symptoms are then helpful in the differential diagnosis.

Other conditions with diffuse or localized thickening can be difficult to differentiate from neoplastic disease. Chronic cholecystitis is a common disease combining gallstones and a hyperechoic wall with a preserved layer structure. The wall is usually uniformly involved, but localized thickening is possible.[125] Adenomyomatosis of the gallbladder is usually considered a benign condition. Thickening of the wall is combined with the presence of small cysts, which usually represent intramural diverticula (dilated Rokitansky–Aschoff sinuses). Ultrasonographically, preservation of the layers is visible in a thickened wall with anechoic areas and sometimes associated with hyperechoic echoes (comet-tail artifact, V-shaped reverberation ultrasound artefact).[103] According to the extent and site of involvement, adenomyomatosis was conventionally classified into three types: localized, generalized, and segmental. The diagnosis is generally easy with conventional US as cancer mimicking adeno-

EUS CHARACTERISTICS AND ETIOLOGY OF GALLBLADDER WALL THICKENING		
Disease	Thickening	Other signs
Acute cholecystitis	Localized or diffuse, layers preserved	Perigallbladder fluid
Chronic cholecystitis	High echogenicity	
Gallbladder carcinoma	Localized, layers inconstantly preserved	Polyp or mass
Adenomyomatosis	Localized or diffuse, layers preserved	Anechoic areas (cysts), hyperechoic echoes, comet tail artifact
Xanthogranulomatous cholecystitis	Localized or diffuse, layers inconstantly preserved	Hyperechoic nodules in gallbladder wall
Portal hypertension, viral hepatitis, ascites, or hypoalbuminemia	Diffuse, layers preserved	
Extrahepatic portal venous obstruction	Localized, layers preserved	Varices inside gallbladder wall
Primary cholangitis	Diffuse, layers preserved	Irregular thickening
Diffuse papillomatosis	Localized or diffuse, layers inconstantly preserved	
Anomalous arrangement of pancreatobiliary duct	Diffuse, layers preserved	Predominantly thickening of hypoechoic layer

Table 18.2 EUS characteristics and etiology of gallbladder wall thickening

myomatosis is exceptional.[126] Nevertheless, some cases can be difficult to diagnose, especially the localized type, and the relationship between segmental adenomyomatosis and gallbladder carcinoma is questionable. Segmental adenomyomatosis appears to be a high-risk condition for gallbladder carcinoma, especially in elderly patients.[127] The other types of adenomyomatosis did not show any significant increase in the incidence of gallbladder carcinoma. Xanthogranulomatous cholecystitis (XGC) is an uncommon form of chronic inflammation of the gallbladder, the clinical presentation of which is similar to that of cholecystitis. In a large 15-year series of cholecystectomy, XGC was present in 1.46% of patients.[128] It was associated with lithiasis in 85%. XGC may simulate gallbladder cancer. EUS can sometimes visualize hyperechoic nodules in the gallbladder wall, probably representing xanthogranulomas.[129]

The role of EUS in the diagnosis of gallbladder wall thickening remains poorly analyzed. Mizuguchi et al.[117] compared EUS, conventional US, CT, and MRI in the differential diagnosis of gallbladder wall thickening (seven gallbladder cancers, nine cases of chronic cholecystitis, five cases of XGC, and four cases of adenomyomatosis). The multiple-layer pattern was demonstrated by EUS more efficiently than by other imaging modalities. Loss of multiple-layer patterns of the gallbladder wall demonstrated by EUS was the most specific finding in diagnosing gallbladder cancer. It is nevertheless not pathognomonic, as this finding can also be seen in XGC.[129]

In other diseases the presence of complementary abnormalities is helpful in making the diagnosis. In sclerosing cholangitis, the gallbladder is involved in 15% of cases.[123] Irregular thickening also involves the extrahepatic ducts with alternating stenosis and dilation.[123,130] In extrahepatic portal venous obstruction, varices are observed inside the gallbladder wall in 43% of cases,[131] and can induce a localized thickening. Perivesicular varices or ascites can also be seen. A diffuse regular thickening can also be observed in patients with anatomic variants of the pancreatobiliary duct.[132,133] Generally it is greater than 4 mm and predominantly involves the hypoechoic layer.[132] It can be confirmed pathologically in as many as 91% of patients when biliary ducts are not dilated.[133] Finally, the diffuse papillomatosis of the biliary tract may also involve the gallbladder, presenting as a thickening with a protruding mass[143] combined with biliary ducts polyps.

Summary

In conclusion, the place of EUS in gallbladder disease remains questionable. US is generally sufficient to determine the diagnosis and treatment. In some patients with gallbladder polyps (5–10 mm in diameter, or greater than 10 mm in those with poor operative status), EUS should be proposed to help define the therapeutic choice. It may also be helpful before surgery in patients with suspected gallbladder cancer or in those with large polyps (>15 mm), to highlight criteria that can guide the surgical choice: a laparoscopic approach in tumors without modification of the structural layer of the wall, extensive resection for tumors causing entire disruption of the layer structure, and open cholecystectomy with adaptation during surgery peroperatively for other cases. Finally, in cases of doubtful diagnosis on abdominal US, EUS could be useful in differentiating benign from malignant lesions in the presence of diffuse wall thickening.

AMPULLARY TUMORS

Tumors of the ampulla of Vater originate from the pancreaticobiliary–duodenal junction, limited by the sphincter of Oddi. The pancreatic duct and common bile duct join in the ampulla of Vater and form a distal common channel in about 85% of individuals. The normal ampulla starts about 2 mm outside the duodenal wall and penetrates the muscularis propria somewhat more distally, forming an intraduodenal segment 9–25 mm in length.[135] A wide variety of tumors arise from the ampulla of Vater, including benign tubular and villous adenoma, carcinoma, and several rare other pathologic types, such as lipoma, fibroma, neurofibroma, leiomyoma, lymphangioma, hemangioma, and various neuroendocrine tumors. Adenomas occur sporadically and in the setting of polyposis syndromes. They are considered as premalignant and the adenoma–carcinoma sequence has been assumed to be the main explanation for the pathogenesis of periampullary cancer.[136] Benign adenomas are being detected more frequently during gastroscopy, and now represent an important proportion of endoscopically treated ampullary tumors.[137] Moreover, endoscopic surveillance programs are recommended for patients with familial adenomatosis polyposis syndrome (FAP), because the abnormal findings of the major duodenal papilla, a common site of extracolonic adenoma or malignancy in these patients, show progression of endoscopic and histologic features during follow-up.[138] Tumors can also be discovered in symptomatic patients presenting with jaundice, abdominal pain, weight loss, pancreatitis, or anemia.

Carcinoma of the ampulla (papillary carcinoma) spreads by extension to contiguous organs and by invasion of lymphatic and/or venous vessels. Most ampullary cancers develop from the mucosa of the ampulla and infiltrate the Oddi muscle going through it. They gradually invade the muscularis propria and the serosa of the duodenum, and grow beyond the serosa towards the pancreas. Nevertheless, compared with pancreatic cancer, ampullary neoplasia has a much better prognosis due to the onset of symptoms at an earlier tumor stage. EUS should be useful in two situations: to confirm the diagnosis of an ampullary tumor and to stage adenocarcinomas.

Diagnosis of an ampullary tumor is not always easy endoscopically. The tumors are macroscopically polypoid or ulcerative. The polypoid form can be visible or unexposed (intramural). Bile stasis may also contribute to gallstone formation. In fact, between 6% and 38% of patients with ampullary neoplasm also have coexistent choledocholithiasis.[139–143] Limitations are due to false-positive results following stone migration, to false-negative findings as a result of endoampullary growth, or to the coexistence of stones leading to diagnostic errors because of similiar clinical manifestations.

These limitations also exist for pathology. First, biopsies can be falsely negative owing to endoampullary growth in 5–38% of cases.[142–146] In these cases endoscopic sphincterotomy is necessary to expose the endoampullary growth and allow secondary positive biopsies. Second, the differential diagnosis between an inflammatory tissue and a low-grade dysplasia (LGD) adenoma can be difficult for the pathologist, and repeated biopsies may be necessary. Finally, standard forceps biopsies are not representative of the overall status of the tumor: benign adenomas may harbor foci of carcinoma that may be either superficial or invasive, just as benign tissue elements may be found in ampullary carcinomas.[147] In fact, biopsies underestimate the presence of adenocarcinoma in 19–30% of cases.[142–146]

Considering these drawbacks, the differential diagnosis between a normal ampulla, an odditis, or a real tumor can be difficult. Whether EUS should be used to diagnose an ampul-

loma when faced with a protruding ampulla without mucosal abnormalities at duodenoscopy is questionable. Few series have addressed this problem. Will et al.[148] reported a series of 133 patients with unclear biliary problems, cholestasis, or tumors of the papilla found by duodenoscopy in which EUS sensitivity and specificity in the detection of malignant lesions of the papilla and the peripapillary region were 92.3% and 75.3%, respectively. This low specificity was confirmed by other series. In 1993, the present authors showed that the only specific signs to confirm the presence of an ampulloma were criteria in favor of an invasive tumor (at least with infiltration of the duodenal muscularis propria) (Fig. 18.16) or the presence of endoluminal growth in the CBD (Fig. 18.17) or the Wirsung duct.[149] The other criteria – echogenicity (Figs 18.18 & 18.19), enlargement of the ampulla, and CBD or Wirsung duct dilation (Fig. 18.20) – were not specific and were possibly seen in sclerosing odditis or even in the normal ampulla. These results were confirmed by Rösch et al.[150] If EUS sensitivity in the detection of an ampullary tumor is high in symptomatic patients, it is certainly lower in asymptomatic ones. It is common in patients with FAP to diagnose ampullary tumors without EUS abnormalities. This emphasizes the fact that, if EUS is a useful tool in the diagnosis of ampulloma in some patients, only biopsy can reliably confirm the diagnosis.

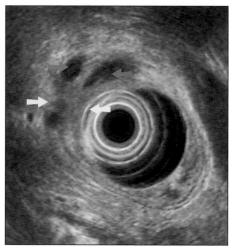

Fig. 18.16 uT3 ampulloma with pancreatic infiltration. Yellow arrow, tumor; green arrow, CBD; blue arrow, pancreatic duct.

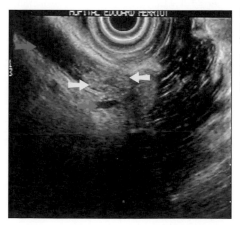

Fig. 18.17 Intraductal (CBD) infiltration. Yellow arrow, tumor; green arrow, CBD; blue arrow, pancreatic duct.

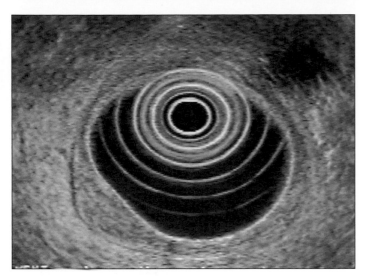

Fig. 18.18 Sclerosing odditis.

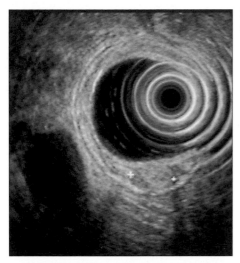

Fig. 18.19 uT1 ampulloma.

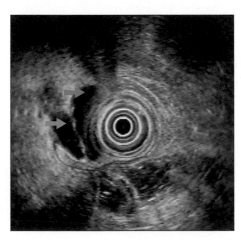

Fig. 18.20 Sclerosing odditis with dilation of the ducts. Green arrow, CBD; blue arrow, pancreatic duct.

Finally, two different situations can be encountered: (1) in patients with a suspicion of ampullary obstruction (clinically, biochemically, or by morphologic examination) but with inconclusive biopsy findings and no specific criteria of ampullary tumor at EUS, endoscopic sphincterotomy with repeated biopsy is needed to differentiate odditis from an early ampullary tumor;

and (2) in asymptomatic patients with a suspicion of early tumor at endoscopy but inconclusive biopsy findings and normal EUS, only follow-up with repeated biopsy can be recommended.

As for other digestive cancers, the aim of staging is to choose the best therapeutic approach and determine the prognosis. For a long time Whipple's operation has been the only potentially curative treatment. In patients with benign tumors or early cancer, the same treatment was generally undertaken. Surgical ampullectomy was rarely done, owing to its morbidity and the impossibility of ascertaining before the pathologic analysis that there was no likelihood of metastatic lymph nodes. During the last decade, progressive developments in endoscopic ampullectomy have allowed the curative treatment of benign adenomas or early cancers in 70–80% of patients.[151–154] Snare ampullectomy has a lower morbidity rate (6–36%[137,142,155–157]) than local surgical excision,[144] and essentially no mortality (0–1%). Nevertheless, morbidity remains significant and careful patient selection is required to avoid an unnecessary endoscopic approach that would need to be completed by a Whipple's operation. Two limitations of the endoscopic curative approach must be considered: tumors with a risk of lymph node metastasis and intraductal invasion inside the pancreatic duct or CBD (technical limitation). This evolution explains the role of pretherapeutic staging, not only to assess the resectability of the tumor but also to determine which tumors may be resected endoscopically (benign adenomas and early cancer without intraductal infiltration).

According to the TNM classification[158] used to stage ampullary tumors, T1 corresponds to tumors not extending beyond the sphincter of Oddi, T2 tumors are those invading the muscularis propria of the duodenal wall, T3 corresponds to tumors invading the adjacent pancreas by less than 2 cm, and T4 tumors invade the pancreas deeply or involve adjacent organs or basic vessels. Nevertheless, this classification is not perfect, as stage T1 includes early cancers invading the mucosa or limited to the sphincter of Oddi but also tumors invading the duodenal submucosa. The Japanese staging system developed by biliary surgeons is more selective. T1 tumors are divided into d0 tumors limited to the sphincter of Oddi and d1 tumors that invade the duodenal submucosa; stage d2 is equivalent to T2. The difference is marked in terms of the risk of lymph node metastasis. Although the risk for T1 tumors ranges from 0% to 20%,[159–161] it is very different for d0 (0%) and d1 (30%) tumors.[162–164] The presence of metastatic lymph nodes is of course greater in more advanced tumors: 55% in T2 and 78% in T3–T4 lesions.[162] Logically, Japanese surgeons consider d0 cancer as an early cancer. In these patients, endoscopic ampullectomy should be used with curative intent.

Various imaging modalities, such as US, CT, angiography, ERCP, MRCP, and EUS, have been used to stage the lesion and evaluate its resectability. These tumors often grow around the ampulla, far from the mesenteric and portal vessels, with rapid symptomatic signs such as jaundice and pancreatitis. It is therefore rare to see a large tumor originating from the ampulla and invading the vessels. The likelihood of the tumor being resectable is then easier to determine than for pancreatic adenocarcinomas. More important is the T staging, which allows the prognosis to be determined and the choice between a surgical or endoscopic resection to be made.

EUS is the most reliable modality for local preoperative staging of these lesions. In the earliest series, EUS was shown to be superior to CT, US, and angiography[69,150] for evaluation of T and N staging, and to determine resectability (95% accuracy in assessing portal venous system involvement[150]). These results have been confirmed in more recent studies comparing EUS (radial or linear) with conventional or helical CT for staging as well as for resectability.[165–167] In the largest series of 50 consecutive patients with ampullary neoplasms, EUS was compared with CT, MRI, and angiography, and found to be more accurate than CT (78% versus 24%, respectively) and MRI (46%) in the overall assessment of T stage.[159] EUS understaging of true T3 lesions or overstaging of true T2 carcinomas accounted for most of the errors in the EUS T-stage assessment, probably due to desmoplastic peritumoral pancreatitis, which cannot easily be differentiated from foci of invasive carcinoma.[160] Nevertheless, this differentiation is not mandatory as the same surgical treatment is used for T2 and T3 tumors. More important is the accuracy of EUS in determining whether or not endoscopic resection can be used with curative intent. The accuracy of EUS in confirming that the T stage is higher than T1 is very good, ranging from 87% to 94% (Table 18.3). Its ability to show an intraductal infiltration also seems to be good, although this has not yet been clearly evaluated in the literature. However, EUS is limited in its ability to show infiltration of the duodenal submucosa, as the sphincter of Oddi is not seen with 7.5 or 12 MHz, even though the infiltration of the third hyperechoic layer of the duodenum sometimes enables the diagnosis of a d1 tumor[168] (Fig. 18.21). EUS also has low accuracy in the detection of lymph node metastases (53–87%), with a negative predictive value of less than 75%, which is insufficient to consider that a T1 tumor is N0.[69,150,159,160,169,170] As EUS-guided FNA is highly accurate in sampling tissue from extraluminal lesions,[171] use of this technique might increase the diagnostic accuracy of preoperative EUS; however, no specific studies regarding ampullary staging

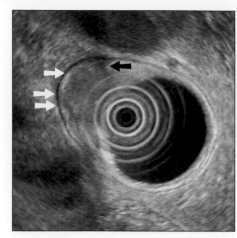

Fig. 18.21 uT1sm ampulloma (black arrow) with disruption of the submucosa (white arrows indicate muscularis propria).

have yet been published. In any case, the accuracy would certainly not be 100%.

EUS can therefore be considered a highly accurate modality in predicting the irresectability of ampullary carcinoma and determining the T stage. Nevertheless, in view of the difficulty of selecting patients correctly for endoscopic ampullectomy, EUS is not sufficient as it does not demarcate the sphincter of Oddi and its negative predictive value for the presence of metastatic lymph nodes is very low. Two complementary explorations, duodenoscopy and intraductal ultrasonography (IDUS), may be useful. On duodenoscopy, ulceration above the roof of the ampulla, separated from the papilla by normal mucosa, indicates a lesion invading the duodenal submucosa and should be considered invasive.[155] For other tumors, IDUS should be proposed. Intraductal catheter probes (Fig. 18.22) employ a higher frequency (20 MHz) and show a marked improvement in resolution compared with the 7.5 or 12 MHz used for conventional EUS. However, they have some restrictions: the ultrasonic probe should be inserted into the tumor via ERCP and the scanning area is smaller than that for EUS, so that N staging is more difficult.[169] However, IDUS is the only imaging modality that can provide an image of Oddi's muscle layer as a distinct layer.[170] The possibility of delineating the sphincter of Oddi and the duodenal submucosa allows the staging of patients as in the Japanese classification, especially

PERFORMANCE OF ULTRASONOGRAPHIC MODALITIES IN THE STAGING OF AMPULLOMA AS A TUMOR ABOVE T1							
Reference	No. of patients	Techniques	Sensitivity (%)	Specificity (%)	PPV (%)	NPV (%)	Accuracy (%)
Tio et al.[26]	32	EUS	100	60	93.1	100	93.7
Menzel et al.[36]	15	IDUS	100	80	90.9	100	93.3
Mukai et al.[31]	23	EUS	92.8	77.8	86.7	87.5	86.9
Itoh et al.[37]	32	IDUS	84.6	100	100	90.5	93.7
Cannon et al.[25]	50	EUS	88.2	100	100	80	90

Table 18.3 Performance of ultrasonographic modalities in the staging of ampulloma as a tumor above T1

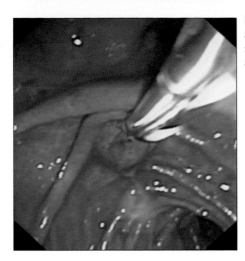

Fig. 18.22 IDUS over a guidewire for staging of ampulloma.

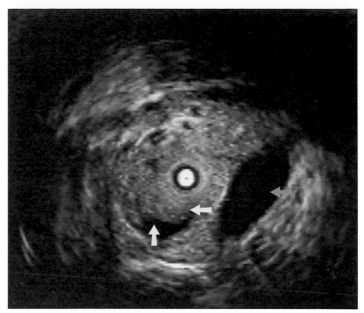

Fig. 18.24 IDUS showing an ampulloma. Yellow arrows, intrabiliary spread; blue arrow, normal pancreatic duct.

in the differentiation of do from d1 tumors (Fig. 18.23). In the first series of 32 patients with cancer of the papilla of Vater, the accuracy of IDUS was 87.5%, and its sensitivity and specificity in assessing lymph node metastases were 66.7% and 91.3%, respectively.[170] The diagnostic accuracy of tumor dissemination was greatest for early tumors, with a rate of 100%, 92.3%, and 100% for do, d1, and d2 lesions, respectively. In the authors' experience,[172] in 31 patients with uT1 No disease without intraductal involvement at EUS, IDUS had an accuracy of 89% for parietal staging (do vs > do) (do vs d1 or d2); in 19% of patients a true infiltration of the submucosa was diagnosed. IDUS was also very accurate in showing intraductal involvement, with 100% accuracy[170,172] (Fig. 18.24).

Considering the respective performances of these investigations, a three-step algorithm could be applied to ascertain whether an ampullary tumor may be treated curatively by endoscopic ampullectomy:

1 EUS – Tumors staged above uT1 and tumors with intraductal infiltration can be selected for a Whipple's resection with no further exploration.

2 Duodenoscopy (for uT1 tumors without intraductal infiltration) – If ulceration is seen above the roof of the ampulla, this indicates submucosal infiltration; a Whipple's resection should be considered.

3 IDUS (for uT1 tumors without intraductal infiltration or duodenal ulceration) – Tumors without submucosal infiltration and intraductal spread should be considered for endoscopic ampullectomy with curative intent (Fig. 18.25).

In the authors' experience, this algorithm is very effective in the selection of patients for endoscopic ampullectomy.[172] In 81% of 24 patients selected using this sequence, the pathologic specimen confirmed that the resection was complete, with no tumoral infiltration of the duodenal submucosa or extension into the ducts. As for local surgical excision, the recurrence rate

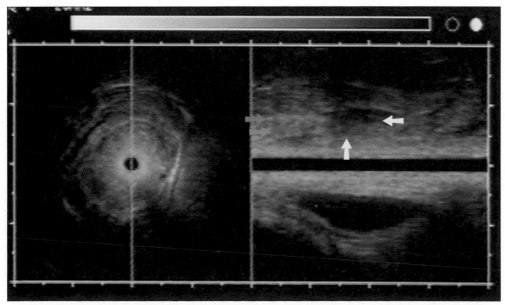

Fig. 18.23 Three-dimensional IDUS showing a d1 ampulloma. Yellow arrows, tumor with disruption of the submucosa; green arrow, normal submucosa; blue arrow, sphincter of Oddi.

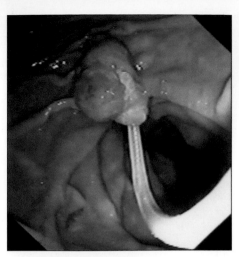

Fig. 18.25
Endoscopic snare resection of an ampullary tumor.

after snare ampullectomy is about 30%.[173] EUS is needed, in combination with endoscopy and biopsy, in the follow-up of patients with ampullary adenomas treated endoscopically, especially to detect intraductal recurrence.

EUS and IDUS staging of ampullary tumors must be performed before any invasive treatment of the ampulla of Vater, particularly prior to diathermic biopsy, endoscopic sphincterotomy, or biliary stent insertion. These procedures may compromise EUS interpretation by introducing air and creating artifacts, as was observed in some series; in the presence of a transpapillary endobiliary stent, EUS T-stage accuracy was reduced from 84% to 72%.[159] This was most prominent in the understaging of T2 and T3 carcinomas. Moreover, the bile duct wall thickness, measured by an intraductal ultrasonographic probe, was more than doubled in patients with an endobiliary drainage catheter in place for as little as 14 days,[79] and could be interpreted as intraductal spread.

Economic studies concerning the value of pretherapeutic staging are rare. Only one series has shown that use of EUS in the selection of patients for local resection may be a cost-effective approach in the management of ampullary tumors.[174]

Summary

EUS can be helpful in the diagnosis of ampullary tumors, especially advanced lesions with no endoscopic abnormalities. It is also of use in the management of ampullary cancer, as it is fairly accurate in the assessment of resectability and prognosis. With the development of curative endoscopic treatment for benign and early cancers of the ampulla, accurate staging is needed for patient selection. A three-step algorithm combining EUS, duodenoscopy, and IDUS is promising. More widespread use of IDUS is now needed.

DIAGNOSTIC CHECKLIST

Ampullary tumors
- Hypoechoic or hyperechoic thickening of the ampulla
- Polypoid intraluminal tumor
- Involvement of vessels, pancreas, or duodenum
- Bile or pancreatic duct dilation

Odditis
- Hypoechoic or hyperechoic thickening of the ampulla
- Duodenal wall layers preserved
- No intraductal polypoid infiltration
- Bile or pancreatic duct dilation

EXAMINATION CHECKLIST

Extrahepatic ducts (CBD, common hepatic duct, cystic duct)
Intrahepatic ducts (dilation, stones?)
Left and right liver lobe
Gallbladder
Ampulla (including IDUS in the case of T1 ampullary lesions)
Pancreas and Wirsung duct
Lymph nodes
Ascites
Portal hypertension

REFERENCES

1 Davis WZ, Cotton PB, Arias A. ERCP and sphincterotomy in the context of laparoscopic cholecystectomy: academic and community practice patterns and results. Am J Gastroenterol 1997; 92:597–601.

2 Loperfido S, Angelini G, Benedetti G. Major early complications from diagnostic and therapeutic ERCP: a prospective multicenter study. Endoscopy 1999; 31:125–130.

3 Freeman ML, Nelson DB, Sherman S, et al. Complications of endoscopic biliary sphincterotomy. N Engl J Med 1996; 335:908–918.

4 Sherman S, Ruffolo TA, Hawes RH, et al. Complications of endoscopic sphincterotomy. Gastroenterology 1991; 101:1068–1072.

5 Lambert ME, Betts CD, Hill J, et al. Endoscopic sphincterotomy: the whole truth. Br J Surg 1991; 78:473–476.

6 Hawes RH, Cotton PB, Vallon AG. Follow up 6–11 years after duodenoscopic sphincterotomy for stones in patients with prior cholecystectomy. Gastroenterology 1990; 98:1008–1012.

7 Bergman JG, van Berkel AM, Groen AK, et al. Biliary manometry, bacterial characteristics, bile composition, and histologic changes fifteen to seventeen years after endoscopic sphincterotomy. Gastrointest Endosc 1997; 45:400–405.

8 Dong B, Chen M. Improved sonographic visualization of choledocholithiasis. J Clin Ultrasound 1987; 15:185–190.

9 Stott MA, Farrands PA, Guyer PB, et al. Ultrasound of the common bile duct in patients undergoing cholecystectomy. J Clin Ultrasound 1991; 19:73–76.

10 Neitlich JD, Topazian M, Smith RC, et al. Detection of choledocholithiasis: comparison of unenhanced helical CT and

endoscopic retrograde cholangiopancreatography. Radiology 1997; 203:753–757.

11 Polkowski M, Palucki J, Regula J, et al. Helical computed tomographic cholangiography versus endosonography for suspected bile duct stones: a prospective blinded study in non-jaundiced patients. Gut 1999; 45:744–749.

12 Napoléon B, Dumortier J, Keriven-Souquet O, et al. Do normal findings at biliary endoscopic ultrasonography obviate the need for endoscopic retrograde cholangiography in patients with suspicion of common bile duct stone? A prospective follow-up of 238 patients. Endoscopy 2003; 35:411–415.

13 Canto MIF, Chak A, Stellato T, et al. Endoscopic ultrasonography versus cholangiography for the diagnosis of choledocholithiasis. Gastrointest Endosc 1998; 47:439–448.

14 Lightdale CJ. Indications, contraindications and complications of endoscopic ultrasonography. Gastrointest Endosc 1996; 43:15–19.

15 Palazzo L, Girollet PP, Salmeron M, et al. Value of endoscopic ultrasonography in the diagnosis of common bile duct stones: comparison with surgical exploration and ERCP. Gastrointest Endosc 1995; 42:225–231.

16 Liu CL, Lo CM, Chan JK, et al. EUS for detection of occult cholelithiasis in patients with idiopathic pancreatitis. Gastrointest Endosc 2000; 51:28–32.

17 Frossard JL, Sosa-Valencia L, Amouyal G, et al. Usefulness of endoscopic ultrasonography in patients with 'idiopathic' acute pancreatitis. Am J Med 2000; 109:196–200.

18 Bret PM, Reinhold C. Magnetic resonance cholangiopancreatography. Endoscopy 1997; 29:472–486.

19 Kay CL. Which test to replace diagnostic ERCP – MRCP or EUS? Endoscopy 2003; 35:426–428.

20 Lambert R. Clinical outcome of EUS in biliary diseases. Endoscopy 2000; 32:558–561.

21 Chan WL, Chan AC, Lam WW, et al. Choledocholithiasis: comparison of MR cholangiography and endoscopic retrograde cholangiography. Radiology 1996; 200:85–89.

22 Mendler MH, Bouillet P, Sautereau P, et al. Value of MR cholangiography in the diagnosis of obstructive diseases of the biliary tree: a study of 58 cases. Am J Gastroenterol 1998; 93:2482–2490.

23 Zidi SH, Prat F, Le Guen O, et al. Use of magnetic resonance cholangiography in the diagnosis of choledocholithiasis: prospective comparison with the reference imaging method. Gut 1999; 44:118–122.

24 Aubé C, Delorme B, Yzet T, et al. MR cholangiopancreatography versus endoscopic sonography in suspected common bile duct lithiasis: a prospective, comparative study. Am J Roentgenol 2005; 184:55–62.

25 Frossard JL, Hadengue A, Amouyal G, et al. Choledocholithiasis: a prospective study of spontaneous common bile duct stone migration. Gastrointest Endosc 2000; 51:175–179.

26 Berdah SV, Orsoni P, Berge T, et al. Follow-up of selective endoscopic ultrasonography and/or endoscopic retrograde cholangiography prior to laparoscopic cholecystectomy: a prospective study of 300 patients. Endoscopy 2001; 33:216–220.

27 Prat F, Amouyal G, Amouyal P, et al. Prospective controlled study of endoscopic ultrasonography and endoscopic retrograde cholangiography in patients with suspected bile duct lithiasis. Lancet 1996; 347:75–79.

28 Buscarini E, Tansini P, Vallisa D, et al. EUS for suspected choledocholithiasis: do benefits outweigh costs? A prospective, controlled study. Gastrointest Endosc 2003; 57:510–518.

29 Scheiman JM, Carlos RC, Barnett JL, et al. Can endoscopic ultrasound or magnetic resonance cholangiopancreatography replace ERCP in patients with suspected biliary disease? A prospective trial and cost analysis. Am J Gastroenterol 2001; 96:2900–2904.

30 De Ledinghen V, Lecesne R, Raymond JM, et al. Diagnosis of choledocholithiasis: EUS or magnetic resonance cholangiography? A prospective controlled study. Gastrointest Endosc 1999; 49:26–31.

31 Materne R, Van Beers BE, Gigot JF, et al. Extrahepatic biliary obstruction: magnetic resonance imaging compared with endoscopic ultrasonography. Endoscopy 2000; 32:3–9.

32 Kohut M, Nowakowska-Dulawa E, Marek T, et al. Accuracy of linear endoscopic ultrasonography in the evaluation of patients with suspected common bile duct stones. Endoscopy 2002; 34:299–303.

33 Seifert H, Wehrmann T, Hilgers R, et al. Catheter probe extraductal EUS reliably detects distal common bile duct abnormalities. Gastrointest Endosc 2004; 60:61–67.

34 Catanzaro A, Pfau P, Isenberg GA, et al. Clinical utility of intraductal EUS for evaluation of choledocholithiasis. Gastrointest Endosc 2003; 57:712–714.

35 Cotton PB, Baillie J, Pappas TN, et al. Laparoscopic cholecystectomy and the biliary endoscopist (editorial). Gastrointest Endosc 1991; 37:94–97.

36 Cotton PB. Endoscopic retrograde cholangiopancreatography and laparoscopic cholecystectomy. Am J Surg 1993; 165:474–478.

37 Abboud PA, Malet PF, Berlin JA, et al. Predictors of bile duct stones prior to cholecystectomy: a meta-analysis. Gastrointest Endosc 1996; 44:450–459.

38 Sugiyama M, Atomi Y. Endoscopic ultrasonography for diagnosing choledocholithiasis: a prospective comparative study with ultrasonography and computed tomography. Gastrointest Endosc 1997; 45:143–146.

39 Sahai AV, Mauldin PD, Marsi V, et al. Bile duct stones and laparoscopic cholecystectomy: a decision analysis to assess the roles of intraoperative cholangiography, EUS and ERCP. Gastrointest Endosc 1999; 49:334–343.

40 Das A, Chak A. EUS. Endoscopic ultrasonography. Endoscopy 2004; 36:17–22.

41 Shea JA, Berlin JA, Escarce JJ, et al. Revised estimates of diagnostic test sensitivity and specificity in suspected biliary tract disease. Arch Intern Med 1994; 154:2573–2581.

42 Ko C, Sekijima J, Lee S. Biliary sludge. Ann Intern Med 1999; 130:301–311.

43 Dill JE, Hill S, Callis J, et al. Combined endoscopic ultrasound and stimulated biliary drainage in cholecystitis and microlithiasis – diagnoses and outcomes. Endoscopy 1995; 27:424–427.

44 Dahan P, Andant C, Levy P, et al. Prospective evaluation of endoscopic ultrasonography and microscopic examination of duodenal bile in the diagnosis of cholecystolithiasis in 45 patients with normal conventional ultrasonography. Gut 1996; 38:277–281.

45 Chak A, Hawes RH, Cooper GS, et al. Prospective assessment of the utility of EUS in the evaluation of gallstone pancreatitis. Gastrointest Endosc 1999; 49:599–604.

46 Liu CL, Lo CM, Chan LK, et al. Detection of choledocholithiasis by EUS in acute pancreatitis: a prospective evaluation in 100 consecutive patients. Gastrointest Endosc 2001; 54:325–330.

47 Shim CS, Joo JH, Park CW, et al. Effectiveness of endoscopic ultrasonography in the diagnosis of choledocolithiasis prior to laparoscopic cholecystectomy. Endoscopy 1995; 27:428–432.

48 Amouyal P, Amouyal G, Levy P, et al. Diagnosis of choledocholithiasis by endoscopic ultrasonography. Gastroenterology. 1994;106: 1062–1067.

49 Gautier G, Pilleul F, Crombe-Ternamian A, et al. Contribution of magnetic resonance cholangiopancreatography to the management of patients with suspected common bile duct stones. Gastroenterol Clin Biol 2004; 28:129–134.

50 Cervi C, Aube C, Tuech JJ, et al. Nuclear magnetic resonance cholangiography in biliary disease. Prospective study in 60 patients. Ann Chir 2000; 125:428–434.

51 Demartines N, Eisner L, Schnabel K, et al. Evaluation of magnetic resonance cholangiography in the management of bile duct stones. Arch Surg 2000; 135:148–152.

52 Kim JH, Kim MJ, Park SI, et al. MR cholangiography in symptomatic gallstones: diagnostic accuracy according to clinical risk group. Radiology 2002; 224:410–416.

53 Stiris MG, Tennoe B, Aadland E, et al. MR cholangiopancreaticography and endoscopic retrograde cholangiopancreaticography in patients with suspected common bile duct stones. Acta Radiol 2000; 41:269–272.

54 Taylor AC, Little AF, Hennessy OF, et al. Prospective assessment of magnetic resonance cholangiopancreatography for noninvasive imaging of the biliary tree. Gastrointest Endosc 2002; 55:17–22.

55 Lahde S. Helical CT in the examination of bile duct obstruction. Acta Radiol 1996; 37:660–664.

56 Park MS, Kim TK, Kim KW, et al. Differentiation of extrahepatic bile duct cholangiocarcinoma from benign stricture: findings at MRCP versus ERCP. Radiology 2004; 233:234–240.

57 Stewart CJ, Mills PR, Carter R, et al. Brush cytology in the assessment of pancreatico-biliary strictures: a review of 406 cases. J Clin Pathol 2001; 54:449–455.

58 Ponchon T, Gagnon P, Berger F, et al. Value of endobiliary brush cytology and biopsies for the diagnosis of malignant bile duct stenosis: results of a prospective study. Gastrointest Endosc 1995; 42:565–572.

59 Schoefl R, Haefner M, Wbra F, et al. Forceps biopsy and brush cytology during endoscopic retrograde cholangiopancreatography for the diagnosis of biliary stenoses. Scand J Gastroenterol 1997; 32:363–368.

60 Farrell RJ, Jain AK, Wang H, et al. The combination of stricture dilation, endoscopic needle aspiration and biliary brushing significantly improves the diagnostic yield of malignant bile duct strictures. Gastrointest Endosc 2001; 54:587–594.

61 de Bellis M, Fogel EL, Sherman S, et al. Influence of stricture dilation and repeat brushing on the cancer detection rate of brush cytology in the evaluation of malignant biliary obstruction. Gastrointest Endosc 2003; 58:176–182.

62 Tamada K, Ueno N, Tomiyama T, et al. Characterization of biliary strictures using intraductal ultrasonography: comparison with percutaneous cholangioscopic biopsy. Gastrointest Endosc 1998; 47:341–349.

63 Tamada K, Kurihara K, Tomiyama T, et al. How many biopsies should be performed during percutaneous transhepatic cholangioscopy to diagnose biliary tract cancer. Gastrointest Endosc 1999; 50:653–658.

64 Deveraux CE, Binmoeller KF. Endoscopic retrograde cholangiopancreatography in the next millennium. Gastrointest Clin N Am 2000; 10:117–133.

65 Fogel EL, Sheman S. How to improve the accuracy of diagnosis of malignant biliary strictures. Endoscopy 1999; 31:758–760.

66 Tio TL, Cheng J, Wijers OB, et al. Endosonographic TNM staging of extrahepatic bile duct cancer: comparison with pathological staging. Gastroenterology 1991; 100:1351–1361.

67 Dancygier H, Nattermann C. The role of endoscopic ultrasonography in biliary tract disease: obstructive jaundice. Endoscopy 1994; 26:800–802.

68 Songur Y, Temucin G, Sahin B. Endoscopic ultrasonography in the evaluation of dilated common bile duct. J Clin Gastroenterol 2001; 33:302–305.

69 Mukai H, Nakajima M, Yasuda K, et al. Evaluation of endoscopic ultrasonography in the preoperative staging of carcinoma of the ampulla of Vater and common bile duct. Gastrointest Endosc 1992; 38:676–683.

70 Rosch T, Meining A, Fruhmorgen S, et al. A prospective comparison of the diagnostic accuracy of ERCP, MRCP, CT, and EUS in the biliary strictures. Gastrointest Endosc 2002; 55:870–876.

71 Menzel J, Poremba C, Dietl KH, et al. Preoperative diagnosis of bile duct strictures –comparison of intraductal ultrasonography with conventional endosonography. Scand J Gastroenterol 2000; 35:77–82.

72 Palazzo L, Roseau G, Gayet B, et al. Endoscopic ultrasonography in the diagnosis and staging of pancreatic adenocarcinoma. Results of a prospective study with comparison to ultrasonography and CT scan. Endoscopy 1993; 25:143–150.

73 Hollerbach S, Klamann A, Topalidis T, et al. Endoscopic ultrasonography (EUS) and fine needle aspiration (FNA) cytology for diagnosis of chronic pancreatitis. Endoscopy 2001; 33:824–831.

74 Gress F, Gotlieb K, Sherman S, et al. Endoscopic ultrasonography-guided fine-needle aspiration biopsy of suspected pancreatic cancer. Ann Intern Med 2001; 134:459–464.

75 Harewood GC, Wiersema MJ. Endosonography-guided fine needle aspiration biopsy in the evaluation of pancreatic masses. Am J Gastroenterol 2002; 97:1386–1391.

76 Byrne MF, Gerke H, Mitchell RM, et al. Yield of endoscopic ultrasound-guided fine-needle aspiration of bile duct lesions. Endoscopy 2004; 36:715–719.

77 Fritscher-Ravens A, Broering DC, Sriram PV, et al. Endoscopic ultrasound-guided fine needle aspiration cytodiagnosis of hilar cholangiocarcinoma: a case series. Gastrointest Endosc 2000; 52:534–540.

78 Lefort C, Napoleon B, Ponchon T, et al. Interest of an intraductal ultrasonographic (IDUS) system in pancreatobiliary tract: results about our 100 first patients (abstract). Endoscopy 2002; 34:A7.

79 Tamada T, Tomiyama T, Ischiyama M, et al. Influence of biliary drainage catheter on bile duct wall thickness as measured by intraductal ultrasonography. Gastrointest Endosc 1998; 47:28–33.

80 Vasquez-Sequeiros E, Baron TH, Clain JE, et al. Evaluation of indeterminate bile duct strictures by intraductal US. Gastrointest Endosc 2002; 56:372–379.

81 Tamada K, Nagai H, Yasuda Y, et al. Transpapillary intraductal US prior to biliary drainage in the assessment of longitudinal spread of extrahepatic bile duct carcinoma. Gastrointest Endosc 2001; 53:300–307.

82 Kuroiwa M, Tsukamoto Y, Naitoh Y, et al. New technique using intraductal ultrasonography for the diagnosis of bile duct cancer. J Ultrasound Med 1994; 13:189–195.

83 Gress F, Chen YK, Sherman S, et al. Experience with a catheter-based ultrasound probe in the bile duct and pancreas. Endoscopy 1995; 27:178–184.

84 Kuroiwa M, Goto H, Hirooka Y, et al. Intraductal ultrasonography for the diagnosis of proximal invasion in extrahepatic bile duct cancer. J Gastroenterol Hepatol 1998; 13:715–719.

85 Tamada K, Tomiyama T, Wada S, et al. Endoscopic transpapillary bile duct biopsy with the combination of intraductal ultrasonography in the diagnosis of biliary strictures. Gut 2002; 50:326–331.

86 Lefort C, Napoléon B, Dumortier J, et al. Intraductal ultrasonography may modify the management of cholangiocarcinomas in diagnosing diffuse papillomatosis (abstract). Endoscopy 2003; 35:A45.

87 Dumortier J, Scoazec JY, Valette PJ, et al. Succesful liver transplantation for diffuse biliary papillomatosis. J Hepatol 2001; 35:542–543.

88 Tamada K, Tomiyama T, Oohashi A, et al. Bile duct wall thickness measured by intraductal US in patients who have not undergone previous biliary drainage. Gastrointest Endosc 1999; 48:199–203.

89 Napoléon B, Lefort C. IDUS: diagnosis of bile duct carcinoma. Dig Endosc 2004; 16:S230–S235.

90 Sato M, Inoue H, Ogawa S, et al. Limitations of transhepatic cholangioscopy for the diagnosis of intramural extension of bile duct carcinoma. Endoscopy 1998; 30:281–288.

91 Tamada K, Ueno N, Ischiyama M, et al. Assessment of pancreatic parenchymal invasion by bile duct cancer using intraductal ultrasonography. Endoscopy 1996; 28:492–496.

92 Tamada K, Ido K, Ueno N, et al. Assessment of hepatic artery invasion by bile duct cancer using intraductal ultrasonography. Endoscopy 1995; 27:579–583.

93 Tamada K, Ido K, Ueno N, et al. Assessment of portal vein invasion by bile duct cancer using intraductal ultrasonography. Endoscopy 1995; 27:573–578.

94 Chen CY, Lu CL, Chang FY, et al. Risk factors for gallbladder polyp in the Chinese population. Am J Gastroenterol 1997; 92:2066–2068.

95 Segawa K, Arisawa T, Niwa Y, et al. Prevalence of gallbladder polyps among apparently healthy Japanese: ultrasonographic study. Am J Gastroenterol 1992; 87:630–633.

96 Sugiyama M, Atomi Y, Kuroda A, et al. Large cholesterol of the gallbladder: diagnosis by means of US and endoscopic US. Radiology 1995; 196:493–497.

97 Kozuka S, Tsubone M, Yasui A, et al. Relation of adenoma to carcinoma in the gallbladder. Cancer 1982; 50:2226–2234.

98 Aldridge MC, Bismuth H. Gallbladder cancer: the polyp–cancer sequence. Br J Surg 1990; 77:363–364.

99 Silverstein B, Cecconello I, Ramos AC, et al. Hemobilia as a complication of laparoscopic cholecystectomy. Surg Laparosc Endosc 1994; 4:301–303.

100 Garcia-Olmo D, Vasquez P, Cifuentes J, et al. Postoperative gangrenous peritonitis after laparoscopic cholecystectomy: a new complication for a new technique. Surg Laparosc Endosc 1996; 6:224–225.

101 Black NA, Thombson E, Sanderson CFB, et al. Symptoms and health status before and 6 weeks after open cholecystectomy: a European cohort study. Gut 1994; 35:1301–1305.

102 Desautels SG, Slivka A, Hutson WR, et al. Post-cholecystectomy pain syndrome: pathophysiology of abdominal pain in sphincter of Oddi type III. Gastroenterology 1999; 116:900–905.

103 Sugiyama K, Atomi Y, Yamato T. Endoscopic ultrasonography for differential diagnosis of polypoid gallbladder lesions: analysis in surgical and follow-up series. Gut 2000; 46:250–254.

104 Shinkai H, Kimura W, Muto T. Surgical indications for small polypoid lesions of the gallbladder. Am J Surg 1998; 175:114–117.

105 Kubota K, Bandai Y, Noie T, et al. How should polypoid lesions of the gallbladder be treated in the era of laparoscopic cholecystectomy? Surgery 1995; 117:481–487.

106 Sadamoto Y, Oda S, Tanaka M, et al. A useful approach to the differential diagnosis of small polypoid lesions of the gallbladder, utilizing an endoscopic ultrasound scoring system. Endoscopy 2002; 34:959–965.

107 Sugiyama M, Xie XY, Atomi Y, et al. Differential diagnosis of small polypoid lesions of the gallbladder. Ann Surg 1999; 229:498–504.

108 Choi WB, Lee SK, Kim MH, et al. A new strategy to predict the neoplastic polyps of the gallbladder based on a scoring system using EUS. Gastrointest Endosc 2000; 52:372–379.

109 Azuma T, Yoshikawa T, Araida T, et al. Differential diagnosis of polypoid lesions of the gallbladder by endoscopic ultrasonography. Am J Surg 2001; 181:65–70.

110 Fujita N, Noda Y, Kobayashi GO, et al. Analysis of the layer structure of the gallbladder wall delineated by endoscopic ultrasound using the pinning method. Dig Endosc 1995; 7:353–356.

111 Fujita N, Noda Y, Kobayashi G, et al. Diagnosis of depth of invasion of gallbladder carcinoma by EUS. Gastrointest Endosc 1999; 50:659–663.

112 Morita K, Nakazawa S, Naito Y, et al. Endoscopic ultrasonography of the gallbladder compared with pathological findings. Jpn J Gastroenterol 1986; 83:86–95.

113 Matsumoto J. Endoscopic ultrasonography diagnosis of gallbladder lesions. Endoscopy 1998; 30(Suppl 1):A120–A127.

114 Kimura K, Fujita N, Noda Y, et al. Differential diagnosis of large-sized pedunculated polypoid lesions of the gallbladder by endoscopic ultrasonography: a prospective study. J Gastroenterol 2001; 36:619–622.

115 Chijiwa K, Sumiyoshi K, Nakayama F. Impact of recent advances in hepatobiliary imaging techniques on the preoperative diagnosis of carcinoma of the gallbladder. World J Surg 1991; 15:322–327.

116 Clair DG, Lautz DB, Brooks DC. Rapid development of umbilical metastases after laparoscopic cholecystectomy for unsuspected gallbladder carcinoma. Surgery 1993; 113:355–358.

117 Mizuguchi M, Kudo S, Fukahori T, et al. Endoscopic ultrasonography for demonstrating loss of multiple layer patterns of the thickened gallbladder wall in the preoperative diagnosis of gllabladder cancer. Eur Radiol 1997; 7:1323–1327.

118 Hermanek P, Hutter VP, Sobin LH, et al. (eds). UICC atlas – illustrated guide to the TNM/pTNM classification of malignant tumors, 5th edn. New York: Springer; 1997.

119 Sadamoto Y, Kubo H, Harada N, et al. Preoperative diagnosis and staging of gallbladder carcinoma by EUS. Gastrointest Endosc 2003; 58:536–541.

120 Fujimoto T, Kato Y, Kitamura T, et al. Hypoechoic area as an ultrasound finding suggesting subserosal invasion in polypoid carcinoma of the gallbladder. Br J Radiol 2001; 74:455–457.

121 Jacobson BC, Pitman MB, Brugge WR. EUS-guided FNA for the diagnosis of gallbladder masses. Gastrointest Endosc 2003; 57:251–254.

122 Fleming ID, Cooper JS, Henson DE, et al. AJCC cancer staging handbook, 5th edn. Philadelphia: Lippincott-Raven; 1998.

123 Vilgrain V, Menu Y. Imagerie du foie, des voies biliaires, du pancréas et de la rate. Médecine Sciences. Paris: Flammarion; 2002.

124 Kim MY, Baik SK, Choi YJ, et al. Endoscopic sonographic evaluation of the thickened gallbladder wall in patients with acute hepatitis. J Clin Ultrasound 2003; 31:245–249.

125 Sato M, Ishida H, Konno K, et al. Segmental chronic cholecystitis: sonographic findings and clinical manifestations. Abdom Imaging 2002; 27:43–46.

126 Ishizuka D, Shirai Y, Tsukada K, et al. Gallbladder cancer with intratumoral anechoic foci: a mimic of adenomyomatosis. Hepatogastroenterology 1998; 45:927–929.

127 Nabatame N, Shirai Y, Nishimura A, et al. High risk of gallbladder carcinoma in elderly patients with segmental adenomyomatosis of the gallbladder. J Exp Clin Cancer Res 2004; 23:593–598.

128 Guzman-Valdivia G. Xanthogranulomatous cholecystitis: 15 years' experience. World J Surg 2004; 28:254–257.

129 Muguruma N, Okamura S, Okahisa T, et al. Endoscopic sonography in the diagnosis of xanthogranulomatous cholecystitis. J Clin Ultrasound 1999; 27:347–350.

130 Palazzo L, Ngo Y, Cellier C. Endosonographic features of primary cholangitis. Study of 23 cases (abstract). Gastrointest Endosc 1997; 45:A611.

131 Palazzo L, Hochain P, Helmer C, et al. Biliary varices on endoscopic ultrasonography: clinical presentation and outcome. Endoscopy 2000; 32:520–524.

132 Tokiwa T, Iwai N. Early mucosal changes of the gallbladder in patients with anomalous arrangement of the pancreaticobiliary duct. Gastroenterology 1996; 110:1614–1618.

133 Tanno S, Obara T, Maguchi H, et al. Thickened inner hypoechogenic layer of the gallbladder wall in the diagnosis of anomalous pancreaticobiliary ductal union with endosonography. Gastrointest Endosc 1997; 46:520–526.

134 Kawakatsu M, Vilgrain V, Zins M, et al. Radiologic features of papillary adenoma and papillomatosis of the biliary tract. Abdom Imaging 1997; 22:87–90.

135 Fockens P. The role of endoscopic ultrasonography in the biliary tract: ampullary tumors. Endoscopy 1994; 26:803–805.

136 Spigelman AD, Talbot IC, Penna C, et al. Evidence for adenoma–carcinoma sequence in the duodenum of patients with familial adenomatous polyposis. J Clin Pathol 1994; 47:709–710.

137 Napoléon B, Barthet M, Saurin JC, et al. Les risques de l'ampullectomie endoscopique sont-ils assez faibles pour en faire une alternative à la chirurgie? Résultats d'une étude rétrospective multicentrique (abstract). Gastrointest Clin Biol 2003; 27:A79.

138 Burke CA, Beck GJ, Church JM, et al. The natural history of untreated duodenal and ampullary adenomas in patients with familial adenomatous polyposis followed in an endoscopic surveillance program. Gastrointest Endosc 1999; 49:358–364.

139 Hayes DH, Bolton JS, Willis GW, et al. Carcinoma of the ampulla of Vater. Ann Surg 1987; 206:572–577.

140 Knox RA, Kingston RD. Carcinoma of the ampulla of Vater. Br J Surg 1986; 73:72–73.

141 Baczako K, Buchler M, Beger H, et al. Morphogenesis and possible precursor lesions of invasive carcinoma of the papilla of Vater: epithelial dysplasia and adenoma. Hum Pathol 1985; 16:305–310.

142 Ponchon T, Berger F, Chavaillon A, et al. Contribution of endoscopy to diagnosis and treatment of tumors of the ampulla of Vater. Cancer 1989; 64:161–167.

143 Kimchi N, Mindrul V, Broide E, et al. The contribution of endoscopy and biopsy to the diagnosis of periampullary tumors. Endoscopy 1998; 30:538–543.

144 Clary B, Tyler D, Dematos P, et al. Local ampullary resection with careful intraoperative frozen section evaluation for presumed benign ampullary neoplasms. Surgery 2000; 127:628–633.

145 Neoptolemos J, Talbot I, Carr-Locke D, et al. Treatment and outcome in 52 consecutive cases of ampullary carcinoma. Br J Surg 1987; 74:957–961.

146 Yamaguchi K, Enjoji M, Kitamura K. Endoscopic biopsy has limited accuracy in diagnosis of ampullary tumors. Gastrointest Endosc 1990; 36:588–592.

147 Sivak MV. Clinical and endoscopic aspects of the tumors of the ampulla of Vater. Endoscopy 1988; 20:211–217.

148 Will U, Meyer F, Erhardt C, et al. Correlation of differential diagnosis between inflammatory and malignant lesions of the papilla of Vater using endosonography with results of histologic investigation (abstract). Gastroenterology 2003; 124(Suppl 1):A440.

149 Keriven O, Napoléon B, Souquet JC, et al. Patterns of the ampulla of Vater at endoscopic ultrasonography (abstract). Gastrointest Endosc 1993; 39:A290.

150 Rösch T, Braig C, Gain T, et al. Staging of pancreatic and ampullary carcinoma by endoscopic ultrasonography. Gastroenterology 1992; 102:188–199.

151 Saurin JC, Chavaillon A, Napoléon B, et al. Long-term follow-up of patients with endoscopic treatment of sporadic adenomas of the papilla of Vater. Endoscopy 2003; 35:402–406.

152 Binmoeller K, Boaventura S, Ramsperger K, et al. Endoscopic snare excision of the benign adenomas of the papilla of Vater. Gastrointest Endosc 1993; 39:127–131.

153 Zadorova Z, Dvokaf M, Hajer J. Endoscopic therapy of benign tumors of the papilla of Vater. Endoscopy 2001; 33:345–347.

154 Norton I, Gostout C, Baron T, et al. Safety and outcome of endoscopic snare excision of the major duodenal papilla. Gastrointest Endosc 2002; 56:239–243.

155 Napoléon B, Pialat J, Saurin JC, et al. Adénomes et adénocarcinomes débutants de l'ampoule de Vater: place du traitement endoscopique à but curatif. Gastroenterol Clin Biol 2004; 28:385–392.

156 Catalano M, Linder J, Chak A, et al. Endoscopic management of adenoma of the major duodenal papilla. Gastrointest Endosc 2004; 59:225–232.

157 Desilets D, Dy P, Ku P, et al. Endoscopic management of tumors of the major duodenal papilla: refined techniques to improve outcome and avoid complications. Gastrointest Endosc 2001; 54:202–208.

158 Hermanek P, Sobin LH (eds); International Union Against Cancer (UICC). TNM classification of malignant tumours, 4th edn. Berlin: Springer;1987.

159 Cannon M, Carpenter S, Elta G, et al. EUS compared with CT, magnetic resonance imaging, and angiography and the influence of biliary stenting on staging accuracy of ampullary neoplasms. Gastrointest Endosc 1999; 50:27–33.

160 Tio TL, Sie LH, Kallimanis G, et al. Staging of ampullary and pancreatic carcinoma: comparison between endosonography and surgery. Gastrointest Endosc 1996; 44:706–713.

161 Yoshida T, Matsumoto T, Shibata K, et al. Patterns of lymph node metastasis in carcinoma of the ampulla of Vater. Hepatogastroenterology 2000; 47:880–883.

162 Yamaguchi K, Enjoji M. Carcinoma of the ampulla of Vater. A clinicopathologic study and pathologic staging of 109 cases of carcinoma and 5 cases of adenoma. Cancer 1987; 59:506–515.

163 Nakao A, Harada A, Nonami T, et al. Prognosis of cancer of the duodenal papilla of Vater in relation to clinicopathological tumor extension. Hepatogastroenterology 1994; 41:73–78.

164 Shirai Y, Tsukada K, Ohtani T, et al. Carcinoma of the ampulla of Vater: histopathologic analysis of tumor spread in Whipple pancreatoduodenectomy specimens. World J Surg 1995; 19:102–107.

165 Rivadeneira DE, Pochapin M, Grobmyer SP, et al. Comparison of linear array endoscopic ultrasonography and helical CT for the staging of periampullary malignancies. Ann Surg Oncol 2003; 10:890–897.

166 Buscail L, Pages P, Bertelemy P, et al. Role of EUS in the management of pancreatic and ampullary carcinoma: a prospective study assessing resectability and prognosis. Gastrointest Endosc 1999; 50:34–40.

167 Midwinter MJ, Beveridge CJ, Wilsdon JB, et al. Correlation between spiral computed tomography, endoscopic ultrasonography, and findings at operation in pancreatic and ampullary tumors. Br J Surg 1999; 86:189–193.

168 Morozumi A, Fujino MA, Sato T, et al. Endosonographic criteria for assessment of the depth of duodenal invasion in carcinoma of the papilla of Vater. Digestive Endosc 2001; 13:149–158.

169 Menzel J, Hoepffner N, Sulkowski U, et al. Polypoid tumors of the major duodenal papilla – preoperative staging with intraductal US, EUS, and CT: a prospective histopathologically controlled study. Gastrointest Endosc 1999; 49:349–357.

170 Itoh A, Goto H, Naitoh Y, et al. Intraductal ultrasonography in diagnosing tumor extension of cancer of the papilla of Vater. Gastrointest Endosc 1997; 45:251–260.

171 Gress FG, Hawes RH, Savides TJ, et al. Endoscopic ultrasound-guided fine-needle aspiration biopsy using linear array and radial scanning endosonography. Gastrointest Endosc 1997; 45:243–250.

172 Napoleon B, Saurin JC, Scoazec JY, et al. Do endoscopic ultrasound and intraductal ultrasonography allow to orientate the treatment of ampullary tumour? (abstract). Endoscopy 2001; 33:A2770.

173 Martin JA, Haber GB. Ampullary adenoma: clinical manifestations, diagnosis, and treatment. Gastrointest Endosc Clin N Am 2003; 13:649–669.

174 Quirk D, Rattner D, del Castillo CF, et al. The use of endoscopic ultrasonography to reduce the cost of treating ampullary tumors. Gastrointest Endosc 1997; 46:334–337.

ANORECTUM

Chapter
19

How to Perform Anorectal EUS

Paul Fockens, Steve Halligan, and Robert H. Hawes

THE PERIANAL AREA

Examination of the perianal area is simplicity itself. Dedicated equipment is preferred (see Ch. 20). No special patient preparation is required. The patient is told that any discomfort will be similar to having a finger in the anus, and likely less uncomfortable than digital rectal examination by a doctor. To the patient, the probe is potentially quite a frightening piece of equipment, so it is worth mentioning that only the distal few centimeters will enter the anus (as opposed to rectal endosonography where insertion is obviously deeper). Some people examine all patients in left lateral position; others prefer to examine women in the prone position. It has been described previously that placing women in the left lateral position can potentially distort anterior perineal anatomy with the result that the asymmetric images obtained are difficult to interpret, especially with respect to perineal scarring.[1] The probe is prepared as necessary for the transducer being used. Some, for example, require the transducer head to be filled with degassed water to achieve acoustic coupling. This is achieved by injection using a syringe via a side port. The probe must be maneuvered during filling so that all air is expelled via a pinhole located at the tip of the cone.

Whether or not water filling is required, the probe tip is lubricated with ultrasound jelly and then covered with a condom, which is itself lubricated to facilitate insertion. The probe is then inserted into the anus and image acquisition started by the operator. The probe is inserted so that its tip lies just in the distal rectum. The probe is then withdrawn gently to examine the anal sphincters. As for all ultrasound examinations, the clinical findings are generally based on the image displayed on the monitor screen in real-time (with the exception of three-dimensional acquisition, in which case the examination in its entirety can be replayed later). However, still images are usually required, and it is convenient to obtain these at three levels: proximal, mid, and distal anal canal. These three anatomic levels are imaged at standard magnification and the examination is then repeated at a higher magnification, so that six images are obtained in total, three at each magnification. The probe is oriented so that anterior (i.e., 12 o'clock) is uppermost, and is then withdrawn. The examination is normally very quick, perhaps only a minute or so for the experienced operator who is familiar with normal and abnormal anatomy, and especially so when the sphincters are normal.

THE RECTUM

EUS of the rectum is mainly performed to examine suspicious rectal polyps or to stage rectal cancer. From country to country, huge differences exist in the utilization of EUS for this indication. Patients should be prepared with an enema or complete bowel preparation in order to evacuate all stools from the area to be investigated. For the start of the examination the patient is usually placed in the left lateral position. The position may be changed during the examination. Sedation is usually not necessary as the rectosigmoid junction is not passed with the instrument.

There can be no standard advice for the equipment to be used. For staging of tumors located very distally in the rectum, rigid radial scanning probes are often used. An alternative is a radial scanning echoendoscope, as also used in the upper gastrointestinal tract. The advantage of echoendoscopes is that they can be advanced higher up into the rectum with help of the (oblique-viewing) optics. Linear echoendoscopes can also be used, with the advantage of being able to perform EUS fine-needle aspiration (FNA) biopsy of extrarectal abnormalities such as lymph nodes or suspected tumor recurrences after surgery. The linear probes sometimes offer a further advantage, as the tumor and mural layers can be followed in the same image. This sometimes makes it easier to determine the exact involvement of the deeper layers. Finally, mini-probes can be used in case of superficial lesions. With 12-MHz mini-probes, a penetration depth of 2 cm is generally possible.

Using a balloon around the tip of the rigid probe or echoendoscope gets rid of the air and allows for good acoustic coupling between probe and tumor. Filling of the rectum with water is sometimes helpful, especially in the case of smaller lesions which may otherwise be compressed with a balloon. After filling the rectum with water, the position of the patient can be changed until the lesion can be seen endoscopically to be completely under water. Complete filling of the rectum with water is usually not possible, and should not be attempted as it is much easier to change the patient's position. When the bowel has been prepared with an enema, care should be taken not to fill the colon extensively with water, as this may mobilize stool located in the proximal colon.

Once the tumor is seen with EUS, the lesion is examined extensively and all layers of the colon wall are followed underneath the tumor. Houston's valves and the rectosigmoid junction make it almost impossible to maintain a perpendicular view of the rectal wall at all times with a radial instrument scan.

Adaptation of the plane of scanning with the controls of the echoendoscope is important to prevent overstaging by non-perpendicular imaging.

After imaging of the tumor, the echoendoscope is advanced to the rectosigmoid junction to look for suspicious perirectal lymph nodes. Although it may be possible to advance the echoendoscope higher up, this is generally not advised. Images of the lesion and all other findings should be made; there are no standard positions at which images should be captured in every examination.

REFERENCES

1 Frudinger A, Bartram CI, Halligan S, et al. Examination techniques for endosonography of the anal canal. Abdom Imaging 1998; 23:301–303.

Chapter
20

EUS in Rectal Cancer

Gavin C. Harewood

INTRODUCTION

Accurate assessment of the extent of rectal cancer has important implications for the management of patients. Conventionally, initial staging is accomplished by means of computed tomography (CT) of the abdomen and pelvis; this serves to exclude distant metastatic (M1) disease. In patients without distant metastases (M0), endoscopic ultrasound (EUS) is the most accurate imaging modality for determining locoregional stage (both T and N stages) of rectal tumors.

Rationale for use of EUS in staging rectal cancer

In 1990, the National Institutes of Health Consensus Conference recommended that patients with locally invasive rectal tumors (T3, T4 N0 or Tx N1–2 or stage II–III) (Fig. 20.1) should receive adjuvant therapy.[1] In large part, these recommendations reflected the findings of the Swedish Rectal Cancer trials, which demonstrated a reduction in recurrence rates among patients with locally advanced disease following the administration of preoperative radiation therapy compared with postoperative radiotherapy.[2,3] Since then, further studies have corroborated these findings,[4–8] confirming an improvement in recurrence-free survival and comparable toxicity when adjuvant therapy is given prior to surgery. This is the rationale for accurately staging rectal tumors with EUS before operation; identification of patients with locally advanced non-metastatic disease permits the selection of a subgroup of patients who will benefit maximally from preoperative neoadjuvant therapy.

TECHNIQUE

Transrectal EUS is conventionally performed with the patient in the left lateral decubitus position; occasionally, repositioning of the patient is necessary to image lesions adequately. In the author's experience, full colonoscopy preparation solution facilitates optimal ultrasonic visualization. This also allows colonoscopy to be performed at the same setting, if necessary; in that case, it is preferable to sequence the EUS first to minimize the introduction of colonic air, which impedes ultrasound imaging.

Equipment

Both radial and linear viewing echoendoscopes are utilized for transrectal EUS. The radial instrument is available in both rigid and flexible models. Although the rigid instrument is cheaper, the flexible version has the advantage of an oblique viewing mechanism, which allows tumor visualization and thereby facilitates traversal of stenotic tumors. The flexible instrument also allows deeper intubation to allow imaging of the iliac lymph nodes. This carries significant clinical implications, as nodal metastases in the iliac region confer M1 status on the patient. Scanning is performed at a frequency of 7.5 or 12 MHz. If suspicious perirectal lymph nodes are detected on radial imaging, the linear scanning instrument is then used to target these nodes for EUS-guided fine-needle aspiration (EUS-FNA). Post-FNA antibiotic prophylaxis may be used to minimize the risk of postprocedure infection, although there is little evidence in the medical literature to support this practice.

STAGING

T staging

The superiority of EUS over other imaging modalities, such as CT and magnetic resonance imaging (MRI), for local tumor (T) and nodal (N) staging has been convincingly demonstrated in multiple clinical studies. As illustrated in Table 20.1, 41 studies evaluating EUS in this setting have been published in the peer-reviewed literature. Overall, the experience in 4118 subjects has reported a mean EUS T-staging accuracy of 85.2% (median 87.5%), a mean sensitivity of 87.5% (median 89.0%), and a mean specificity of 83.5% (median 86%). This compares to an accuracy of 65–75% for CT and 75–85% for MRI.[9–12]

With the growing importance of outcomes research, it is important to note not only that EUS demonstrates superior staging performance but that this translates into a change in patient management. In a prospective clinical study of 80 consecutive patients with non-metastatic rectal cancer, it was found that the incremental staging information provided by EUS resulted in a change in management in 31% of patients – usually the addition of neoadjuvant treatment.[13] This was often the result of these rectal tumors being understaged by pelvic CT; when local invasion was missed by CT, candidates were not offered preoperative neoadjuvant therapy. Decision-analysis studies have also demonstrated that the most cost-effective strategy for evaluation of proximal rectal cancer is the combination of initial abdominal CT (to exclude distant metastatic disease) in conjunction with EUS (for local staging) in patients without distant disease.[14]

A concern exists that patients with early-stage disease (T1–2 N0) may be erroneously overstaged by EUS, thereby

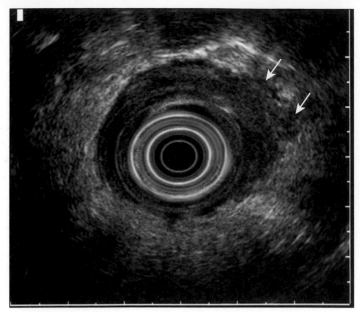

Fig. 20.1   T3 rectal tumor with extension of tumor through muscularis propria (arrows)

leading to administration of unnecessary preoperative treatment (Fig. 20.2). However, in the study by Harewood et al.[13] no patients were overstaged by EUS, and other investigators have demonstrated similar findings.[15] This reassuringly indicates that EUS-based treatment decisions will rarely expose patients to unnecessary overtreatment.

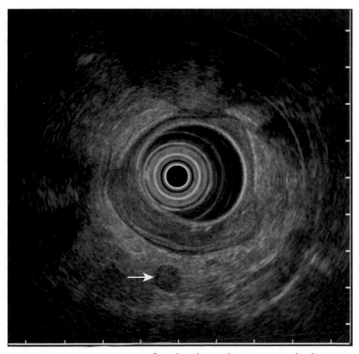

Fig. 20.2   T1 N1 tumor confined within submucosa and adjacent perirectal lymph node (arrow).

		Accuracy (%)	
Reference no.	No. of patients	T stage	N stage
33	88	90	75
34	79	89	–
35	100	93	83
36	122	78	–
37	102	72	81
38	113	–	78
39	76	82	70
40	118	89	80
41	154	86	81
42	100	85	–
43	160	77	83
44	70	76	69
45	121	92	65
46	154	96	72
47	545	69	64
48	422	63	–
49	44	91	–
50	45	89	79
51	85	91	76
52	70	89	–
53	131	75	–
11	21	83	–
54	38	76	–
55	63	83	66
56	164	79	76
57	10	100	83
58	89	90	54
59	26	77	76
60	48	89	85
61	67	88	73
62	18	89	–
13	80	91	82
10	37	88	80
63	13	85	–
64	14	100	86
65	23	87	–
66	29	93	–
67	25	92	–
68	356	85	66
69	63	81	70
70	35	79	73

STUDIES REPORTING THE ACCURACY OF EUS IN STAGING RECTAL CANCER

Table 20.1 Studies reporting the accuracy of EUS in staging rectal cancer
From Harewood GC. Assessment of publication bias in the reporting of EUS performance in staging rectal cancer. Am J Gastroenterol 2005; 100:808–816. With permission of Blackwell Publishing Ltd.

N staging

The medical literature has not demonstrated convincing superiority for EUS over other imaging modalities in assessing the nodal (N) stage of rectal cancer. Twenty-seven studies have addressed EUS performance in N-stage evaluation. Overall, the mean N-staging accuracy is 75.0% (median 76.0%), with a mean sensitivity of 68.1% (median 72.0%) and specificity of 81.5% (median 82.0%). This is not significantly superior to the accuracy of CT and MRI.

The incorporation of FNA into EUS represented a promising advance in N staging of tumors elsewhere in the gastrointestinal tract.[16–24] The major benefit of FNA is the high specificity of this sampling technique; false-positive aspirates are rarely, if ever, obtained from benign lymph nodes. A theoretical concern exists that traversing tumor tissue when accessing peritumoral lymph nodes may yield a false-positive result. For this reason, FNA of peritumoral lymph nodes is generally avoided.

An important practical consideration to bear in mind relates to the EUS appearance of perirectal lymph nodes. Generally, perirectal nodes are not visualized in healthy patients. Therefore, visualization of perirectal nodes alone is sufficient to warrant sampling by FNA. This contrasts with benign lymph nodes in, for example, the periesophageal region, which can be seen by EUS. In that context, we rely on the echocharacteristics of the node to determine malignancy (size, shape, border, echogenicity). All visualized perirectal nodes should be considered suspicious and sampled (Fig. 20.3).

LEARNING CURVE

An important aspect that appears to influence EUS performance in any region of the gastrointestinal tract is the level of experience of the endoscopist. Experienced endosonographers demonstrate superior performance, underscoring the learning

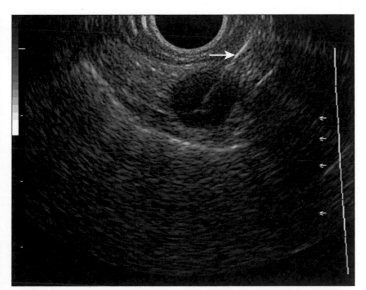

Fig. 20.3 Perirectal node with malignant-appearing features (large, round, hypoechoic, sharp border) being sampled by FNA needle (arrow).

curve that exists for mastering EUS. Transrectal EUS is no exception. The improvement with experience was shown by Orrom et al.,[25] who found that the staging accuracy of rectal cancer increased from 58% in the initial 12 examinations to 88% for the subsequent 24 procedures.

RECURRENT RECTAL CANCER

Rectal cancer recurrence rates generally range from 20% to 50%, with higher rates in patients with a more advanced initial tumor stage. One of the challenging aspects of rectal cancer recurrence is its occasional extraluminal nature, hindering early endoscopic detection.[26,27] Because of its ability to discern extramucosal structures, EUS may play an important role in this setting. Two studies have demonstrated superior performance characteristics of EUS when compared with pelvic CT in the detection of local recurrence of rectal cancer.[28,29] The sensitivity of EUS for detecting recurrence was higher (100%) in both studies compared with CT (82% and 85%).

One limitation of EUS in the postradiation setting is the inflammatory soft tissue changes induced by radiotherapy. These changes often obscure the detail of mucosal layers and diminish EUS sensitivity.[28] For this reason, FNA may offer greater utility in the detection of recurrent rectal cancer. By sampling any suspicious areas, histologic examination overcomes the limitation of relying on EUS appearance alone. Hunerbein et al.[30] evaluated 312 patients with a history of rectal cancer and demonstrated a significantly improved accuracy for EUS-FNA (92%) in the detection of tumor recurrence compared with EUS (75%). Predictably, this superiority was primarily a reflection of the better specificity of FNA. Similarly, Lohnert et al.[31] documented the superiority of EUS-FNA in the detection of rectal cancer recurrence in a cohort of 116 patients (100% versus 79% for EUS alone).

Follow-up after resection

Although EUS, especially EUS-FNA, offers a benefit in the detection of rectal tumor recurrence, there is no consensus regarding the standard practice for postresection surveillance. In the study by Lohnert et al.[31] EUS was performed at 3-month intervals for 2 years and subsequently at 6-month intervals for a further year postsurgery. Generally, recurrence rates are related to initial tumor stage; therefore, it would appear prudent to perform the most aggressive surveillance in patients with locally advanced tumor stage at the outset, as such patients have the highest risk of recurrence.[32]

EXAMINATION CHECKLIST

Examination of primary tumor, especially the relationship with the prostate or vagina, and the distance from the anal canal

Scan peritumoral area for lymph nodes

REFERENCES

1   National Institutes of Health consensus conference. Adjuvant therapy for patients with colon and rectal cancer. JAMA 1990; 264:1444–1450.

2   Pahlman L, Glimelius B. Pre- or postoperative radiotherapy in rectal and rectosigmoid carcinoma. Report from a randomized multicenter trial. Ann Surg 1990; 211:187–195.

3   Frykholm GJ, Glimelius B, Pahlman L. Preoperative or postoperative irradiation in adenocarcinoma of the rectum: final treatment results of a randomized trial and an evaluation of late secondary effects. Dis Colon Rectum 1993; 36:564–572.

4   Swedish Rectal Cancer Trial. Improved survival with preoperative radiotherapy in resectable rectal cancer. N Engl J Med 1997; 336:980–987.

5   Medical Research Council Rectal Cancer Working Party. Randomised trial of surgery alone versus radiotherapy followed by surgery for potentially operable locally advanced rectal cancer. Lancet 1996; 348:1605–1610.

6   Minsky BD. Adjuvant therapy for rectal cancer–a good first step. N Engl J Med 1997; 336:1016–1017.

7   Grann A, Feng C, Wong D, et al. Preoperative combined modality therapy for clinically resectable uT3 rectal adenocarcinoma. Int J Radiat Oncol Biol Phys 2001; 49:987–995.

8   Hyams DM, Mamounas EP, Petrelli N, et al. A clinical trial to evaluate the worth of preoperative multimodality therapy in patients with operable carcinoma of the rectum: a progress report of National Surgical Breast and Bowel Project Protocol R-03. Dis Colon Rectum 1997; 40:131–139.

9   Kwok H, Bissett IP, Hill GL. Preoperative staging of rectal cancer. Int J Colorectal Dis 2000; 15:9–20.

10 Thaler W, Watzka S, Martin F, et al. Preoperative staging of rectal cancer by endoluminal ultrasound vs. magnetic resonance imaging. Preliminary results of a prospective, comparative study. Dis Colon Rectum 1994; 37:1189–1193.

11 Meyenberger C, Huch Boni RA, Bertschinger P, et al. Endoscopic ultrasound and endorectal magnetic resonance imaging: a prospective, comparative study for preoperative staging and follow-up of rectal cancer. Endoscopy 1995; 27:469–479.

12 Guinet C, Buy JN, Ghossain MA, et al. Comparison of magnetic resonance imaging and computed tomography in the preoperative staging of rectal cancer. Arch Surg 1990; 125:385–388.

13 Harewood GC, Wiersema MJ, Nelson H, et al. A prospective, blinded assessment of the impact of preoperative staging on the management of rectal cancer. Gastroenterology 2002; 123:24–32.

14 Harewood GC, Wiersema MJ. Cost-effectiveness of endoscopic ultrasonography in the evaluation of proximal rectal cancer. Am J Gastroenterol. 2002; 97:874–882.

15 Hawes RH. New staging techniques. Endoscopic ultrasound. Cancer 1993; 71(Suppl):4207–4213.

16 Wiersema MJ, Kochman ML, Cramer HM, et al. Endosonography-guided real-time fine-needle aspiration biopsy. Gastrointest Endosc 1994; 40:700–707.

17 Chang KJ, Nguyen P, Erickson RA, et al. The clinical utility of endoscopic ultrasound-guided fine-needle aspiration in the diagnosis and staging of pancreatic carcinoma. Gastrointest Endosc 1997; 45:387–393.

18 Rodriguez J, Kasberg C, Nipper M, et al. CT-guided needle biopsy of the pancreas: a retrospective analysis of diagnostic accuracy. Am J Gastroenterol 1992; 87:1610–1613.

19 Gress FG, Savides TJ, Sandler A, et al. Endoscopic ultrasonography, fine-needle aspiration biopsy guided by endoscopic ultrasonography, and computed tomography in the preoperative staging of non-small-cell lung cancer: a comparison study. Ann Intern Med 1997; 127:604–612.

20 Wiersema MJ, Vilmann P, Giovannini M, et al. Endosonography-guided fine-needle aspiration biopsy: diagnostic accuracy and complication assessment. Gastroenterology 1997; 112:1087–1095.

21 Giovannini M, Seitz JF, Monges G, et al. Fine-needle aspiration cytology guided by endoscopic ultrasonography: results in 141 patients. Endoscopy 1995; 27:171–177.

22 Williams DB, Sahai AV, Aabakken L, et al. Endoscopic ultrasound guided fine needle aspiration biopsy: a large single centre experience. Gut 1999; 44:720–726.

23 Catalano MF, Alcocer E, Chak A, et al. Evaluation of metastatic celiac axis lymph nodes in patients with esophageal carcinoma: accuracy of EUS. Gastrointest Endosc 1999; 50:352–356.

24 Giovannini M, Monges G, Seitz JF, et al. Distant lymph node metastases in esophageal cancer: impact of endoscopic ultrasound-guided biopsy. Endoscopy 1999; 31:536–540.

25 Orrom WJ, Wong WD, Rothenberger DA, et al. Endorectal ultrasound in the preoperative staging of rectal tumors. A learning experience. Dis Colon Rectum 1990; 33:654–659.

26 Mascagni DCL, Urciuoli P, De Matteo G. Endoluminal ultrasound for early detection of local recurrence of rectal cancer. Br J Surg 1989; 76:1176–1180.

27 Ramirez J, Mortensen NJ, Takeuchi N, et al. Endoluminal ultrasonography in the follow-up of patients with rectal cancer. Br J Surg 1994; 81:692–694.

28 Novell F, Pascual S, Viella P, et al. Endorectal ultrasonography in the follow-up of rectal cancer. Is it a better way to detect early local recurrence? Int J Colorectal Dis 1997; 12:78–81.

29 Rotondano G, Esposito P, Pellecchia L, et al. Early detection of locally recurrent rectal cancer by endosonography. Br J Radiol 1997; 70:567–571.

30 Hunerbein M, Totkas S, Moesta KT, et al. The role of transrectal ultrasound-guided biopsy in the postoperative follow-up of patients with rectal cancer. Surgery 2001; 129:164–169.

31 Lohnert M, Doniec JM, Henne-Bruns D. Effectiveness of endoluminal sonography in the identification of occult local rectal cancer. Dis Colon Rectum 2000; 43:483–491.

32 Mellgren A, Sirivongs P, Rothenberger DA, et al. Is local excision adequate therapy for early rectal cancer? Dis Colon Rectum 2000; 43:1064–1071.

33 Saitoh N, Okui K, Sarashina H, et al. Evaluation of echographic diagnosis of rectal cancer using intrarectal ultrasonic examination. Dis Colon Rectum 1986; 29:234–242.

34 Feifel G, Hildebrandt U, Dhom G. Assessment of depth of invasion in rectal cancer by endosonography. Endoscopy 1987; 19:64–67.

35 Beynon J, Foy DM, Temple LN, et al. The endosonic appearances of normal colon and rectum. Dis Colon Rectum 1986; 29:810–813.

36 Yamashita Y, Machi J, Shirouzu K, et al. Evaluation of endorectal ultrasound for the assessment of wall invasion of rectal cancer. Report of a case. Dis Colon Rectum 1988; 31:617–623.

37 Rifkin MD, Ehrlich SM, Marks G. Staging of rectal carcinoma: prospective comparison of endorectal US and CT. Radiology 1989; 170:319–322.

38 Hildebrandt U, Klein T, Feifel G, et al. Endosonography of pararectal lymph nodes. In vitro and in vivo evaluation. Dis Colon Rectum 1990; 33:863–868.

39 Cho E, Nakajima M, Yasuda K, et al. Endoscopic ultrasonography in the diagnosis of colorectal cancer invasion. Gastrointest Endosc 1993; 39:521–527.

40 Herzog U, von Flue M, Tondelli P, et al. How accurate is endorectal ultrasound in the preoperative staging of rectal cancer? Dis Colon Rectum 1993; 36:127–134.

41 Glaser F, Kuntz C, Schlag P, et al. Endorectal ultrasound for control of preoperative radiotherapy of rectal cancer. Ann Surg 1993; 217:64–71.

42 Nielsen MB, Qvitzau S, Pedersen JF, et al. Endosonography for preoperative staging of rectal tumours. Acta Radiol 1996; 37:799–803.

43 Sailer M, Leppert R, Kraemer M, et al. The value of endorectal ultrasound in the assessment of adenomas, T1- and T2-carcinomas. Int J Colorectal Dis 1997; 12:214–219.

44 Nishimori H, Sasaki K, Hirata K, et al. The value of endoscopic ultrasonography in preoperative evaluation of rectal cancer. Int Surg 1998; 83:157–160.

45 Norton SA, Thomas MG. Staging of rectosigmoid neoplasia with colonoscopic endoluminal ultrasonography. Br J Surg 1999; 86:942–946.

46 Akasu T, Kondo H, Moriya Y, et al. Endorectal ultrasonography and treatment of early stage rectal cancer. World J Surg 2000; 24:1061–1068.

47 Garcia-Aguilar J, Pollack J, Lee SH, et al. Accuracy of endorectal ultrasonography in preoperative staging of rectal tumors. Dis Colon Rectum 2002; 45:10–15.

48 Marusch F, Koch A, Schmidt U, et al. Routine use of transrectal ultrasound in rectal carcinoma: results of a prospective multicenter study. Endoscopy 2002; 34:385–390.

49 Beynon J, Mortensen NJ, Foy DM, et al. Pre-operative assessment of local invasion in rectal cancer: digital examination, endoluminal sonography or computed tomography? Br J Surg 1986; 73:1015–1017.

50 Boyce GA, Sivak MV Jr, Lavery IC, et al. Endoscopic ultrasound in the pre-operative staging of rectal carcinoma. Gastrointest Endosc 1992; 38:468–471.

51 Massari M, De Simone M, Cioffi U, et al. Value and limits of endorectal ultrasonography for preoperative staging of rectal carcinoma. Surg Laparosc Endosc 1998; 8:438–444.

52 Adams DR, Blatchford GJ, Lin KM, et al. Use of preoperative ultrasound staging for treatment of rectal cancer. Dis Colon Rectum 1999; 42:159–166.

53 Spinelli P, Schiavo M, Meroni E, et al. Results of EUS in detecting perirectal lymph node metastases of rectal cancer: the pathologist makes the difference. Gastrointest Endosc 1999; 49:754–758.

54 Kaneko K, Boku N, Hosokawa K, et al. Diagnostic utility of endoscopic ultrasonography for preoperative rectal cancer staging estimation. Jpn J Clin Oncol 1996; 26:30–35.

55 Osti MF, Padovan FS, Pirolli C, et al. Comparison between transrectal ultrasonography and computed tomography with rectal inflation of gas in preoperative staging of lower rectal cancer. Eur Radiol 1997; 7:26–30.

56 Akasu T, Sugihara K, Moriya Y, et al. Limitations and pitfalls of transrectal ultrasonography for staging of rectal cancer. Dis Colon Rectum 1997; 40(Suppl):S10–S15.

57 Ramana KN, Murthy PV, Rao KP, et al. Transrectal ultrasonography versus computed tomography in staging rectal carcinoma. Indian J Gastroenterol 1997; 16:142–143.

58 Kim JC, Yu CS, Jung HY, et al. Source of errors in the evaluation of early rectal cancer by endoluminal ultrasonography. Dis Colon Rectum 2001; 44:1302–1309.

59 Gualdi GF, Casciani E, Guadalaxara A, et al. Local staging of rectal cancer with transrectal ultrasound and endorectal magnetic resonance imaging: comparison with histologic findings. Dis Colon Rectum 2000; 43:338–345.

60 Shami VM, Parmar KS, Waxman I. Clinical impact of endoscopic ultrasound and endoscopic ultrasound-guided fine-needle aspiration in the management of rectal carcinoma. Dis Colon Rectum 2004; 47:59–65.

61 Hsieh PS, Changchien CR, Chen JS, et al. Comparing results of preoperative staging of rectal tumor using endorectal ultrasonography and histopathology. Chang Gung Med J 2003; 26:474–478.

62 Starck M, Bohe M, Simanaitis M, et al. Rectal endosonography can distinguish benign rectal lesions from invasive early rectal cancers. Colorectal Dis 2003; 5:246–250.

63 Waizer A, Powsner E, Russo I, et al. Prospective comparative study of magnetic resonance imaging versus transrectal ultrasound for preoperative staging and follow-up of rectal cancer. Preliminary report. Dis Colon Rectum 1991; 34:1068–1072.

64 Pappalardo G, Reggio D, Frattaroli FM, et al. The value of endoluminal ultrasonography and computed tomography in the staging of rectal cancer: a preliminary study. J Surg Oncol 1990; 43:219–222.

65 Romano G, de Rosa P, Vallone G, et al. Intrarectal ultrasound and computed tomography in the pre- and postoperative assessment of patients with rectal cancer. Br J Surg 1985; 72(Suppl):S117–S119.

66 Kramann B, Hildebrandt U. Computed tomography versus endosonography in the staging of rectal carcinoma: a comparative study. Int J Colorectal Dis 1986; 1:216–218.

67 Hildebrandt U, Feifel G. Preoperative staging of rectal cancer by intrarectal ultrasound. Dis Colon Rectum 1985; 28:42–46.

68 Mackay SG, Pager CK, Joseph D, et al. Assessment of the accuracy of transrectal ultrasonography in anorectal neoplasia. Br J Surg 2003; 90:346–350.

69 Marone P, Petrulio F, de Bellis M, et al. Role of endoscopic ultrasonography in the staging of rectal cancer: a retrospective study of 63 patients. J Clin Gastroenterol 2000; 30:420–424.

70 Sentovich SM, Blatchford GJ, Falk PM, et al. Transrectal ultrasound of rectal tumors. Am J Surg 1993; 166:638–641, discussion 641–642.

Chapter 21

EUS in the Evaluation of Anal Sphincter Abnormalities

Steve Halligan

KEY POINTS

- Anal endosonography (AES) is simple to perform and visualizes the anal sphincter complex, notably the external and internal anal sphincters.

- AES is able to image sphincter tears and defects.

- AES can also characterize sphincter morphology and determine muscular quality.

- AES is the single most important investigation in patients with anal incontinence.

INTRODUCTION

First described in 1989,[1] anal endosonography (AES) was the first technique to visualize the anal sphincter complex with spatial resolution sufficient to resolve the individual components of the sphincter mechanism. Most importantly, this precipitated a significant reappraisal of the causes of anal incontinence (and its treatment), which had hitherto been thought to be due mainly to pelvic neuropathy.[2] However, when incontinent patients were studied with AES it rapidly became clear that occult sphincter disruption was present in many cases. At the time of writing, AES has become the pivotal examination in the clinical decision-making process for these patients, displacing physiologic tests. Patients with disrupted sphincters undergo surgery that aims to restore integrity to the sphincter ring, whereas those whose sphincters are intact or whose muscles are thought to be of poor quality can be channeled towards conservative measures or alternative surgical approaches. Although AES is probably utilized most following obstetric injury, it has also facilitated the anatomic characterization of other causes of fecal incontinence. For example, it is able to identify neurogenic incontinence by way of specific patterns of sphincter atrophy, and can identify occult and unintended sphincter damage following anal surgical procedures.

EQUIPMENT

It is possible to perform AES using an echoendoscope, but in the author's experience the best results by far are obtained using a dedicated anal probe. The anus is a very superficial structure, and an endoscope is cumbersome in comparison with a probe designed specifically for the purpose, and also more expensive. AES first employed a 7.5-MHz transducer that had been designed initially for rectal cancer staging and prostatic imaging. The transducer was covered by a rubber balloon, inserted through the anus into the rectum, the balloon inflated with degased water, and the transducer rotated mechanically to produce 360° images of the rectal wall. Professor Clive Bartram of St Mark's Hospital, London, realized that simply by replacing the soft rubber balloon with a rigid plastic cone, the rotating transducer could be safely withdrawn right into the anus.[1] This maneuver was previously impossible because the balloon was torn when compressed by the anus against the rotating metal transducer. The modern equivalent uses a 10-MHz transducer, but is pretty much the same piece of equipment (Fig. 21.1A). Recent developments include probes that have integral three-dimensional (3-D) capacity. The transducer and all the moving parts necessary for 3-D acquisition are permanently sealed within the probe head, thereby avoiding the need for complex withdrawal jigs; the probe is merely held stationary within the anus while the transducer moves craniocaudally within the probe head, acquiring the 3-D data set. Not only can this type of information aid interpretation, but the examination can be performed by a technician and read by the supervising radiologist later, as the whole volume of data around the anus is acquired rather than a series of individual axial slices.

ANAL SPHINCTER ANATOMY

Clearly, a grasp of basic anal anatomy is a prerequisite for accurate interpretation of endosonographic findings. There are two anal sphincters: the external anal sphincter (EAS) is composed of striated muscle, whereas the internal anal shincter (IAS) is smooth muscle. These form two cylindrical layers, with the IAS innermost (Fig. 21.2).

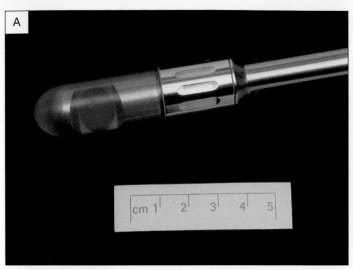

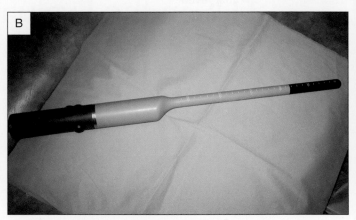

Fig. 21.1 Probes for anal endosonography. **A,** B-K Medical type 1850, 10-MHz transducer probe. External diameter 17 mm. **B,** B-K Medical type 2050, 6–16-MHz transducer probe. This probe has a built-in 3-D acquisition system with all moving parts enclosed, so that 3-D acquisitions are possible without having to alter the transducer position.

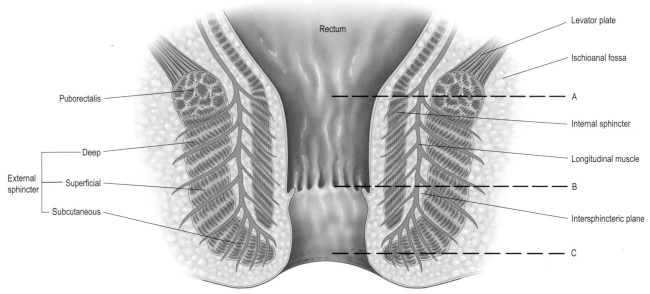

Fig. 21.2 Coronal diagrammatic representation of important anal canal structures, with scan levels indicated corresponding to Fig. 21.3A–C.

The EAS arises from the striated muscles of the pelvic floor and is composed of three cylindrical bundles lying one on top of the other (deep, superficial, and subcutaneous); in practice, these are difficult to distinguish from one another. The deep portion is fused with the puborectalis (or pubococcygeus) muscle, which itself merges with the levator plate of the pelvic floor. The EAS extends approximately 1 cm distal to the IAS, where it forms the subcutaneous part of the EAS muscle. Anteriorly the EAS is closely related to several surrounding structures, such as the superficial transverse muscle of the perineum and the perineal body. Posteriorly it is continuous with the anococcygeal ligament, a structure that is often more

prominent in men and should not be mistaken for a posterior sphincter defect. It is important to note that the EAS is much shorter anteriorly in women than in men, and this feature should not be confused with a sphincter defect.

The IAS is the distal termination and condensation of the circular smooth muscle of the gut tube and extends from the anorectal junction to approximately 1–1.5 cm below the dentate line (Fig. 21.2). The longitudinal muscle of the gut tube also terminates in the anal canal, but is less obvious than the IAS. The longitudinal muscle interdigitates between the EAS and IAS, and terminates in the subcutaneous EAS and subcutaneous anus. Its exact sphincteric action, if any, is much less clear than that of the EAS and IAS, and it is thought that the main purpose of the longitudinal muscle is to brace the anus, preventing anal eversion during defecation.[3] Lying between the EAS and longitudinal muscle is a potential plane, the 'intersphincteric space', which may contain fat. The components of the anal sphincter are surrounded by the ischioanal space (often referred to as the ischiorectal fossa), which contains fat predominantly.

Directly anterior to the anal sphincter is the central perineal tendon or perineal body. In men this lies posterior to the bulbospongious and corpus cavernosum and their related muscles, whereas in women it lies within the anovaginal septum. Many structures insert fibers into the perineal body, such as the EAS, deep and superficial transverse muscles of the perineum, bulbocavernous muscle, and puborectalis muscle. These structures should not be confused with sphincter defects. For example, normal variants of anal sphincter anatomy have been identified, such as differing relationships between the superficial transverse perineal muscle and EAS.[4]

The distal anal canal is lined with stratified squamous epithelium, richly supplied by sensory receptors that are most concentrated at the dentate line, which demarcates the junction with proximal columnar epithelium. The anal subepithelial tissues are relatively thick, and this lining and its underlining vascular spaces (the anal cushions) also play a role in maintaining continence.

NORMAL ENDOSONOGRAPHIC FINDINGS

Because the anus and surrounding sphincter muscles are cylindrical, a 360° field of view is optimal, and the axial plane is also the most relevant surgically. As stated above, the author finds it convenient to obtain baseline images at three levels: proximal, mid, and distal anal canal.

The proximal anal canal is identified primarily by the puborectalis and transverse perineal muscles. The puborectalis slings around the anorectal junction and can be distinguished from the EAS, with which it blends imperceptibly, because its anterior ends splay outwards as they travel towards their fusion with the pubic arch (Fig. 21.3A). The internal sphincter is visible as a continuous hypoechoic ring, and is generally the easiest structure to differentiate from other adjacent anal canal components because it is normally very hyporeflective – the subepithelial tissues, EAS, and longitudinal muscle all normally show varying degrees of hyperreflectivity and their margins can often be difficult to define precisely, although direct comparisons with endoanal magnetic resonance imaging (MRI) have helped tremendously.[5] Increases in transducer frequency that improve spatial resolution have also helped to clarify the sonographic anatomy,[6] as has 3-D work.[7] Sultan et al.[8] carefully imaged cadaveric specimens following sequential histologic dissection of anal layers, thereby validating the sonographic appearances. Importantly, they found that the

Arterior

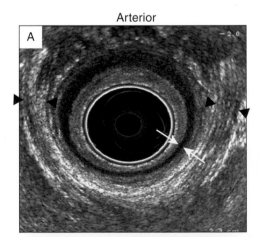

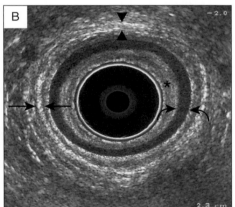

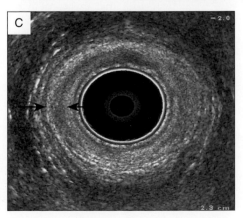

Fig. 21.3   Normal endosonographic anatomy of the anal canal in a woman, obtained using a 10-MHz 360° probe. **A,** Proximal anal canal level. The anterior ends of puborectalis muscle are well seen bilaterally (between arrowheads) as its fibers course forwards towards the pubis. The hyporeflective internal anal sphincter is also well seen (between arrows). **B,** Mid anal canal level. The external sphincter (superficial part) forms a complete ring around the anal canal, notably anteriorly (between arrowheads). The internal sphincter is also at its thickest (between curved arrows). The intersphincteric plane and longitudinal muscle (between straight arrows) lie between the external and internal sphincters. The subepithelial tissues (asterisk) lie medial to the internal sphincter. **C,** Distal anal canal level. The predominant muscle is the subcutaneous external sphincter (between arrows), because the scan plane is caudal to the termination of the internal sphincter.

echogenicity of normal muscle changed as its orientation was altered with respect to the transducer. Thus, normal variant striated muscle slips may appear hypoechoic depending on their orientation to the transducer, and should not be confused with sphincter tears or scars.

If the probe is withdrawn about 1 cm from the proximal anal canal position, the anterior ends of the puborectalis muscle will converge anteriorly as they segue imperceptibly into the EAS. The mid anal canal is thus defined where the EAS forms a complete ring anteriorly (Fig. 21.3B). The IAS is also normally thickest and best seen at this location also. At this level, the intersphincteric plane and longitudinal muscle may be resolved as two distinct layers, the latter forming distinct bundles of smooth muscle fibers.

Withdrawing the probe a little more will move the field of view into the subcutaneous EAS (Fig. 21.3C). This is below the termination of the IAS, so this muscle is either not visualized or only partially visualized if its termination is irregular (a common normal variant). It is usually impossible to visualize the longitudinal muscle reliably at this level because it thins out as it interdigitates into the EAS and is composed mainly of fibroelastic tissue rather than the smooth muscle found more proximally.

Correct interpretation of AES is possible only if the operator has a firm grasp of the normal sonographic anatomy described above. Pathology is defined by either muscular discontinuity (i.e., sphincter tears or lacerations, which may be due to a variety of causes) or abnormal muscular quality (usually due to neuromuscular atrophy or degeneration). To appreciate muscular quality correctly, it is important to realize that normal sonographic appearances are contingent on both age and sex. Frudinger et al.[6] examined 150 nulliparous women using high-frequency AES in order to define normal age-related differences in sphincter morphology, and found that there was a highly significant positive correlation between IAS thickness and increasing age, whereas the EAS showed a highly significant negative correlation with age. There was also some evidence that the reflectivity of the IAS increased with age. There was no significant correlation between age and thickness of sub-epithelial tissues, the longitudinal muscle, or puborectalis muscle.[6] On average, the IAS is 2–3 mm thick (measured at either 3 o'clock or 9 o'clock in the mid anal canal) in normal adults, but it is important to realize that a thin IAS has more significance in an older person with symptoms (see below). It should also be noted that, although the IAS can be measured easily because it contrasts against adjacent structures, other muscles may be more difficult to measure and are subject to more interobserver variation. Gold et al.[9] measured anal canal structures in 51 consecutive referrals and found that, although intraobserver agreement was superior to interobserver agreement, the 95% limits of agreement for EAS measurements spanned 5 mm, whereas those for the IAS spanned 1.5 mm. More importantly from a diagnostic viewpoint, interobserver agreement for diagnosis of sphincter disruption and internal

sphincter echogenicity was very good (κ=0.80 and 0.74, respectively).[9]

It should also be noted that there are clear sonographic differences between men and women with respect to the dimensions of anal canal structures and their sonographic appearances. Most importantly, the anterior complete ring of the EAS is shorter in women. This has been widely appreciated for some time, and Williams et al.[7] used 3-D AES to show that the craniocaudal length of the EAS was approximately 17 mm in women as opposed to 30 mm in men. It should also be appreciated that the various muscular components in men have a generally more striated appearance (Fig. 21.4).

ANAL SPHINCTER FUNCTION

The vast majority of patients referred for AES complain of anal incontinence, either to gas alone or to both gas and feces. Because of this, it is important to have some basic understanding of normal anal sphincter function. The anal sphincter is the most complex sphincter in the human body, and continence is maintained by a complex interrelationship between anal and pelvic floor musculature, integrating somatic and autonomic nervous pathways, the effects of which must be temporarily overcome during the act of defecation. The IAS is innervated via sympathetic presacral nerve fibers and is not under conscious control. It is primarily responsible for closing the anal canal at rest, at which time it is in a state of continuous involuntary contraction. Despite being striated muscle, the puborectalis and EAS also display some resting tone and can contract rapidly without conscious control in response to any sudden increase in intra-abdominal pressure in order to prevent anal incontinence. The EAS is innervated via the pudendal nerves (S2, S3, and S4).

Defecation is initiated by colonic smooth muscle contractions, which are provoked by waking and eating. These contractions propel stool from the sigmoid colon into the normally empty rectum and stimulate rectal sensory nerves, producing an urge to defecate. These nerves are also able to determine the nature of rectal content (i.e., solid, liquid, or gas). The sensation of a

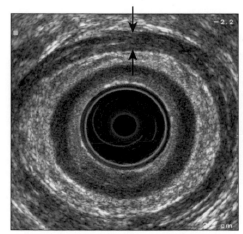

Fig. 21.4 AES at mid anal canal in an asymptomatic man. Note the generally more striated appearance in comparison with Fig. 21.3. The external sphincter (between arrows), in particular, is relatively hyporeflective.

full rectum, and the ability to discriminate gaseous, liquid, and solid content, are important components of continence, in addition to sphincter integrity. Interestingly, sensation is retained after rectal excision, suggesting that some sensory receptors reside in the pelvic floor itself.[10] Rectal filling causes reflex IAS relaxation (the rectoanal inhibitory reflex), rectal contraction, and contraction of the puborectalis and EAS, both of which are heavily modulated by conscious control. Stool within the anal canal contacts sensory receptors concentrated at the dentate line and greatly intensifies the urge to defecate, which is resisted by vigorous striated muscle contraction until the circumstances for defecation are appropriate. When this is so, pelvic floor relaxation and increased intra-abdominal pressure create a positive pressure gradient from rectum to anus to allow evacuation. It is interesting to note that the normal function and contribution of the EAS and IAS to anal continence can be used to predict which muscles are abnormal in incontinent patients. For example, IAS abnormality generally results in passive incontinence (i.e., the patient is unaware that leakage is about to occur), whereas EAS abnormality is more frequently manifest as urge incontinence (i.e., the patient is unable consciously to defer defecation).[11]

ANORECTAL PHYSIOLOGIC TESTING

Before the advent of AES, sphincter integrity and function was determined via anorectal physiologic testing, which tests nervous integrity, conduction, and muscular performance. Few physiologic tests are absolutely diagnostic and most need to be considered together with symptoms, clinical findings, and imaging. However, they provide valuable complementary information and continue to be requested in combination with AES. Because of this, endosonographers working in this field need to be aware of them. Normal values vary between laboratories.

Manometry

Because digital assessment is unreliable, manometry is used to determine rectal and anal pressures. The systems used vary in complexity, from simple balloons connected to a pressure transducer to perfused multichannel catheters capable of measuring pressure at several sites simultaneously, and even ambulatory systems that record over 24 h or more. The pressure recorded will rise when a rectal catheter is withdrawn into the anus, falling again when it reaches the anal margin, and therefore reflecting functional anal canal length (as opposed to anatomic length, which is usually shorter). The high-pressure zone generated at the anus is frequently diminished in incontinent patients. A static anal catheter can measure resting anal canal pressure, and predominantly reflects IAS function. Reduced resting pressure points to IAS pathology. In contrast, the squeeze pressure is the incremental rise over resting pressure elicited when the patient is asked to contract their anus voluntarily, and reflects EAS function. This is frequently reduced when incontinence is due to external sphincter

laceration, as occurs with obstetric injury. Dual sphincter pathology is implicated when both resting and squeeze pressures are abnormal.

Pudendal nerve latency

The pudendal nerve terminal motor latency can be determined from the time taken for a digitally delivered pudendal nerve stimulus to elicit anal sphincter contraction. This is achieved using a disposable glove with a stimulating electrode at the fingertip coupled with a pressure sensor at its base.[12] The nerve is stimulated near the ischial spine and has both sensory and motor components. Slow conduction is thought to be due predominantly to stretch-induced injury. This may follow childbirth[13,14] or chronic straining,[15] and can even be demonstrated transiently in normal individuals when they are asked to strain excessively. The clinical relevance of pudendal neuropathy remains unclear, especially because the degree of neuropathy, pelvic floor descent, and anal sensation should be directly related, but studies cannot demonstrate this.[16] Nevertheless, in patients with abnormal latencies but intact sphincters the incontinence is usually attributed to neuropathic sphincter degeneration, and sphincter repair is less successful if there is underlying neuropathy.[17]

Electromyography

A needle electrode inserted into the EAS can determine both its activity and muscular quality. Sphincter denervation is followed by reinnervation via neighboring healthy axons; this can be quantified electromyographically because the recorded action potentials become polyphasic. Until the advent of AES, electromyography was the only reliable way to diagnose sphincter tears before surgery. The needle was passed into the suspected defect, which was confirmed if no muscular potentials could be recorded subsequently (also possible if the needle tip missed the normal muscle). Needle passes were then made circumferentially around the anus until normal potentials were encountered, 'mapping' the sphincter defect. Electromyography is painful because local anesthetic interferes with recording. Fortunately, AES is superior for detecting sphincter defects when the two modalities are compared directly.[18]

SONOGRAPHIC FINDINGS IN ANAL INCONTINENCE

As mentioned above, the vast majority of clinical referrals for AES are patients complaining of anal incontinence. Anal incontinence may be due to a variety of factors, many of which relate to the integrity and quality of the sphincter mechanism, and it is for assessment of this that AES has assumed the central role in diagnostic work-up. This is because AES can reliably identify those patients who have a sphincter tear, selecting individuals likely to benefit from surgery that aims to restore integrity to the sphincter ring. Physical examination cannot reliably detect anal sphincter defects and, although anal canal pressures can help determine whether sphincter function is normal or not, they cannot indicate whether this is due to loss of sphincter integrity or neuropathy.

Anal incontinence is common, especially in women, and its prevalence increases with age; 2% of the general population older than 45 years have anal incontinence,[19] rising to 7% in those over the age of 65 years.[20] In retirement homes or hospitals, approximately one-third of individuals have anal incontinence.[19] The prevalence is also likely to be higher, because of underreporting. Anal incontinence has considerable economic impact. A 1988 study estimated that more than $400 million annually was spent on incontinence appliances in the USA alone, and anal incontinence was the second commonest cause for placement in a nursing home.[21] Several clinical grading systems for anal incontinence have been developed.

Obstetric injury

Childbirth is a common cause of anal incontinence, either directly, as a result of anal sphincter laceration, or indirectly, via damage to sphincter innervation. Until the advent of AES it was assumed that neuropathy was the primary cause of obstetric-related incontinence, as impaired pudendal nerve conduction can be demonstrated after vaginal delivery, presumably due to stretch-induced injury.[14] Anal sphincter laceration was thought to be a relatively rare event, because it could be identified clinically in only 1 per 200 vaginal deliveries.[22] However, AES revealed that anal sphincter tears were far commoner than initially assumed. An early study of 11 women with a diagnosis of neurogenic fecal incontinence revealed that four had also sustained unsuspected anal sphincter tears,[23] and a further study of 62 women whose incontinence was related to childbirth found EAS tears in 56 (90%).[24] In a landmark study, Sultan et al.[25] investigated 202 unselected consecutive women before and after vaginal delivery using AES, and found anal sphincter tears in 28 (35%) of 79 of primiparous subjects and in 21 (44%) of 48 of multiparous subjects. Furthermore, endosonographic evidence of sphincter laceration was associated with symptoms of anal incontinence 6 weeks after delivery and also evidence of physiologic impairment, namely reduced anal resting and squeeze pressures. No primiparous woman had a sphincter defect before childbirth, and no subject undergoing cesarian section developed a new defect, confirming that sphincter injury was related to vaginal delivery, especially forceps extraction. Moreover, the study confirmed that clinical examination of the perineum immediately after vaginal delivery misses the vast majority of sphincter tears. Anal incontinence may occur immediately after delivery if trauma is marked, but many women present much later, presumably because cumulative effects of multiple deliveries, progressive neuropathy, aging, and the menopause overcome their compensatory mechanisms. Many women are also too embarrassed to complain, or they (or their doctors) believe that the condition is incurable. The accuracy of endosonography has been validated both histologically[8] and during surgery,[18] and accuracy approaches

95%.[23,26,27] For example, a study of 44 patients found that all 23 EAS defects, and 21 of 22 IAS defects visualized on preoperative AES were subsequently confirmed surgically.[26]

The sphincters are cylindrical structures and discontinuity is diagnostic of a sphincter tear. A break in the hypoechoic IAS ring indicates an internal sphincter defect, whereas EAS defects are defined by discontinuity of the more heterogeneous EAS, located peripheral to the intersphincteric plane and longitudinal muscle. Obstetric injury is practically always anterior, since this is where the vagina lies. Because the EAS and IAS are in close proximity, it is usual for obstetric injury to involve both sphincters – isolated EAS injury is relatively ucommon and isolated IAS injury is probably never due to obstetric injury alone. In severe disruptions the entire sphincter mechanism is completely absent anteriorly, with a cloacal defect between the vagina and anal canal (Fig. 21.5). However, it is usual for a primary repair of some sort to have been performed immediately after childbirth, closing the perineum to a variable degree. The competence with which these repairs are performed varies enormously. Scar tissue forms between the sphincter ends, creating a sonographic 'defect' (Figs 21.6–21.8). It is unclear how symptoms relate to the sonographic extent of the injury. For example, a study of 330 women found that, although

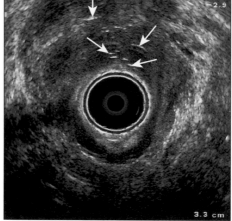

Fig. 21.5 Obstetric injury. Anterior cloacal defect in a woman following vaginal delivery of a 5-kg baby. Note there is no external or internal sphincter anteriorly, and air within the defect (arrows) extends right to the probe surface.

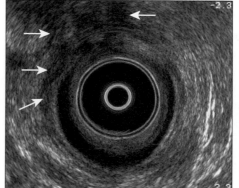

Fig. 21.6 Typical anterior obstetric injury affecting both the external and internal sphincter in a 29-year-old woman who was completely asymptomatic and examined as part of a research study. The primary repair following delivery has opposed the external sphincter to some degree, but a sonographic defect remains (arrows).

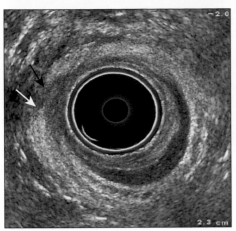

Fig. 21.7 Typical anterior obstetric injury affecting both the external and internal sphincter. The sphincters have been reasonably well approximated (arrows) by primary repair, but the patient complained of anal incontinence immediately after childbirth.

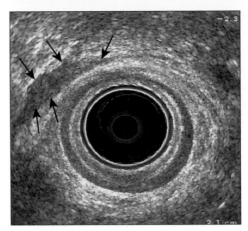

Fig. 21.9 Endosonography following vaginal delivery revealed a right anterior quadrant perineal scar (arrows) in this asymptomatic woman.

women with an EAS tear had lower basal squeeze pressures than those without, beyond this there was no consistent relationship between the morphology of the tear (in terms of both the longitudinal and circumferential extent) and either symptoms or impaired anal pressures.[28] It is also important to realize that patients may only present several years after the initial injury (Fig. 21.8), and some patients with large defects may be entirely asymptomatic initially (Fig. 21.6). Supporting this, a prospective study found that some women with clear evidence of sphincter disruption on AES were entirely asymptomatic following delivery,[29] and a study of 124 consecutive women with late-onset anal incontinence after vaginal delivery found that 71% has sonographic sphincter defects that were believed to be the cause of symptoms despite the temporal separation between childbirth and symptoms.[30] It also seems that perineal tears that do not involve the sphincter mechanism directly are much less likely to be associated with immediate symptoms (Fig. 21.9). A prospective study of 55 nulliparous women using 3-D AES found postpartum trauma in 29%, but those whose damage was limited to the puboanalis or transverse perineal muscles

did not have symptoms and there was no association with reduced anal pressures.[31] It is also possible that anal canal morphology may change postpartum without any direct tearing of the perineum or sphincters. In particular, both 2-D and 3-D studies have found that the anterior EAS may shorten following vaginal delivery but without any sonographic evidence of a tear.[32,33] At the other extreme, AES may be used to examine women who have an anovaginal fistula following delivery, as gas within the fistula is highly reflective, allowing delineation of the track and its relationship to the sphincter mechanism (Fig. 21.10).

Perineal and sphincter trauma following vaginal delivery is generally repaired immediately afterwards, usually under local anesthesia unless a significant disruption has been detected clinically. Such sphincter surgery is known as a 'primary' repair and considerable attention has been focused on the sonographic assessment of such repairs. It is clear that many of these women suffer symptoms of anal incontinence subsequently, despite recognition of the tear and attempted surgery. A study of 156 such women found that 40% of respondents were anally incontinent and that this was associated with a persistent sphincter defect on AES.[34] Another study found that 44 (79%) of 56 women who had undergone primary sphincter repair for a clinically recognized EAS tear following vaginal delivery had persistent sphincter defects on AES and were more sympto-

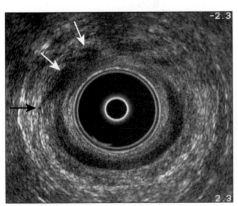

Fig. 21.8 Typical anterior obstetric injury affecting both the external and internal sphincter in a 55-year-old woman whose symptoms of anal incontinence developed several years after vaginal delivery. It would be easy to ascribe this deterioration to progressive neuropathy, but endosonography clearly reveals a sonographic defect centered on the right anterior quadrant (arrows).

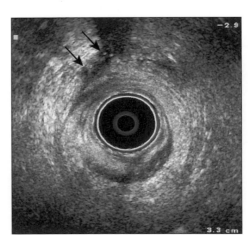

Fig. 21.10 Anterior anovaginal fistula (arrows) in a woman following prolonged vaginal delivery.

matic than those whose repair showed no sonographic defect,[35] findings confirmed by other workers.[36] Primary sphincter repair aims to restore intergrity to the sphincter ring, but seems unable to achieve this in a significant proportion of cases (Fig. 21.11). This may be because the perineum is very edematous and bruised immediately after vaginal delivery, factors that may conspire against successful repair. A study of 48 women 2–7 days after primary repair found that 90% had sonographic defects, with many of these confined to the proximal anal canal, suggesting that the initial repair had been incomplete.[37] The authors concluded that inadequate repair was due to surgical inexperience rather than the extent of sphincter damage, because many such repairs are undertaken by junior doctors or midwives.

If symptoms remain after primary repair and there is clear sonographic evidence of a persistent sphincter defect, patients may be offered a formal sphincter repair. An increasingly common option is to perform an anterior overlap repair, in which the disrupted external sphincter ends are mobilized, overlapped (thus tightening the anal canal), and then sutured together. Symptoms improve in approximately 85% of women immediately afterwards, but this is not maintained and drops to approximately 50% at 5 years.[38] The cause of this deterioration is unclear, but concomitant progressive neuropathy is implicated, possibly due to pudendal damage, or perhaps sphincter denervation and ischemia during the surgical procedure. However, it is also clear that repeated attempts at secondary sphincter repair are possible and can improve symptoms, even after many previous attempts, and that delayed sphincter repair is also possible with good symptomatic outcome.[39,40] Endosonography has also assumed a role for assessment of such secondary repairs. For example, it is recognized that the sonographic integrity of the repair correlates with symptoms and improved physiologic status.[41] Endosonography following a good anterior sphincter repair will reveal sphincter ends that are well overlapped (Fig. 21.12), whereas poor repairs are revealed by persistent sphincter defects (Fig. 21.13). It should be noted that only the EAS is repaired, as attempts at IAS repair have not been successful. Residual IAS defects in the face of a good EAS repair may underpin persistent symptoms, especially those of passive incontinence.

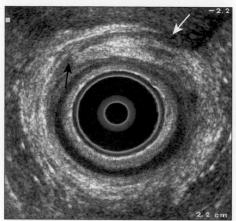

Fig. 21.12 Good sonographic appearances following anterior overlapping sphincter repair. The external sphincter ends are well overlapped (arrows) and there is no residual defect.

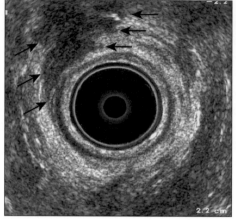

Fig. 21.13 Poor sonographic appearances in a woman who remained symptomatic following a formal sphincter repair. There is a large persistent defect (arrows).

Endosonography has also been used to predict those women most at risk of obstetric injury. For example, some authors have suggested that AES should be used routinely following vaginal delivery in order to identify women with clinically occult sphincter tears whose sphincter may be at further risk from subsequent deliveries,[42] as this is known to increase the risk of cumulative damage.[43,44] Endosonography has also been used to determine which routinely collected obstetric information best indicates the likelihood of associated sphincter disruption. A study of 159 women found no correlation between sonographic tears and head circumference, baby weight, episiotomy, or the duration of active pushing.[45] However, forceps delivery was strongly associated with sphincter tears,[45] an association that has been recognized by other workers.[25,46] Other workers have been able to identify a link between sphincter tears and a second stage of labor prolonged by epidural anesthesia, which increased the risk of disruption by an odds ratio of 2.1.[46] Where access to AES is limited, it may be possible to identify women who harbor sphincter tears by administering a simple incontinence questionnaire after delivery. Frudinger et al. found that such an approach was able to identify 60% of women who sustained EAS tears following vaginal delivery.[29]

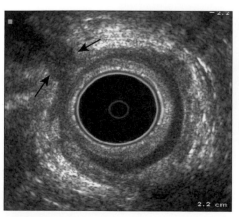

Fig. 21.11 AES following primary repair of a clinically recognized third-degree tear following vaginal delivery. There is a persistent external sphincter defect (arrows).

AES has revolutionized the management of women who sustain sphincter damage following vaginal delivery, but it is fair to say that some controversy persists regarding the exact incidence of EAS tears. For example, although the landmark study by Sultan et al.[25] found an incidence of 35% in primiparous women, Varma et al.[47] suggested the true incidence was nearer 9%, and others have suggested 17%.[48] In an attempt to resolve this uncertainty, a recent meta-analysis of 717 vaginal deliveries found a 27% incidence of sphincter defects in nulliparous women; 30% of these were symptomatic, with the authors concluding that the probability of postpartum anal incontinence being due to sphincter disruption was in the order of 80%.[49]

Idiopathic IAS degeneration and EAS atrophy

Not all anal incontinence is due to sphincter disruption. Many incontinent patients have intact sphincters, but the functional quality of the sphincter muscle is impaired due to neuromuscular degeneration. Vaizey et al.[50] reported on 52 patients with anal incontinence who had an intact EAS and IAS on endosonography but whose IAS was thinned and hyperreflective. Resting pressures, reflecting IAS function, were significantly lowered in this group, but squeeze pressures and pudendal nerve latencies were normal. The authors concluded that a discrete and isolated primary degeneration of the IAS was likely responsible for anal incontinence in these patients. Because the IAS normally thickens with age,[6] IAS thinning is relatively easy to diagnose using EAS, and the diagnosis should be considered in any older patient whose IAS is 1 mm thick or less (Fig. 21.14). A rare cause of isolated IAS thinning is systemic sclerosis (scleroderma).[51]

It is also clear that the EAS may degenerate, a process termed 'atrophy'. This phenomenon was first recognized using endoanal MRI because the striated fibers of the EAS contrast strongly against ischioanal fat.[52] Although the mechanisms are unclear, possibly being due to longstanding pudendal neuropathy, EAS atrophy is important because it adversely affects sphincter surgery. Briel et al.[52] found that surgery for concomitant EAS defects in this group was unsuccessful because the functional quality of the EAS was compromised by atrophy. Using both endoanal MRI and AES, Williams et al.[53] were able to define the sonographic features of EAS atrophy.

They found that EAS imaging in these patients was patchy and poorly defined; in particular, the lateral edge of the EAS was indistinct and the muscle thinner than normal. It should be noted that IAS degeneration and EAS atrophy may be combined in the same patient, and these are probably the sonographic features of what has long been termed 'neurogenic' fecal incontinence (Fig. 21.15). Although endoanal MRI is likely superior to AES for the diagnosis of EAS atrophy, both modalities are equivalent for diagnosing sphincter tears, and AES is particularly good for the diagnosis of IAS degeneration, because the IAS is normally so well visualized during endosonography and is thin in these patients, whereas it is normally thicker in older people.[54] External sphincter atrophy is more difficult to diagnose reliably on AES, not only because the sphincter is difficult to define, but because the normal EAS also tends to thin with age.[6]

Iatrogenic sphincter injury and anal trauma

Unfortunately, iatrogenic damage is a relatively common cause of anal incontinence in the author's practice. A study of 50 patients following a variety of anal surgical procedures found subsequent sphincter defects in 46%.[55] Although some procedures aim to divide the sphincter mechanism (most obviously IAS sphincterotomy), others should not normally involve any sphincter damage. An association between unintentional sphincter division and hemorrhoidectomy is now well recognized (Fig. 21.16). A study of 16 patients undergoing hemorrhoidec-

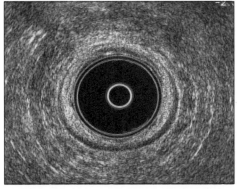

Fig. 21.15   AES in a 50-year-old-woman complaining of anal incontinence. Both sphincters are intact but very poorly seen. The lateral margins of the EAS are indistinct, suggesting EAS atrophy, and the IAS is very thin, suggesting degeneration.

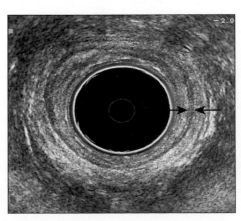

Fig. 21.14   AES in a 69-year-old woman with passive anal incontinence. The internal sphincter (between arrows) is intact but barely visible, and measured 0.7 mm at its thickest. The findings suggest idiopathic IAS degeneration.

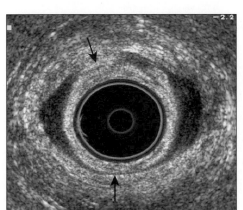

Fig. 21.16 Endosonography in a man who became incontinent following hemorrhoidectomy revealed extensive internal sphincter division, with large anterior and posterior defects (arrows).

tomy found subsequent sphincter defects in 50%.[56] In the author's experience, quadrantic IAS division is relatively common is symptomatic patients, but occasionally the incision has been sufficiently deep to lacerate the longitudinal muscle and EAS as well. The IAS may also be damaged in patients who have undergone procedures that require anal dilatation. In these cases the appearances tend to be those of generalized IAS fragmentation around its circumference (Fig. 21.17). Anal stretch (Lord's procedure) for anal fissure is a common cause of such disruption, as is manual evacuation of the rectum for intractable constipation, if not performed carefully.[57] Transanal stapling instruments, such as those used for low anterior resection, may also unintentionally incorporate the IAS in their firing path, resulting in IAS defects and subsequent passive incontinence.[58,59] Although the IAS is purposefully divided during lateral sphincterotomy, the intention is usually to divide the muscle for only one-third of its length. However, prospective sonographic studies of IAS morphology following this procedure have revealed that division is often more extensive than intended, notably in women, probably because their anatomic anal canal is shorter than that of men.[60] The converse is also true: sonographic studies have revealed that patients whose anal fissure persists after sphincterotomy may not actually have had any muscle divided during the procedure.[61]

SONOGRAPHIC FINDINGS IN OTHER ANAL PATHOLOGIES

Although the main role for AES is in anal incontinence, there are other useful applications. The most prominent of these is probably for imaging fistula-in-ano. Surgeons operating on these patients need to know the relationship of the fistula tract to the anal sphincter mechanism, because treatment is usually effected by cutting down onto the fistula and laying it open, so that infection can drain and subsequent healing can occur. This nearly always necessitates a degree of unavoidable sphincter division, which may be predicted by AES.

Early attempts to use AES for preoperative assessment of fistula-in-ano were relatively disappointing, and assessment was no better than that achieved with digital examination by an experienced colorectal surgeon.[62] However, more recent studies using 10-MHz AES have been more optimistic. A recent study of 108 fistulas in 104 patients found that AES correctly classified the primary fistula tract in 81%, compared with 61% for digital examination by an experienced surgeon.[63] Endosonography was particularly adept at correctly predicting the site of the internal enteric opening in the anal canal, achieving this in 91% of cases.[63] This is because the internal opening is inevitably close to the transducer surface and is thus visualized with high spatial resolution. However, there are undoubtedly several areas where AES suffers specific disadvantages. For example, insufficient penetration beyond the EAS, especially with high-frequency transducers, limits the ability to resolve tracts and abscesses that are remote from the anal canal. Unfortunately these are especially common in patients with recurrent disease.[64] In addition, AES cannot reliably distinguish infection from fibrosis, as both appear hypoechoic. This causes particular difficulties in patients with recurrent disease, as active tracts and fibrotic scars are frequently combined. Attempts have been made to clarify the course of patent tracts by injecting hydrogen peroxide or ultrasound contrast agents into the external opening during examination.[65] AES is also disadvantaged by an inability to image in the surgically important coronal plane, so that it may be difficult to distinguish supralevator from infralevator extensions. Some workers have attempted to overcome this disadvantage by employing 3-D acquisition[66,67] (Fig. 21.18), but this remains relatively experimental. However, there is little doubt that MRI is a superior technique overall and, given this, the major role of AES in fistula disease is probably to assess the degree of sphincter disruption in patients who become anally incontinent following surgery for the fistula. AES also has a particular role in patients who might have a small intersphincteric abscess that could be difficult to resolve using standard body or surface-coil MRI (Fig. 21.19).

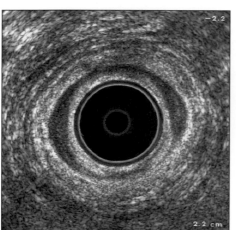

Fig. 21.17 Endosonography reveals internal sphincter fragmentation in this woman who had anal dilatation for an anal fissure, and then complained of anal incontinence.

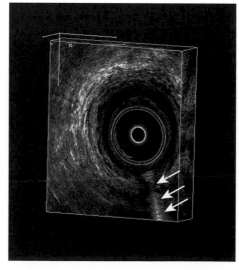

Fig. 21.18 Three-dimensional anal endosonography following hydrogen peroxide injection through the external opening of a fistula-in-ano. There is echogenic gas within an intersphincteric tract (arrows).

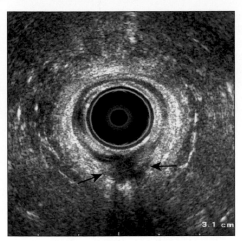

Fig. 21.19 Endosonography clearly revealed a posterior intersphincteric abscess (arrows) in this patient with anal pain, in whom digital examination had been normal.

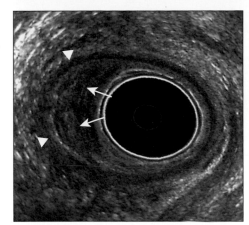

Fig. 21.21 Endosonography in a man with an anal tumour revealed a right-sided mass (arrows) that remained confined by the internal sphincter (arrowheads).

Endosonography has also revealed sphincter abnormalities in patients who are severely constipated, although the significance of these findings remains largely uncertain. For example, patients with solitary rectal ulcer syndrome are known to have an abnormally thickened IAS (Fig. 21.20),[68] and this finding has been correlated with the presence of high-grade prolapse of rectal mucosa.[69] IAS hypertrophy has also been demonstrated by AES in children with intractable constipation,[70] and a study of 144 constipated children found that this correlated with the duration and severity of symptoms, size of megarectum, and amplitude of rectal contraction.[71] The authors suggested that

IAS thickening was due to hypertrophy resulting from chronic stimulation owing to the presence of feces in the rectum.[71] Endosonography may also be useful when it is necessary to determine the correct anatomic position of the neoanus with respect to any residual musculature in children with imperforate anus and, unlike MRI, can be performed easily during operation.[72,73]

Endosonography may also be used to stage anal tumors locally, as it can determine the depth of penetration into surrounding tissues (Fig. 21.21).[74] However, some authors have found the technique less useful in the detection of local recurrence: all 14 recurrences in a series of 82 patients were detected by visual inspection and digital examination alone.[75]

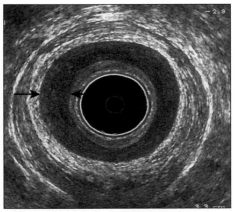

Fig. 21.20 Solitary rectal ulcer syndrome. The internal sphincter (between arrows) measured 7.5 mm, far greater than normal for a man.

EXAMINATION CHECKLIST

Use of a dedicated anal probe is recommended

No patient preparation is necessary

Place patient in optimal position – men in left lateral and women in prone position

Acquire still image in proximal, mid, and distal anal canal

Obtain at least two image sets, one at standard magnification and one at high magnification

REFERENCES

1 Law PJ, Bartram CI. Anal endosonography: technique and normal anatomy. Gastrointest Radiol 1989; 14:349–353.

2 Snooks SJ, Setchell M, Swash M, et al. Injury to the innervation of the pelvic floor sphincter musculature in childbirth. Lancet 1984; ii:546–550.

3 Lunniss PJ, Phillips RK. Anatomy and function of the anal longitudinal muscle. Br J Surg 1992; 79:882–884.

4 Stoker J, Rociu E, Zwamborn AW, et al. Endoluminal MR imaging of the rectum and anus: technique, applications, and pitfalls. Radiographics 1999; 19:383–398.

5 Williams AB, Bartram CI, Halligan S, et al. Endosonographic anatomy of the normal anal canal compared with endocoil magnetic resonance imaging. Dis Colon Rectum 2002; 45:176–183.

6 Frudinger A, Halligan S, Bartram CI, et al. Female anal sphincter: age-related differences in asymptomatic volunteers with high-frequency endoanal US. Radiology 2002; 224:417–423.

7 Williams AB, Bartram CI, Halligan S, et al. Multiplanar anal endosonography – normal anal canal anatomy. Colorectal Dis 2001; 3:169–174.

8   Sultan AH, Nicholls RJ, Kamm MA, et al. Anal endosonography and correlation with in vitro and in vivo anatomy. Br J Surg 1993; 80:508–511.

9   Gold DM, Halligan S, Kmiot WA, et al. Intraobserver and interobserver agreement in anal endosonography. Br J Surg 1999; 86:371–375.

10 Lane RH, Parks AG. Function of the anal sphincters following colo-anal anastomosis. Br J Surg 1977; 64:596–599.

11 Engel AG, Kamm MA. Relationship of symptoms in faecal incontinence to specific sphincter abnormalities. Int J Colorectal Dis 1995; 10:152–155.

12 Rogers J, Henry MM, Misiewicz JJ. Disposable pudendal nerve stimulator: evaluation of the standard instrument and new device. Gut 1988; 29:1131–1133.

13 Kiff ES, Swash M. Slowed conduction in the pudendal nerves in idiopathic (neurogenic) faecal incontinence. Br J Surg 1984; 71:614–616.

14 Snooks SJ, Setchell M, Swash M, et al. Injury to innervation of pelvic floor sphincter musculature in childbirth. Lancet 1984; ii:546–550.

15 Parks AG, Porter NH, Hardcastle JD. The syndrome of the descending perineum. Proc R Soc Med 1966; 59:477–482.

16 Jorge JMN, Wexner SD, Ehrenpreis ED, et al. Does perineal descent correlate with pudendal neuropathy? Dis Colon Rectum 1993; 36:475–483.

17 Gilliand R, Altomare DF, Moreira H, et al. Pudendal neuropathy is predictive of failure following anterior overlapping sphincteroplasty. Dis Colon Rectum 1998; 41:1516–1522.

18 Sultan AH, Kamm MA, Talbot IC, et al. Anal endosonograpy for identifying external sphincter defects confirmed histologically. Br J Surg 1994; 81:463–465.

19 Denis P, Bercoff E, Bizien MF. Etude de la prevalence di l'incontinence anale chez l'adulte. Gastroenterol Clin Biol 1992; 16:344–350.

20 Talley NJ, O'Keefe EA, Zinsmeister AR, et al. Prevalence of gastrointestinal symptoms in the elderly: a population based study. Gastroenterology 1992; 102:895–901.

21 Lahr CJ. Evaluation and treatment of incontinence. Pract Gastroenterol 1988; 12:27–35.

22 Sultan AH, Kamm MA, Hudson CN, et al. Third degree obstetric tears: risk factors and outcome of primary repair. BMJ 1994; 308:887–891.

23 Law PJ, Kamm MA, Bartram CI. Anal endosonography in the investigation of faecal incontinence. Br J Surg 1991; 78:312–314.

24 Burnett SJD, Spence-Jones C, Speakman CTM, et al. Unsuspected sphincter damage following childbirth revealed by anal endosonography. Br J Radiol 1991; 64:225–227.

25 Sultan AH, Kamm MA, Hudson CN, et al. Anal sphincter disruption during vaginal delivery. N Engl J Med 1993; 329:1905–1911.

26 Deen KI, Kumar D, Williams JG, et al. Anal sphincter defects: correlation between endoanal ultrasound and surgery. Ann Surg 1993; 218:201–205.

27 Sentovich SM, Wong WD, Blatchford GJ. Accuracy and reliability of transanal ultrasound for anterior anal sphincter injury. Dis Colon Rectum 1998; 41:1000–1004.

28 Voyvodic F, Rieger NA, Skinner S, et al. Endosonographic imaging of anal sphincter injury: does the size of the tear correlate with the degree of dysfunction? Dis Colon Rectum 2003; 46:735–741.

29 Frudinger A, Halligan S, Bartram CI, et al. Assessment of the predictive value of a bowel symptom questionnaire in identifying perianal and anal sphincter trauma after vaginal delivery. Dis Colon Rectum 2003; 46:742–747.

30 Oberwalder M, Dinnewitzer A, Baig MK, et al. The association between late-onset fecal incontinence and obstetric anal sphincter defects. Arch Surg 2004; 139:429–432.

31 Williams AB, Bartram CI, Halligan S, et al. Anal sphincter damage after vaginal delivery using three-dimensional endosonography. Obstet Gynecol 2001; 97:770–775.

32 Frudinger A, Halligan S, Bartram CI, et al. Changes in anal anatomy following vaginal delivery revealed by anal endosonography. Br J Obstet Gynaecol 1999; 106:233–237.

33 Williams AB, Bartram CI, Halligan S, et al. Alteration of anal sphincter morphology following vaginal delivery revealed by multiplanar anal endosonography. Br J Obstet Gynaecol 2002; 109:942–946.

34 Poen AC, Felt-Bersma RJ, Strijers RL, et al. Third-degree obstetric perineal tear: long-term clinical and functional results after primary repair. Br J Surg 1998; 85:1433–1438.

35 Davis K, Kumar D, Stanton SL, et al. Symptoms and anal sphincter morphology following primary repair of third-degree tears. Br J Surg 2003; 90:1573–1579.

36 Savoye-Collet C, Savoye G, Koning E, et al. Endosonography in the evaluation of anal function after primary repair of a third-degree obstetric tear. Scand J Gastroenterol 2003; 38:1149–1153.

37 Starck M, Bohe M, Valentin L. Results of endosonographic imaging of the anal sphincter 2–7 days after primary repair of third- or fourth-degree obstetric sphincter tears. Ultrasound Obstet Gynecol 2003; 22:609–615.

38 Malouf AJ, Norton CS, Engel AF, et al. Long-term results of overlapping anterior anal-sphincter repair for obstetric trauma. Lancet 2000; 355:260–265.

39 Pinedo G, Vaizey CJ, Nicholls RJ, et al. Results of repeat anal sphincter repair. Br J Surg 1999; 86:66–69.

40 Giordano P, Renzi A, Efron J, et al. Previous sphincter repair does not affect the outcome of repeat repair. Dis Colon Rectum 2002; 45:635–640.

41 Felt-Bersma RJ, Cuesta MA, Koorevaar M. Anal sphincter repair improves anorectal function and endosonographic image. A prospective clinical study. Dis Colon Rectum 1996; 39:878–885.

42 Faltin DL, Boulvain M, Irion O, et al. Diagnosis of anal sphincter tears by postpartum endosonography to predict fecal incontinence. Obstet Gynecol 2000; 95:643–647.

43 Fines M, Donnelly V, Behan M, et al. Effect of second vaginal delivery on anorectal physiology and faecal continence: a prospective study. Lancet 1999; 354:983–986.

44 Faltin DL, Sangalli MR, Roche B, et al. Does a second delivery increase the risk of anal incontinence? Br J Obstet Gynaecol 2001; 108:684–688.

45 Varma A, Gunn J, Lindow SW, et al. Do routinely measured delivery variables predict anal sphincter outcome? Dis Colon Rectum 1999; 42:1261–1264.

46 Donnelly V, Fynes M, Campbell D, et al. Obstetric events leading to anal sphincter damage. Obstet Gynecol 1998; 92:955–961.

47 Varma A, Gunn J, Gardiner A, et al. Obstetric anal sphincter injury: prospective evaluation of incidence. Dis Colon Rectum 1999; 42:1537–1543.

48 Abramowitz L, Sobhani I, Ganansia R, et al. Are sphincter defects the cause of anal incontinence after vaginal delivery? Results of a prospective study. Dis Colon Rectum 2000; 43:590–596, discussion 596–598.

49 Oberwalder M, Connor J, Wexner SD. Meta-analysis to determine the incidence of obstetric anal sphincter damage. Br J Surg 2003; 90:1333–1337.

50 Vaizey CJ, Kamm MA, Bartram CI. Primary degeneration of the internal anal sphincter as a cause of passive faecal incontinence. Lancet 1997; 349:612–615.

51 Engel AF, Kamm MA, Talbot IC. Progressive systemic sclerosis of the internal anal sphincter leading to passive faecal incontinence. Gut 1994; 35:857–859.

52 Briel JW, Stoker J, Rociu E, et al. External anal sphincter atrophy on endoanal magnetic resonance imaging adversely affects continence after sphincteroplasty. Br J Surg 1999; 86:1322–1327.

53 Williams AB, Bartram CI, Modhwadia D, et al. Endocoil magnetic resonance imaging quantification of external anal sphincter atrophy. Br J Surg 2001; 88:853–859.

54 Malouf AJ, Williams AB, Halligan S, et al. Prospective assessment of accuracy of endoanal MR imaging and endosonography in patients with fecal incontinence. AJR Am J Roentgenol 2000; 175:741–745.

55 Felt-Bersma RJ, van Baren R, Koorevaar M, et al. Unsuspected sphincter defects shown by anal endosonography after anorectal surgery. A prospective study. Dis Colon Rectum 1995; 38:249–253.

56 Abbasakoor F, Nelson M, Beynon J, et al. Anal endosonography in patients with anorectal symptoms after haemorrhoidectomy. Br J Surg 1998; 85:1522–1524.

57 Gattuso JM, Kamm MA, Halligan SM, et al. The anal sphincter in idiopathic megarectum: effects of manual disimpaction under general anesthetic. Dis Colon Rectum 1996; 39:435–439.

58 Ho YH, Tsang C, Tang CL, et al. Anal sphincter injuries from stapling instruments introduced transanally: randomized, controlled study with endoanal ultrasound and anorectal manometry. Dis Colon Rectum 2000; 43:169–173.

59 Farouk R, Duthie GS, Lee PW, et al. Endosonographic evidence of injury to the internal anal sphincter after low anterior resection: long-term follow-up. Dis Colon Rectum 1998; 41:888–891.

60 Sultan AH, Kamm MA, Nicholls RJ, et al. Prospective study of the extent of internal anal sphincter division during lateral sphincterotomy. Dis Colon Rectum 1994; 37:1031–1033.

61 Garcia-Granero E, Sanahuja A, Garcia-Armengol J, et al. Anal endosonographic evaluation after closed lateral subcutaneous sphincterotomy. Dis Colon Rectum 1998; 41:598–601.

62 Choen S, Burnett S, Bartram CI, et al. Comparison between anal endosonography and digital examination in the evaluation of anal fistulae. Br J Surg 1991; 78:445–447.

63 Buchanan GN, Halligan S, Bartram CI, et al. Clinical examination, endosonography, and magnetic resonance imaging for preoperative assessment of fistula-in-ano: comparison to an outcome based reference standard. Radiology 2004; 233:674–681.

64 Buchanan G, Halligan S, Williams A, et al. Effect of MRI on clinical outcome of recurrent fistula-in-ano. Lancet 2002; 360:1661–1662.

65 Kruskal JB, Kane RA, Morrin MM. Peroxide-enhanced anal endosonography: technique, image interpretation, and clinical applications. Radiographics 2001; 21:173–189.

66 Buchanan GN, Bartram CI, Williams AB, et al. Value of hydrogen peroxide enhancement of three-dimensional endoanal ultrasound in fistula-in-ano. Dis Colon Rectum 2005; 48:141–147.

67 West RL, Zimmerman DD, Dwarkasing S, et al. Prospective comparison of hydrogen peroxide-enhanced three-dimensional endoanal ultrasonography and endoanal magnetic resonance imaging of perianal fistulas. Dis Colon Rectum 2003; 46:1407–1415.

68 Halligan S, Sultan A, Rottenberg G, et al. Endosonography of the anal sphincters in solitary rectal ulcer syndrome. Int J Colorectal Dis 1995; 10:79–82.

69 Marshall M, Halligan S, Fotheringham T, et al. Predictive value of internal anal sphincter thickness for diagnosis of rectal intussusception in patients with solitary rectal ulcer syndrome. Br J Surg 2002; 89:1281–1285.

70 Hosie GP, Spitz L. Idiopathic constipation in childhood is associated with thickening of the internal anal sphincter. J Pediatr Surg 1997; 32:1041–1043, discussion 1043–1044.

71 Keshtgar AS, Ward HC, Clayden GS, et al. Thickening of the internal anal sphincter in idiopathic constipation in children. Pediatr Surg Int 2004; 20:817–823.

72 Jones NM, Humphreys MS, Goodman TR, et al. The value of anal endosonography compared with magnetic resonance imaging following the repair of anorectal malformations. Pediatr Radiol 2003; 33:183–185.

73 Yamataka A, Yoshida R, Kobayashi H, et al. Intraoperative endosonography enhances laparoscopy-assisted colon pull-through for high imperforate anus. J Pediatr Surg 2002; 37:1657–1660.

74 Tarantino D, Bernstein MA. Endoanal ultrasound in the staging and management of squamous-cell carcinoma of the anal canal: potential implications of a new ultrasound staging system. Dis Colon Rectum 2002; 45:16–22.

75 Lund JA, Sundstrom SH, Haaverstad R, et al. Endoanal ultrasound is of little value in follow-up of anal carcinomas. Dis Colon Rectum 2004; 47:839–842.

EUS-GUIDED FINE-NEEDLE ASPIRATION

Chapter 22

How to Perform EUS-Guided FNA

Anand V. Sahai and Promila Banerjee

KEY POINTS

- As movement of the needle is easier when the echoendoscope is straight, the endosonographer should try to achieve a position in which there is minimal up/down and left/right tip angulation and no elevator is required.

- Before inserting a needle, scan the needle pathway using color Doppler mode.

- Never use excessive force to pass the needle sheath past an acute bend in the endoscope tip.

- Keep the needle in the visual plane at all times during EUS-FNA.

- When aspirating cysts without a mass component, fully aspirate all fluid, make only one pass, use antibiotics, and do not try to perform aspiration cytology from the cyst wall.

INTRODUCTION

Fine-needle aspiration (FNA) provides some of the most clinically powerful information that endoscopic ultrasound (EUS) has to offer: pathologic confirmation of the presence (or absence) of malignancy and/or metastasis to secondary sites ('histologic staging'). Like any procedure, proficiency requires adequate experience, but EUS-FNA is not a universally difficult technique to master. Some cases are more technically demanding than others. Sampling a 5-mm pancreatic nodule buried deep in the uncinate process is certainly more challenging than sampling a 4-cm subcarinal lymph node. Interestingly, some of the easiest cases provide information that can have a tremendous impact on patient management, such as prevention of surgery by documentation of mediastinal node involvement in a patient with non-small cell lung cancer.

This chapter provides a detailed description of a generic EUS-FNA technique that can be applied to the great majority of lesions. Special situations are also discussed.

EUS-FNA can be broken down into a series of steps. Proper execution of each step will make the procedure easier and probably increase the yield for malignancy. Experts likely have varying opinions of the best way to perform EUS-FNA, but there are few or no data that show clearly which procedural variables predict success.

STEPS FOR EUS-FNA

Verify the indication

Before performing EUS-FNA, the indication should be clear and the endoscopy suite and team adequately prepared. Like any test, EUS-FNA does not need to 'change management' to be useful. However, before considering EUS-FNA in any patient, it should be clear that the information obtained has a reasonable chance of being clinically useful (to those managing the patient and/or to the patient). If the endosonographer is not in charge of the patient's management, his or her opinion as to the value of the information need not affect the decision to perform EUS-FNA, unless there is compelling evidence that the risks of the procedure will likely far outweigh the possible benefits. If there is any doubt, these issues should be addressed with the referring physician before the procedure (or even during the procedure) if necessary.

Localize the lesion and position the echoendoscope

Optimal positioning of the echoendoscope with respect to the lesion should make EUS-FNA easier, safer, and more effective. Once the lesion has been identified, it should be positioned as much as possible within the natural path of the needle (i.e., the path taken by the needle when no elevation is applied). This varies depending on the instrument used. If this is not possible, the lesion should be positioned within the range of deflection offered by the elevator (if present) (Fig. 22.1). The elevator can be used to increase the angle formed between the echoendoscope shaft and the needle. It cannot reduce this angle. The effectiveness of the elevator is also diminished if the distance that the sheath of the needle extends beyond the opening of the biopsy channel is excessively long. Depending on the needle used, this distance can be adjusted using a system integrated into the needle or by using spacers that luer-lock on to the opening of the biopsy channel.

When elevator adjustment is required, it may be helpful first to lock the up/down dial to immobilize the endoscope tip. If no elevator is available or the tip deflection obtainable using the elevator is insufficient, the angle can also be increased by implanting the needle tip into the gut wall and then gently advancing the echoendoscope (Fig. 22.2).

Movement of the EUS-FNA needle is always easier when it is straight. Any bend in the needle induced by the echoendo-

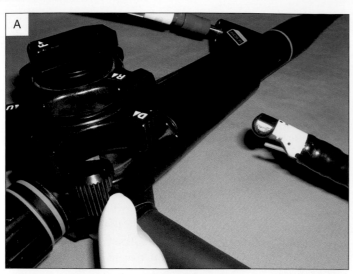
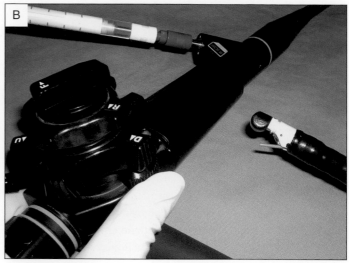

Fig. 22.1   Elevator range of movement. **A,** No elevator. **B,** Maximum deflection of elevator.

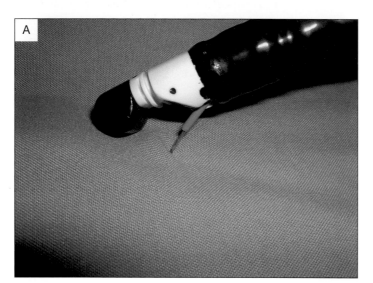
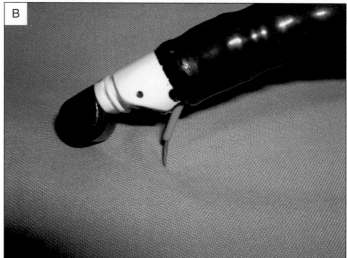

Fig. 22.2   Planting and pushing to deflect the needle, **A,** Planting the needle. **B,** Advancing the echoendoscope

scope position and/or the elevator increases the resistance in the needle system and makes needle movement more difficult. This is problematic primarily when sampling lesions with the probe in the bulb or the duodenal sweep. However, wedging the echoendoscope in the bulb (which requires a long, bent scope) provides a mechanical advantage when trying to puncture indurated lesions in the region of the pancreatic head. Conversely, when the scope is in a short, straight position in the second duodenum, it may limit the ability to exert strong force in the direction of the lesion when advancing the needle, because the needle is well out of the long axis of the echoendoscope shaft. Therefore, finding the most effective position may require some compromise between maintaining a fairly straight needle and not losing the mechanical advantage provided by the long echoendoscope position.

Given the risks inherent to needle puncture of any retroperitoneal structure, it is logical to assume that limiting the distance the needle must travel to reach the target will reduce the risk of

complications relating to trauma of the surrounding tissues and organs. One should also avoid puncturing undrained, obstructed ducts, owing to the risk of inducing cholangitis or pancreatitis. Although not proven, it is also logical to assume that, if a liquid-containing structure such as a blood vessel or bile duct is punctured, the risk of leakage is lower if the needle enters perpendicular to the vessel or duct wall and produces only a pinhole defect; as opposed to passing tangentially and causing a linear laceration. Therefore, contact with all vessels should be avoided, but particularly when passing the needle laterally to a vessel. Before inserting the needle, it is reasonable always to scan the biopsy path with the Doppler function to identify any significant blood vessels in the vicinity.

Insert the EUS-FNA needle into the echoendoscope

Whether or not the needle system is inserted into the biopsy channel before or after the echoendoscope is positioned for FNA is a matter of personal preference. However, it should be noted that, once the echoendoscope is in position, it may be difficult or impossible to pass the needle system completely into position if the echoendoscope is not sufficiently straight. In this situation, the sheath may become stuck in bending portion of the instrument near the tip. Excessive force should never be used to push the sheath past an excessive bend at this location, as the needle sheath may perforate the inner sheath of the biopsy channel. Instead, the echoendoscope should be withdrawn into a straight configuration before attempting to reinsert the needle system completely.

In some cases, a lesion that was clearly visible before the needle deployment may become difficult to see once the needle assembly is in place. The needle/sheath may produce artifact or may slightly reduce complete coupling between the ultrasound probe and the gut wall, producing air artifact. Slight repositioning of the echoendoscope, use of suction, or reinsertion of the needle assembly may help to correct the problem.

Prepare the needle

Once the needle assembly and lesion are in a good position, tissue sampling may begin. The goal is to insert the needle into the lesion under constant real-time ultrasound guidance and to make repetitive thrusting movements to shear off cells and collect them within the needle lumen. This requires that the needle be kept in the ultrasound imaging plane and that thrusting movements be deliberate, but not so fast as to make the needle difficult to see. Care should be taken to ensure that the needle does not leave the confines of the lesion during sampling. This will avoid clogging the needle with tissue other than that from the target lesion.

Use of the stopping device

If the needle system includes a stopping device, this can be set so as to limit the maximum distance that the needle can travel (Fig. 22.3). This can be helpful in instances when inserting the needle beyond the limits of the target lesion would be

dangerous, for example when the target lies directly over a vascular structure. Once the target lesion is in position on the screen, the caliper function can be used to measure the distance between the ultrasound probe and the center of the target lesion. The stopping device can then be set to this distance.

Stylet issues

All commercially available EUS-FNA systems include a removable stylet. It is believed that the stylet helps prevent clogging of the needle by gut wall tissue, which could limit the ability to aspirate cells from the target lesion. This is a logical assumption, but there are no data demonstrating clearly that the use of a stylet increases the yield of EUS-FNA. Why is this question important? Manipulation of the stylet increases the time and energy required to perform EUS-FNA and it likely increases the costs of EUS-FNA needle systems.

In some circumstances, the stylet may actually make EUS-FNA impossible. Occasionally, it may be impossible to advance or remove the stylet once the target has been punctured. This tends to occur only when the echoendoscope is bent (particularly when sampling from the bulb or duodenal sweep) and a large (19 gauge) needle is being used. In this situation, consideration should be given to removing the stylet completely before attempting to perform EUS-FNA.

Depending on the needle system, stylet adjustment may be required before puncturing the target lesion. The stylet tip may be pointed or blunt, and may or may not protrude beyond the tip of the hollow needle. If the stylet is flush with the needle tip, it can be left in place. If it protrudes beyond the needle tip (i.e., the stylet is longer than the needle) and is blunt, the stylet must be withdrawn into the needle lumen to expose the sharp tip of the needle (Fig. 22.4). Even if the stylet tip is pointed, it may help to withdraw it into the needle, as the stylet tip may be less effective at puncturing the gut wall than the beveled needle tip; for example, it may be less pointed and may become dull more easily after multiple passes.

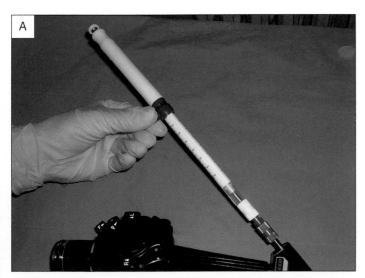
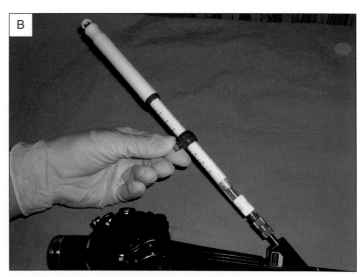

Fig. 22.3   Stopper adjustment. **A,** Stopper off. **B,** Stopper on.

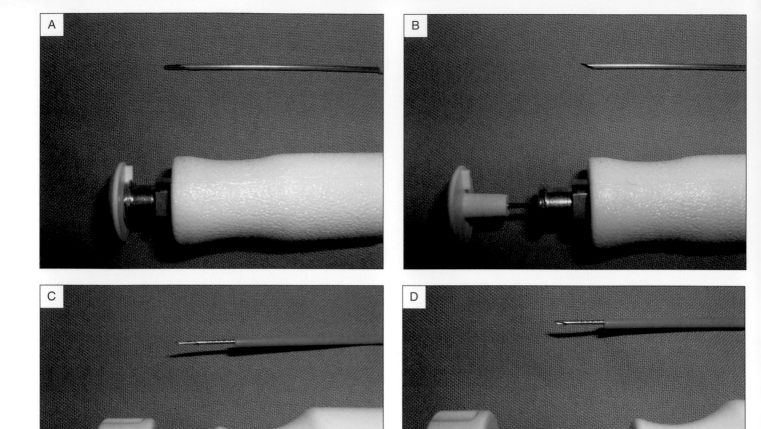

Fig. 22.4   Stylets. **A,** Stylet blunt and longer than needle. **B,** Blunt stylet withdrawn to expose needle tip. **C,** Stylet pointed and longer than needle. **D,** Pointed stylet withdrawn to expose needle.

How to hold the needle

The fixed component of the needle handle should be grasped between the palm and the last three fingers of the right hand (Fig. 22.5). The movable portion should be held with the thumb and index finger. This allows either fine or vigorous needle movements to be performed, but with control. Any method that does not allow such control should be avoided.

Puncture the lesion

As stated above, it is reasonable to look for blood vessels using the Doppler function before inserting the needle. Before beginning to move the needle, firm upward tip deflection should be applied using the up/down dial. This tends to bring the lesion closer to the echoendoscope and reduces the tendency of the ncedle to push the ultrasound probe away from the gut wall, which can reduce the ultrasound image quality by allowing air to seep in between the probe and the gut wall. It also provides a mechanical advantage when trying to puncture an indurated lesion.

The needle should first be advanced slowly a few millimeters out of the sheath – just enough to localize the tip in the ultrasound field. Once the tip has been identified, the needle can be advanced into the lesion under ultrasound guidance. If, for some reason, the needle tip can no longer be seen once the lesion has been punctured, all forward movement of the needle should be stopped. Continuing to advance the needle in the hope that the tip will become visible is a mistake and can result in inadvertent puncture of structures deep to the target lesion. Instead, the first reflex should be slowly to withdraw the needle. This will help to localize the tip without risking puncture of deep structures. If this is ineffective, slow left and right movement of the shoulders can help bring the needle into the ultrasound imaging plane. If both of these techniques fail, the needle should be withdrawn completely from the lesion into the sheath. If it is possible that the scope position could have caused the needle to be bent, the needle assembly should be removed from the echoendoscope and the needle straightened, if needed (see below). The puncture can then be attempted again.

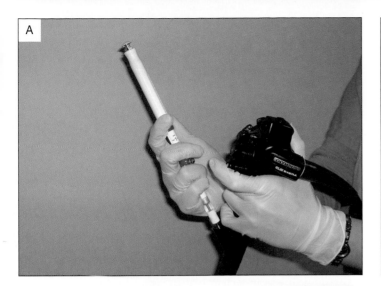

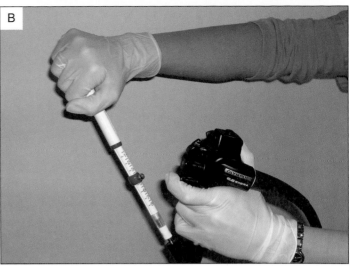

Fig. 22.5 How to hold the needle. **A,** Correct method. **B,** Incorrect method. **C,** Another incorrect method.

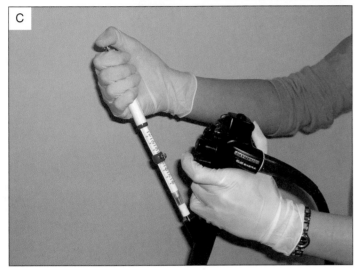

Once the needle is in the lesion and the tip can be seen clearly, the needle is moved back and forth several times, with adequate thrusting force to shear off cells. Care should be taken to stay within the confines of the lesion at all times. In some cases, movement of the needle will tend to separate the ultrasound transducer from the gut wall and reduce needle visibility due to air artifact. To correct this, slight inward pressure should be applied to the shaft of the echoendoscope to push the probe against the gut wall. It may also be helpful to have an assistant prevent the echoendoscope from coming out by bracing the shaft as it exits the patient's mouth (to do this, it is probably best for the assistant to stand on the opposite side of the bed from the echoendoscopist.)

If elevator deflection was used to adjust the needle angle, once the needle is well inside the lesion it may be helpful to return the elevator to the relaxed position, thus allowing the needle to move more freely. In some cases (e.g., soft masses or nodes), manipulation of the elevator and/or up/down tip deflection may be used to guide the needle into different regions of the target lesion or to orient the needle into the long axis of an oval or oblong lesion.

Use of suction

The use of continuous suction during movement of the needle does not appear to increase the yield of EUS-FNA, and may actually hinder adequate cytologic analysis by causing aspirates to become diluted with blood.[1] Adequate samples can be obtained in many cases with no suction. However, if in-room cytologic analysis of aspirates obtained initially without suction shows inadequate cellularity, it may be helpful to apply 5–10 ml of suction for a few seconds immediately before withdrawing the needle from the lesion, or to use continuous suction.

Withdraw the needle and process the aspirate

Once a pass has been completed, withdraw the needle completely into the sheath. If a locking device is present, slide it to the highest position and lock it, to prevent the needle from coming out of the sheath accidentally during removal of the needle assembly from the operating channel.

To avoid clotting in the needle, the aspirate should be expressed from the needle as quickly as possible with a 10-ml air-filled syringe. If the needle appears blocked, the aspirate can be forced out by inserting the stylet. Once the clot has been expressed into an appropriate receptacle (e.g., slide, container), the syringe should be used to express any remaining material. The needle can also be flushed with alcohol, but this should not be done until the last pass because, in some cases, insertion of the stylet becomes difficult or impossible once the lumen has been in contact with alcohol.

Prepare the needle for subsequent passes

The same needle can be used for several passes and need not be changed unless it malfunctions or the needle tip becomes too dull. If previous aspirates were bloody, it may be helpful to rinse the lumen with water and then air before reinserting the stylet.

If the needle is bent, it must be straightened; otherwise it will deflect out of the ultrasound beam on subsequent passes. To straighten the needle, push it completely out of the sheath, then use your fingers to straighten it manually (Fig. 22.6). An alcohol swab can be used to clean the outer surface of the needle.

If a cytologist is available, passes should be performed until adequate material or a diagnosis is obtained. If not, the available data suggest that three to seven passes should be sufficient to obtain a diagnosis (if cancer is indeed present).[1,2]

There is no absolute limit to the number of passes that can be performed with the same needle. However, it should be changed if it malfunctions, becomes too difficult to reinsert the stylet, etc.

SPECIAL ISSUES

Biopsy of multiple lesions

When there are several potential biopsy sites or lesions in an individual patient (e.g., pancreatic mass, celiac node, liver lesion, mediastinal node), biopsies should be performed starting with the lesion that, if positive, will confirm the most advanced stage. If the first lesion is negative, the lesion offering the next highest stage should be sampled. If a metastatic lesion

is confirmed, the primary lesion need not necessarily be biopsied, unless there is a compelling reason to do so. If the above sequence of biopsy sites is employed (i.e., from distant lesions towards the primary lesion), then several lesions can be sampled using a single EUS-FNA needle. If not, a new needle should be used for each lesion, to avoid the risk of creating false-positive results and/or seeding distant sites.

EUS-FNA of cystic lesions

Cystic lesions may be punctured for cyst fluid analysis, biopsy of the cyst wall, and/or treatment. The primary concerns relate to the risk of infection and bleeding. Bleeding is alarming, but rarely serious, as it is usually contained by the cyst cavity. Infections, however, can lead to serious morbidity and death. Therefore, perhaps more than with other lesions, cysts should not be punctured unless it is clear that the information obtained will likely be useful to someone.

Unless there is clear evidence of a mass component, it is the author's opinion that sampling of the wall is rarely productive and serves only to increase the risk of bleeding. Likewise, cyst fluid cytology is almost always negative. Therefore, for cysts without a significant mass component, the primary goal should be to aspirate sufficient fluid to perform tumor marker analysis. Conversely, if there is a significant mass component, it is reasonable to perform EUS-FNA of the mass alone, and avoid the risks of cyst puncture. Biochemistry laboratory personnel should be consulted to determine the minimum quantity of cyst fluid required to perform the desired analyses.

For larger-diameter lesions (>1–2 cm), the author prefers to use a 19-G needle rather than a smaller gauge needle to allow for more rapid and complete cyst fluid aspiration (especially when the fluid is viscous). Always use a new needle to puncture a cyst and, if possible, perform only one pass. If more than one pass is required, change to a new needle. Before introducing the needle, some authors 'clean' the puncture site by injecting an antiseptic solution into the biopsy channel and on to the gut wall.

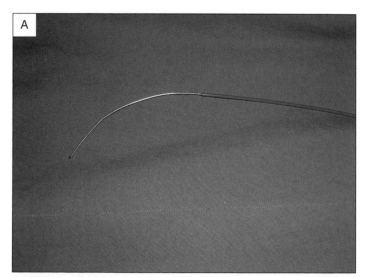
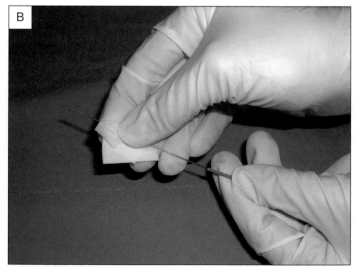

Fig. 22.6   Straightening the needle. **A,** Bent needle. **B,** Straightening the needle.

Many experts believe that the risk of infection is lower if the cyst is drained completely, so this is probably a reasonable goal. However, in the case of a multiloculated cyst, it may be safer to focus on draining only a single, superficial loculation – one that appears to contain sufficient fluid for marker analysis.

Once the cyst has been punctured, try to place the needle tip in the center of the cavity before aspirating. During aspiration and as the cyst collapses, the needle should be repositioned as necessary to stay away from the wall or any debris that may clog the needle lumen. If the needle clogs before the cyst has collapsed completely, suction may be halted and an attempt made to reposition the needle gently, without removing it from the cyst. When the cyst is almost completely collapsed, drainage frequently stops and it often becomes difficult to locate the needle tip. Attempts to reposition the needle to obtain 'every last drop' should probably be avoided, as this may lead to bleeding. Once adequate fluid has been obtained for analysis, the remaining fluid can be drained by repeatedly filling a syringe or by connecting the aspiration port of the needle to wall suction. After drainage of the cyst, it should be observed for a short time to look for early recurrence or bleeding.

Mobile lesions

Lesions that are not fixed (e.g., retroperitoneal nodes) can be difficult to puncture because they tend to bounce off the needle tip. This may be compounded when the lesion is not directly adjacent to the gut wall, is small, or there is excessive respiratory movement. To puncture these lesions effectively, it may be helpful first to focus on traversing the gut wall with the needle. Once the needle tip is in the extraluminal space, the focus can turn to puncturing the lesion.

To puncture the lesion, advance the needle tip so that it abuts the lesion wall. Coordination with respiratory movement may be required. To enter the lesion, use a single rapid thrust to stab the lesion effectively. It may be necessary to pass the needle completely through lesion. If this occurs, the lesion will be effectively immobilized and the needle tip can then be slowly withdrawn until it is within the confines of the lesion.

Indurated lesions

Occasionally, it may be difficult to penetrate a lesion because it is indurated. When a lesion is difficult to penetrate, it must first be verified that the needle is functioning correctly. The needle tip may have become dull, for example due to multiple previous passes, or may not be exiting the sheath effectively. The stylet tip may also be too dull or, if it is blunt, may not have been withdrawn sufficiently to expose the needle tip.

If the needle is functioning properly, the lesion can be punctured by using more forceful stabbing maneuvers. However, this should be a last resort as it is difficult to stab forcefully while at the same time controlling the depth of penetration. Instead, firm upward tip deflection should be applied, the needle tip should be placed against the leading edge of the lesion, and firm, progressively increasing, pressure applied to the needle. If this fails, it may be helpful to apply force by advancing the echoendoscope (assuming the echoendoscope is in a position that enables pressure to be applied in the same axis as the needle).

Tumor seeding

Tumor seeding is definitely possible with EUS-FNA.[3] If the biopsy track will not be included in the surgical specimen (e.g., gastric wall in the case of a pancreatic body lesion), EUS-FNA should not be performed unless absolutely necessary. Instead, if at all possible, an attempt should be made to perform biopsies through a part of the gut wall that will be removed should the patient proceed to surgery (e.g., lesions of the pancreatic genu should be biopsied through the duodenum if possible).

To avoid seeding extraluminal sites (e.g., nodes), EUS-FNA should never be performed through an area of the gut wall that is overtly or possibly infiltrated by malignancy or dysplasia.

CONCLUSION

EUS-FNA is a powerful clinical tool. It can be technically challenging, but is often straightforward if the lesion can be located, is sufficiently large, and can be brought into the needle path with the echoendoscope in a fairly straight position. The primary goal of the needle puncture is to shear off sufficient cells for cytologic analysis, while limiting the amount of dilution with blood. In the interest of safety and optimizing the yield, emphasis should be placed on always moving the needle in a controlled fashion and under constant, real-time ultrasound guidance.

REFERENCES

1 Wallace MB, Kennedy T, Durkalski V, et al. Randomized controlled trial of EUS-guided fine needle aspiration techniques for the detection of malignant lymphadenopathy. Gastrointest Endosc 2001; 4:441–447.

2 LeBlanc JK, Ciaccia D, Al Assi MT, et al. Optimal number of EUS-guided fine needle passes needed to obtain a correct diagnosis. Gastrointest Endosc 2004; 4:475–481.

3 Shah JN, Fraker D, Guerry D, et al. Melanoma seeding of an EUS-guided fine needle track. Gastrointest Endosc 2004; 7:923–924.

Chapter
23

A Cytology Primer for Endosonographers

Cynthia Behling

KEY POINTS

- Core biopsy and cytology each has its advantages and disadvantages. For some applications, cytology is considered a more sensitive diagnostic method.

- Technical aspects of the fine-needle aspiration (FNA) procedure, such as needle size and use of suction, influence the quantity and quality of cells obtained.

- Use of complementary cytologic preparations, such as air-dried Romanowsky-stained slides, alcohol-fixed slides, and cell block, optimize the diagnostic yield.

- A cytologic diagnosis is based on a composite of microscopic features including microarchitecture and nuclear and cytoplasmic characteristics of the cells.

INTRODUCTION

EUS-guided fine-needle aspiration (EUS-FNA) is a highly effective technique for obtaining a tissue diagnosis from a variety of organs in proximity to the gastrointestinal tract. Optimal results require the cooperation of two professional services: gastroenterology and pathology. The endoscopist localizes and characterizes the lesion, and obtains biopsy material, which is then prepared and interpreted in the laboratory. In a sense, the endosonographer acts as a 'conduit to the pathologist', and understanding the issues involved in obtaining and interpreting cytologic specimens optimizes the diagnostic yield. The goal of this chapter is to help the endosonographer learn technical aspects of cytology procedures and understand basic principles of interpretive cytopathology diagnosis.

This chapter is divided into two parts. The first portion of the chapter reviews the technical aspects of EUS-FNA that influence cytology outcomes. The second portion of the chapter introduces basic cytologic features of benign and malignant lesions commonly sampled by EUS-FNA.

There is a limited amount of EUS-specific literature addressing cytology topics. In some instances, the opinions in general cytology literature differ from those in existing EUS or FNA literature. This may be due to the small number of EUS studies, relatively small sample sizes, or possibly the specifics of the technique, individual endoscopists, and pathologists. Many technical factors are site and lesion specific, and further study will help to optimize the procedural issues specific to EUS-FNA.

TECHNICAL ASPECTS OF EUS THAT IMPROVE DIAGNOSTIC YIELD

Preliminary planning

Ideally, an interested or responsible pathologist or cytotechnologist should be involved in the development of the EUS-FNA service from the earliest stages of the planning process. A number of factors need to be considered, including the manner in which the cells will be prepared, personnel involved, scheduling, use of immediate cytologic evaluation for determination of adequacy, and the role of the procedure in the patient care algorithm (Table 23.1).

The type of tissue specimen preparation (direct smear, liquid-based cytologic preparation, cell block, core biopsy, or a combination) depends on institutional practice, staffing, and the physical distance between the pathologist and endoscopy suite, in addition to the relative sensitivity, specificity, and diagnostic accuracy of the various choices. At some institutions a trained laboratory technician or cytotechnologist is called to the GI suite to handle the specimen directly, make direct smears, or further process the specimen. Elsewhere, GI suite staff may be trained to handle the specimen. EUS-FNA procedures should be scheduled so that laboratory services are available to process the specimens in a timely manner for culture, flow cytometry, or molecular studies. Preliminary planning should also include a discussion of whether a pathologist will attend the FNA procedure to provide immediate cytologic interpretation of adequacy and triage of the specimen. Further planning should detail ordering of supplies, stocking, and provision of the FNA cart or cabinet.

For the pathologist and laboratory staff, a comprehensive understanding of their direct role in the EUS procedure and the patient care algorithm ensures appropriate support.[1] Pathologist and endosonographer should understand the indications for the procedure. Diagnostic strategies depend on whether the procedure is a screening test, a diagnostic test in a patient who may not undergo further diagnostic workup, or to procure material for flow cytometry, microbiologic, or other studies.

Communication between pathologist and endosonographer is one key to the success of the procedure. As one cytopathologist noted: 'There is some truth in the statement that the results of cytology are inversely proportional to the square of the distance between the cytologist and clinician ... and the best results are achieved by those clinicians who really believe in

Table 23.1 Factors to consider in preliminary planning for cytology services

FACTORS TO CONSIDER IN PRELIMINARY PLANNING FOR CYTOLOGY SERVICES	
Factor	Details
Type of biopsy	Needle core or cytology (fine needle)
Size of needle	25, 22, 20 G or other
Fixation or processing for cores	Formalin, other
Type of preparation of cells for FNA	Direct smears, transport media (proprietary, culture media (RPMI-1640), formalin, other
Type of smear	Air dried, alcohol fixed, or both
Personnel	GI suite staff, laboratory staff, training
On-site assessment of adequacy	Pathologist, cytopathologist, other, not performed
Database Archives for Cytology Information	Diagnosis, number of passes, pathologist, type of smears prepared, cell block available, special studies

cytology for their own patients and who work in close cooperation with their "own" cytologist'.[2]

A further preliminary planning step is consideration of database archives of cytology and diagnostic data. In combination with the EUS characteristics of lesions and other clinical information, these data can provide valuable feedback regarding diagnostic accuracy, individual practitioner competency, utility of immediate cytologic evaluation, and other quality assurance measures.

Professional staff should be properly trained and understand the limitations of their expertise and of the technique. In the USA, both the technical and interpretive services in the cytology laboratory are regulated at state and federal levels by the provisions of the Clinical Laboratory Improvement Amendments of 1988 (CLIA 1988), the Laboratory Accreditation Program of the College of American Pathologists (CAP), and others. These mandatory and voluntary standards ensure high-quality laboratories.[3] Specific details of practice guidelines and other standards are available from the College of American Pathologists[4] and American Society of Cytopathology.[5]

The following sections discuss technical factors that may improve diagnostic yield for EUS biopsy procedures, including needle type and size, use of heparin in the needle, suction or 'capillary' aspiration, number of passes, and direction of passes. These factors are listed in Table 23.2.

Histology (core biopsy) versus cytology (FNA)

Typical (non-EUS) needle core biopsies are obtained with relatively large (14–18 G) cutting needles. For some applications, even larger needles are used, such as those with 11- and 9-G cores used for some breast lesions.[6,7] Material obtained from needles of this size maintains its structure within the hollow of the needle, and is placed intact into fixative and subsequently

TECHNICAL ASPECTS THAT MAY POSITIVELY INFLUENCE DIAGNOSTIC YIELD		
Technical feature	Advantage	Disadvantage
Preliminary planning	Optimal laboratory support	None
Endoscopist skill	More likey to procure adequate specimen	None
Pathologist skill	Few if any false-positive or 'atypical' diagnoses	None
Core biopsy	Histologic diagnosis	Possibly more tissue injury
	Tissue for special stains	No capacity for on-site evaluation for adequacy
	Does not require on site laboratory personnel for specimen processing or evaluation	
Aspiration biopsy	More cells	Few disadvantages
		Risk of inadequate sample for some lesions or sites
Smaller needle size	Less tissue injury	Relatively fewer cells
Heparinized needle	Biopsy material not bound in blood clot	Too much heparin may cause cytologic artifact
Suction	Retrieves more cells	Increases bleeding in tissue
		May compromise some cell features
More passes	More cells	Injury to tissue
Cytopathologist in room	Specimens adequate for diagnosis	Time and cost
Air-dried and alcohol-fixed smears	Complementary stains yield optimal nuclear and cytologic detail	Increased technical effort required
Cell block	Tissue available for special stains	Not a stand-alone preparation; best in combination with smears

Table 23.2 Technical aspects that may positively influence diagnostic yield

embedded in paraffin or plastic tissue blocks and sectioned with a microtome. Sections made from these core biopsies are thin, 3–5-μm slices of the tissue, and, when stained and viewed microscopically, show cells or portions of cells within their intact tissue stroma – the familiar appearance of histology slides.

A 'fine' needle is 22 G or smaller, and procures a 'cytology' specimen.[8] Fine-needle biopsies are used widely for EUS, computed tomography, or other image-guided biopsies or percutaneous biopsies of palpable masses. Material obtained from a fine needle is generally dispersed as single and small groups of cells, rather than the intact tissue core obtained with larger needles. The drops and fragments of material contained within a fine needle are usually smeared onto slides in a manner similar to blood smears, resulting in a monolayer of cells to be fixed and/or dried and stained. As the preparation is not sectioned, the cells represented on an aspirate smear are intact, and round up or splay out depending on how they are treated in further processing steps. The monolayer smear created from a fine-needle biopsy allows resolution of microarchitecture and details of the nucleus and cytoplasm.

For a given lesion, the interpretive approach and diagnostic criteria differ between cytology smears and histology tissue sections. Cytology preparations emphasize details of individual cells. The criteria for diagnosis of well differentiated pancreatic ductal adenocarcinoma provide an example. Common to both cytology and histology is a fourfold or greater nuclear size variation between duct epithelial cells; however, major histologic criteria for diagnosis of a well differentiated pancreatic adenocarcinoma include identification of incomplete ductal lumens and an overall disorganized distribution of ducts within the stroma, features not identifiable in cytology preparations.[9] Rather, in fine-needle aspirates of well differentiated pancreatic adenocarcinoma, the cytologic criteria for malignancy include nuclear membrane irregularities, nuclear crowding, and overlapping, as well as variation in nuclear size.[10,11]

For a number of reasons – rational and not – some clinicians and pathologists believe that a tissue core yields unequivocally 'better' diagnostic material. Possible advantages of a core biopsy in EUS procedures include elimination of the need for an on-site pathologist, availability of tissue in a paraffin block for marker studies, and the possibility of obtaining tissue with fewer needle passes.[12] Core biopsies provide information on tissue architecture, which is important for the traditional diagnostic criteria of lymphomas, in the distinction of in situ from invasive malignancies, and may help to resolve difficult lesions such as well differentiated malignancies. Furthermore, many pathologists are more familiar with tissue sections.[13]

Use of core biopsies in EUS has limitations, however. Needle biopsies (Tru-Cut or Menghini) sometimes fail to obtain tissue.[14–16] In a prospective study of Tru-Cut biopsies of pancreatic masses, pancreatic tissue was obtained in only 17 of 23 patients, with an overall diagnostic accuracy of 61%.[14] Similarly, an inadequate specimen was obtained in 3 of 18

patients biopsied with EUS guidance with a 19-G Tru-Cut needle, with no inadequate specimens in the FNA group.[15] One possible explanation for the failure of core needles to sample the lesion may be attributes of the lesion itself, as the larger needle may deflect from the surface of firm or rubbery lesions.

In addition, a Tru-Cut biopsy represents a single pass into the tissue and is not able to sample the lesion widely without further passes into the tissue. Larger-sized needles increase the risk of bleeding and complications, although the risks remain very low.[15,17,18]

Studies directly comparing core biopsies and fine-needle aspirates raise additional issues. Core biopsies contain fewer tumor cells than a fine-needle aspirate.[19] The overall quantity of tumor cells is important when immunohistochemistry, microbiology, flow cytometry, or molecular diagnostic studies are warranted. FNA specimens are more likely to be adequate for evaluation.[15] In 100 cases of pancreas biopsies comparing core and FNA samples from needles of the same size, histologic diagnoses had lower interobserver and intraobserver variation (κ value of 0.70 versus 0.61), but cytologic specimens produced more consistent diagnoses of malignancy and fewer inadequate samples.[20]

In addition, technical limitations of the currently available EUS-guided Tru-Cut biopsy equipment limit the anatomic regions that can be biopsied successfully.[14]

The decision to obtain cores instead of, or in addition to, aspirates rests on a number of factors including the available equipment and personnel, training and expertise of the pathologists and staff, and endoscopist preference. Each type of biopsy has advantages and disadvantages that must be considered for individual lesions or patients. Overall, FNA is considered a more sensitive diagnostic method, which can be complemented by core biopsy or cell block.[21]

Needle size for fine-needle biopsy

Within the range of fine-needle biopsies (22 G or less), the choice of needle size also influences cytology findings. In a study designed to determine the optimum needle size and number of passes to obtain material for RNA quantitation, the number of cells obtained from needles of varying sizes was counted. With ten needle excursions into a tumor, 32 000 cells were obtained with a 25-G needle and 195 900 cells with a 20-G needle.[19] Although large numbers of cells are important for some tests, such as RNA extraction, it is generally accepted that diagnoses can be made on smears containing fewer than 100 cells. Specific evaluation of diagnostic adequacy in 25-G needle aspirations showed that 92% of 26 image-guided pulmonary aspirations performed with a 25-G needle were adequate, with a definitive diagnosis in 88% of cases, based on quick staining of material at the time of the aspiration alone.[22]

A smaller needle size decreases potential complications such as bleeding into the tissue, and hemodilution or obscuring of the cytology sample by excessive blood.[22] Smaller needles also cause less tissue damage, and thus possibly less risk of pancreatitis.

Given the trade-off between more cells but more complications with larger fine needles, the choice of needle size should be based on the site and type of lesion to be aspirated. Indications for a smaller needle (e.g., 25 G) include patients with coagulopathy, organs where leakage of fluid or air may occur, organs where tissue trauma may increase complications (pancreas), and vascular organs or lesions. Lesions for which there is less risk of complication, or for which large numbers of cells are required for classification such as lymphomas, can be approached with a larger needle, such as 22 G.[22]

Use of heparin

One of the technical problems encountered with fine-needle biopsies is clotting of blood and material within the needle. Clotting is a particular problem in EUS-FNA, given the extreme length of the needle. Clotting may be particularily troublesome with 25-G needles. Cells bound up in a fibrin or red cell clot may be trapped in the needle and, if expelled, cannot be thinly dispersed onto a slide – and thus are unavailable for viewing. Clotting may also lead to artifactual groupings of cells. Two techniques may circumvent this problem. Often practiced but little documented in the cytology literature is the use of heparin in the needle.[23] Ideally, the heparin forms a thin coat on the luminal surface of the needle and does not fill the needle lumen. Its purpose is to 'lubricate' the needle lumen so that material does not stick to the wall, and to reduce blood clotting within the needle. However, too much heparin in the needle is problematic, because excessive heparin can alter cell features, create artifacts, and dilute the specimen. Ideally, the heparin is aspirated into the needle and the needle then flushed with air.

A less desirable, but useful, salvage of material is gentle microdissection of the clot or fragment with a small scalpel blade or separate needle tip. The fragments are then lifted from the slide and placed in formalin for subsequent cell block preparation. Forceful smearing of the clot to disperse the cells may cause significant crush artifact and render the cells uninterpretable.

Use of suction

For many fine-needle biopsies, suction is applied to the needle to attempt to increase cell yield. This is the origin of the term 'fine-needle aspirate', which is often used more generally for any fine-needle biopsy. The purpose of suction is not to draw the cells into the needle, but to 'hold' the tissue against the cutting edge of the needle.[24] Suction is turned off before withdrawing the needle. This is done to prevent drying artifact of the cells caused by the rush of air into the needle as it is withdrawn, and to prevent the material from passing into the syringe, from which it is difficult to remove. Theoretically, release of suction before withdrawing the needle also prevents contamination of the needle track with tumor cells. (Although needle track seeding from FNA has been reported, the incidence is very low, and may be less in EUS than for percutaneous biopsies.[25,26])

If suction is not applied to the needle, the lumen is filled with cells by the direct force of the needle through the tissue and/or capillary action. In a large group of fine-needle biopsies of the breast, similar diagnostic results were obtained with or without suction.[27] A study of 670 superficial and deep lesions biopsied with a fine needle without suction showed that diagnostic material was obtained in more than 90% of cases.[28] A study of image-guided fine-needle biopsies of 50 intra-abdominal sites, including liver, adrenal, retroperitoneum, and pancreas found no difference in aspiration and non-aspiration techniques in regard to numbers of cells, amount of blood, or artifact; however, aspiration biopsies had a higher positive predictive value.[29] In another study, however, capillary biopsy (without suction) performed poorly for pancreatic fine-needle biopsies.[30] Material obtained without suction may result in higher-quality preparations with better preservation of cytologic fine detail and less artifact.[31,32] However, fewer insufficient specimens are generated when suction is used and smaller (higher gauge) and longer needles yield less material without suction.[33,34]

Specific to EUS-FNA, a study by Wallace et al.[35] found no difference in suction versus no suction in terms of overall diagnostic yield for lymph nodes, but noted excess blood in the specimens to which suction was applied.

In general, applying suction to the needle increases cellular yield but potentially increases artifact and blood, especially in vascular organs or lesions. Suction is commonly used, however, because the increased cellular yield of specimens often outweighs the disadvantages. Some attempt up to three passes without suction, adding further passes with suction if the cellular yield is low.

Number of passes

A 'pass' is the placement of the needle into the lesion. For EUS this constitutes penetrating the lesion and then moving the needle back and forth throughout the lesion. A pass usually comprises ten or more needle excursions, or movement of the needle to and fro once it is within the lesion. The number of passes needed to obtain diagnostic material depends on the quality of the pass, cellularity of the lesion, type of lesion, and risk of complications. More passes into a lesion increases diagnostic yield to a certain degree. The general FNA literature advocates two to three passes, with diminishing returns after three passes; however, some EUS-specific studies recommend more.

In studies that specifically address EUS-FNA, the optimal number of passes needed again varies by site, type of lesion, and institution. For example, LeBlanc et al.[36] determined that at least seven passes were needed in pancreatic lesions to obtain a sensitivity and specificity of 83% and 100%, respectively, although only five passes were needed in lymph node aspirates for a sensitivity and specificity of 77% and 100%. Wallace et al.[35] deemed two to three passes sufficient for mediastinal lymph nodes. In a retrospective study of transesophageal FNA,[37] diagnostic cells were present in the first pass in 42% of cases, and in the second pass in 58%. Four passes would have produced a diagnosis in 95% of cases, and all cases were diagnostic by the sixth pass.[37] Klapman et al.[38] reported one to seven passes per procedure when immediate cytologic evaluation was used.

In a study in which a cytopathologist was present at the time of the FNA, Erickson et al.[39] demonstrated that only tumor site and differentiation influenced the number of passes. The retrospective transesophageal study discussed above reached a similar diagnosis-specific conclusion, with benign diagnoses requiring more passes than malignant ones.[37]

Directed passes

A well known advantage of image-guided biopsies, especially EUS, is the ability to direct the needle to a small point of interest.[40] Selection of the exact site of biopsy may influence the cytologic yield. Biopsy of the necrotic center of a tumor may be non-diagnostic, whereas the edge may contain viable tumor cells. Conversely, biopsy of the edge of a pancreatic carcinoma may show only chronic pancreatitis, a common reactive change in the surrounding pancreatic tissue.

Depending on the anatomic site, directing the needle to specific portions of the lesion may not always be advantageous. Metastatic tumor in lymph nodes may be histologically more apparent in the subcapsular sinus, but in 46 lymph node aspirates evaluated by EUS-FNA, aspiration at the edge of the node did not increase the likelihood of a correct diagnosis.[35] Nonetheless, as EUS allows visualization of the lesion, biopsy of a necrotic area can be avoided and, as discussed below, on-site evaluation of the specimen can provide guidance to another location if the first is necrotic.

A chief advantage of the FNA technique is the wide sampling of a lesion by directing the needle in different directions with each to and fro movement. Small redirections of the needle to make a fan shape result in sampling of new areas of the lesion each time. Repeated needle excursions in the same direction, along the same needle track, result in biopsy of the blood or fluid that fills the needle track space, rather than more sampling of the lesion.

FACTORS ASSOCIATED WITH IMPROVED CYTOLOGIC PREPARATION

The material from an EUS-guided biopsy can be prepared in many different ways, each of which has advantages and disadvantages. A number of the preparations are complementary, and two or three are often prepared from the same biopsy. The following sections define preparation of air-dried and alcohol-fixed smears, cell block, and the stains used for highlighting various cell features.

Cytology smears or histology cell block

A smear slide is the standard method of preparing cells obtained from a fine-needle biopsy for viewing. Like a blood smear, the biopsy material is dispersed or 'smeared' onto a glass slide, stained, and viewed as individual cells. For EUS-FNA, after the needle is removed from the endoscope, the tip is placed near the frosted end of a labeled slide, and a single small drop expressed onto the slide by slowly advancing the stylet into the needle. Dropping the material from a distance, squirting, or spraying it onto the slide can result in drying of the specimen and unwanted artifact. A second slide is then drawn over the drop of material, pulling the material into a monolayer. The technique requires practice. When the smear is too thick, the cells are obscured by one another or by background cells; if too much pressure is applied, the cells are artificially disrupted from their normal microarchitecture or are lysed. Imperfect smears may reduce diagnostic yield.

In contrast to smears, a cell block is a preparation in which the cells are placed into a liquid medium or fixative, transported to the laboratory, spun into a pellet, formalin fixed, paraffin embedded, and sectioned for standard hematoxylin and eosin (H&E) staining.[41] This routine formalin fixation and paraffin embedding is not optimal for preserving cytologic detail[42] and, although convenient and familiar to pathologists, cell block preparation of FNA material is limited as a primary or stand-alone preparation. A cell block is often made from leftover material rinsed from the needle, and this too is of value only as an adjunct to the smears.[43] Material aliquoted for cell block cannot be assessed for adequacy at the time of the procedure.

However, intentionally placing representative biopsy material from the needle into fixative for cell block or procuring additional passes for cell block is highly recommended for lesions that may require special stains.

One means of assuring representative diagnostic material on the smears and cell block is to alternate drops of material between the slides for smears and the fixative or medium for cell block. Once four to six slides have been prepared, the remaining material can be rinsed from the needle to add to the cell block. Special studies, such as immunoperoxidase staining, can be performed on the sections from the block.[44]

Overall, cell block should be considered complementary to the smears and useful for defining or classifying lesions, rather than a primary diagnostic preparation.

Air-dried or alcohol-fixed smears

Two types of smear can be prepared from FNA material: air dried and alcohol fixed. After the cells are smeared onto the slides, they are either left to dry in air or fixed immediately in alcohol, by either immersion or spray. Air-dried smears are stained rapidly (using a modified Romanowsky stain, for example Diff-Quik™) and typically used for immediate cytologic evaluation. The cells spread out as they dry, and the result is an exaggeration of pleomorphism if present. Diff-Quik™-stained, air-dried smear preparations highlight intracytoplasmic material and extracellular substances. The Diff-Quik™ stain is similar to those used for bone marrow aspirates and blood smears, a feature helpful when evaluating lymph node aspirates.

Alcohol fixation causes cells to shrink and round up, but preserves nuclear features and is followed by Papanicolau (Pap) or H&E stains. The Pap stain highlights nuclear detail and chromatin quality, as well as demonstrating keratinization of squamous cells. The cytoplasm appears more transparent in Pap-stained slides. Slides can be fixed in preparation for a Pap stain by immersing or spraying them with alcohol. Some cells may be lost into the fixative when the smears are fixed by immersion into the alcohol; however, spray fixation is more time consuming and inconsistent, leading to artifacts.[45]

The Pap and Diff-Quik™ stains are complementary, and optimal cytologic detail is provided when both alcohol-fixed and air-dried smears are prepared from the FNA (Fig. 23.1).

Liquid-based preparations

Liquid-based cytology is a relatively new procedure in which the sample is placed into a proprietary fixative and slides are prepared by an automated process designed to minimize the technical problems associated with manual preparation of smears. There are currently two Food and Drug Administration-approved methods: ThinPrep (Cytyc Co., Marlborough, MA, USA) and SurePath (TriPath Inc., Burlington, NC, USA). There are slight differences between the two methodologies,[46] but the advantages of both include highly consistent cell preservation and a uniform monolayer dispersion of cells into a confined area of the slide. This decreases technical problems due to poor fixation, poor smear technique, air drying, and interpretive problems caused by cell overlap. There is an increase in the overall cellularity and quantity of diagnostic material on the slide.[47] In addition, the smaller area in which the cells are placed decreases the amount of time required to screen the slides for diagnostic cells.

Liquid-based fixatives may allow optimal preservation of cells when quality preparation of smears is not possible.[48] Liquid-based preparations are becoming a method of choice for cervical (Pap) smears.[49] Disadvantages include increased cost and, specifically for FNA procedures, inability to provide immediate cytologic assessment (ICE) at the time of the procedure (unless the sample is split). Interpretive disadvantages include disaggregation of cells (loss of architecture) and alteration of some cytologic details. Although decreased background is an advantage of the procedure for most applications, the loss of a mucinous background may be problematic for aspirations of cystic pancreatic lesions, where identification of mucin is an important diagnostic clue. Some of the proprietary liquid fixatives contain methanol, a coagulative fixative (rather than a protein cross-linking fixative such as formalin), which may lead to suboptimal fixation for immunohistochemistry.

de Luna et al.[50] compared conventional preparations with liquid-based preparations for 67 pancreatic EUS-FNAs. Specimens were split, so that conventional smears were prepared first, and the remainder of the material was expressed into the vial of fixative. Although the conventional smears were significantly better by 'diagnostic index', the study demonstrated proof of principle for this application of liquid-based cytology. Future studies of 'direct to vial' preparations (in which the entire specimen is placed in the vial) compared with conventional smears may provide a more definitive comparison.

The above study also illustrates the alterations in cytologic features typical of liquid-based preparations. The pancreatic

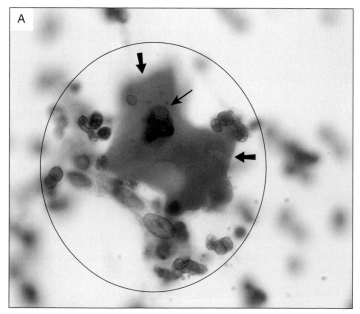
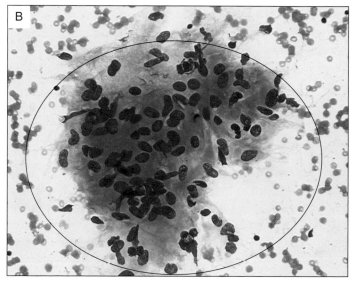

Fig. 23.1 Comparison of alcohol-fixed, Papanicolaou-stained cells with air-dried Diff-Quik™-stained cells. **A,** Papanicolaou stain provides clear detail of the markedly irregular nuclear membrane (thin arrow) and keratinization of the cytoplasm of this malignant squamous cell (thick arrow) (transduodenal aspirate of pancreatic adenosquamous carcinoma). **B,** Diff-Quik™ stain demonstrates uniformity of nuclei and abundant granular cytoplasm of benign histiocytes in a granulomatous lymph node (transesophageal aspirate of enlarged mediastinal nodes).

aspirates had smaller cell clusters and more single cells, more prominent and conspicuous nucleoli, and diminished or absent mucin.

Given the smalll number of studies of liquid-based EUS-FNA samples, more data are required to assess fully the relative merits of this methodology. However, the ability to fix cells immediately and optimally in real time during an FNA procedure may make it advantageous for endoscopists who do not have access to technical help.

A detailed model of an optimized EUS-FNA procedure is given in Table 23.3.

Cytology interpretation

Evaluation of the biopsy begins the moment material is expressed from the needle onto a slide or into fixative. A 'good' aspirate, or one that is likely to yield a diagnosis, is cellular, so that when placed on the slides and smeared out a finely granular quality is apparent, in contrast to a hypocellular or

OPTIMIZED EUS-FNA MODEL TECHNIQUE	
Stage	**Description**
Preparation	When the procedure is scheduled, arrangements are made for the cytology technician and pathologist to be at the site. Clinical findings are discussed with the pathologist at the start of the procedure. The locations of the lesions or other details are noted on previous imaging studies. Conscious sedation is provided to the patient with intravenous meperidine and midazolam.
Needle preparation	The stylet is removed completely from a 22-G EUS-FNA needle and the needle flushed with heparin. Air is then flushed through the needle to expel the excess heparin. The stylet is replaced and the needle is ready for use. Needle preparation and heparin flush should be performed before every pass. The needle may also be straightened manually between passes if necessary.
Radial EUS	A radial echoendoscope is first used for an overview of appropriate anatomic landmarks. The location of lesions are noted.
Linear-array EUS-FNA	The radial echoendoscope is replaced with a linear-array echoendoscope. The scope is advanced to the distance at which the lesion of interest was identified with radial endosonography. The lesion is visualized, and color Doppler used if there is concern about intervening blood vessels. The EUS-FNA needle is inserted and fastened to the biopsy channel of the echoendoscope, and then advanced just slightly beyond the scope into the gut lumen. At this point, the stylet is retracted about 1 cm. The needle is passed into the lesion. The stylet is replaced into the needle to expel any tissue from normal structures and then removed completely and a suction syringe attached. Sampling is performed with and without suction. The needle is moved into various locations throughout the lesion ('fanning the lesion') in order to improve sampling. After approximately 20 back and forth movements, the suction is turned off, the needle retracted back into the catheter, and the entire assembly removed.
Expressing material on slide	A dedicated cytology technician holds the end of the catheter over a labeled glass slide. The needle is advanced approximately 1 cm from the catheter by the endoscopy technician, and the stylet slowly advanced back into the needle. This produces a controlled passage of drops of material out from the tip. The cytology technician alternately places drops onto a slide and into RPMI-1640 medium. Finally, the needle is flushed with a few milliliters of saline and then air to expel any remaining material into the RPMI. RPMI-1640 is a cell culture transport medium used to preserve the cells until they are made into a cell block or sent for flow cytometry or other special study.
Preparing and staining cytologic material	Up to six slides are prepared depending on the amount of material. As rapidly as possible, the drops of aspirated material are spread downward onto the slides using another clean glass slide. Half of the slides are air dried and the remainder immediately immersed in 95% ethyl alcohol for later Papanicolaou staining. The air-dried slides are stained with a Diff-Quik™ stain for immediate cytologic evaluation by the pathologist (see below). When the procedure is finished, the material in RPMI-1640 is transported to the laboratory and a cell block prepared. The material in RPMI cell suspension is centrifuged into a pellet, to which thrombin is added. The pellet is resuspended and the resulting clot removed, wrapped in lens paper, placed in a tissue cassette, fixed in formalin, and routinely processed for paraffin embedding and H&E or immunostaining. If indicated, material for flow cytometric immunophenotyping or other studies is removed from the RPMI before the cell block is prepared. The alcohol-fixed slides are stained with a standard Papanicolau stain.
Immediate cytologic evaluation	A pathologist microscopically examines the air-dried Diff-Quik™-stained slides prepared at the site. The purpose of the immediate cytologic evaluation is to determine adequacy and triage the specimen for special studies. A preliminary diagnosis is often provided. If the lesion shows granulomas or infection is suspected, material is sent for culture; if atypical lymphoid cells are present, material is set for flow, etc. More material from a pass or entire additional passes can be directed to the RPMI if warranted.
Total time	Most cases for EUS-FNA in the authors' unit involve between three to six FNA passes. It takes 1 h for the complete examination and all cytologic evaluation.

Table 23.3 Optimized EUS-FNA model technique

purely bloody smear in which the thin sheen of material is smooth (Fig. 23.2). When placed in fixative, visible particulate matter or cloudiness is usually present. Mucus, pus, and necrosis may also be apparent grossly.

Adequacy

Once under the microscope, the smear is first assessed for adequacy. For an aspirate to be interpretable, it must be free of technical artifacts and contain cells for evaluation. A global assessment of cellularity as a measure of adequacy, however, may be misleading in FNA, as the number of cells relates to the lesion. For example, aspiration of neuroendocrine tumors usually yields highly cellular smears, whereas aspiration of a gastrointestinal stromal tumor (GIST) may yield few cells, but be equally as adequate for diagnosis.

Adequacy criteria for screening cytology tests, such as the cervical (Pap) smear, include documentation of the number and type of each cell and the presence of limiting factors such as excessive blood, inflammation, or air drying. These criteria are codified in the well known Bethesda System.[51]

For diagnostic, non-gynecologic cytology specimens, a sample is adequate when it explains the clinical scenario or lesion. The issue of adequacy has been discussed for other types of FNA, such as breast FNAs, and this literature provides some relevance for EUS. In 1997, the National Cancer Institute issued guidelines entitled 'The Uniform Approach to Breast Fine-Needle Aspiration Biopsy'. These guidelines state that an adequate specimen is one that leads to the resolution of a problem presented by a lesion in a particular patient.[52,53] The aspirator must be certain that the lesion has been sampled and the pathologist must be able to interpret the slides. The concept of the 'triple test' is applicable to EUS-FNA. The clinical, imaging, and FNA findings should agree and correlate on whether the lesion is benign or malignant.[54] A malignant cytologic finding should be further investigated in the face of low clinical suspicion; a clinically suspicious mass should be rebiopsied regardless of an initial benign aspirate.

A problematic area in EUS-FNA is definitive benign diagnoses in transesophageal aspirates of mediastinal nodes for lymphadenopathy in the absence of a lung mass. Identification of benign lymph node elements is necessary, but there are no guidelines regarding quantity or types of cells that guarantee benignity. Some advocate a requirement for a certain number or type of cells to be applied to aspirates with non-specific findings.[52] When immediate cytologic evaluation is used, pathologists request more passes when only benign material is identified.[37] EUS-FNA of chronic pancreatitis may pose a similar problem.[55,56]

Benign tumors such as granular cell tumors or granulomatous inflammation are exceptions, as these have easily identifiable specific cytologic features.

Immediate cytologic evaluation

One way to ensure adequate material from a FNA procedure is the use of immediate cytologic evaluation (ICE).[38,57,58] The goal of ICE is to provide real-time feedback about the content and quality of the smears, in order to reduce the number of non-diagnostic or atypical biopsies and maximize the efficiency of the procedure.[39] ICE also yields a highly reliable preliminary diagnosis.[58] In a direct comparison of EUS-FNA procedures performed by the same endoscopist at two institutions, with and without a pathologist present at the procedure, ICE was more likely to result in a definitive diagnosis and less likely to involve an inadequate specimen.[38] Most false-negative EUS procedures are due to inadequate sampling, which may necessitate a second procedure.[11,54,59,60] The most effective way to reduce sampling error is by ICE.[58]

Although ICE clearly improves diagnostic yield, this practice is variable in the USA and is not common in Europe. The

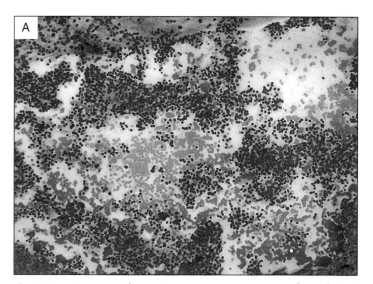
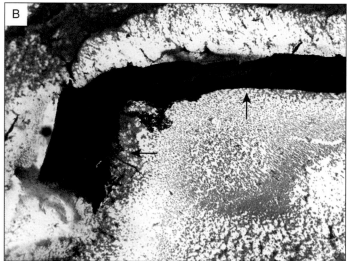

Fig. 23.2 Smear quality. **A,** Low-power assessment of a technically good smear reveals numerous cells spread thinly over the slide (transduodenal aspirate of a pancreatic neuroendocrine tumor). **B,** Poor quality smears are hypocellular, too thick, or marred by blood clots (arrows), which obscure the cells.

practice of ICE is influenced by the physical locations of the laboratory and GI suite, personnel, and cost issues. Reluctance of a pathologist to attend EUS-FNA procedures may relate to inadequate reimbursement for the time investment required.[61] The institution, however, may realize significant cost savings by reducing the number of procedures that need to be repeated because of an inadequate specimen.[57]

When ICE is performed, selected air-dried slides are stained in the endoscopy suite or an adjacent room and reviewed immediately by a pathologist, so that feedback can be given to the endoscopist regarding the adequacy of the pass. If diagnostic material is present, no additional passes are made and the procedure is stopped. If the smears are non-diagnostic, further passes are made. If there are no cells or only necrosis, the needle can be redirected for the next pass and the procedure continued until adequate material for diagnosis is obtained. Consequently, ICE results in a wide range in the number of passes per procedure.[38]

In addition to minimizing the number of passes needed to obtain diagnostic material, another advantage of ICE is the triage of specimens for special studies. Additional passes can be made for flow cytometry when the initial smears favor lymphoma,[62] for culture when the initial smears show granulomas or an abscess, or for cell block when the initial smears show a tumor that may need classification by immunohistochemistry, in situ hybridization, or other studies.

Compromise procedures can be developed to gain the advantages of ICE with less time investment. A cytotechnologist could replace the pathologist for the initial screening of adequacy (but not diagnosis), 'runners' could be used to carry the slides to the pathology laboratory for evaluation, or the pathologist could be called only once several passes are ready to be reviewed.

In institutions where ICE is not available, the initial assessment of the gross cellularity of the slides becomes important. The ability to recognize a 'good' slide may improve yield. However, a visual inspection of the slides for particulate matter alone does not ensure that the cells present represent the lesion. One study calculated how many procedures would be diagnostic if stopped after a gross estimation of moderate to high cellularity. When this estimate was applied to transesophageal aspirates of 73 mediastinal lymph nodes, diagnostic material would have been obtained from only 75% of the nodes sampled.[37]

Regardless of whether ICE is used or not, an adequate sample is the foundation of a diagnosis. The needle must be placed into the lesion, technical aspects of the sampling optimized to obtain cells for evaluation, and the smears free of crush, drying, staining, or other artifact and obscuring blood, inflammation, or necrosis.

Diagnostic evaluation of the slide

Whether on-site or in the laboratory, once the smear is deemed to be free of technical artifacts and to possess cells for evaluation, the cytotechnologist or pathologist begins the screening or diagnostic evaluation, respectively, by assessing the types, arrangement, and features of the cells on the smear. Central to a cytology diagnosis is the appearance of the nuclear and cytoplasmic features of individual cells; these are quite distinct, depending on the lesion sampled (Fig. 23.3).

No single feature is diagnostic of malignancy, but rather the composite picture of cell type, microarchitecture, and nuclear and cytoplasmic characteristics determines the diagnosis. It is useful to know the common pathologic diagnoses as well as the characteristic of the normal tissue in the region sampled (Table 23.4).

As in histologic sections, order and esthetics reign in cytologic preparations of benign tissue. The cell groups are regularly

COMMON EUS CYTOLOGIC DIAGNOSES IN SPECIFIC SITES

Site	Cytologic diagnoses
Mediastinum and mediastinal nodes	
Granulomatous disease	Sarcoid Tuberculosis Fungal infection (Coccidiodes immitis, Histoplasma capsulatum)
Lung cancer	Adenocarcinoma Squamous carcinoma Small cell carcinoma
Lymphoma	
Neurogenic tumors	Ganglioneuroma Gangliomeuroblastoma, peripheral nerve sheath tumors (schwannoma) Neurofibroma
Esophagus	Squamous carcinoma Adenocarcinoma Granular cell tumors Leiomyoma or other spindle cell tumor (GIST or neurofibroma)
Stomach	Carcinoid GIST Lymphoma
Pancreas	Ductal adenocarcinoma Intraductal papillary mucinous neoplasms (IPMNs) and cystic mucinous neoplasms Serous cystadenomas Neuroendocrine tumors Chronic pancreatitis Rare tumors: solid pseudpapillary tumor, pancreatoblastoma, acinar cell carcinoma, benign cysts, metastatic tumors
Rectum and perirectal lymph nodes	Metastatic adenocarcinoma or squamous carcinoma GIST
Liver	Metastatic carcinoma, melanoma, sarcoma Lymphoma Primary hepatocellular tumors

Table 23.4 Common EUS cytologic diagnoses in specific sites
GIST, gastrointestinal stromal tumor; IPMN, intraductal papillary mucinous neoplasm.

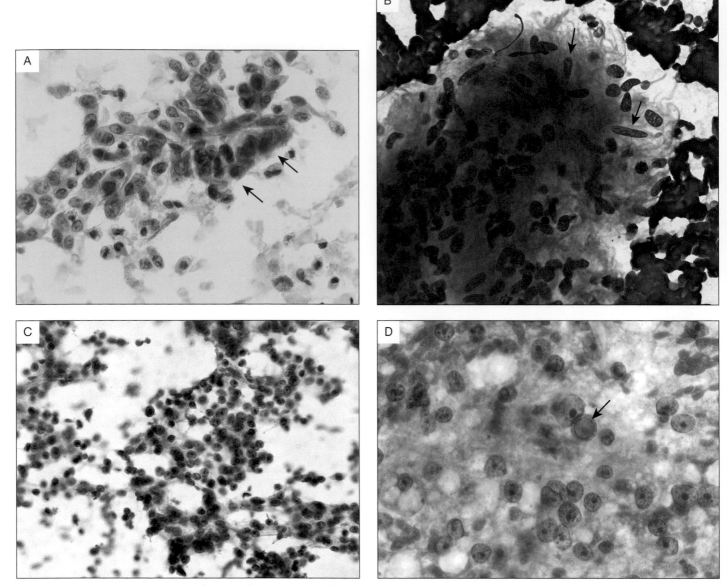

Fig. 23.3   Distinctive appearance of various lesions sampled by EUS-FNA: diagnostic cytologic features of a variety of neoplasms sampled by EUS-FNA. **A,** Adenocarcinoma is characterized by columnar cells with enlarged, overlapping, hyperchromatic nuclei (arrows) (transduodenal aspirate of a pancreatic head adenocarcinoma). **B,** Spindle cells with blunt end nuclei and abundant cytoplasm (arrows) are features of a gastrointestinal stromal tumor (transgastric aspirate of a submucosal nodule). **C,** Neuroendocrine tumors show a spectrum of changes. In this smear, there are relatively small cells with scant cytoplasm arranged in loosely cohesive groups (transgastric aspirate of a pancreatic tail mass). **D,** Dyshesive round cells with granular cytoplasm, prominent nucleoli, and intranuclear cytoplasmic inclusions (arrow) are consistent with a metastatic hepatocellular carcinoma (transesophageal aspirate of enlarged mediastinal lymph node).

arranged and similar in size, shape, and overall appearance, and have bland nuclei (Fig. 23.4). The appearance and composition of a benign aspirate reflects the various cell populations in normal tissue. Epithelial cells are round to oval, have moderate to abundant cytoplasm, and are cohesive. Benign epithelial cells show evidence of differentiation. Squamous cells acquire keratin as they mature, whereas their nuclei become progressively smaller and darker (pyknotic). A benign superficial squamous cell exfoliated from the esophagus has a large polyhedral shape, with a small, uniformly dark, nucleus described as an 'ink dot'.[63–66] The cytoplasm is orange–pink to blue, depending on the degree of keratin accumulation. Benign, mature squamous cells appear singly, unless they are from the deeper layers of the epithelium, in which case they may remain together as large sheets of cells with less keratinization of the cytoplasm. Benign glandular epithelium from the stomach, intestine, and pancreas also demonstrates an orderly arrangement of differentiated cells with organ-specific variations. In smears, duodenal epithelium consists of folded or draped sheets of columnar cells, with interspersed goblet cells appearing as clear spaces amongst the absorptive cells. Glandular cells are polarized, with the nucleus present at one end of each cell in

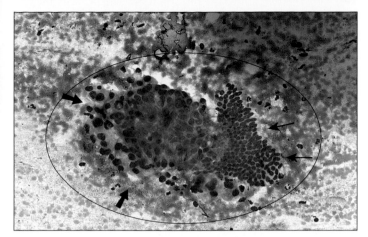

Fig. 23.4   Arrangement of benign and malignant ductal cells. Benign ductal epithelium is composed of small uniform cells arranged in regularly ordered rows (thin arrows), in contrast to the enlarged, disorganized sheet of cells in the adjacent malignant epithelium (thick arrows) (transduodenal aspirate of pancreatic head adenocarcinoma).

the sheet of epithelium. The cytoplasm may be filled with a single mucin droplet (the goblet cell), smaller more finely divided vacuoles, or other secretory products such as zymogen granules. Classically, benign columnar epithelium has a honeycomb pattern. Changing the microscopic plane of focus reveals the hexagonal borders of the apical cytoplasm and polarized, orderly nuclei at the base of the honeycomb sheet. In contrast, benign stromal or mesenchymal cells have elongate nuclei and usually abundant cytoplasm. Fat appears as large round, clear cells with thin, crescent-shaped nuclei pushed to one side. Occasionally, small vascular structures are visible in smears of benign tissue.

The cells represented in an aspirate of normal tissue are proportionate to their mixture in the organ. For example, benign pancreatic tissue is composed mostly of acini, with relatively few ductal structures and islets, a histologic fact that should be represented on FNA smears. In contrast, a smear from pancreatic ductal adenocarcinoma consists almost exclusively of ductal cells with few or no acinar structures present. A benign reactive lymph node contains a polymorphic mixture of cell types, with large and small lymphocytes, macrophages, and sometimes identifiable germinal centers, whereas a lymphoid malignancy is usually monomorphic.

In EUS procedures, because the needle passes through normal tissues it is common to find benign 'contaminants' in the smears (Fig. 23.5). Benign, mature squamous cells are frequently identified in transesophageal lymph node aspirates, and sheets of duodenal or gastric cells in a pancreatic FNA. This occasionally becomes an interpretive problem, but attention to strict diagnostic criteria and correlation with clinical findings may resolve the issue.

In contrast to the order inherent in benign tissue, malignant cells deviate in their organization, cell–cell attachments (cohesion), and microarchitecture.

Normal epithelial cells exhibit cohesion. Malignant epithelial cells are loosely aggregated or single cells. The degree of dyshesion is relative and an important criterion in the overall assessment of malignancy (Fig. 23.6). Dyshesion in a well differentiated carcinoma may be subtle, with fraying of the edges of the cell groups and only occasional single cells, whereas cells from poorly differentiated carcinomas may dissociate completely. Epithelial cohesion explains the reluctance of some benign lesions to yield cells when aspirated. Some tissue types are normally dyshesive. FNA of lymphoid tissue demonstrates unattached single cells widely scattered over the smear, but benign nodes are composed of mostly small and maturing lymphocytes and may have aggregation of cells in follicles or germinal centers with debris containing (tangible body) macrophages. Although both are dyshesive, the polymorphous features of a benign node will not be apparent in monomorphic aspirates of lymphoma. Of note, an overzealous smearing technique may artifactually separate cells and lead to overestimation of dyshesion.

Malignant cells also exhibit disorganization of their normal arrangement or polarity. The loss of polarity is a particular diagnostic feature in lesions arising in columnar epithelium. An important EUS-FNA example is the diagnosis of atypia or malignancy in mucinous neoplasms of the pancreas. Loss of polarity in a mucinous tumor is popularly described as a 'drunken' honeycomb, and this disorganization is a typical feature of well differentiated mucinous tumors.

Once the low-power assessment of the general characteristic of the smear has been evaluated for cell types, overall organization, and cohesion, detailed analysis of the nucleus and cytoplasm allows characterization of a cell as benign or malignant. Specific nuclear features determine malignancy, whereas cytoplasmic features and microarchitecture demonstrate differentiation of the cell.

Nuclear features

Nuclear features include relative and absolute size of the nucleus, nuclear shape and contour, quantity and quality of chromatin, and the presence or number of nucleoli (Fig. 23.7). Nuclei inadvertently removed from their cytoplasm by the process of aspiration or smearing the cells may show marked abnormalities and be misleading. These so-called 'naked nuclei' should not be interpreted, although the presence of markedly atypical bare nuclei warrants further sampling of a lesion.

Nuclear size is determined by comparing the nucleus to cells or nuclei of known size. On fixed slides, a red cell is approximately 7 µm, a neutrophil 10–14 µm, and a macrophage or endothelial cell nucleus 15–20 µm. Normal or reactive nuclei may enlarge but have a concomitant increase in their cytoplasm or a preserved nucleus to cytoplasm (N/C) ratio. Tumor cell nuclei may be markedly enlarged. Giant tumor cells, known as tombstone cells, are a characteristic finding in some pancreatic carcinomas, where occasional nuclei may be ten times larger than those in the surrounding cells.

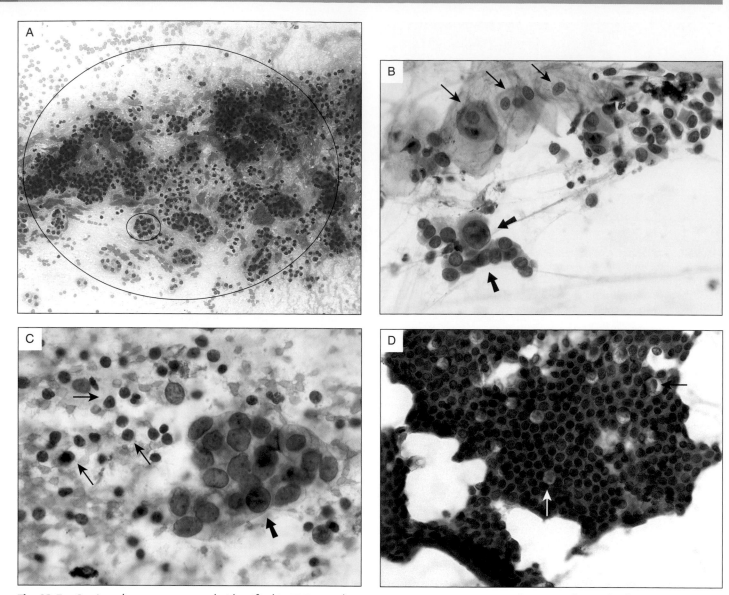

Fig. 23.5 Benign elements commonly identified in EUS samples. **A,** Benign pancreatic acinar cells are small round cells with abundant granular cytoplasm arranged in small, uniform acini (small circle) (transduodenal aspirate). **B,** Benign esophageal squamous cells are polyhedral and have abundant cytoplasm with small, uniform nuclei (thin arrows), in contrast to the adjacent cells from a non-small cell carcinoma (thick arrows) (transesophageal aspirate of mediastinal lymph nodes in a patient with non-small cell lung cancer). **C,** Benign lymph node elements (thin arrows) indicated that this sample was from a lymph node. The large cells with irregular nuclear borders and scant cytoplasm (thick arrow) represent an adenocarcinoma from a lung primary (transesophageal aspirate of mediastinal lymph nodes). **D,** Benign sheet of duodenal epithelium showing absorptive cells with interspersed goblet cells (arrows) (transduodenal aspirate).

Variation in the size of the nucleus from cell to cell within a group of similar-type cells (anisonucleosis) is also an important feature of malignancy. This finding is particularly important in pancreatic and bile duct lesions.[10]

Nuclear membrane contour or shape has been colorfully described as cemetery flowers, cat's claws, bud-like, shark's teeth, or popcorn.[2] The shape of the nucleus of a malignant cell may be irregular with sharp creases or indentations, whereas a benign nucleus should be round or oval, regular, and free of indentations. Chromatin may aggregate thickly on the inner surface of the nuclear membrane, adding to its irregular appearance.

Chromasia is a feature of cytologic evaluation that reflects the amount and distribution of DNA and DNA-related proteins, or chromatin. The dyes used to color the cells stain the nuclear material in direct proportion to the amount present, so the more DNA and associated protein, the darker the color of the nucleus. Hyperchromasia (increased color) reflects an increase in the amount of chromatin in the nucleus of the cell.

The structure of chromatin is best seen in alcohol-fixed, Pap-stained smears. Heterochromatin is inactive and appears as clumps or condensations, whereas euchromatin is pale and represents areas of active RNA synthesis. Normal cells have an even distribution of euchromatin and heterochromatin, and so

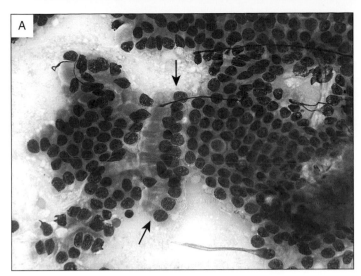
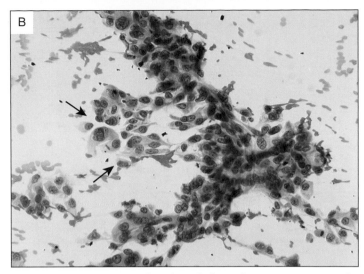

Fig. 23.6   Cohesive benign epithelium versus dyshesive group in adenocarcinoma. **A,** Benign ductal epithelium demonstrates a regular arrangement of polarized cells (arrows) that are tightly cohesive. **B,** In constrast, ductal adenocarcinoma cells are loosely aggregated or dyshesive, with clearly visible spaces between cells, fraying of the cells from the sheet at the edge, and some single cells (arrows). (Both cases represent transduodenal aspirates of the pancreas.)

have light and dark areas, with the dark heterochromatin evenly divided among the quadrants of the nucleus and clumping mainly around the nuclear membrane. In malignant cells, the chromatin is irregularly clumped and distributed. Chromocenters are larger aggregates of heterochromatin that must be distinguished from nucleoli. Degenerating nuclei may be quite hyperchromatic, but are small and have indistinct chromatin.[8]

The cell's nucleolus represents RNA accumulation. Nucleoli are present in benign, reactive, and malignant cells. The differences between nucleoli in benign and malignant cells are relative, but variably sized, multiple, or irregular nucleoli are signs of malignancy. A nucleolus with sharp edges is almost never benign, nor is a very large (macro) nucleolus. Some tumors, such as breast and prostate cancer, have characteristic marked nucleolar enlargement.

Mitotic figures may be seen in both benign and malignant epithelium, but highly abnormal mitotic figures, such as tripolar mitoses or those that clearly have more than 46 chromosomes or abnormal mitotic spindles, are indicative of aneuploidy and malignancy. For some tumors, such as GIST and sarcoma, assessment of a mitotic rate is useful in predicting clinical outcome. As the cells in a smear are variably thick, a standardized mitotic count cannot be performed; however, markers such as Ki-67 (Mib1) can demonstrate a relative proliferative index.

Other nuclear details that may be observed in cytologic preparations include intranuclear cytoplasmic inclusions. Intranuclear inclusions are clear, round, well defined spaces within the nucleus, and are characteristic features of some malignancies such as malignant melanoma.

Cytoplasmic differentiation

The cytoplasm of the cell reflects its differentiation (Fig. 23.8). Malignant cells have less cytoplasmic volume in relation to nuclear size (higher N/C ratio), and may have eccentric placement of the nucleus. Malignant squamous cells have keratinized cytoplasm which appears hyaline or somewhat refractile and is orangeophilic on Pap-stained smears. There is often a sharp or hard edge to the cytoplasm. Some malignant squamous cells develop an exaggerated 'tadpole' shape. In contrast, the cytoplasm from an adenocarcinoma contains mucins that impart a slight foamy quality to the cytoplasm or may coalesce into discrete globules. The signet ring cell is a typical example of a well defined, round, intracytoplasmic mucin droplet that displaces the nucleus to one edge of the cell. In poorly differentiated tumors, special stains may be required to demonstrate cytoplasmic mucin. Cells included within the cytoplasm of another cell (cannibalism) are never normal. Occasionally, other inclusions or pigments may be noted in cytologic preparations. Melanin and iron pigment are fine granules within the cytoplasm. Melanin is often a dusky, powdery grey–brown, whereas hemosiderin occurs as larger, more refractile, and irregular golden brown pigment. Neuroendocrine granules are fine and may appear red (metachromatic) on Diff-Quik™ staining, but their presence is usually confirmed with a panel of immunostains, neuron-specific enolase, synaptophysin, and/or chromogranin.

Immunohistochemistry

Immunohistochemical stains are widely used for identification of cytoplasmic or nuclear differentiation. A monoclonal or polyclonal antibody binds to its specific epitope in the cell and

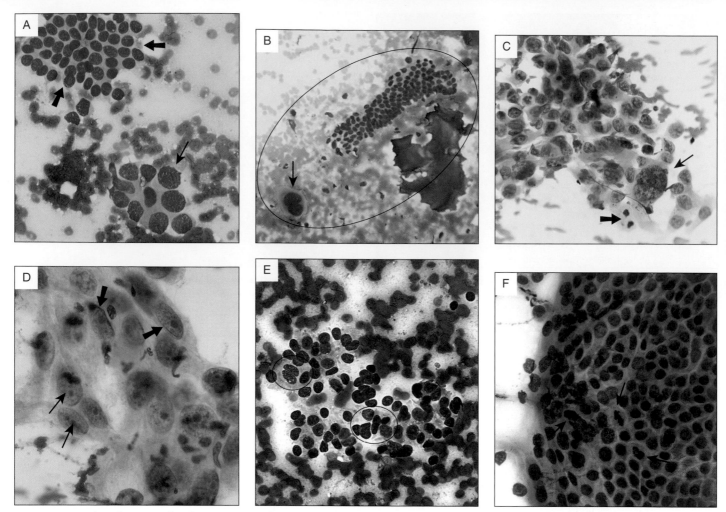

Fig. 23.7 Nuclear features of malignancy. **A,** Malignant nuclei (thin arrows) are enlarged compared with benign nuclei (thick arrows) (transduodenal aspirate of breast cancer metastatic to the pancreas). **B,** Marked nuclear enlargement (arrow) is characteristic of pancreatic ductal adenocarcinoma. Benign duct is on the right (transduodenal aspirate of a pancreatic head mass). **C,** Marked variation in nuclear size (thin arrow) as well as nuclear membrane irregularities, coarse chromatin, and a mitosis (thick arrow) are identifiable in this sheet of malignant cells from a pancreatic ductal carcinoma (transduodenal aspirate of a pancreatic head mass). **D,** Coarse chromatin, thickened nuclear membrane (thick arrows), and prominent nucleoli (thin arrows) are features of carcinoma (transesophageal aspirate of mediastinal lymph nodes). **E,** Nuclear molding (circles) is present in neuroendocrine tumors including carcinoids, islet cell tumors, small cell carcinoma, and others. Neuroendocrine tumors also may show rosette formations (transgastric aspirate of islet cell tumor). **F,** Increased mitotic rate may be seen in malignant tumors (arrows) (transduodenal aspirate of an ill defined pancreatic mass that showed more obvious malignant features in other passes).

is subsequently labeled with a chromogen. A panel of immuno-peroxidase stains can be used to identify a tumor type, characterize a lesion, or provide information used for prognosis or treatment. Immunoperoxidase stains are particularly useful in determining the cell type of poorly differentiated tumors and the primary site of metastatic lesions. Immunoperoxidase stains can be applied to fixed smears, although cell block material is usually more reliable. A limitation of performing special stains on smears is the variability in the number of tumor cells from slide to slide. The small number of smear slides per case also limits the number of stains that can be performed on direct smears. Sections from the cell block can be used with routine immunoperoxidase methodology for formalin-fixed, paraffin-embedded material and numerous slides made (Fig. 23.9).

Immunoperoxidase stains should almost always be used as a panel selected to yield pertinent positive and negative results. Although some immunostains are reasonably sensitive and specific, none is perfect. Poorly differentiated tumors frequently exhibit unusual staining patterns, and the type and length of fixation, antigen retrieval process, and other technical factors influence results. A comprehensive review is beyond the scope of this primer and for more introductory information about immunoperoxidase stains the reader is referred to basic textbooks of cytology or pathology. In-depth information can be found through web resources or specific texts.[64–66] Like cytologic features on routine stains, immunohistochemical stains must be interpreted in the context of the other clinical and pathologic findings.

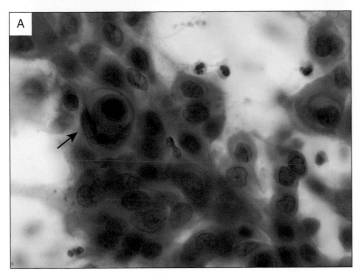

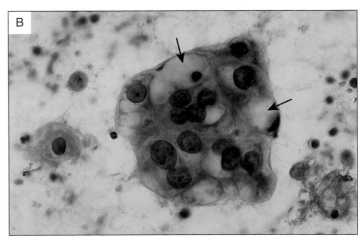

Fig. 23.8   Cytoplasmic evidence of differentiation. **A,** Papinocolaou stain of malignant cells reveals keratinization of the cells as well as a cell within a cell, characteristic of squamous cell carcinoma (arrow) (transesophageal aspirate of a mediastinal lymph node). **B,** Well formed mucin droplets (arrows) are present within a tightly cohesive group of cells, diagnostic of adenocarcinoma (transesophageal aspirate of a mediastinal mass).

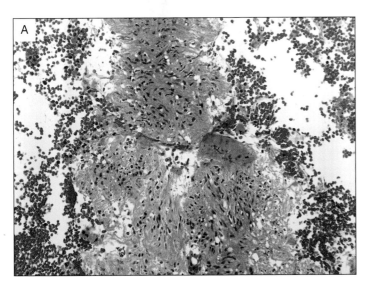

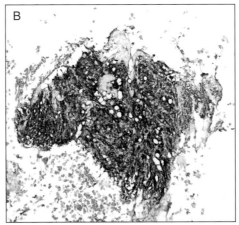

Fig. 23.9   Cell block preparation and immunoperoxidase stain. **A,** Characteristic cellular fragments of spindle cells are present in the cell block of a gastrointestinal stromal tumor (transgastric aspirate of a submucosal mass). **B,** Immunoperoxidase stain for CD177 (c-kit) shows strong staining of the tumor cells.

Microarchitecture

The microarchitecture of tumor cells yields clues as to the type of malignancy and its differentiation (Fig. 23.10). Carcinomas may form sheets, glands or acini, papillae, pseudopapillae, ducts, fragments, or pearls. Papillae are epithelial cells lining a true vascular core.

Acini are cells arranged in a ball around a lumen. Ducts are also luminal structures, but cylindrical rather than spherical. Molding is an arrangement of cells in which the contours of the nucleus and cytoplasm change to fit the contour of the next cell. Each of these patterns represents a diagnostic clue to the type of malignancy.

Frequently, the cells or extracellular material in the background of the slide form a context for interpretation (Fig. 23.11). Smear backgrounds may be bloody, necrotic, or inflammatory. Extracellular material may include necrosis, mucin, lipid, psammoma bodies, and calcifications. These changes are easily identifiable on conventional smears, but reduced in slides made from liquid-based preparations. Although mucolytic and hemolytic agents eliminate obscuring background material, they can also eliminate helpful background material such as mucin. Specific cytologic features of common types of malignancy are detailed in Table 23.5.

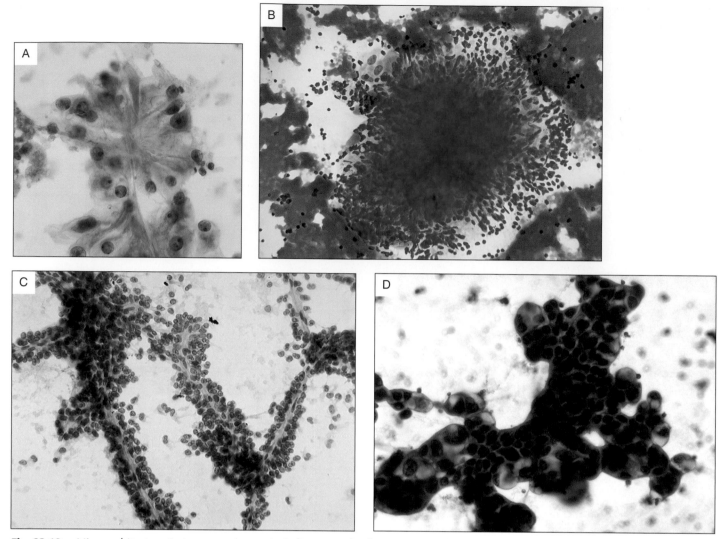

Fig. 23.10   Microarchitecture in tumor aspirates. **A,** Delicate renal cell carcinoma cells form a flower-like arrangement around a central point. **B,** Well organized palisading histiocytes form a granuloma. Scattered small lymphocytes are seen in the periphery. (**A & B,** Transesophageal aspirates of mediastinal lymph nodes.) **C,** Thin, fine, papillary fronds are characteristic of solid pseudopapillary tumors. **D,** Disorganized micropapillae are a structural characteristic of some intraductal papillary mucinous neoplasms. (**C & D,** Transduodenal aspirates of pancreatic masses.)

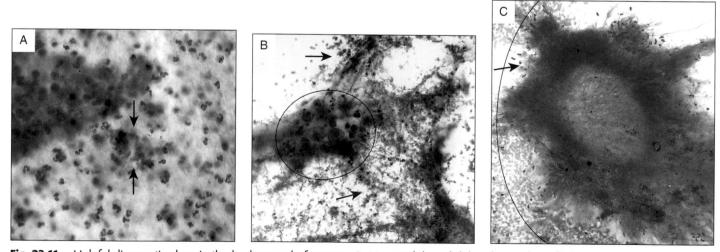

Fig. 23.11   Helpful diagnostic clues in the background of smears. **A,** Neutrophils and debris (arrows) are features in the background of inflammation or an abscess (transduodenal aspirate of liver lesion). **B,** Necrotic material (arrows) present in the background of a malignant mucinous tumor (circle) (transduodenal aspirate of a pancreatic mass). **C,** Abundant mucin (arrow) from a mucinous pancreatic neoplasm (transgastric aspirate of a cystic pancreatic lesion).

CYTOLOGIC FEATURES OF COMMON LESIONS

Lesion	Cytologic features	Comment
Granulomas	Epithelioid histiocytes arranged as sheets or in a palisade	May represent infectious disease (mycobacteria or fungi) or sarcoidosis
Benign or reactive lymph nodes	Mixture of cell types with lymphocytes in varying degrees of activation, plasma cells, histiocytes, or macrophages, which may contain phagocytic debris. These debris-containing cells correspond to the tingible body macrophages seen in germinal centers	Lymphoglandular bodies, small fragments of degenerating lymphoid cells may be seen in reactive or malignant nodes
Adenocarcinoma	Large cuboidal to columnar cells with high N/C ratios arranged in small, loose, three-dimensional clusters, sometimes forming acini or glands. Well differentiated pancreatic carcinoma may show subtle features of crowding or overlapping nuclei, irregular nuclear contour, irregular chromatin	Signet ring cells may mimick macrophages
Squamous cell carcinoma	Variably cellular aspirates with loose sheet-like arrangements of cells with defined cell borders and keratinized cytoplasm. Nuclei markedly pleomorphic. Papanicolaou stain is especially useful for demonstrating keratinization of the cytoplasm	Focal evidence of squamous differentiation is commonly found in others tumors, such as pancreatic adenocarcinoma
Small cell carcinoma	Very cellular but sometimes bloody smears composed of markedly atypical small malignant cells. Many single cells or small groups. Cells overlap, have indistinct borders, and exhibit the key feature of nuclear molding. Chromatin is coarse	Cells appear larger in air-dried preparations. Cells are also fragile and crush easily
Spindle cell lesions, benign	Variably cellular, composed of spindle cells with abundant cytoplasm. Differential diagnosis includes leiomyoma, GIST, neural tumors. Cytologic features of malignant lesions below.	Immunoperoxidase stains required for definitive identification of cells
GIST	Hypercellular; spindle cells arranged in groups	Diagnosis depends on identification of specific markers
Carcinoid	Uniform population of cells with moderate amount of cytoplasm; regular, even chromatin	
Spindle cell lesions, malignant	Sarcomas are cellular spindle cell lesions that may show fat, fibrous, myogenic, or neural differentiation, each of which has a corresponding cytologic appearance. Low-grade sarcomas may be similar in appearance to their benign tissue counterparts, whereas high-grade lesions appear as anaplastic cells with no apparent distinguishing features. Cytologic features of benign spindle cell lesions above	Immunoperoxidase stains are useful in the classification of sarcomas
Lymphoma	Monomorphic population of lymphoid cells. Specific features depend on type. May have coarse, marginated chromatin, nuclear membrane irregularities. May have prominent nucleoli	Cells in a large cell lymphoma sometimes clump, imitating cohesion and an epithelial malignancy
Acute pancreatitis	Smears from acute pancreatitis show necrotic debris, neutrophils, and calcifications	Rarely aspirated
Chronic pancreatitis	Key features include identification of fibrotic acinar tissue, fibrous tissue, and calcific debris. There may be mild inflammation and hemosiderin-laden macrophages. Ductal epithelium, if present, should have minimal atypia or appear reactive; sheets of cohesive, organized ductal cells with little variation in size with or without small nucleoli	Smears may be paucicellular. A cytologic diagnosis of chronic pancreatitis does not rule out carcinoma
Mucinous neoplasms	Cytologic features vary from bland to highly atypical. All are characterized by abundant cytoplasmic mucin. Tumor cells are sometimes 'floating' in pools of mucin	Benign-appearing lesions may have more atypical areas which are missed by sampling
Islet cell tumors	Cellular tumors composed of monotonous small to medium-sized cells arranged in loose groups. May have rosettes or perivascular arrangements of tumor cells. Nuclei are central with a fine 'salt and pepper' chromatin pattern	Cytologic findings may not help distinguish the malignant potential of islet cell tumors
Melanoma	Melanoma is characterized by large anaplastic cells that generally occur in loose sheets or singly. They have markedly abnormal nuclei, with binucleate cells sometimes exhibiting a double mirror-image appearance, prominent nucleoli, and possibly intranuclear inclusions. Pigment may be noted as fine brown granules on Papanicolaou-stained smears, or blue gray granules on Diff-Quik™ staining	Metastatic tumor seen in lymph nodes, liver, and pancreas

Table 23.5 Cytologic features of common lesions
GIST, gastrointestinal stromal tumor.

REFERENCES

1 Jhala NC, Jhala DN, Chhieng DC, et al. Endoscopic ultrasound-guided fine-needle aspiration. A cytopathologist's perspective. Am J Clin Pathol 2003; 120:351–367.

2 Lopes-Cardozo P. Atlas of clinical cytology. Leiden: Targa b.v.'s Hertogenbosch; 1976:14.

3 The Papanicolaou Society of Cytopathology Task Force on Standards of Practice. Guidelines of the Papanicolaou Society of Cytopathology for fine needle aspiration procedure and reporting. Mod Pathol 1997; 10:739–747.

4 College of American Pathologists. Online. Available: http://www.cap.org

5 American Society of Cytopathology. Online. Available: http://www.cytopathology.org

6 Gregory N, Rebner M. Very large core needle biopsies of the breast: a review. Breast Dis 2001; 13:59–66.

7 Pandelidis S, Heiland D, Jones D, et al. Accuracy of 11-gauge vacuum-assisted core biopsy of mammographic breast lesions. Ann Surg Oncol 2003; 10:43–47.

8 DeMay RM. The art and science of cytopathology. Chicago: American Society of Clinical Pathologists; 1996:465.

9 Hyland C, Kheir SM, Kashlan MB. Frozen section diagnosis of pancreatic carcinoma: a prospective study of 64 biopsies. Am J Surg Pathol 1981; 5:179–191.

10 Lin F, Staerkel G. Cytologic criteria for well differentiated adenocarcinoma of the pancreas in fine-needle aspiration biopsy specimens. Cancer 2003; 99:44–50.

11 Ylagan LR, Edmundowicz S, Kasal K, et al. Endoscopic ultrasound guided fine-needle aspiration cytology of pancreatic carcinoma: a 3-year experience and review of the literature. Cancer 2002; 96:362–369.

12 Levy MJ, Jondal ML, Clain J, et al. Preliminary experience with an EUS-guided trucut biopsy needle compared with EUS-guided FNA. Gastrointest Endosc 2003; 57:101–106.

13 Stewart CJ, Coldewey J, Stewart IS. Comparison of fine needle aspiration cytology and needle core biopsy in the diagnosis of radiologically detected abdominal lesions. J Clin Pathol 2002; 55:93–97.

14 Larghi A, Verna EC, Stavropoulos SN, et al. EUS-guided trucut needle biopsies in patients with solid pancreatic masses: a prospective study. Gastrointest Endosc 2004; 59:185–190.

15 Varadarajulu S, Fraig M, Schmulewitz N, et al. Comparison of EUS-guided 19-gauge Trucut needle biopsy with EUS-guided fine-needle aspiration. Endoscopy 2004; 36:397–401.

16 Binmoeller KF, Thul R, Rathod V, et al. Endoscopic ultrasound-guided, 18-gauge, fine needle aspiration biopsy of the pancreas using a 2.8 mm channel convex array echoendoscope. Gastrointest Endosc 1998; 47:121–127.

17 Adler DG, Jacobson BC, Davila RE, et al. ASGE guideline: Complications of EUS. Gastrointest Endosc 2005; 61:8–12.

18 Zech CJ, Helmberger T, Wichmann MW, et al. Large core biopsy of the pancreas under CT fluoroscopy control: results and complications. J Comput Assist Tomogr 2002; 26:743–749.

19 Centeno BA, Enkemann SA, Coppola D, et al. Classification of human tumors using gene expression profiles obtained after microarray analysis of fine-needle aspiration biopsy samples. Cancer 2005; 105:101–109.

20 Glenthoj A, Sehested M, Torp-Pederson S. Utrasonically guided histological and cytological fine needle biopsies of the pancreas. Reliability and reproducibility of diagnosis. Gut 1990; 31:930–933.

21 Stewart CJ, Stewart IS. Immediate assessment of fine needle aspiration cytology of lung. J Clin Pathol 1996; 49:839–843.

22 vanSonnenberg E, Goodacre BW, Wittich GR, et al. Image-guided 25-gauge needle biopsy for thoracic lesions: diagnostic feasibility and safety. Radiology 2003; 227:414–418.

23 Kasugai H, Tatsuta YR, Okano Y, et al. Value of heparinized fine needle aspiration biopsy in liver malignancy. AJR Am J Roentgenol 1985; 144:243–244.

24 Thomson HD. Thin needle aspiration biopsy. Acta Cytol 1982; 26:262–263.

25 Weynand B, Deprez P. Endoscopic ultrasound guided fine needle aspiration in biliary and pancreatic diseases: pitfalls and performances. Acta Gastroenterol Belg 2004; 67:294–300.

26 Smith EH. Complications of percutaneous abdominal fine-needle biopsy. Radiology 1991; 178:253–258.

27 Zajdela A, Zillhardt P, Voillemot N. Cytological diagnosis by fine needle sampling without aspiration. Cancer 1987; 59:1201–1205.

28 Kate MS, Kamal MM, Bobhate SK, et al. Evaluation of fine needle capillary sampling in superficial and deep-seated lesions. An analysis of 670 cases. Acta Cytol 1998; 42:679–684.

29 Kinney TB, Lee MJ, Filomena CA, et al. Fine-needle biopsy: prospective comparison of aspiration versus nonaspiration techniques in the abdomen. Radiology 1993; 186:549–552.

30 Hopper KD, Abendroth CS, Sturtz KW, et al. Fine needle aspiration biopsy for cytopathologic analysis: utility of syringe hand semiautomated guns and the nonsuction method. Radiology 1993; 185:819–824.

31 Mair S, Dunbar F, Becker PJ, et al. Fine needle cytology – is aspiration suction necessary? A study of 100 masses in various sites. Acta Cytol 1989; 33:809–813.

32 Kamal MM, Arjune DJ, Kulkarni HR. Comparative study of fine needle aspiration and fine needle capillary sampling of thyroid lesions. Acta Cytol 2002; 46:30–34.

33 Hopper KD, Grenko RT, Fisher AI, et al. Capillary versus aspiration biopsy: effect of needle size and length on the cytopathological specimen quality. Cardiovasc Intervent Radiol 1996; 19:341–344.

34 Savage CA, Hopper KD, Abendroth CS, et al. Fine-needle aspiration biopsy versus fine-needle capillary (nonaspiration) biopsy: in vivo comparison. Radiology 1995; 195:815–819.

35 Wallace MB, Kennedy T, Durkalski V, et al. Randomized controlled trial of EUS-guided fine needle aspiration techniques for the detection of malignant lymphadenopathy. Gastrointest Endosc 2001; 54:441–447.

36 LeBlanc JK, Ciaccia D, Al-Assi MT, et al. Optimal number of EUS-guided fine needle passes needed to obtain a correct diagnosis. Gastrointest Endosc 2004; 59:475–481.

37 Emery SC, Savides TJ, Behling CA. Utility of immediate evaluation of endoscopic ultrasound-guided transesophageal fine needle aspiration of mediastinal lymph nodes. Acta Cytol 2004; 48:630–634.

38 Klapman JB, Logrono R, Dye CE, et al. Clinical impact of on site cytopathology interpretation on endoscopic ultrasound guided fine needle aspiration. Am J Gastroenterol 2003; 98:1289–1294.

39 Erickson RA, Sayage-Rabie L, Beissner RS. Factors predicting the number of EUS-guided fine needle passes for diagnosis of pancreatic malignancies. Gastrointest Endosc 2000; 51:184–190.

40 Jhala NC, Jhala D, Eltoum I, et al. Endoscopic ultrasound-guided fine-needle aspiration biopsy: a powerful tool to obtain samples from small lesions. Cancer 2004; 102:239–246.

41 Koss LG. Diagnostic cytology and its histopathologic basis, 3rd edn, vol. 2. Philadelphia: JB Lippincott; 1979.

42 Nithyanda NA, Narayan E, Smith MM, et al. Cell block cytology. Improved preparation and its efficacy in diagnostic cytology. Am J Clin Pathol 2000; 114:559–606.

43 Henry-Stanley MJ, Stanley MW. Processing of needle rinse material from fine needle aspirations rarely detects malignancy not identified in smears. Diag Cytopathol 1992; 8:538–540.

44 Chhieng DC, Benson E, Eltoum I, et al. MUC1 and MUC2 expression in pancreatic ductal carcinoma obtained by fine-needle aspiration. Cancer 2003; 99:365–371.

45 Safneck JR, Kutryk E, Chrobak A, et al. Fixation techniques for fine needle aspiration biopsy smears prepared off site. Acta Cytol 2001; 45:365–371.

46 Michael CW, McConnel J, Pecott J, et al. Comparison of ThinPrep and TriPath PREP liquid-based preparations in nongynecologic specimens: a pilot study. Diagn Cytopathol 2001; 25:177–184.

47 Jhala N, Jhala D. Gastrointestinal tract cytology: advancing horizons. Adv Anat Pathol 2003; 10:261–277.

48 Lee KR, Papillo JL, St John R, et al. Evaluation of the ThinPrep processor for fine needle aspiration specimens. Acta Cytol 1996; 40:895–899.

49 Fremont-Smith M, Marino J, Griffin B, et al. Comparison of the SurePath liquid-based Papanicolaou smear with the conventional Papanicolaou smear in a multisite direct-to-vial study. Cancer 2004; 102:269–279.

50 de Luna R, Eloubeidi MA, Sheffield MV, et al. Comparison of ThinPrep and conventional preparations in pancreatic fine-needle aspiration biopsy. Diagn Cytopathol 2004; 30:71–76.

51 Solomon D, Davey D, Kurman R, et al. The 2001 Bethesda System: terminology for reporting results of cervical cytology. JAMA 2002; 287:2114–2119.

52 Sneige N. Should specimen adequacy be determined by the opinion of the aspirator or by the cells on the slides. Cancer Cytopathol 1997; 81:3–5.

53 National Cancer Institute Fine-Needle Aspiration of Breast Workshop Subcommittees. The uniform approach to breast fine-needle aspiration biopsy. Diagn Cytopathol 1997; 16:295–311.

54 Shin HJ, Lahoti S, Sneige N. Endoscopic ultrasound guided fine needle aspiration in 179 cases: the M. D. Anderson Cancer Center experience. Cancer Cytopathol 2002; 96:174–180.

55 Stelow EB, Bardales RH, Lai R, et al. The cytologic spectrum of chronic pancreatitis. Diagn Cytopathol 2005; 32:65–69.

56 Hollerbach S, Klamann A, Topalidis T, et al. Endoscopic ultrasonography (EUS) and fine-needle aspiration (FNA) cytology for diagnosis of chronic pancreatitis. Endoscopy 2001; 33:824–831.

57 Nasuti JF, Gupta PK, Baloch ZW. Diagnostic value and cost effectiveness of on site evaluation of fine needle aspiration specimens: review of 5688 cases. Diagn Cytopathol 2002; 27:1–4.

58 Logrono R, Waxman I. Interactive role of the cytopathologist in EUS guided fine needle aspiration: an efficient approach. Gastrointest Endosc 2001; 54:485–490.

59 Harewood GC, Wiersema LM, Halling AC, et al. Influence of EUS training and pathology interpretation on accuracy of EUS-guided fine needle aspiration of pancreatic masses. Gastrointest Endosc 2002; 55:669–673.

60 David O, Green L, Reddy V, et al. Pancreatic masses: a multi-institutional study of 364 fine-needle aspiration biopsies with histopathologic correlation. Diagn Cytopathol 1998; 19:423–427.

61 Lui K, Dodge R, Glasgow BJ, et al. Fine needle aspiration: comparison of smear, cytospin and cell block preparations in diagnostic and cost effectiveness. Diagn Cytopathol 1998; 19:70–74.

62 Ribeiro A, Vazquez-Sequeiros E, Wiersema LM, et al. EUS-guided fine-needle aspiration combined with flow cytometry and immunocytochemistry in the diagnosis of lymphoma. Gastrointest Endosc 2001; 53:485–491.

63 Ramzy I. Clinical cytopathology and aspiration biopsy: fundamental principles and practice. Connecticut: Appleton & Lange; 1990.

64 Dabbs DJ. Diagnostic immunohistochemistry. Pittsburgh: Churchill Livingstone; 2002.

65 Rosai J. Rosai and Ackerman's surgical pathology (9th edn). Edinburgh: CV Mosby; 2004.

66 Weidner N, Cote RJ, Suster S, et al. Modern surgical pathology. Philadelphia: Saunders; 2003.

THERAPEUTIC EUS

Fine-Needle Injection Therapy

Phuong T. Nguyen

KEY POINTS

- Celiac plexus neurolysis is effective in providing long-term pain relief in 70–90% of patients with intra-abdominal malignancy.

- Endosonography-guided fine-needle injection (EUS-FNI) can be used to tattoo small pancreatic lesions (e.g., neuroendocrine tumors); this may increase the efficiency of surgical resection.

- A needle can be placed across the gut wall and into the common bile duct or dilated pancreatic duct lumen using EUS guidance, and can be used to inject dye for diagnosis or to place a stent to facilitate drainage.

- EUS-guided injection of antitumor therapy remains promising, but the key is finding a safe and efficacious agent.

INTRODUCTION

Over the years, EUS has evolved from an imaging to an interventional modality with fine-needle injection (FNI) therapy. Initially, with the development of the linear-array echoendoscope and EUS-guided fine-needle aspiration (EUS-FNA), tissue diagnosis became possible. Subsequently, the diagnosis and staging of gastrointestinal and pancreatic malignancies with EUS and EUS-FNA became the standard of care. As FNA can be performed safely and as a minimally invasive procedure, FNI therapy with EUS guidance emerged (EUS-FNI).

Initially, EUS-FNI delivered botulinum toxin to patients with achalasia. EUS-guided celiac plexus block or neurolysis (CPB/N) was then described in patients with pain from pancreatic cancer and chronic pancreatitis. EUS-FNI has also been used to tattoo tumors with ink, deliver sclerosant to varices, and place dye into the bile duct for cholangiography. Subsequently, once the feasibility and safety of EUS-FNI had been demonstrated, the technique was applied to the delivery of antitumor agents in patients with locally advanced cancer, such as pancreatic and esophageal tumors. The use of this technique in tumor therapy adds a host of potential new applications. This chapter reviews the current and emerging applications of EUS-FNI.

EUS-GUIDED CELIAC PLEXUS BLOCK OR NEUROLYSIS

Upper abdominal pain from chronic pancreatitis or pancreatic cancer is typically treated with medications, pancreatic enzymes, and celiac plexus neurolysis (CPN).[1,2] Celiac plexus block (CPB) is the term used when a steroid and/or a local anesthetic is injected rather than a neurolytic agent, such as alcohol, used for CPN. These two terms are often used interchangeably without differentiation. Initially described in 1914,[3] CPN can be performed with a percutaneous technique (fluoroscopically guided or CT-guided) or at the time of surgery.

A recent meta-analysis of the effectiveness of CPN for intra-abdominal malignancy using the percutaneous route showed that it provided long-term pain relief in 70–90% of patients.[4] This result was noted regardless of the percutaneous technique employed and the use of radiologic guidance. Adverse events noted were common (local pain, diarrhea, hypotension), but mild and transient. Severe adverse events were uncommon, occurring in less than 2%.[4,5] CPN performed at the time of surgery was reported in a randomized placebo-controlled study of 137 patients with unresectable pancreatic cancer to improve pain control at 6 months' follow-up.[6] In the treatment of pain from chronic pancreatitis, a limited number of studies with inadequate sample sizes have suggested that CPN and CPB may have short-term effect.[7,8]

In 1996, Wiersema and Wiersema[9] first reported the use of EUS in guiding the delivery of CPN in patients with pancreatic cancer. As the celiac trunk is easily identified on EUS and is in close proximity to the gastric wall, EUS-guided CPN has the potential advantage of easy delivery. Also, in patients with unresectable pancreatic cancer diagnosed on EUS, EUS-guided CPN can be conveniently performed at the time of diagnostic EUS, with therapeutic intent. In this pilot study of 30 patients (25 with pancreatic malignancy), these authors reported a 79–88% improvement in pain score at a median follow-up of 10 weeks. This same group later reported on a larger prospective series of 58 patients with inoperable pancreatic cancer who underwent CPN for pain control[10] (Table 24.1). Interestingly, a multivariate analysis showed that patients had sustained pain relief for 24 weeks independent of morphine use or adjuvant therapy; however, patients who received adjuvant therapy had additional benefit.

In a prospective randomized trial, Gress et al.[11] compared EUS-guided with CT-guided CPB in 18 patients with chronic pancreatitis pain. They found that 50% of patients in the EUS-guided group had a reduction in pain score and medication use, compared with 25% in the CT-guided group. These authors later updated their experience in 90 patients with chronic pancreatitis treated with EUS-guided CPB[12] (Table 24.1). Patients over 45 years of age and those who had never undergone pancreatic surgery were more likely to experience pain relief.

The technique of EUS-guided CPN/CPB is performed with a linear-array echoendoscope and a 22-gauge needle, as used for EUS-guided fine-needle aspiration (EUS-FNA). From the posterior gastric body, the aorta is identified on EUS and followed to the celiac trunk, which is the first major branch off the aorta below the diaphragm (Fig. 24.1). The needle is primed with the injectate solution and then placed through the biopsy channel. Under EUS guidance, the tip of the needle is placed immediately anterior and lateral to the celiac trunk take-off from the aorta. Aspiration is performed to rule out vessel penetration prior to each injection. In patients with pancreatic cancer, 3–10 ml (0.25%) bupivacaine is injected, followed by 10 ml (98%) dehydrated alcohol.[10,13] For CPB in patients with chronic pancreatitis, a steroid (triamcinolone 40 mg each side, bilaterally) is substituted in place of alcohol.[12] An echogenic cloud is seen on EUS at the site of the injection (Fig. 24.2). The patient may experience discomfort with the injection, despite sedation. The process is then repeated on the opposite side of the celiac take-off from the aorta. With celiac lymphadenopathy or tumors in the area, visualization of the celiac take-off may be difficult and the entire solution may be injected midline rather than on either side of the celiac trunk. No study has been performed to compare EUS-guided injection at the midline with injection lateral to the celiac trunk, but the author has noted similar results. Before the procedure, and again before hospital discharge, the patient is evaluated for orthostatic hypotension.

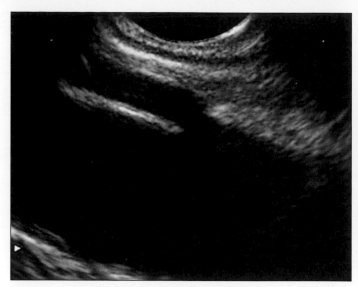

Fig. 24.1 The celiac trunk is seen as the first major vessel take-off from the aorta, as seen from the stomach.

There are several potential advantages to using EUS guidance compared with percutaneous routes for performing CPN and CPB. EUS provides continuous real-time visualization of the celiac area, and Doppler imaging to assess the vasculature before needle placement; this may reduce the complication rate. In addition, EUS approaches the celiac area anteriorly, avoiding the retrocrural space, and may reduce the risk of neurologic complications.[14] However, these theoretical advantages have not been demonstrated in any comparative studies between EUS and percutaneous approaches.

In a recent review of EUS-guided CPN, it was concluded that, despite limited data, EUS-guided CPN appeared to be as effective and safe as other approaches providing CPN for pain control in patients with pancreatic cancer.[13] The EUS approach may be most cost-effective when CPN is performed at the time of a diagnostic EUS. Regardless of the method of delivery,

EUS-GUIDED CELIAC PLEXUS NEUROLYSIS OR BLOCK				
	n	Injectate	Patients with reduction in pain score ≥3 on visual analog scale	Complications
EUS-guided CPN in pancreatic cancer[10]	58	3–6 ml (0.25%) bupivacaine + 10 ml (98%) alcohol	78%	Hypotension (20%) Diarrhea (17%) Pain exacerbation (9%)
EUS-guided CPB in chronic pancreatitis[12]	90	10 ml (0.25%) bupivacaine + 3 ml (40 mg) triamcinolone	55%	Diarrhea (5%) Peripancreatic abscess (1%)

Table 24.1 EUS-guided celiac plexus neurolysis or block
CPN, celiac plexus neurolysis; CPB, celiac plexus block.

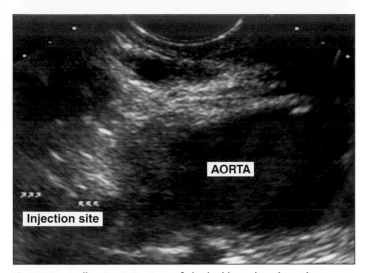

Fig. 24.2 Following injection of alcohol lateral to the celiac trunk, an echogenic cloud is noted at the injection site (arrows).

because of the conflicting data regarding risks and benefits, CPB should be considered only investigational in patients with chronic pancreatitis.

EUS-GUIDED BOTULINUM TOXIN INJECTION

Endoscopic injection of botulinum toxin (botox) into the lower esophageal sphincter (LES) in patients with achalasia is a safe and widely used technique. Initially successful in the majority of patients, the benefit lasts for only 6–9 months on average.[15] Long-term success may be higher in elderly patients and in those without very high LES pressures prior to therapy.[16,17] A randomized controlled trial comparing pneumatic dilatation with a single botox injection showed a better long-term outcome for dilatation.[18] Because the endoscopic injection of botox is 'blind', a possible explanation of the relatively short-term response in some patients is that the botox may not have been delivered entirely into the LES muscle.

EUS has the theoretical advantage of providing direct visualization of the LES to guide the delivery of botox. Hoffman et al.[19] first reported the application of EUS-guided botulinum toxin injection in four patients with achalasia. They demonstrated that the technique was feasible and provided improvement in dysphagia scores, with a follow-up of less than 13 months. On EUS, the LES appeared as a thickened hypoechoic area (approximately 4 mm wide), continuous with the muscularis propria of the distal esophagus. The FNA needle was passed through the biopsy channel of the echoendoscope and advanced into the hypoechoic LES under real-time EUS guidance. As in the endoscopic approach, four 1-ml injections (80 units in total) of botulinum toxin were made in different quadrants of the LES. Similarly, in a smaller series of three patients, Maiorana et al.[20] observed a sustained response. There have been no prospective randomized controlled trials comparing EUS-guided injection with endoscopy, and it is not clear whether this technique provides more sustained relief

from dysphagia. However, this approach may be considered in patients who fail to respond to the endoscopic technique of botulinum toxin injection.

EUS-GUIDED FINE-NEEDLE INJECTION FOR TATTOOING

EUS is a highly sensitive and specific test in the preoperative localization of pancreatic endocrine tumors.[21,22] In patients with negative findings on transabdominal ultrasonography (US) and computed tomography (CT), EUS has been shown to be superior to angiography in the preoperative detection of small pancreatic endocrine tumors.[22] In addition, specifically in the detection of insulinomas, EUS was reported as a more sensitive test than somatostatin receptor scintigraphy, US, and CT.[23] Intraoperative palpation and intraoperative US are complementary techniques, frequently used for the detection of insulinomas, with high sensitivity.[24] However, these techniques may prolong the operating time.

Preoperative endoscopic colonic tattooing has been used increasingly to localize small lesions in order to facilitate surgical resection, with minimal risks. EUS-guided fine-needle tattooing (EUS-FNT) is a new technique, described by Gress[25] in a case report as safe and useful in the preoperative localization of an insulinoma. The patient had a 1.9-cm insulinoma between the splenic artery and vein, detected only by EUS and confirmed with FNA. Given the negative results of other imaging studies and the hope of tumor enucleation at surgery, EUS-FNT was performed with 4 ml India ink (PMT Permark, Chanhassen, MN, USA). The injection was commenced in the center of the lesion and continued until the needle had exited the pancreas. At the time of laparotomy, the tattooed area was easily identified and resected.

The author has performed EUS-FNT in three patients with small insulinomas diagnosed only on EUS (unpublished findings) (Fig. 24.3). One of these patients went on to have laparoscopic enucleation of the tumor (Fig. 24.4). This technique shortened the operating time because it obviated the need to localize the tumor by intraoperative palpation and US. EUS-FNT may facilitate minimally invasive surgery including enucleation and the laparoscopic resection of these tumors. Larger and prospective studies are needed to determine the usefulness of this technique in the preoperative evaluation of these patients.

EUS-GUIDED CHOLANGIOPANCREATOGRAPHY

In 1996, Wiersema et al.[26] first described EUS-guided cholangiopancreatography as a diagnostic alternative in two patients with failed endoscopic retrograde cholangiopancreatography (ERCP). Under EUS guidance, the FNA/I needle was placed into the bile duct or the pancreatic duct, transduodenally or transgastrically; dye was injected and images were obtained similar to ERCP. The technique was shown to be feasible; however, it may not be necessary for diagnostic purposes, with

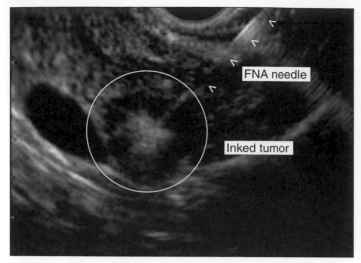

Fig. 24.3   EUS-guided fine-needle tattooing of a 1.2-cm insulinoma diagnosed only on EUS. The whitish cloud is seen within the tumor after injection.

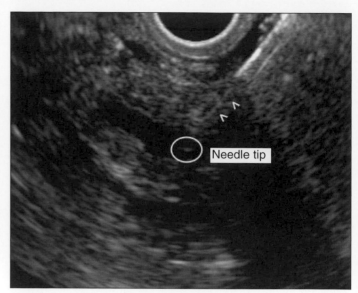

Fig. 24.5   EUS-guided pancreatography. The needle (arrows) was placed transgastrically into a dilated pancreatic duct.

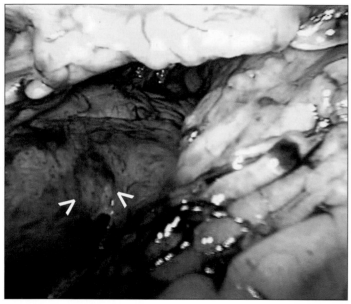

Fig. 24.4   The India ink tattoo of the insulinoma (arrows) was seen at laparoscopy.

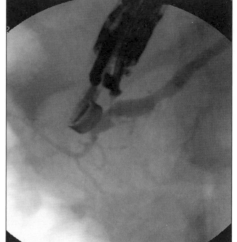

Fig. 24.6   EUS-guided pancreatogram showing the FNA needle in the pancreatic duct.

the current availability of other modalities such as magnetic resonance cholangiopancreatography (MRCP) and EUS. Two other case reports have described the application of EUS-guided pancreatography (Figs 24.5 & 24.6).[27,28]

Recent reports have demonstrated the feasibility of EUS-guided cholangiography or pancreatography with stent placement in patients with failed cannulation at ERCP as an alternative to percutaneous approaches to drainage. Burmester et al.[29] performed successfully EUS-guided cholangiography with biliary drainage (enterobiliary) in three of four patients with malignant pancreatobiliary strictures in whom ERCP was not possible because of altered anatomy and tumor infiltration. The technique was a modification of the method used for endoscopic pseudocyst drainage and involved the formation of a fistulous track through the bowel wall under EUS guidance, followed by transmural stent placement. The advantage of this technique was the proximity of the EUS transducer to the dilated extrahepatic or intrahepatic ducts, which permitted direct puncture of the duct. Another potential advantage was better patient quality of life from the internal placement of the biliary stent, compared with percutaneous techniques. One of these patients developed a local peritonitis, which was treated successfully. A limitation of the technique was that the echoendoscope used at the time of the publication allowed the passage of only a 8.5-Fr stent. In another series of five patients, a similar technique of EUS-guided cholangiography and biliary access permitted the use of a 'rendezvous' procedure.[30] In three of the five patients, a transduodenal procedure was used to guide placement of a transpapillary guidewire, which permitted subsequent successful ERCP.

When transpapillary access to a dilated portion of the main pancreatic duct could not be obtained, EUS-guided pancreaticogastrostomy was reported in a series of four patients with strictures secondary to chronic pancreatitis.[31] Gastropancreatic duct stents were placed directly through the gastric wall into markedly dilated pancreatic ducts. The procedure was successful in these patients, with no early complications. In another series, Kahaleh et al[32] performed EUS-guided pancreatography with gastropancreatic duct stent placement in two patients with pancreatic duct strictures from complicated pancreatitis in whom surgical reconstruction precluded access to the papilla. One of the patients developed upper gastrointestinal bleeding 24 h later, and was treated endoscopically. It is important to note that these reports described injection into the markedly dilated pancreatic ducts of patients with established chronic pancreatitis, where it may be technically easier to drain and the risk of iatrogenic pancreatitis may be less. In one report of EUS-guided pancreatography and rendezvous drainage of smaller-sized pancreatic ducts (<5 mm), success was seen in only one of four patients.[33]

These case reports demonstrated that EUS-guided cholangiopancreatography and duct decompression, whether with enteroductal or transpapillary stents, can be performed successfully in patients in whom ERCP has failed. Larger studies with long-term follow-up are needed to determine the safety and efficacy of these techniques.

EUS-GUIDED SCLEROTHERAPY

Recurrence of esophageal varices and rebleeding after initial obliteration by endoscopic band ligation is not uncommon, but data on the prediction of recurrent varices are limited. In one report, 40 patients who underwent endoscopic band ligation for esophageal variceal bleeding were studied by EUS within 4 weeks after obliteration of varices. Patients with large paraesophageal varices were found to have a higher risk of developing recurrent varices and rebleeding.[34] The perforating veins connecting the paraesophageal varices are believed to play a vital role in the development of esophageal varices. Lahoti et al.[35] first reported EUS-guided sclerotherapy as primary prevention, with non-bleeding esophageal varices in five patients and variceal obliteration in a mean of 2.2 sessions. By using EUS guidance, sclerosant can be delivered directly into the varix at the level of the perforating veins until seen to be completely thrombosed by Doppler US. These authors concluded that the confirmation of obliteration of varices, together with the ability to obliterate the perforating veins (which is not possible with standard sclerotherapy or banding techniques) might decrease the number of sessions needed and variceal recurrence.

It is not known whether secondary prevention of esophageal variceal bleeding by EUS-guided FNI or sclerotherapy of perforating veins and paraesophageal varices improves patient morbidity and mortality rates.

EUS-GUIDED ANTITUMOR INJECTION THERAPY

The author's group first reported their phase I clinical trial of EUS-guided injection of allogenic mixed lymphocyte culture (cytoimplant) in eight patients with advanced pancreatic cancer.[36] FNI was performed with a linear echoendoscope, and a 22-gauge needle was advanced into the bulk of the tumor. Escalating doses of cytoimplant cells were injected into the tumor, in a slow, steady fashion as the needle was withdrawn. Tumor response (Figs 24.7 & 24.8), defined as tumor regression, was monitored by follow-up imaging (CT and/or EUS) every 3 months for the first year, with a final evaluation at 24 months (Table 24.2). Although this was a small study, it demonstrated that the injection of antitumor agents in pancreatic cancer was feasible and safe.

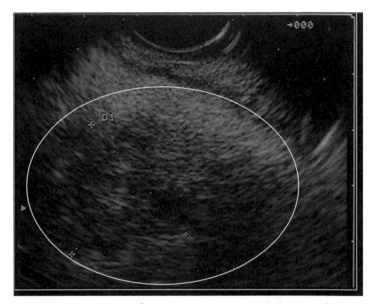

Fig. 24.7   EUS image of a 3.1×2.2-cm pancreatic tumor in the head of the pancreas prior to use of cytoimplant.[36]

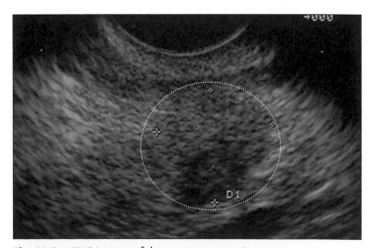

Fig. 24.8   EUS image of the same pancreatic tumor, demonstrating a reduction in tumor size to 1.5×1.6 cm.[36]

NOVEL THERAPY FOR UNRESECTABLE PANCREATIC CANCER						
	n	No. of injection sessions	Complications	Adjuvant therapy	Response	Median survival (months)
Cytoimplant[36]	8	1	Low-grade fever (7), transient gastrointestinal toxicity (3), reversible hyperbilirubinemia (3)	None	Partial (2) Minor (1)	13.2
Onyx-015[37]	21	8	Sepsis (2), duodenal perforation (2)	Gemcitabine	Partial (2) Minor (2) Stable (6)	7.5
TNFerade[38]	37 (17 by EUS)	5	Fatigue, nausea, abdominal pain (24%)	5-FU + radiation	Tumor stable at 3 months (73%)	–

Table 24.2 Novel therapy for unresectable pancreatic cancer
5-FU, 5-fluorouracil.

A second phase I/II trial in 21 patients with unresectable pancreatic carcinoma was recently reported by Hecht et al.[37] They performed EUS-guided injection of ONYX-015, an adenovirus that selectively replicates and kills malignant cells. Patients received intratumoral injections of 1ml ONYX-015, with up to ten injections per session depending on tumor size, for a total of eight sessions. Two patients had duodenal perforations and with adjustments in the protocol to the transgastric route of injection, this was avoided. This study showed that repeated injections of antitumoral agents by EUS-FNI were feasible and generally well tolerated.

More recently, a phase I multicenter clinical trial of a novel gene transfer therapy (TNFerade) was reported, for irresectable, locally advanced, pancreatic adenocarcinoma delivered by EUS-FNI or percutaneously by CT or US guidance.[38] TNFerade is a replication-deficient adenovector containing the human *TNFα* gene, regulated by a radiation-inducible promoter, Egr-1. Patients received weekly intratumoral injections of TNFerade with up to four injections per session, in a fan-like distribution by EUS or a single injection using the percutaneous approach (Table 24.2). The study endpoints were safety and tumor control as demonstrated by spiral CT. Three of the 37 enrolled patients underwent surgical resection after therapy, and one patient in the EUS group had a complete pathologic response. The authors concluded that TNFerade plus chemoradiation was well tolerated, with clinical activity as demonstrated by local tumor control, and was safe to deliver by EUS or percutaneously. A phase II trial involving locally advanced pancreatic cancer will shortly be enrolling patients, and trials of TNFerade in patients with locally advanced esophageal cancer are currently ongoing.

POTENTIAL FUTURE EUS-FNI APPLICATIONS

EUS-guided brachytherapy

Although no published data are available, EUS-guided brachytherapy of recurrent malignancies and irresectable cancers detected only by EUS has a potential future application. Similar to brachytherapy for prostate cancer, the author has performed EUS-guided brachytherapy in a patient with squamous cell esophageal carcinoma recurrent in perigastric lymph nodes (Figs 24.9 & 24.10) (in press) and in a patient with irresectable cholangiocarcinoma. Radioactive seeds of iodine-125 or palladium-103 were loaded into the FNI needle, and injected or implanted into the lymph nodes or tumor. Nodal and tumor shrinkage was noted on follow-up EUS. Larger series of EUS-guided brachytherapy may demonstrate a role for this technique in the palliation of patients with irresectable cancers such as cholangiocarcinoma.

EUS-guided ethanol injection

A case of EUS-guided injection of 95% ethanol into a gastrointestinal stromal tumor (GIST) has been described previously.[39]

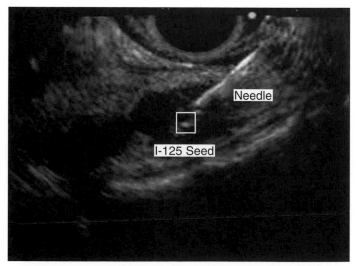

Fig. 24.9 Recurrent esophageal cancer in perigastric lymph nodes treated by EUS-guided brachytherapy. Radioactive iodine seeds were placed into the nodes, with complete ablation.

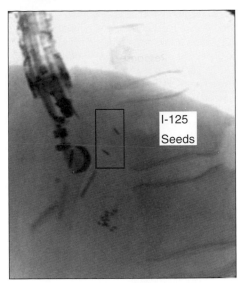

Fig. 24.10
Fluoroscopic image of radioactive seeds implanted into perigastric lymph nodes under EUS guidance and fine-needle injection.

I-125 Seeds

The patient was considered to be unfit for surgery because of severe chronic obstructive lung disease. The tumor was 40 mm in diameter, and 1.5 ml ethanol was injected in a single session under EUS guidance, with complete tumor ablation. This method might be used as an alternative to endoscopic or surgical resection in selected patients with GIST.

Other potential targets for EUS-guided therapy include tumors in close proximity to the stomach, as in the left lobe of the liver. Percutaneous intralesional injection of absolute ethanol is an accepted non-surgical alternative for treating hepatic tumors.

One case report described EUS-guided ethanol injection of a solid hepatic metastasis in which ablative therapy could not be administered safely by the percutaneous route.[40] EUS localized the metastatic lesion precisely, and guided multiple sessions of ethanol injection. The authors noted a reduction in tumor size and in tumor marker levels, suggesting that the treatment was effective in controlling the tumor burden. No major complications resulted from the multiple EUS-guided hepatic tumor injections, and the procedure was well tolerated. With the encouraging results in these single cases, further study is warranted, especially in patients with tumors that are difficult to treat by conventional methods.

Conclusion

Initially a diagnostic modality, the development of EUS-guided FNA and subsequently FNI has broadened the field of endosonography. EUS-guided CPN has been shown to be effective in patients with pancreatic cancer pain. EUS-guided FNT, EUS-guided cholangiopancreatography, and EUS-guided sclerotherapy are all EUS-FNI procedures with clinical application in specific situations. Currently, our understanding and interest is increasing most widely in the use of EUS-FNI to deliver antitumor agents. Clinical trials have thus far demonstrated that EUS-guided FNI delivery of antitumor agents is safe and feasible. EUS-guided FNI-directed therapy with its minimal invasiveness and low complication rates will continue to have great clinical impact in the treatment of benign and malignant diseases.

REFERENCES

1 Reidenberg MM, Portenoy RK. The need for an open mind about the treatment of chronic nonmalignant pain. Clin Pharmacol Ther 1994; 55:367–369.
2 Ventafridda V, Caraceni AT, Sbanotto AM, et al. Pain treatment in cancer of the pancreas. Eur J Surg Oncol 1990; 16:1–6.
3 Kappis M. Erfahrungen mit local anasthesie bie bauchoperationen. Vehr Dtsch Gesellsch Chir 1914; 43:87–89.
4 Eisenberg E, Carr DB, Chalmers TC. Neurolytic celiac plexus block for treatment of cancer pain: a meta-analysis. Anesth Analg 1995; 80:290–295.
5 Davies DD. Incidence of major complications of neurolytic coeliac plexus block. J R Soc Med 1993; 86:264–266.
6 Lillemoe KD, Cameron JL, Kaufman HS, et al. Chemical splanchnicectomy in patients with unresectable pancreatic cancer. A prospective randomized trial. Ann Surg 1993; 217:447–457.
7 Leung JW, Bowen-Wright M, Aveling W, et al. Coeliac plexus block for pain in pancreatic cancer and chronic pancreatitis. Br J Surg 1983; 70:730–732.
8 Wong GY, Sakorafas GH, Tsiotos GG, et al. Palliation of pain in chronic pancreatitis. Use of neural blocks and neurotomy. Surg Clin North Am 1999; 79:873–893.
9 Wiersema MJ, Wiersema LM. Endosonography-guided celiac plexus neurolysis. Gastrointest Endosc 1996; 44:656–662.
10 Gunaratnam NT, Saram AV, Norton ID, et al. A prospective study of EUS-guided celiac plexus neurolysis for pancreatic cancer pain. Gastrointest Endosc 2001; 54:316–324.
11 Gress F, Schmitt C, Sherman S, et al. A prospective randomized comparison of endoscopic ultrasound- and computed tomography-guided celiac plexus block for managing chronic pancreatitis pain. Am J Gastroenterol 1999; 94:900–905.
12 Gress F, Schmitt C, Sherman S, et al. Endoscopic ultrasound-guided celiac plexus block for managing abdominal pain associated with chronic pancreatitis: a prospective single center experience. Am J Gastroenterol 2001; 96:409–416.
13 Levy MJ, Wiersema MJ. EUS-guided celiac plexus neurolysis and celiac plexus block. Gastrointest Endosc 2003; 57:923–930.
14 De Conno F, Caraceni A, Aldrighetti L, et al. Paralegia following coeliac plexy block. Anesthesia 1991; 46:862–863.
15 Pasricha PJ, Rai R, Ravich WJ, et al. Botulinum toxin for achalasia: long-term outcome and predictors of response. Gastroenterology 1996; 110:1410–1415.
16 Neubrand M. Long-term results and prognostic factors in the treatment of achalasia with botulinum toxin. Endoscopy 2002; 34:519–523.
17 D'Onofrio V, Miletto P, Leandro G, et al. Long-term follow-up of achalasia patients treated with botulinum toxin. Dig Liver Dis (Italy) 2002; 34:105–110.
18 Bansal R. Intrasphincteric botulinum toxin versus pneumatic balloon dilation for treatment of primary achalasia. J Clin Gastroenterol 2003; 36:209–214.
19 Hoffman BJ, Knapple WL, Bhutani MS, et al. Treatment of achalasia by injection of botulinum toxin under endoscopic ultrasound guidance. Gastrointest Endosc 1997; 45:77–79.

20 Maiorana A, Fiorentino E, Genova EG, et al. Echo-guided injection of botulinum toxin in patients with achalasia: initial experience. Endoscopy 1999; 31:S2–S3.

21 Lightdale CJ, Botet JF, Woodruff JN, et al. Localization of endocrine tumors of the pancreas with endoscopic ultrasonography. Cancer 1991; 68:1815–1820.

22 Rösch T, Lightdale CJ, Botet JF, et al. Localization of pancreatic endocrine tumors by endoscopic ultrasonography. N Engl J Med 1992; 326:1721–1726.

23 Zimmer T, Stölzel U, Bäder M, et al. Endoscopic ultrasonography and somatotatin receptor scintigraphy in the preoperative localization of insulinomas and gastrinomas. Gut 1996; 39:562–568.

24 Galliber AK, Reading CC, Charboneau JW, et al. Localization of pancreatic insulinoma: comparison of pre- and intraoperative US with CT and angiography. Radiology 1988; 166:405–408.

25 Gress FG. Preoperative localization of a neuroendocrine tumor of the pancreas with EUS-guided fine needle tattooing. Gastrointest Endosc 2002; 55:594–597.

26 Wiersema MJ, Sandusky D, Carr R, et al. Endosonography-guided cholangiopancreatography. Gastrointest Endosc 1996; 43:102–106.

27 Harada N, Kozu T, Arima M. Endoscopic ultrasound-guided pancreatography: a case report. Endoscopy 1995; 27:612–615.

28 Gress F, Ikenberry S, Sherman S, et al. Endoscopic ultrasound-directed pancreatography. Gastrointest Endosc 1996; 44:736–739.

29 Burmester E, Niehaus J, Leineweber T, et al. EUS-cholangio-drainage of the bile duct: report of 4 cases. Gastrointest Endosc 2003; 57:246–251.

30 Kahaleh M, Yoshida C, Kane L, et al. Interventional EUS cholangiography: report of 5 cases. Gastrointest Endosc 2004; 60:138–142.

31 Francois E, Kahaleh M, Giovannini M, et al. EUS-guided pancreaticogastrostomy. Gastrointest Endosc 2002; 56:128–133.

32 Kahaleh M, Yoshida C, Yeaton P. EUS antegrade pancreatography with gastropancreatic duct stent placement: review of two cases. Gastrointest Endosc 2003; 58:919–923.

33 Mallery S, Matlock J, Freeman M. EUS-guided rendezvous drainage of obstructed biliary and pancreatic ducts: report of 6 cases. Gastrointest Endosc 2004; 59:100–107.

34 Leung VKS, Sung JJY, Ahuja AT, et al. Large paraesophageal varices on endosonography predict recurrence of esophageal varices and rebleeding. Gastroenterology 1997; 112:1811–1816.

35 Lahoti S, Catalano MF, Alcocer E, et al. Obliteration of esophageal varices using EUS-guided sclerotherapy with color Doppler. Gastrointest Endosc 2000; 51:331–333.

36 Chang KJ, Nguyen PT, Thompson JA, et al. Phase 1 clinical trial of allogeneic mixed lymphocyte culture (cytoimplant) delivered by endoscopic ultrasound-guided fine needle-injection in patients with advanced pancreatic carcinoma. Cancer 2000; 88:1325–1335.

37 Hecht JR, Bedford R, Abbruzzese JL, et al. A phase I/II trial of intramural endoscopic ultrasound injection of ONYX-015 with intravenous gemcitabine in unresectable pancreatic carcinoma. Clin Cancer Res 2003; 9:555–561.

38 Chang KJ, Senzer N, Chung T, et al. A novel gene transfer therapy against pancreatic cancer (TNFerade) delivered by endoscopic ultrasound (EUS) and percutaneously guided fine needle injection (FNI). Digestive Disease Week, oral presentation 2004; 59: pAB92.

39 Gunter E, Lingenfelser T, Eitelbach F, et al. EUS-guided ethanol injection for treatment of a GI stromal tumor. Gastrointest Endosc 2003; 57:113–115.

40 Barclay R, Perez-Miranda M, Giovannini M. EUS-guided treatment of a solid hepatic metastasis. Gastrointest Endosc 2002; 55:266–270.

Chapter 25

EUS-Guided Drainage and Anastomosis

Annette Fritscher-Ravens

KEY POINTS

- EUS-guided therapeutic interventions are still mostly experimental, with the exception of pseudocyst drainage.

- Only pseudocysts existing for 6 weeks or more and with a minimal size of 6 cm should be considered for drainage.

- In patients with a pseudocyst in the setting of acute pancreatitis, waiting more than 6 weeks is not dangerous if the cyst does not increase in size.

- The EUS-guided technique allows for drainage of non-bulging cysts.

- Techniques for performing EUS-guided anastomoses are under development but not yet ready for general use.

INTRODUCTION

During the last decade existing diagnostic imaging techniques, in particular computed tomography (CT), magnetic resonance imaging (MRI), and positron emission tomography (PET), have been developed and refined, competing with radial endoscopic ultrasound (EUS) to provide reliable imaging and TNM staging of upper gastrointestinal malignancies. With the introduction of linear-array echoendoscopy, imaging parallel to the shaft of the endoscope has become possible and has enabled real-time visualization of any tool or instrument pushed out of the biopsy channel into a target lesion in or beyond the gut wall. This has allowed the development of EUS-guided fine-needle aspiration (EUS-FNA) for tissue diagnosis and has changed the role of EUS from being exclusively an imaging modality into a simultaneous imaging and tissue sampling technique. The possibility of placing a needle precisely into a lesion and sampling material has also provided the opportunity to reverse this process and deliver materials into an organ, thereby providing treatment under real-time visualization. Interventional procedures being developed for therapeutic use include cyst drainage and celiac axis block injection of cytoimplants,[1] radiofrequency ablation,[2] and ethanol injection (see Ch. 24).[3,4]

Recently, more refined procedures for EUS-guided treatment have been developed, including fistula formation. Even more advanced techniques that may be classified as EUS-guided endosurgery (EUGE) have also been attempted. EUS-guided therapy and EUGE have opened up new routes for the non-surgical treatment of diseases that have previously required open or laparoscopic surgery, thus expanding the role of endoscopy. Most of these new techniques are still experimental, with only a few case reports available. They should be performed only in specialist centers under study conditions.

There are no randomized studies available comparing EUS-guided therapies with other minimally invasive or surgical techniques, making evaluation of the true benefit of EUS-assisted interventions rather difficult. However, there is clearly great potential as EUS allows the endoscopist to see beyond the lumen into structures adjacent to the bowel.

This chapter attempts to provide an overview of the newest therapeutic interventions, although it focuses on the most commonly performed and first EUS-guided therapeutic approach: the drainage of pancreatic pseudocysts. It compares the different techniques, provides the available results, and gives a description of how to perform EUS-guided cyst drainage, as well as some newer therapies such as the formation of anastomoses.

DRAINAGE OF PANCREATIC PSEUDOCYSTS

The treatment of pancreatic pseudocysts in a non-surgical fashion has fascinated physicians of different disciplines including radiologists, ultrasonographers, and endoscopists. Percutaneous ultrasound (US) and CT-guided procedures have been well described. When an endoscopic approach was introduced in 1985 by Kozarek et al.,[5] it was thought that this might overcome some of the complications, such as cutaneous fistula formation, that occur with the percutaneous route. The recent introduction of EUS-guided drainage combines the advantages of both techniques, allowing internal drainage but avoiding the risk of inadvertent puncture of other organs or blood vessels.

The proximity of the EUS transducer to the gut wall and pancreas in combination with the high resolution of EUS imaging afforded by high-frequency (5–10 MHz) transducers allows excellent visualization of the gut wall and nearby structures. Vessels within or just beyond the wall are visualized, and verified by color Doppler US. This is especially valuable when assessing interposed vessels and, if the cyst is small enough, aneurysms.

Before describing the technique it is necessary to understand the percutaneous and endoscopic approach, the results obtained, and any shortcomings. It is also important to understand the various cystic structures related to the pancreas and their pathologies, so as not to approach the wrong kind of cyst at the wrong time using the wrong procedure.

Terminology

Definition

Pseudocyst formation is a well known complication of acute or chronic pancreatitis or of pancreatic trauma. It is a collection of pancreatic juice enclosed by a wall within the pancreas or peripancreatic area. Pseudocysts are usually round or ovoid and have a well defined wall of fibrous or granulation tissue.[6] Formation of a pseudocyst requires at least 4 weeks from the onset of acute pancreatitis. The cyst is usually rich in pancreatic enzymes; bacteria may be present, but the cyst is most often sterile. When pus is present, it is defined as a pancreatic abscess. In acute pancreatitis pseudocysts consist of inflammatory exudate, whereas in chronic pancreatitis the cyst develops following an acute exacerbation of pancreatitis, or is the result of an obstructed duct. Detailed definitions and terminology should be used according to the recommendations of the International Symposium on Acute Pancreatitis 1992.[6]

Cysts are mainly single, but multiple cysts may develop in 10–20% of cases.[7–9] About 30–60% are stable with no complications, and resolve spontaneously.[7,8,10–12] Pancreatic pseudocysts are a complication of acute pancreatitis in 10% of patients, and chronic pancreatitis in 20%.[13,14] Depending on their size and location, pseudocysts can produce a wide range of clinical problems: duodenal and biliary obstruction, fistula formation into adjacent viscera or pleural space, spontaneous infection, and severe complications such as rupture with shock and peritonitis, or pseudoaneurysm.[15,16]

US features and characterization

On US, pancreatic pseudocysts, like fluid-filled organs such as the gallbladder, present as echo-poor, nearly echo-free, structures surrounded by a wall. This structure is defined as a 'simple cyst' (Fig. 25.1A).[17] Occasionally it may contain some echogenic material, representing debris or blood (Fig. 25.1B). Abnormality of the pancreatic duct and/or parenchyma may help to diagnose underlying acute or chronic pancreatitis. In general, a clear wall, smooth contour, round or oval shape, with

or without a thin septum defines a pseudocyst.[17] Other signs include peripancreatic inflammation and/or calcification.[18] Despite these features, it is not possible reliably to differentiate a pseudocyst from a cystic tumor or other pathologic cystic structure (Fig. 25.1C).[17,19,20] Irregularity of the wall, thick septations, areas of microcysts, or a larger area of solid material make a tumor more likely. The accuracy of EUS in diagnosing cystic neoplasms versus pseudocysts has a wide variation of 40–93%, even for experienced endosonographers,[19] and underlines the impossibility of diagnosing a pancreatic pseudocyst solely on the basis of echo features (see Ch. 17). In a recent study of 341 patients, analysis of cystic fluid for carcinoembryonic antigen (CEA) proved to be significantly more accurate than evaluation of EUS morphology.[20]

Indication for drainage

Early data suggest that pseudocysts larger than 6 cm, persisting for more than 6 weeks, are unlikely to resolve spontaneously and have an increased risk of complications after 13 weeks.[8] To avoid these complications, intervention has been thought to be appropriate after 6 weeks of observation. Newer data are controversial and may justify a more differentiated approach. In 9% of patients serious complications such as pseudoaneurysm, perforation, and spontaneous infection were seen, the majority occurring within the first 2 months.[12,21] These data support clinical follow-up in patients who have no complications, constant size of cyst, and are symptom-free even after 6 weeks of observation.

Cyst drainage is recommended for cyst complications such as unrelenting symptoms, significant abdominal pain, pseudocyst expansion, or the more serious complications described in Table 25.1. The majority of patients require drainage therapy because of mass symptoms such as pain due to an increase in cyst size or gastric outlet obstruction. Patients with pancreatic duct disruption are suitable for transpapillary drainage or a combined approach, and those with underlying necrosis may need surgical and/or extensive and aggressive repeat endoscopic treatment.[22–24] Patients with severe bleeding or cyst rupture may still need surgery.

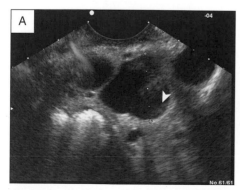 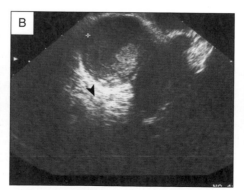 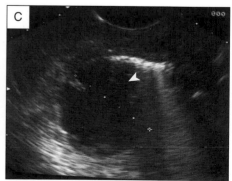

Fig. 25.1 **A,** 2-cm, nearly echo-free pseudocyst. The blurry echoes represent artifacts (arrowhead). **B,** Echo-poor cyst with echogenic material representing debris (arrowhead). **C,** Echo-poor cystic lesion mimicking a pseudocyst. This lesion turned out to be a duodenal diverticulum. Note the air in the lesion (arrowhead).

COMPLICATIONS OF PANCREATIC PSEUDOCYST	
Type	Complication
Frequent	Abdominal pain
	Gastric or duodenal bulge
	Gastric outlet obstruction
	Infection
	Hemorrhage
	Portal or splenic vein thrombosis
Severe	Cyst rupture (shock, peritonitis)
	Splenic rupture
	Erosion of gastroduodenal or splenic artery
Occasional	Fistulae: stomach, duodenum, colon, pelvis
	Obstruction: stomach, duodenum, colon, pelvis, CBD, ureter
	Pleural effusion
	Pseudoaneurysm

Table 25.1 Complications of pancreatic pseudocyst

Sterile cysts smaller than 4–6 cm have a high rate of spontaneous resolution and should be watched carefully.[12,15,16,21,25]

It is recommended that endoscopic drainage should not be performed if the interface between the cyst and the gut wall is greater than 1 cm, as this might increase the complication rate.[5,23,26,27] This is also widely accepted for the EUS-guided approach.

The presence of a pseudoaneurysm, which may be seen in 10% of pseudocysts, represents an absolute contraindication for endoscopic drainage, because multidisciplinary treatment is required in this situation.[28,29]

Conventional non-surgical drainage

Traditionally, pseudocyst drainage has been primarily surgical, in the form of cystenterostomy. Although effective, there is a significant morbidity rate of about 15%, with a postoperative recurrence rate of approximately 10% and a mortality rate of more than 5%.[16,25,30] Consequently, non-surgical interventional options such as percutaneous or endoscopic cyst drainage have been favored since the first non-surgical drainage was performed in the 1970s.

Percutaneous drainage

Percutaneous cyst aspiration can be performed for diagnosis. Even if the cyst is completely emptied, the recurrence rate is as high as 60%.[15,31] If therapy is warranted, continuous drainage is required. Percutaneous drainage, performed mainly by transabdominal US, was the first non-surgical approach, introduced in 1976 by Hancke and Pedersen.[31] This technique avoided the need for surgery, was easy to perform, and did not require general anesthesia or much sedation. However, for successful treatment, external prolonged catheter drainage was needed. In a review of this technique, the recurrence rate was only 7% in 246 patients from nine studies, with a failure rate of 16% and a complication rate of 18%. The mortality rate ranged between 0.6% and 2%, with the most of the later publications reporting no deaths.[15]

The most common complication is infection or the development of cystocutaneous fistulae owing to the necessary external prolonged catheter drainage. To avoid the latter and the inconvenience to the patient of having to carry a percutaneous catheter, a transabdominal transgastric approach was favored.[15]

This technique included the US-guided placement of a percutaneous transcystic guidewire into the gastric lumen. This guidewire, once seen to be in the stomach endoscopically, would facilitate the transabdominal placement of a stent or pigtail from the cyst to the stomach under endoscopic view. When the guidewire was removed, the cyst would drain through the stent into the stomach with no percutaneous connections.[32] A modification of this technique was performed by a combination of transabdominal US and gastroscopy. It included the endoscopic rather than percutaneous placement of the stent over the percutaneously placed guidewire.[33]

Using these techniques, several groups have published encouraging results with a success rate of 70–100% and a complication rate of 10–18%.[33,34]

Endoscopic drainage

Since Hershfield[35] and Kozarek et al.[5] published their first endoscopic cystenterostomies, endoscopic drainage has been considered an attractive alternative to the percutaneous route. Percutaneous guidewire placement requires expertise in transabdominal US or the assistance of an US expert. Under certain circumstances, for instance when the bulge of the cyst can be seen in the gut lumen, internal endoscopic drainage can be achieved blindly without the need for that specific knowledge. Growing experience in interventional endoscopy has made the development of two types of endoscopic drainage procedure possible, providing three different options for drainage: (1) the blind endoscopic puncture of the cyst through the stomach or duodenal wall, using the bulge of the cyst as a guide; (2) the transpapillary approach during endoscopic retrograde cholangiopancreatography (ERCP) in the case of communication of the cyst and the pancreatic duct; or (3) a combination of both.

Transmural drainage

Endoscopic transgastric or transduodenal drainage of pseudocysts, although simple, is technically challenging. An ideal but necessary prerequisite is that the pseudocyst impinges on the stomach or duodenum. Prior US or CT imaging is necessary to confirm adherence of the cyst to the gut wall. In the absence of a visible 'bulge', or if the distance between the cyst and the stomach/duodenum exceeds 1 cm on imaging, the complication rate increases and endoscopic drainage should not be performed. About 40% of pseudocysts have been reported to fulfil these criteria.[36]

Once a 'bulge' is present, and stomach and cyst are proven to have a common wall, a gastric or duodenal incision is made using diathermy on a needle-knife papillotome or cystotome, and the cyst is punctured. When the resistance of solid structures is overcome and the knife is felt to be within the cyst lumen, a gush of fluid is often visible in the stomach or duodenum. Fluid should be aspirated to prove the intracystic location and for microbiologic and cytologic examination. In addition, contrast medium can be injected to define the anatomy of the cyst. The diathermy needle can be removed and replaced by a guidewire, leaving the outer catheter within the cyst lumen. After dilatation of the tract, preferably with a balloon catheter, a pigtail or nasocystic drainage tube can be passed into the cyst. The stent should be kept in the cyst for at least 1 month, or until the cyst has resolved. Modifications of the technique and design of tools have been reported, including cyst puncture and drainage without diathermy.[37]

Analysis of various series has proven transmural endoscopic drainage to be feasible in 80–100% of patients who fulfilled the criteria for a positive 'bulge',[16,27,38,39] with a recurrence rate of about 20%[22,27,36–45] (Table 25.2). However, significant complications have been reported in up to 20%, most commonly bleeding, due mainly to inadvertent puncture of a vessel within or between the gut wall and the cyst, and infection[41] (Table 25.2). Other complications include perforation and severe bleeding due to unrecognized pseudoaneurysm, which carries the greatest risk of death. The outcome differs among patients with acute or chronic pancreatic pseudocysts or pancreatic necrosis.[22,23]

Transpapillary drainage

Transpapillary drainage is technically the most demanding procedure and should be performed in all patients with pancreatic duct disruption, whenever feasible. It carries the lowest risk of bleeding and perforation, and is performed using the standard technique of pancreatic duct stenting during endoscopic retrograde pancreatography (ERP). Once a communication of the cyst with the pancreatic duct has been established, a guidewire is advanced along the pancreatic duct deep into the cyst, and a stent placed after papillotomy.

In a review of published series, a success rate greater than 80%, with a recurrence rate of about 10% and a complication rate of about 12%, was reported.[46] Pancreatitis and infection are the most frequent complications. Overall, the success rate reaches 70–100%, with a recurrence rate of up to 37% and a complication rate of up to 26%[38,42–45,47–49] (Table 25.3).

Transmural and transpapillary draining methods are equally effective, although the complication rate is lower with the transpapillary approach. Combinations of the procedures, or modified combinations such a stenting of the pancreatic duct plus endoscopic drainage, are possible depending on the anatomy of the pseudocyst.[38,44]

All endoscopic methods combined have a success rate of 94%, with cyst resolution of 90% and a recurrence rate of 16%, but there is a high complication rate of up to 20% and some deaths have been reported. Nevertheless, these results may still be better than those achieved with the surgical approach.[50] Endoscopic cyst drainage has emerged as the preferred method in centers with expertise in the non-surgical management of patients with pancreatic pseudocysts who do not have an absolute indication for surgery such as severe bleeding or perforation.[51] To evaluate whether the relatively high complication rate could be further reduced, EUS was introduced into this field as a high-resolution imaging technique that can be performed during endoscopy.

RESULTS OF LARGER SERIES OF ENDOSCOPIC TRANSMURAL CYST DRAINAGE				
Reference	n	Success rate (%)	Complication rate (%)	Recurrence rate (%)
Cremer et al.[27]	33	82	6	12
Grimm et al.[40]	18	88	13	0
Dohmoto et al.[43,a]	42	89	17	14
Smits et al.[38,a]	17	84	31	–
Sharma et al.[39]	38	100	13	16
De Palma et al.[45]	30	90	21	20
Libera et al.[42]	25	70	16	4.2
Beckingham et al.[36]	34	71	?	7
Binmoeller et al.[44]	20	94	11	23
Mönkemüller et al.[37]	94	93	7–15[b]	–
Baron et al.[22]	138	82	17–37[b] (1 death)	16

Table 25.2 Results of larger series of endoscopic transmural cyst drainage
No differentiation was made in relation to the kind of pseudocyst (acute versus chronic pancreatitis versus pancreatic necrosis).
[a]Transmural and transpapillary drainage.
[b]Complications related to different kinds of cyst.

RESULTS OF LARGER SERIES USING TRANSPAPILLARY DRAINAGE				
Reference	n	Success rate (%)	Complication rate (%)	Recurrence rate (%)
Smits et al.[38]	19	70	16	5
Binmoeller et al.[44]	33	94	11	23
Dohmoto et al.[43]	9	94	0	0
Kozarek et al.[49]	18	100	22	15
De Palma et al.[45]	19	84	26	37
Catalano et al.[48]	21	76	5	5
Barthet et al.[47]	20	76	15	10
Libera et al.[42]	25	70	16	4.2

Table 25.3 Results of larger series using transpapillary drainage

EUS and pseudocysts

The fact that transmural imaging can be achieved out of the gut lumen to visualize nearby intra-abdominal structures such as the pancreas gives EUS an edge over other imaging techniques. EUS can thus provide highly detailed images of the gut wall and the vessels within it or just beyond, as well as visualization of the pancreas and peripancreatic structures. These characteristics appear to be nearly ideal to help prevent complications of endoscopic cyst drainage such as bleeding from vessels within or just beyond the gut wall, or failure to localize a suitable puncture site for cysts that do not produce a 'bulge'. However, the high-frequency imaging is associated with limited tissue penetration, and pancreatic pseudocysts can be seen in detail only when 7 cm or less from the bowel wall. CT provides a better overview of the pancreatic pseudocyst and its various relations to other organs and major vessels, and is mandatory before any EUS-guided intervention is performed.

The information provided by the combination of EUS and CT also helps in the planning of appropriate cyst management, as EUS can identify features of fluid collections that may help to differentiate a pseudocyst from a cystic tumor, which is the reason for cyst formation in 10–13% of cases.[52,53] Other features include septations, irregularities of the wall, and debris (see above), which can also lead to other diagnoses and consequently to modified investigations and treatment.[17,18] The downside of EUS is that, in the presence of a cyst, it cannot provide sufficient information about the entire pancreatic duct to exclude a connection between the pancreatic duct and the fluid collection, and so is not a substitute for ERP.

In summary, EUS imaging can provide:

- Detailed images of the pancreas
- Visualization of the cyst, its contents, and neighboring structures (within 7 cm)
- Morphologic criteria for the differentiation of various cysts
- Exact measurement of the distance between the cyst and the gut wall
- Detection of intervening vessels.

Early data reported an accuracy of 92% for EUS in the detection of pancreatic cysts.[54] The higher resolution enabled the detection of more pseudocysts by EUS than by CT (89% versus 74%), an advantage that was obvious only in cysts less 2 cm in diameter (83% versus 33%). ERCP detected the lowest proportion of pseudocysts (23%).[55]

In a study performed by Fockens et al.[56] evaluating the efficacy of EUS, a series of 32 patients referred for endoscopic cyst drainage was analyzed. Only 63% were found to have a cyst suitable for drainage by EUS. In 16% no clear cyst could be identified. In 26% of patients with visible cysts, drainage was not performed because of the distance between the gut and the cyst, interposing varices or pancreatic parenchyma.[56] EUS evaluation was facilitated with radial endoscopes, which neither have a color Doppler facility nor allow puncture under direct vision, and the optimal drainage site was not marked. On subsequent endoscopic transmural puncture, these authors observed bleeding from the mucosal incision in two patients. They concluded that synchronous EUS including color Doppler imaging might have prevented bleeding. Other investigators have marked the selected puncture site with biopsy forceps. This has proved helpful, especially when there was no 'bulge' in the gut wall.[57–60] Finally, it should be noted that in cases of clearly visible 'bulging', some authors have considered that EUS may not be necessary to guide cyst drainage.[39]

EUS-guided drainage – available instruments

Drainage through small-channel linear echoendoscopes

With the development of linear echoendoscopes with a view parallel to the axis of the shaft, cysts could be punctured through the echoendoscope under direct vision. This enabled:

- EUS imaging, evaluation, and guided cyst drainage during the same procedure
- Precise puncture of cysts without 'bulging'
- Bypassing of intervening vessels
- Reduction in the risk of perforation.

Thus, EUS-guided drainage using a linear echoendoscope should avoid some of the complications reported with other non-surgical drainage procedures, as it would add the dimension of 'views through the gut wall' to the endoscopic approach.

In 1992, Grimm et al.[40] reported the first EUS-guided cyst drainage with a linear echoendoscope containing a 2-mm accessory channel in a patient with chronic pancreatitis complicated by a pancreatic tail pseudocyst without 'bulging' at a distance of 6 mm from the gastric wall. Access to the cyst was obtained with diathermy on a needle-knife within a 5-Fr Teflon catheter. Subsequently, the needle was removed from the catheter and exchanged for a guidewire. The echoendoscope was withdrawn, leaving the guidewire within the cyst. It was exchanged for a large-channel duodenoscope, through which a 10-Fr pigtail was inserted into the cyst cavity.[40]

The main drawback of this two-step technique was the necessity of switching endoscopes to allow a large enough stent to be placed, in the course of which guidewires would frequently slip out of the cyst. Being cumbersome, this technique was used in only a few centers with expertise in interventional endoscopy and EUS.[40,61,62]

As a consequence, data on cyst drainage with the two-step exchange mode described above are scarce. Binmoeller and Soehendra[61] reported successful cyst drainage in nine patients with symptomatic pseudocysts (mean diameter 11 cm), two of which involved no bulging of the gut wall. After 3–12 months' follow-up, disappearance of the cyst was seen in five patients, and small residual cysts remained in four.[61] In another series, EUS-guided cyst drainage was successful in 10 of 11 patients in whom transpapillary drainage was not possible. No complications were reported, but there were two recurrences.[62]

Drainage through large-channel echoendoscopes

In 1996, Wiersema[59] reported the first EUS-guided one-step cyst drainage with a 4-cm 6-Fr double-pigtail using a prototype 2.4-mm channel linear echoendoscope in a patient with a large cyst associated with perigastric venous collaterals. Giovannini et al.[63] reported one-step drainage using therapeutic echoendoscopes with 2.4–3.2-mm accessory channels. Six patients without pseudocyst 'bulging' were treated with 7- or 8-Fr nasocystic tubes or stents. In 1998, a case report was published of cyst drainage with a prototype 3.7-mm accessory channel endoscope and a newly developed delivery system for a 8.5-Fr stent.[64] In a further six patients, Seifert et al.[65] used a custom-made 7-Fr one-step stenting device through a 3.2-mm accessory channel of a linear therapeutic echoendoscope, and three patients were drained with a different 7-Fr one-step drainage system.[66] In a larger series of 35 patients, one-step EUS-guided cyst drainage was performed using 8.5-Fr stents, with no major complication and a success rate of 88.5%. Four patients with abscesses underwent surgery.[67]

The development of electronic linear echoendoscopes with larger working channels of 3.7 or 3.8 mm allowed the placement of larger-caliber 10-Fr stents;[68,69] this is mandatory for successful cyst drainage as smaller tubes have a high rate of occlusion and subsequent cyst infection.

A comparison of EUS-guided cyst drainage with the standard endoscopic technique indicated favorable initial and long-term success rates for the EUS technique (100% and 85% respectively, versus 84% and 74% for the standard technique), with a complication rate of 5% versus 10%, respectively.[70] This, however, is the only comparison available to date. Further and larger studies are necessary to evaluate the true potential of the EUS-guided technique alone and in relation to the standard approach. A summary of results achieved for drainage with large-channel echoendoscopes is provided in Table 25.4.

EUS-guided drainage – practical considerations

Evaluation of suitability

The first step is to detect the cyst with EUS. Despite being previously identified on CT, the cyst may not be visible with EUS, in which case the procedure is abandoned. Possible reasons for a cyst not being visible are that the lesion mimicked a pseudocyst on CT and was in fact solid, represented a fluid-filled duodenal diverticulum (Fig. 25.1C), or was a misinterpreted focal enlargement of the pancreatic or common bile duct.[18,20,56] The cyst may be present but located in the mesentery rather than the pancreatic region, and beyond the range of EUS.

Once the cyst has been detected, its morphologic appearance has to be evaluated and its suitability for drainage assessed.[71] In a recent study the collection of cyst fluid for CEA analysis proved to be significantly more accurate than evaluation of EUS morphology.[20] In consequence, cyst fluid should be aspirated for further tests once the cyst has been assessed, to

RESULTS OF PSEUDOCYST DRAINAGE USING LARGE-CHANNEL ECHOENDOSCOPES				
Reference	n	No. of successful procedures	No. with complications	No. with recurrence
Wiersema et al.[59]	1	1	0	0
Giovannini et al.[63]	6	6	0	1
Seifert et al.[65]	6	6	1 (septicemia)	0
Inui et al.[66]	3	3	0	1
Giovannini et al.[67]	35	31	1	NA
Seifert et al.[68]	4	4	0	NA
Wiersema et al.[69]	1	1	0	NA

Table 25.4 Results of pseudocyst drainage using large-channel echoendoscopes NA, data not available.

rule out pathology other than an inflammatory pseudocyst (see above and Ch. 17).

Ideally, prior to any endoscopic or image-guided drainage, diagnostic ERP should be performed, as it may have a crucial impact on the method of treatment. ERP is able to detect a possible connection of the cyst with the pancreatic duct, or other underlying reason for the pseudocyst such as a ductal stricture.[23,72] In these cases, transmural EUS-guided drainage may not be the sole best treatment for the pseudocyst, and transpapillary drainage alone or pancreatic stenting in addition to the transgastric or transduodenal drainage may be required. At present, this might be the optimal endoscopic approach for these patients, and may prevent further complications or setbacks, such as non-resolving cysts despite treatment or early recurrence following drainage. A transpapillary diagnostic or therapeutic approach may not be possible if there is gastric outlet obstruction, making it impossible to advance a duodenoscope to the papilla.

Some authors, however, have suggested that ERCP should not be performed in every possible patient as infection and pancreatitis might be induced. They recommend ERP only in patients without bulging, with symptoms after drainage, following recurrence, and when common bile duct stones are suspected.[39]

Preparation

Patients suitable for drainage should be selected carefully according to the criteria given above and in Table 25.5. It is advisable to perform cyst drainage under broad-spectrum antibiotic cover as the procedure is non-sterile and bacteria are brought into the cyst cavity. If at all possible, the procedure should be carried out under general anesthesia and with careful monitoring of the patient. Prior to cyst drainage, the stomach and duodenum should be inspected carefully for a 'bulge' or pathology such as varices. The procedure is best performed with large-channel (if available) linear echoendoscopes and fluoroscopy.

WHEN TO DRAIN A CYST	
Management	Clinical findings
Drainage indicated	>6 weeks' observation, ·6 cm, with symptoms
	Complications
	Connection between cyst and pancreatic duct
Drainage contraindication	Pseudoaneurysm
	Space between cyst and gut >1 cm
	Intervening vessels
Observation	Sterile cysts of diameter 4–6 cm
	<6 weeks' observation, >6 cm, no symptoms
	Constant size
	No complications

Table 25.5 When to drain a cyst

Technique

The techniques of EUS-guided cyst drainage and conventional endoscopic drainage share many similarities. However, it should be noted that the distal end of the accessory channel of the echoendoscope opens at a different angle to the channel of both the gastroscope and duodenoscope, and does not allow puncture perpendicular to the gut wall, which would be the optimal approach.

Small-channel echoendoscopes

If only a small-channel echoendoscope is available, the puncture can be made using a needle-knife within a 5-Fr Teflon catheter. The catheter tip is tapered to reduce the step between the catheter and the inner wire. Alternatively the puncture can be made using the 5-Fr Teflon catheter with a stiff wire or inner stylet of an EUS needle (Fig. 25.2). Once the cyst has been

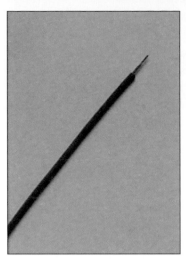

Fig. 25.2 5-Fr Teflon catheter with the inner stylet consisting of a stiff wire, which is the stylet of an EUS needle. This represents an early custom-made EUS puncture device.

visualized with EUS and the optimal puncture site selected, the needle-knife or wire can be advanced (2–3 mm should be sufficient). Electrocautery is used to guide the knife or wire and catheter through the gastric or duodenal wall into the cyst. Entry into the cyst can be felt by a sudden 'give' in resistance.[61] Successful puncture should be apparent on US (Fig. 25.3A) and can be confirmed fluoroscopically with contrast (Fig. 25.3B,C). Some 5–20 ml contrast should be sufficient, depending on the size of the cyst. The position of the catheter can also be confirmed by aspirating fluid, or saline can be injected through the catheter causing obvious turbulence in the cyst on US. Fluoroscopy may not be necessary if the needle is easily seen on US within the cyst and aspiration through the catheter demonstrates cyst fluid. Occasionally the US image is misleading, and fluid should always be aspirated to prove the catheter to be definitively within the cyst cavity. Regardless of the imaging method, the cyst should be aspirated to obtain fluid for biochemical, cytologic, and bacteriologic analysis.

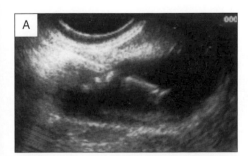

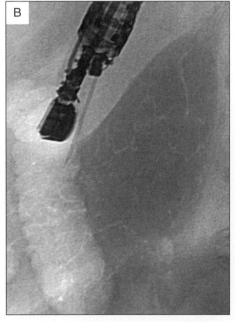

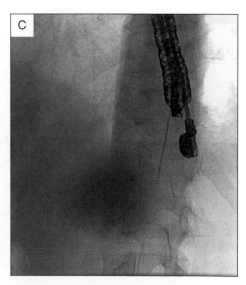

Fig. 25.3 **A,** Successful puncture of a cyst. On the EUS image the needle can be seen deep within the cyst cavity. Successful puncture (**B**) is proven fluoroscopically by injecting contrast (**C**).

Once the puncture has been performed, correct catheter placement confirmed, and fluid aspirated, a 0.035-inch guidewire is inserted via the catheter well into the cyst cavity.

Early linear echoendoscopes have an accessory channel size of only 2 mm, which is not large enough for direct stent placement. Consequently, the echoendoscope has to be exchanged over a guidewire for a 4.2-mm channel therapeutic gastroscope or duodenoscope. This should be done under fluoroscopic control to prevent losing the position of the guidewire. This exchange is the most critical part of the procedure, and failure most often occurs at this point.

After the large-channel gastroscope or duodenoscope has been advanced over the guidewire to the puncture site, one or multiple 10-Fr stents, pigtails, and/or a nasocystic catheter can be advanced into the cyst (Fig. 25.4).

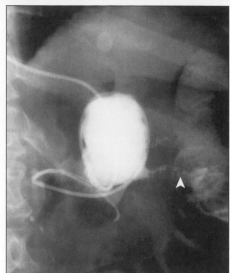

Fig. 25.4 A nasocystic drain has been placed into a large pseudocyst. Contrast has proven correct placement, but also communication between the cyst and the colon (arrowhead).

Large-channel EUS-guided cyst drainage

With large-channel echoendoscopes of 3.7 mm, now commercially available, the first part of the procedure is identical. The cyst is localized and evaluated as with the small-channel scope. A suitable site for puncture is selected. The distance between the bowel and the cyst is measured, and color Doppler imaging used to identify intervening vessels. The cyst is then punctured with an EUS needle or needle-knife (see Fig. 25.3A,B). To use the needle-knife, the inner needle is exposed a few millimeters beyond its protective sheath. Using electrocautery under direct vision, the bowel wall is penetrated and the needle-knife advanced into the cyst cavity. Visualization of the needle with US in real time allows the operator to stop when the needle is far enough into the cyst (see Fig. 25.3A). The needle is then removed, leaving the protecting sheath in place. The cyst should be aspirated to confirm correct placement and for analysis. At this stage, depending on the appearance of the fluid, a decision is made to place either a stent

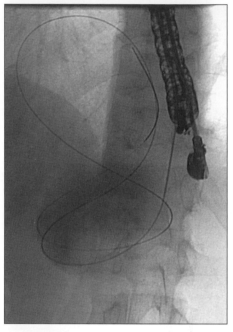

Fig. 25.5 A 0.035-inch guidewire is advanced via the catheter and coiled in the cavity.

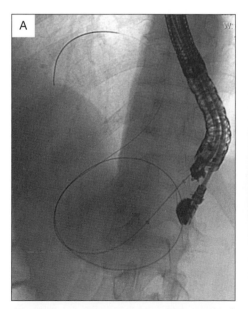

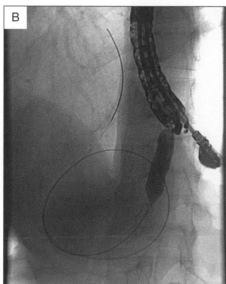

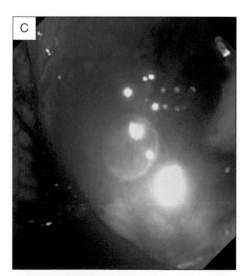

Fig. 25.6 **A,** To permit easy placement of stents of larger diameter (10–12 Fr), the needle track needs to be dilated. A balloon is advanced over the guidewire. Radio-opaque markers on the catheter make the position visible. **B,** The balloon is fully inflated. **C,** Inflation of the balloon can also be seen endoscopically. Once the balloon is inflated, the endoscopic view of the puncture site will be blurred because of the balloon material.

or a nasocystic tube. Although not essential, some physicians would perform a contrast study with fluoroscopy to obtain further information, for example to assess potential communications between the cyst and pancreatic duct or other organs (Fig. 25.4).

With the catheter still in the cyst, a 0.035-inch guidewire is advanced and coiled in the cavity (Fig. 25.5). The catheter is then withdrawn, leaving the guidewire in place. 7-Fr stents or catheters can be introduced without further preparation (see Fig. 25.4), but in general placement of larger-diameter devices is preferred. For this, the needle track needs to be dilated, which is best achieved with a 4–8-mm balloon (Fig. 25.6). Once the balloon is removed, stents of up to 12 Fr can be deployed. By repeating this procedure, several stents can be placed to obtain a larger communication between the cyst and the gut (Figs 25.8 & 25.9), and maintain drainage into the stomach or duodenum. This is particularly important when the cyst is infected or debris is found.

Although with large-channel echoendoscopes no exchange of scopes is necessary, there are still a number of steps to

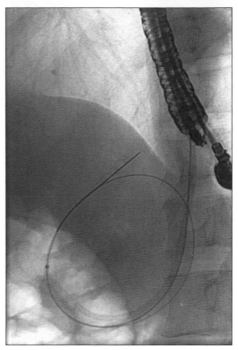

Fig. 25.7   A stent has been deployed over the guidewire. By repeating this procedure, several stents can be placed to obtain a larger communication between the cyst and the gut.

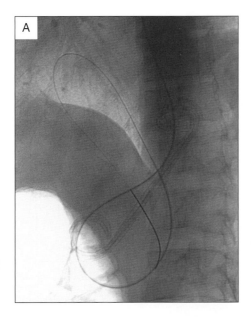

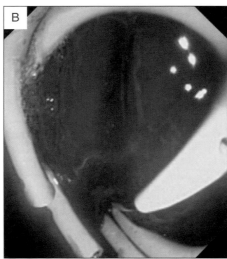

Fig. 25.8   **A,** Placement of several stents and a nasocystic tube into an infected cyst. **B,** Endoscopic view: two stents have been placed and a nasocystic tube is on its way into the cyst cavity; it can be seen running over the guidewire.

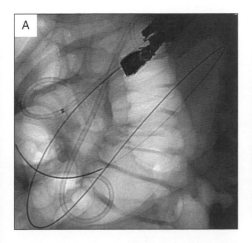

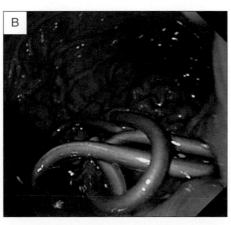

Fig. 25.9   **A,** Radiographic image of several stents that have been placed to obtain a larger communication between the cyst and the gut; the guidewire is in the cavity to enable placement of another stent. **B,** Endoscopic view of several pigtails that are draining a pseudocyst, passing through the gastric wall.

cyst drainage (Table 25.6). This has led to varying designs of drainage sets, enabling all the steps to be performed without removing the wire or protecting catheter. Vilmann et al.[64] and Seifert et al.[65,68] have reported the development and use of custom-made puncture–drainage sets. In one, the needle was loaded with a 7-Fr Teflon pusher and a modified 7-Fr stent that had two side-holes and four flaps to prevent dislocation. A thread attached the stent to the pusher and could be released by removal of the puncture needle (Fig. 25.10).[68]

Giovannini et al.[63] reported a single-step drainage using a needle-knife, Teflon catheter, and guidewire, allowing placement of an 8.5-Fr stent. A similar drainage set is commercially available (Giovannini needle wire oasis; Cook, Limerick, Ireland). This is an all-in-one stent introduction system, containing a needle-wire, guiding catheter, and pushing catheter with a back-loaded stent (Fig. 25.11). This device can be used through a 3.2-mm accessory channel of an echoendoscope without the need for any exchanges.

This system improves the ease of EUS-guided pseudocyst drainage for routine use, although at present it is the only commercially available device, and still has its shortcomings. More and other appropriate and commercially available tools need to be developed to make this method accessible to the echoendoscopy community at large.

THE STEPS OF CYST DRAINAGE
1 Find cyst with EUS
2 Find optimal puncture site
• Gastric or duodenal – distance of cyst <1 cm
• No intervening vessels
3 Puncture cyst through gut wall using electrocautery
4 Remove needle or wire, leave protecting catheter in place
5 Aspirate cyst fluid
• Collect fluid for further analysis
• Decide between nasocystic drainage or stenting
6 Advance guidewire
7 Dilate tract over guidewire
8 Advance stent or drainage catheter

Table 25.6 The steps of cyst drainage

DRAINAGE OF THE PANCREATIC AND COMMON BILE DUCTS

Developments and results

Recently, therapeutic approaches using EUS guidance for interventional techniques have been explored and attempts

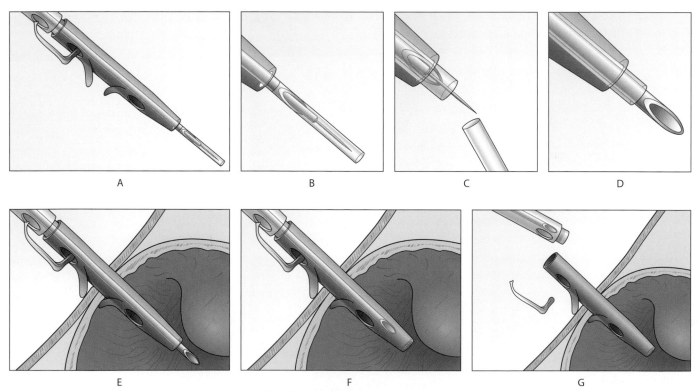

Fig. 25.10 Custom made single step device suitable for 3.7 mm accessory channel: **A,** 10F pusher and stent placed over a 6F catheter, which holds a 1 mm steel needle with stylet. A piece of tubing **(B)** covers the needle, and is released by retraction of the needle against the catheter **(C)**. By withdrawing the inner stylet the system is ready for use **(D)**. The examiner can puncture the cyst and push the stent into its final position **(E, F)**. By withdrawing the inner needle, the stent is released from the catheter **(G)**. From Seifert H, Faust D, Schmitt T, Dietrich C, Caspary W, Wehrmann T. Transmural drainage of cystic peripancreatic lesions with a new large-channel echo endoscope. Endoscopy 2001; 33:1022–1026, with permission from Georg Thieme Publishers.

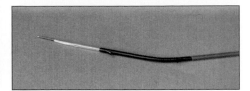

Fig. 25.11 Giovannini needle wire oasis. This is an all-in-one stent introduction system, containing a needle-wire, guiding catheter, pushing catheter, and back-loaded stent.

made to cannulate and drain organs or structures other than pancreatic pseudocysts. Owing to the close proximity to the upper gastrointestinal tract, the common bile duct, the left intrahepatic ducts, and the main pancreatic duct can be visualized well with EUS. EUS-guided transgastric or transduodenal drainage of these ducts, when ERCP or endoscopic approaches were not possible, seemed a logical development.

In 1995 the first case of EUS-guided pancreatography was published,[73] followed by another case report of a patient with surgically altered anatomy.[74] In 1996, EUS-guided transduodenal cholangiography and transgastric pancreatography were reported in two patients who had failed ERCP,[75] and recently case reports of EUS-guided rendezvous drainage of obstructed biliary and pancreatic ducts were published.[76]

An animal study demonstrated the feasibility of performing EUS-guided hepaticogastrotomy for the palliation of obstructive jaundice.[77] The study was performed in five pigs with laparoscopically ligated bile ducts. EUS was used as a guide for the location, puncture, and stenting of dilated left-sided intrahepatic bile ducts through the gastric fundus. In three of the five pigs stenting was possible over a guidewire. Owing to the small channel size of the echoendoscope (2 mm), only 5-Fr stents could be deployed without exchanging the endoscopes. Although complications of cholangitis and migration were reported, this method offered a potentially useful alternative to percutaneous drainage or surgery for palliation of obstruction in patients with pancreatic or bile duct cancer.

In 2001, Giovannini et al.[78] demonstrated the feasibility of this technique in humans in a patient with biliary obstruction from pancreatic cancer. Attempts to access the duct by the transpapillary route had failed. The common bile duct (CBD) was punctured through the duodenum under EUS guidance with a 5-Fr needle-knife and the echoendoscope exchanged over a guidewire for a large-channel duodenoscope. After dilatation, a 10-Fr stent was inserted.[78] Burmester et al.[79] reported on a further four patients, in three of whom transmural EUS-guided bile duct drainage was performed. Two patients had partial gastrectomies with Bilroth II reconstructions. Larger-channel echoendoscopes (3.2 mm accessory channel) were available in this study, and a single-step technique was possible, which enabled the application of 8.5-Fr stents without the need to exchange endoscopes. Transmural drainage was achieved by transduodenal or transgastric access to the CBD or left intrahepatic bile ducts.[79] In another case a self-expandable metal stent was introduced to form a palliative hepaticogastrostomy.[80]

Bile leakage into the peritoneal cavity is a risk.[77,79] In an attempt to overcome the possibility of leakage, a stent system has been developed and tested in animals, and provides a spring force onto the drainage stent and route. This enables the stomach to be kept in direct proximity to the liver (duodenum to CBD), to avoid leakage into the peritoneal cavity.[81] This system and device needs further testing in patients.

Successful drainage of the pancreatic duct has also been reported. Pancreaticogastrostomy for ductal decompression was performed in four patients with chronic pancreatitis, providing an interesting alternative method of drainage where ERP fails to access the occluded pancreatic duct.[82]

It may be noted that all of these methods require technically highly experienced endoscopists with additional expertise in EUS. They should be performed only under study conditions, and reserved for patients in whom ERCP has failed.

Although EUS-guided drainage of the intrahepatic and extrahepatic bile ducts or the pancreatic duct has been demonstrated to be technically feasible, only these few case reports have been published to date. Possible complications such as biliary peritonitis, pancreatitis, stent migration, and bleeding need to be evaluated in larger numbers of patients in long-term follow-up studies. Although transmural drainage through these fistulae follow a pressure gradient from the obstructed duct to the larger bowel lumen, it is most likely that they need to be kept open by stenting, and the frequency of stent exchange due to occlusion or migration remains unknown. As the fistulae do

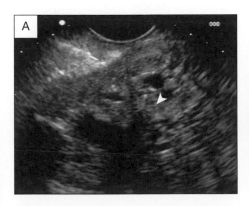

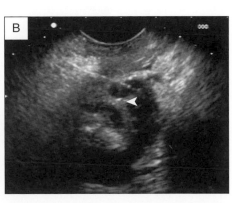

Fig. 25.12 **A,** The EUS needle has punctured a dilated left-sided intrahepatic bile duct from the stomach. The needle can be seen within the duct (arrowhead). **B,** The stylet has been removed and replaced with a guidewire (arrowhead).

not follow an anatomic drainage route, it is possible that closure of this route, once wanted, may be difficult and may make surgery necessary. Further and larger studies are needed to evaluate the true potential of this technique.

Technique of EUS-guided bile duct and pancreatic duct drainage

EUS-guided drainage of the pancreatic, common bile, or intra-hepatic ducts is similar to pancreatic pseudocyst drainage. Although the CBD is assessed from the duodenum, the main pancreatic and intrahepatic bile ducts are approached from the stomach. The procedure has to be performed in a fluoroscopy suite, if possible under general anesthesia and with antibiotic cover. A 22- or 19-gauge EUS-needle is used to access the duct (Fig. 25.12A,B). Once the needle is seen to be within the required duct, the inner stylet can be withdrawn and contrast injected. The pancreatogram or cholangiogram can be visualized under fluoroscopy (Fig. 25.13). If drainage is required, a guidewire is advanced into the duct as deeply as possible (see Fig. 25.12B).

Depending on the size of the echoendoscope accessory channel, drainage is performed with a two-step or single-step technique. If only echoendoscopes with a 2.0–3.2-mm channel size are available and stents larger than 5–8.5 Fr are required, the echoendoscope has to be exchanged for a larger-channel duodenoscope over the guidewire.

When drainage is attempted through the gastric wall, stability and resistance of the echoendoscope may be a problem. As a large, stretchable, hollow organ, the stomach does not provide any abutment to resist the force on the tip of the echoendoscope when a needle-knife, dilator, or stent is being pushed through the gastric wall. To achieve abutments, echoendoscopes can be pushed into a long loop against the greater curve of the stomach to return to the lesser curve. This maneuver may provide better stability and enables greater force to be used on materials pushed through the accessory channel. It may also be useful for a nurse to hold the echoendoscope at the patient's mouth and to push it further into the gut to provide more stability.

Once the duodenoscope is in place, a 6.5-Fr catheter with a metal tip for electrocautery can be used to enlarge the channel between the required duct and the stomach or duodenum. The sheath is withdrawn and the required stent positioned under fluoroscopy (Fig. 25.14 & 25.15). This procedure is particularly useful in cases where the papilla is no longer accessible (Fig. 25.15).

If the channel size of the echoendoscope is 3.7 or 3.8 mm, no exchange is necessary and the whole procedure can be performed as a single step.

Drainage of the pancreatic duct can be achieved in the same way, as depicted in Fig. 25.16. A fluoroscopic image of EUS-guided 5-Fr stent placement into the pancreatic duct is shown in Fig. 25.17.

EUS-GUIDED ANASTOMOSIS FORMATION

In recent years physicians have extended the field of endoscopy and have been developing 'transluminal endosurgery' for more invasive endoscopic examinations, in which endoscopes are deliberately pushed across the wall of the gastrointestinal tract. Examples are retroperitoneal endoscopic debridement for

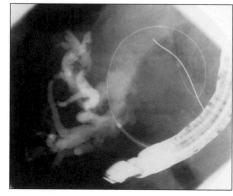

Fig. 25.14   The cholangio-stent is positioned under fluoroscopic control.

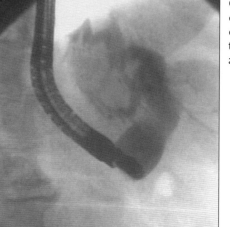

Fig. 25.13 Cholangiogram obtained by means of an EUS-guided transgastric approach.

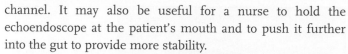

Fig. 25.15   Patient with pancreatic cancer who had previously had a transpapillary stent inserted. The stent was occluded and no longer accessible because of duodenal stenosis. Drainage was achieved by means of a transgastric biliary approach. The stent is being placed with the transpapillary stent still in situ. Gift from E. Burmester.

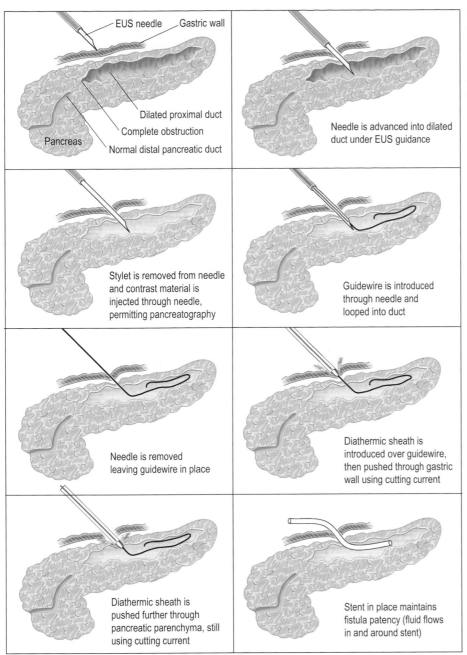

Fig. 25.16 A–H, EUS-guided pancreatic drainage. Reprinted from Gastrointestinal endoscopy, 56, Francois E, Kahaleh M, Giovannini M et al, EUS-guided pancreaticogastrostomy, 128–133, 2002, with permission from the American Society for Gastrointestinal Endoscopy.[82]

infected peripancreatic necrosis and transgastric gastrojejunal anastomosis formation.[83,84]

Simultaneous with the development of endoscopic transgastric methods, new types of EUS-guided interventions for therapy have been explored, and are resulting in the new field of therapeutic EUS-guided endosurgery (EUGE) and in the development of procedures similar to transgastric endoscopic endosurgery. Both of these methods represent moves into areas and techniques that have been purely surgical for many years. One new and so far experimental EUGE method is the creation of anastomoses between various kinds of organs and the stomach to palliate the complications of malignant diseases or to provide therapy in patients deemed to have inoperable disease.

Endoscopic transgastric procedures involve the penetration of non-sterile endoscopes into sterile abdominal areas to reach target organs such as the small bowel loops. This is achieved mainly by cutting the peritoneal or retroperitoneal cavity through the gastric wall. To date, it is not known which complications will arise and whether bacteremia or sepsis will present an insurmountable obstacle, or whether sterility can be achieved.

EUS can be used to visualize some otherwise endoscopically inaccessible organs, such as small bowel loops, the gallbladder, or intrahepatic bile ducts, through the gastric wall. It can assist in the guidance of needles and other tools to these organs, and help to deploy devices with precision beyond the gut wall without the need to cut a direct and unsterile passage through it.

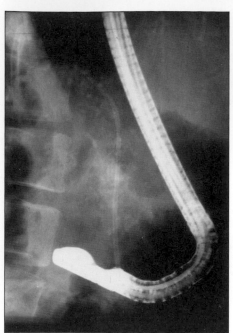

Fig. 25.17
Radiographic image showing EUS-guided placement of a 5-Fr stent into the pancreatic duct.

It may provide non-surgical access to these organs without the risk of soiling the peritoneal or mediastinal cavity. As a consequence, EUS guidance may overcome some obstacles of the transgastric endoscopic approach without the need to abandon the procedures. However, new tools and devices for such EUS-guided operations still need to be developed.

Anastomosis suture system

To perform an anastomosis, it is necessary to place sutures and attach different organs to one another under EUS guidance. A prototype suturing system has been developed for the placement of stitches within or beyond the gut wall under EUS guidance.[85]

A metal anchor attached to a 2-m thread (Fig. 25.18A) can be loaded into the hollow tip of a commercially available 19-G flexible EUS needle (Echotip; Wilson Cook, Winston-Salem, NC, USA) once its inner stylet has been withdrawn (Fig. 25.18B,C). Under EUS control, this needle assembly can be guided from the gut lumen into any structure or hollow organ within 5 cm of the endoscope tip under direct vision. Once it has reached its target, the withdrawn stylet can be pushed forward to eject the anchor with thread. The metal anchor appears as a hyperechoic structure with some reflections on the ultrasound screen. When the needle is withdrawn, the thread will appear out of the gut wall and be visible endoscopically. Once gentle traction is put on the thread, the anchor will pull the target organ into which it was ejected to the gut wall. Subsequently, the thread can either be securely locked as a stitch against the gut wall or be pulled back with the endoscope

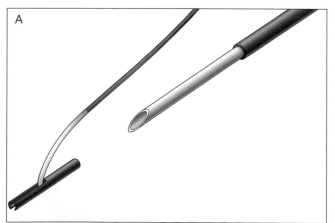

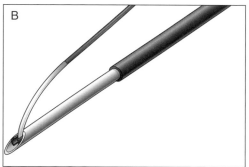

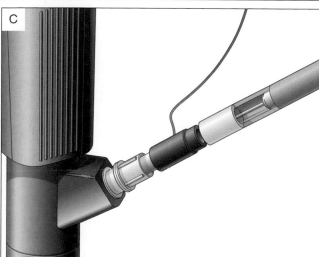

Fig. 25.18   A & B, A metal anchor attached to a 2-m thread is being back-loaded into the hollow tip of a commercially available 19-gauge flexible EUS needle with its inner stylet withdrawn. **C,** Before the needle is advanced through the accessory channel, an interface piece with a hole is screwed onto the needle to allow the thread to be guided freely out of the accessory channel.

through the patient's mouth to allow manipulation from the outside.[86] A specially designed locking and cutting mechanism enables secure connection between different organs and/or structures.[85–88]

How to perform an anastomosis

An anastomosis is created by pushing the 19-G EUS needle hosting the suturing system from the stomach, etc. into the desired organ (Fig. 25.19). The anchor is ejected and pulled at,

or locked, to appose securely, for instance, the small bowel to the gastric wall. Once the inner hollow part of the needle has been emptied from the anchor, a 0.035-inch guidewire is advanced into the small bowel loop and the needle withdrawn (Fig. 25.20). This can be used to guide segments of a 7-Fr Teflon catheter joined by a thread into the lumen of the small bowel. Once the thread is pulled back, the fragments of catheter come together to form a cross (Fig. 25.21), providing a counter-pressure from the small bowel for a compression device, which

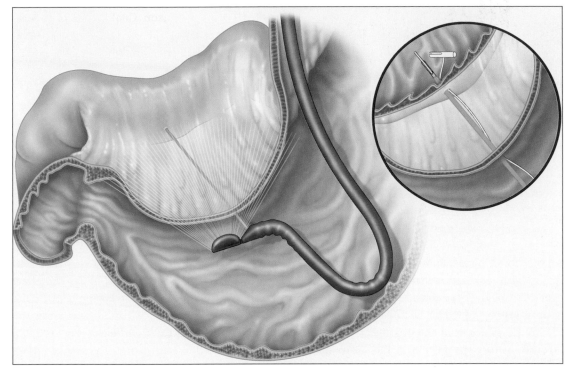

Fig. 25.19   Under EUS guidance the needle hosting the suturing system has been pushed from the stomach into the small bowel and the tag ejected (see window).

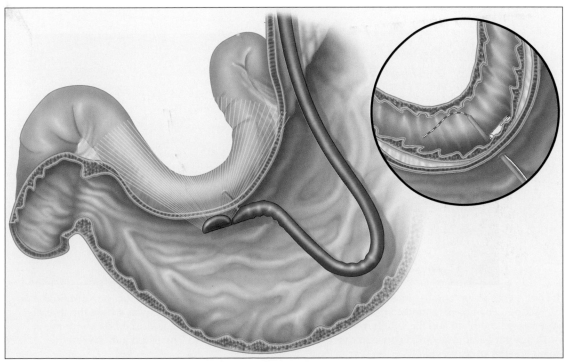

Fig. 25.20   By pulling on the thread (attached to the anchor) outside the endoscope, the small bowel is pulled towards the gastric wall. The ejected anchor has emptied the hollow needle, leaving room for a 0.035-inch guidewire, which is advanced into the small bowel (see window).

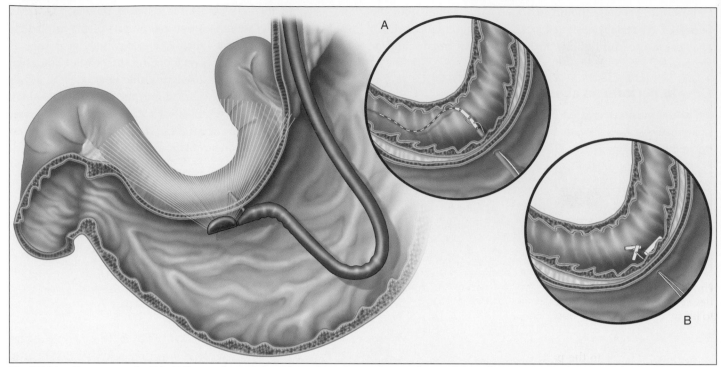

Fig. 25.21   Segments of a 7-Fr Teflon catheter joined by a thread are advanced over the guidewire into the lumen of the small bowel (window A). Once the guidewire is withdrawn and the thread pulled back, the catheter fragments assume a cruciform configuration (window B).

is deployed endoscopically from the stomach side. Subsequently, a plate to spread the force, spring, and locking mechanism is back-loaded onto the tip of a gastroscope over the thread holding the counterpressure. The gastroscope is guided by the thread to the point of its emergence from the gastric wall and pushed against it, to compress the spring against the plate and the counterpressure system in the small bowel (Fig. 25.22A,B). It forces the two walls of the different organs together with a pressure high enough to cause ischemia to the tissue in between, and is then locked in place (Fig. 25.22C). The effect can be directly seen while compressing the spring because the gastric tissue turns a whitish color, which differs from the natural color of the surrounding gastric mucosa (Fig. 25.22C). An opening will be formed in approximately 2–5 days (Fig. 25.23). Additional maneuvers are necessary to keep the fistula open and for enlargement to allow easy passage of food.

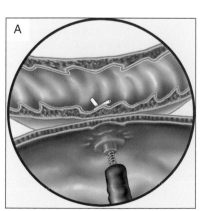
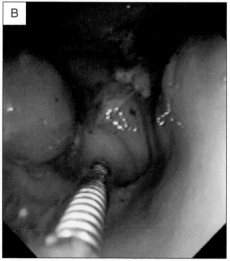
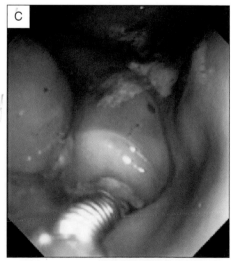

Fig. 25.22   **A,** Once the guidewire is withdrawn and the thread pulled back, the catheter fragments assume a cruciform configuration to provide an abutment. A gastroscope with a back-loaded compression device is pushed against the gastric wall, where the thread emerges, to compress the spring against the plate and the counterpressure system in the small bowel. **B,** Endoscopic view of the compression device. The spring is not yet compressed. **C,** Endoscopic view of the compressed spring. The tissue in between the compression parts appears white as a sign of ischaemia.

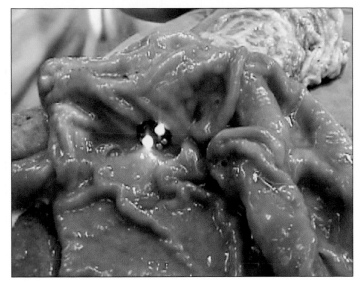

Fig. 25.23   Autopsy finding of an animal in which a compression device had been placed. The anastomosis formed is large enough to be passed by a gastroscope.

As an alternative to the parts of catheter forming a cross, a balloon can be pushed over the guidewire and inflated once in the small bowel (Fig. 25.24).[89] Because the anastomosis obtained is larger, this has become the preferred method.

The technique described above may also be used to access the gallbladder, which is in direct proximity to the wall of the antrum and therefore within easy reach of EUS for approximation to the gastric wall. With a direct connection between the gallbladder and stomach, easy access to gallstones would

enable them to be extracted with a Dormia basket. Animal studies have been performed successfully and studies in humans are awaited.[87,89]

CONCLUSIONS

This chapter has spanned from cyst drainage, the most frequently performed routine therapeutic intervention, to anastomosis formation, currently the most experimental one. EUS-guided interventional procedures are highly dependent on the personal skills, training, and tools available. They are likely, although not certain, to expand with new young enthusiastic endoscopists joining the current teams. With this enthusiasm, the long learning curve, expense of the equipment, and somewhat limited availability of linear-array EUS training facilities, combined with the conservatism of some EUS practitioners, might be overcome, and future generations of endosonographers supported by their teachers may be stimulated to push back the current limits.

An ideal therapeutic technique has been described as having a high success rate, few complications, a low mortality rate, and to be universally applicable and cost effective.[15] However, although new, experimental and under development, the survival of EUS-guided interventional techniques will depend on demonstration of their superiority over existing, proven techniques, and they will have to achieve appropriate benchmarks. The minimally invasive nature of EUS-guided interventional techniques and the short period of hospitalization, resulting in lower costs, have already been demonstrated. There also

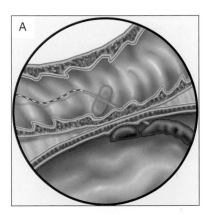
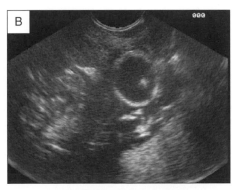
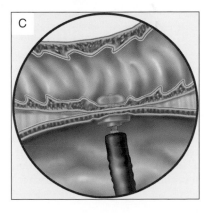
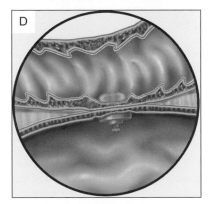

Fig. 25.24   **A,** A balloon, advanced over the guidewire into the small bowel, can be inflated and serve as a counterpressure device. **B–D,** Once the second balloon has been deployed and presses against the small bowel balloon, a spring can be locked in place and the catheter cut.

appears to be a low associated mortality rate together with a high success rate. Only applicability remains to be shown – and this may be only a matter of time.

The potential of future therapeutic indications for EUS is great and has been barely explored. Some new ideas and interventions have started to become reality but much more remains to be done … let's do it!

ACKNOWLEDGMENTS

The author wishes to thank Omar Vakharia for his extraordinary drawings, Mark Pelling, Peter Milla, and Kamini Patel for their relentless corrections in style and grammar, and Jan-Werner Poley and Eike Burmester for their excellent imaging support.

EXAMINATION CHECKLIST

For EUS-guided pseudocyst drainage:
- Adminster prophylactic antibiotics
- Use a large-channel linear EUS endoscope and fluoroscopy
- After entering the cyst, aspirate fluid for CEA level, amylase, and cytology
- In case of multiple stent insertion, dilate tract with a balloon or 10-Fr electrocautery device (Cystotome; Cook, Limerick, Ireland).

REFERENCES

1 Chang KJ, Nguyen PT, Thompson JA, et al. Phase I clinical trial of allogeneic mixed lymphocyte culture (cytoimplant) delivered by endoscopic ultrasound-guided fine-needle injection in patients with advanced pancreatic carcinoma. Cancer 2000; 88:1325–1335.

2 Goldberg SN, Mallery S, Gazelle GS, et al. EUS-guided radiofrequency ablation in the pancreas: preliminary results in a porcine model. Gastrointest Endosc 1999; 50:392–401.

3 Barclay RL, Perez-Miranda M, Giovannini M. EUS-guided treatment of solid hepatic metastasis. Gastrointest Endosc 2002; 55:266–270.

4 Gunter E, Lingenfelser T, Eitelbach F, et al. EUS-guided ethanol injection for treatment of GI stromal tumor. Gastrointest Endosc 2003; 57:113–115.

5 Kozarek RA, Brayko CM, Harlan J, et al. Endoscopic drainage of pancreatic pseudocysts. Gastrointest Endosc 1985; 31:322–327.

6 Bradley EL III. A clinically based classification system for acute pancreatitis. Arch Surg 1993; 128:586–590.

7 Bradley EL III, Consalez AC, Clements JL. Acute pancreatic pseudocysts. Incidence and implication. Ann Surg 1976; 184:734–737.

8 Bradley EL, Clements JL, Gonzales AC. The natural history of pancreatic pseudocysts: a unified concept of management. Am J Surg 1979; 137:135–141.

9 Fedorak IJ, Rao R, Prinz RA, et al. The clinical challenge of multiple pancreatic pseudocysts. Am J Surg 1994; 168:22–28.

10 Warshaw AL, Rattner DW. Timing of surgical drainage for pancreatic pseudocysts. Ann Surg 1985; 202:720–724.

11 Beebe DS, Burbrinck MP, Onstad GR, et al. Management of pancreatic pseudocysts. Surg Gynecol Obstet 1984; 159:562–564.

12 Yeo CJ, Bastida JA, Lynch-Nyhan A, et al. The natural history of pancreatic pseudocysts documented by computed tomography. Surg Gynecol Obstet 1990; 170:411–417.

13 Amman RW, Akovbiantz A, Largiader F, et al. Course and outcome of chronic pancreatitis. Longitudinal study of a mixed medical–surgical series of 245 patients. Gastroenterology 1984; 86:820–828.

14 O'Malley VP, Cannon JP, Postie RG. Pancreatic pseudocysts: cause, therapy, and results. Am J Surg 1985; 150:680–682.

15 Gumaste VV, Pitchumoni CS. Pancreatic pseudocyst. Gastroenterologist 1996; 4:33–43.

16 Howell DA, Elton E, Parsons WG. Endoscopic management of pseudocyst of the pancreas. Gastrointest Endosc Clin N Am 1998; 8:143–161.

17 Koito K, Namieno T, Nagakawa T, et al. Solitary cystic tumor of the pancreas: EUS–pathologic correlation. Gastrointest Endosc 1997; 45:268–276.

18 Brugge WR. Evaluation of pancreatic cystic lesions with EUS. Gastrointest Endosc 2004; 59:698–707.

19 Ahmad NA, Kochman ML, Brensinger C, et al. Interobserver agreement among endosonographers for the diagnosis of neoplastic versus non-neoplastic pancreatic cystic lesions. Gastrointest Endosc 2003; 58:59–64.

20 Brugge WR, Lewandrowski K, Lee-Lewandowski E, et al. Diagnosis of pancreatic cystic neoplasms: a report of the cooperative pancreatic cyst study. Gastroenterology 2004; 126:1330–1336.

21 Vitas GJ, Sarr MG. Selected management of pancreatic pseudocysts. Operative versus expectant management. Surgery 1992; 111:123–130.

22 Baron TH, Thaggard WG, Morgan DE, et al. Endoscopic therapy for organized pancreatic necrosis. Gastroenterology 1996; 111:755–764.

23 Baron TH, Harewood GC, Morgan De, et al. Outcome differences after endoscopic drainage of pancreatic necrosis, acute pancreatic pseudocysts, and chronic pancreatic pseudocysts. Gastrointest Endosc 2002; 56:7–17.

24 Hariri M, Slivka A, Carr-Locke DL, et al. Pseudocysts drainage predisposes to infection when pancreatic necrosis is unrecognized. Am J Gastroenterol 1994; 89:1781–1784.

25 Grace PA, Williamson RCN. Modern management of pancreatic pseudocysts. Br J Surg 1993; 80:573–581.

26 Sahel J. Endoscopic treatment of pancreatic cysts and pseudocysts. In: Beger HG, Buechler M, Malfertheiner P (eds). Standards in pancreatic surgery. Berlin: Springer; 1993:526–532.

27 Cremer M, Deviere J, Engelholm L. Endoscopic management of cysts and pseudocysts in chronic pancreatitis: long term follow-up after 7 years of experience. Gastrointest Endosc 1989; 35:1–9.

28 Adams DB, Anderson MC. Percutaneous catheter drainage compared with internal drainage in the management of pancreatic pseudocyst. Ann Surg 1992; 215:571–576.

29 Marshall GT, Douglas DA, Hanson BL, et al. Multidisciplinary approach to pseudoaneurysms complicating pancreatic pseudocysts. Arch Surg 1996; 131:278–283.

30 Kohler H, Schafmeyer A, Ludtke FE, et al. Surgical treatment of pancreatic pseudocysts. Br J Surg 1987; 74:813–815.

31 Hancke S, Pedersen JF. Percutaneous puncture of pancreatic cysts. Guided by ultrasound. Surg Gynecol Obstet 1976; 142:551–552.

32 Hancke S, Henriksen FW. Percutaneous pancreatic cystogastrostomy by ultrasound scanning and gastroscopy. Br J Surg 1985; 72:916–917.

33 Dunkin BJ, Ponsky JL, Hale JC. Ultrasound directed percutaneous endoscopic cyst gastrostomy for the treatment of pancreatic pseudocyst. Surg Endosc 1998; 12:1426–1429.

34 White SA, Sutton CD, Berry DP, et al. Experience of combined endoscopic percutaneous stenting with ultrasound guidance for drainage of pancreatic pseudocysts. Ann R Coll Surg Engl 2000; 82:11–15.

35 Hershfield NB. Drainage of pancreatic pseudocyst. Gastrointest Endosc 1984; 30:269–270.

36 Beckingham IJ, Krige JE, Bornman PC, et al. Long term outcome of endoscopic drainage of pancreatic pseudocysts. Am J Gastroenterol 1999; 94:71–74.

37 Mönkemuller KE, Baron TH, Morgan DE. Transmural drainage of pancreatic fluid collections without electrocautery using the Seldinger technique. Gastrointest Endosc 1998; 48:195–199.

38 Smits ME, Rauws EA, Tytgat GN, et al. The efficacy of endoscopic treatment of pancreatic pseudocysts. Gastrointest Endosc 1995; 42:202–207.

39 Sharma SS, Bhargawa N, Govil A. Endoscopic management of pancreatic pseudocyst: a long term follow-up. Endoscopy 2002; 34:202–207.

40 Grimm H, Binmoeller KF, Soehendra N. Endosonography guided drainage of a pancreatic pseudocyst. Gastrointest Endosc 1992; 38:170–171.

41 Donelly PK, Lavelle P, Carr-Locke DL. Massive haemorrhage following endoscopic transgastric drainage of pancreatic pseudocyst. Br J Surg 1990; 77:758–759.

42 Libera ED, Siqueira ES, Morais M, et al. Pancreatic pseudocysts transpapillary and transmural drainage. HPB Surg 2000; 11:333–338.

43 Dohmoto M, Akiyama K, Tioka Y. Endoscopic and endosonographic management of pancreatic pseudocyst: follow-up. Rev Gastroenterol Peru 2003; 23:269–275.

44 Binmoeller KF, Seifert H, Walter A, et al. Transpapillary and transmural drainage of pancreatic pseudocysts. Gastrointest Endosc 1995; 42:219–224.

45 De Palma GD, Galloro G, Puzziello A, et al. Endoscopic drainage of pancreatic pseudocysts: a long term follow-up study of 49 patients. Hepatogastroenterology 2002; 49:1113–1115.

46 Beckingham IJ, Krige JE, Bornman PC, et al. Endoscopic management of pancreatic pseudocysts. Br J Surg 1997; 84:1638–1645.

47 Barthet M, Sahel J, Bodiou-Bertei C, et al. Endoscopic transpapillary drainage of pancreatic pseudocysts. Gastrointest Endosc 1995; 42:208–213.

48 Catalano MF, Geenan JE, Schmalz MJ, et al. Treatment of pancreatic pseudocysts with ductal communication by transpapillary pancreatic duct endoprosthesis. Gastrointest Endosc 1995; 42:214–218.

49 Kozarek RA, Ball TJ, Patterson DJ, et al. Endoscopic transpapillary therapy for disrupted pancreatic duct and peripancreatic fluid collections. Gastroenterology 1991; 100:1362–1370.

50 Lo SK, Anderson R. Endoscopic management of pancreatic pseudocysts. Gastroenterologist 1997; 5:10–25.

51 Chak A. Spearing pseudocysts with Seldinger and sonography. Gastrointest Endosc 1998; 48:221–223.

52 Becker WF, Welsh RA, Pratt HS. Cystadenoma and cystadenocarcinoma of the pancreas. Ann Surg 1965; 161:845–860.

53 Norton ID, Clain JE, Wiersema MJ, et al. Utility of endoscopic ultrasound in endoscopic drainage of pancreatic pseudocysts in selected patients. Mayo Clin Proc 2001; 76:794–798.

54 Roesch T, Lorenz R, Neuhaus H, et al. The value of endoscopic ultrasound in chronic pancreatitis. Gastrointest Endosc 1991; 37:A254.

55 Wiersema MJ, Kochman ML, Hawes RN, et al. Endoscopic ultrasound compared with CT and ERCP in the evaluation of pancreatic pseudocysts. Gastrointest Endosc 1993; 39:A336.

56 Fockens P, Johnson TG, van Dullemen HM, et al. Endosonographic imaging of pancreatic pseudocysts before endoscopic transmural drainage. Gastrointest Endosc 1997; 46:412–416.

57 Chan AT, Hellet SJ, Van Dam J, et al. Endoscopic cystgastrostomy: role of endoscopic ultrasonography. Am J Gastroenterol 1996; 91:1622–1625.

58 Gerolami R, Giovannini M, Laugier R. Endoscopic drainage of pancreatic pseudocysts guided by endosonography. Endoscopy 1997; 27:106–108.

59 Wiersema MJ. Endosonography-guided cystoduodenostomy with a therapeutic ultrasound endoscope. Gastrointest Endosc 1996; 44:614–617.

60 Vosoghi M, Sial S, Garrett B, et al. EUS-guided pancreatic pseudocyst drainage: review and experience at Harbor-UCLA Medical Center. MedGenMed 2002; 4:2.

61 Binmoeller K, Soehendra N. Endoscopic ultrasonography in the diagnosis and treatment of pancreatic pseudocysts. Gastrointest Endosc Clin N Am 1995; 5:805–816.

62 Pfaffenbach B, Langer M, Strabenow-Lohbauer U, et al. Endosonographisch geführte transgastrale Drainage von Pankreaspseudozysten. Dtsch Med Wschr 1998; 123:1439–1442.

63 Giovannini M, Bernardini D, Seitz JF. Cystogastrostomy entirely performed under endosonography guidance for pancreatic pseudocyst: results in 6 patients. Gastrointest Endosc 1998; 48:200–203.

64 Vilmann P, Hancke S, Pless T, et al. One-step endosonography-guided drainage of a pancreatic pseudocyst: a new technique of stent delivery through the echoendoscope. Endoscopy 1998; 30:730–733.

65 Seifert H, Dierich C, Schmitt T, et al. Endoscopic ultrasound-guided one-step transmural drainage of cystic abdominal lesions with a large channel echoendoscope. Endoscopy 2000; 32:255–259.

66 Inui K, Yoshino J, Okushima K, et al. EUS-guided one-step drainage of pancreatic pseudocysts: experience in 3 patients. Gastrointest Endosc 2001; 54:87–89.

67 Giovannini M, Pesenti C, Rolland AL, et al. Endoscopic ultrasound-guided drainage of pancreatic pseudocysts or pancreatic abscesses using a therapeutic echoendoscope. Endoscopy 2001; 33:473–477.

68 Seifert H, Faust D, Schmitt T, et al. Transmural drainage of cystic peripancreatic lesions with a new large-channel echo endoscope. Endoscopy 2001; 33:1022–1026.

69 Wiersema MJ, Baron TH, Chari ST. Endosonography-guided pseudocyst drainage with a new large channel linear scanning echoendoscope. Gastrointest Endosc 2001; 53:811–813.

70 Catalano MF, George S, Thomas M, et al. EUS-guided pancreatic pseudocyst drainage: comparison with standard endoscopic cystenterostomy. Gastrointest Endosc 2004; 59:AB202 (Abstract).

71 Warshaw AL, Rutledge PL. Cystic tumors mistaken for pancreatic pseudocysts. Ann Surg 1987; 205:393–398.

72 Hawes RH. Enoscopic management of pseudocysts. Rev Gastroenterol Disord 2003; 3:135–141.

73 Harada N, Kouzu T, Arima M, et al. Endoscopic ultrasound guided pancreatography: a case report. Endoscopy 1995; 27:612–615.

74 Gress F, Ikenberry S, Sherman S, et al. Endoscopic ultrasound directed pancreatography. Gastrointest Endosc 1996; 44:736–739.

75 Wiersema MJ, Sandusky D, Carr R, et al. Endosonography-guided cholangiopancreatography. Gastrointest Endosc 1996; 43:102–106.

76 Mallery S, Matlock J, Freeman ML. EUS-guided rendezvous drainage of obstructed biliary and pancreatic ducts: reports of 6 cases. Gastrointest Endosc 2004; 50:100–107.

77 Sahai AV, Hoffman BJ, Hawes RH. Endoscopic ultrasound guided hepatico-gastrotomy to palliate obstructive jaundice: preliminary results in pigs. Gastrointest Endosc 1998; 47:AB37 (Abstract).

78 Giovannini M, Moutardier B, Presenti C, et al. Endoscopic ultrasound guided bilioduodenal anastomosis: a new technique for biliary drainage. Endoscopy 2001; 33:898–900.

79 Burmester E, Niehaus J, Leineweber T, et al. EUS-cholangiodrainage of the bile duct: report of 4 cases. Gastrointest Endosc 2003; 57:246–250.

80 Giovannini M, Dotti M, Borries E, et al. Hepaticogastrostomy by echo-endoscopy as a palliative treatment in a patient with metastatic biliary obstruction. Endoscopy 2003; 35:1076–1078.

81 Fritscher-Ravens A, Mukherjee D, Mosse A, et al. Push me pull you flexible plastic stents. Gastrointest Endosc 2002; 55: AB176.

82 Francois E, Kahaleh M, Giovannini M, et al. EUS-guided pancreaticogastrostomy. Gastrointest Endosc 2002; 56:128–133.

83 Seifert H, Wehrmann T, Schmitt T, et al. Retroperitoneal endoscopic debridement for infected peripancreatic necrosis. Lancet 2000; 356:653–655.

84 Kalloo A, Kantsevoy S, Jagannath S, et al. Endoscopic gastrojejunostomy with long term survival in a porcine model. Gastrointest Endosc 2002; 55:AB96 (Abstract).

85 Fritscher-Ravens A, Mosse CA, Mills TN, et al. A through-the-scope device for suturing and tissue approximation under EUS control. Gastrointest Endosc 2002; 56:737–742.

86 Fritscher-Ravens A, Mosse CA, Mukherjee D, et al. Transgastric gastropexy and hiatus hernia repair for gastro-esophageal reflux disease under endoscopic ultrasound control: an experimental study in a porcine model. Gastrointest Endosc 2004; 59:89–95.

87 Fritscher-Ravens A, Mosse CA, Mukherjee D, et al. Transluminal endosurgery: single lumen access anastomosis device for flexible endoscopy. Gastrointest Endosc 2003; 58:585–591.

88 Fritscher-Ravens A, Park PO, Swain CP. Esophageal patches and valves: material, design and endoscopic attachment methods. Gastrointest Endosc 2003; 57:AB83.

89 Fritscher-Ravens A, Mosse CA, Mukherjee D, et al. Balloon compression anastomosis at flexible endoscopy. Gastrointest Endosc 2003; 57:AB6 (Abstract).

Index